Spinal Cord Disease
Basic Science, Diagnosis and Management

Springer-Verlag London Ltd.

Edmund Critchley and Andrew Eisen (Eds)

Spinal Cord Disease
Basic Science, Diagnosis and Management

With 118 Figures

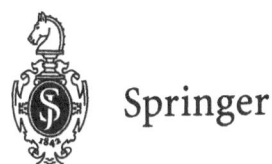 Springer

Edmund Critchley, DM, FRCP
Royal Preston Hospital, Department of Neurology
Sharoe Green Lane, Preston PR2 4HT, UK

Andrew Eisen, MD, FRCP(C)
Vancouver General Hospital
855 West 12th Avenue, Vancouver, BC V5Z 1M9, Canada

Consulting Editor
Michael Swash, MD, FRCP, MRCPath
The London Hospital, Neurology Department
Whitechapel, London E1 1BB, UK

ISBN 978-1-85233-121-4

British Library Cataloguing in Publication Data
Spinal cord disease : basic science, diagnosis and
     management
     1. Spinal cord - Diseases
     I. Critchley, E. M. R. (Edmund Michael Rhys)   II. Eisen,
     Andrew, 1936-
     616.8'3
ISBN 978-1-85233-121-4   ISBN 978-1-4471-0569-5 (eBook)
DOI 10.1007/978-1-4471-0569-5

Library of Congress Cataloging-in-Publication Data
A catalog record for this book is available from the Library of Congress

Typeset by EXPO Holdings, Malaysia

28/3830-54321 Printed on acid-free paper

Contents

Preface

Spinal Cord Injury or disease can happen to anyone at any time and the effects can be devastating. I found this out personally when I was thrown from the back of a pick up truck at age 15 was left paralyzed from the waist down.

It was during my recuperation as a young teenager that I first gained insight into the importance of rehabilitation. My family, doctors, nurses, fellow patients and researchers who were dedicated to helping me overcome my personal tragedy helped me pull through. Today, rehabilitation medicine is taking great strides and empowering the person with the injury to take control of their future, overcome their setbacks and, through collaborative support, reach their personal goals and potential.

Since 1987 the Legacy raised by my Man in Motion World Tour (24 901 miles wheeled around the world March 1985–May 1987) has provided over $13 million dollars to research and rehabilitation in the areas of spinal cord injury. I hope that in some small way this funding has contributed to the development of the vital programmes that supported me and many others.

The effects of spinal cord injury are traumatic and life-shattering and require a skilled interdisciplinary approach. I congratulate those who have contributed to this book and challenge each one of you to *never* give up on your dreams to find the answers to the optimum treatment of spinal cord injury and disease.

Rick Hansen

Contributors

M.J. Aminoff, MD, FRCP
Professor of Neurology, School of Medicine, Department of Neurology M-794, University of California, San Francisco, CA 94143-0114, USA

L.A. Bindoff, MSc, MBBS, MRCP, MD
Consultant Neurologist, Middlesborough General Hospital, Ayresome Green Lane, Middlesborough, Cleveland, TS5 5AZ, UK

E.M.R. Critchley, DM, FRCP
Professor of Neurology, Preston Royal Hospital, Sharoe Green Lane, Preston, PR2 4HT, UK

G.R. Critchley, MA, FRCS
Registrar in Neurosurgery, Department of Neurosurgery, Hope Hospital, Stott Lane, Salford, Greater Manchester, UK

C.H.G. Davis, FRCS
Consultant Neurosurgeon, Royal Preston Hospital, Sharoe Green Lane, Preston, PR2 4HT, UK

J.P.R. Dick
Consultant Neurologist, The Royal London Hospital, Whitechapel, London, E1 1BB, UK

M. Dvorak
3rd Floor, 910 West 10th Avenue, Vancouver, British Columbia, V5Z 4E3, Canada

A.A. Eisen, MD, FRCP(C)
Professor of Neurology, Vancouver General Hospital, Neuromuscular Disease Unit, 855 West 12th Avenue, Vancouver, BCV5Z 1M9, Canada

R.D. Fealey, MD
Department of Neurology, Mayo Clinic, 200 First Street Southwest, Rochester, Minnesota 55905, USA

D.I. Graham
Professor of Neuropathology, Institute of Neurological Sciences, 1345 Govan Road, Glasgow, G51 4TF, UK

B.A. Green

Professor of Neurological Surgery, Orthopaedics and Rehabilitation, and Co-Director of the Acute Spinal Cord Injury Service,
University of Miami School of Medicine/Jackson Memorial Hospital, Attending Physician at the Veterans Administration Hospital, President and Director of Clinical Research at the Miami Project
to Cure Paralysis, 1501 NorthWest 9th Avenue, Miami, Florida, 33136, USA

R. Guiloff, MD, FRCP

Professor, Neuromuscular Unit, Ground Floor Room, South Wing, Charing Cross Hospital, Fulham Palace Road, London, W6 8RF, UK

N.T. Gurusinghe

Consultant Neurosurgeon, Royal Preston Hospital, Sharoe Green Lane, Preston, PR2 4HT, UK

A. Hill

Head of Division of Paediatric Neurology, BC Children's Hospital, 1D18 4480 Oak Street, Vancouver, BC V6H 3VH, Canada

M.T. Isaac

Consultant and Senior Lecturer in Psychiatry, Suite 6, Lewisham Hospital, Lewisham High Street, London, SE13 6LH, UK

J.R. Johnson, MBBS, FRCS

Consultant Orthopaedic Surgeon, St Mary's Hospital, Praed Street, Paddington and Royal National Orthopaedic Hospital, Brockley Hill, Stanmore, Middlesex, UK

R.A. Johnston

Consultant Neurosurgeon, Institute of Neurological Sciences, 1345 Govan Road, Glasgow, G51 4TF, UK

J.S. Lapointe

Associate Professor of Radiology, University of British Columbia, Neuroradiologist, Vancouver General Hospital, Vancouver, British Columbia, V5Z 4E3, Canada

T.T. Lee

Department of Neurological Surgery, University of Miami School of Medicine, Miami, Florida 33101, USA

R.W. McGraw

Professor and Head of Orthopaedics, 3rd Floor, 910 West 10th Avenue, Vancouver, British Columbia, V5Z 4E3, Canada

R.A. Metcalfe
Consultant Neurologist, Institute of Neurological Sciences, 1345 Govan Road, Glasgow, G51 4TF, UK

J.D. Mitchell, MD, FRCP
Consultant Neurologist and Honorary Professor of Clinical Neurology, Preston
Royal Hospital, Sharoe Green Lane, Preston, PR2 4HT, UK

R.R. Pearson
18 Poynings Place, St Nicholas Street, Old Portsmouth, Hampshire, PO1 2PB,
UK

K. Rajamani, MD, DM
Registrar in Neurology, Department of Neurology, Preston Royal Hospital,
Sharoe Green Lane, Preston, PR2 4HT, UK

C.S. Savant, MD, DNB
Registrar, Department of Neurology, Preston Royal Hospital, Sharoe Green
Lane, Preston, PR2 4HT, UK

R.A. Shakir, MBchB, MSc, FRCP, FRCP(E), FRCP(G)
Consultant Neurologist, Department of Neurology, Charing Cross Hospital,
Fulham Palace Road, London, W6 8RF, UK

M. Swash, MD, FRCP, FRCPath
Consultant Neurologist, Department of Neurology, The Royal London Hospital,
Whitechapel, London, E1 1BB, UK

J.D. Steeves
University of British Columbia, Vancouver General Hospital, Vancouver, BC
V5Z 4E3, Canada

R.J. Weber, MD
Professor and Chairman, Department of Physical Medicine and Rehabilitation,
SUNY Health Science Centre, 750 East Adams Street, Syracuse, New York 13210,
USA

T. Zwimpfer
University of British Columbia, Vancouver General Hospital, Vancouver, BC
V5Z 4E3, Canada

Chapter 1

Introduction

E.M.R. Critchley and A.A. Eisen

The first treatise devoted entirely to the spinal cord, *Anatome Medullae Spinalis et Nervorum* (Gerard Blasius, Amsterdam, C. Commelinum), was published in 1666. The separate origin of the anterior and posterior roots, dorsal root ganglia and the differentiation between the grey and the white matter of the spinal cord were illustrated. Despite this early description, the spinal cord has remained, until recently, the Cinderella of the nervous system, receiving relatively scant attention.

In adults, the spinal cord is approximately 40 cm long and extends from the foramen magnum to the lower margin of the body of the first lumbar vertebra. For a long time the ability to localize lesions longitudinally within the spinal cord had been very limited. Sir David Ferrier's "golden guinea test" used a guinea piece to demonstrate the upper limit of spinal compression. If a coin is run down the back of the spine, a weal is produced in the skin above the level of the lesion, but at most a white mark occurs below the lesion where sweating the vital reactions are in abeyance (Critchley 1957). Sir Ludwig Guttmann (Guttmann 1946) deserves special credit for changing the traditionally nihilistic view of spinal cord trauma. Today neurophysiologists are concerned with the feasibility of inducing functional spinal cord regeneration (Aguayo 1987) and innovative biomedical engineering has made it possible for the paraplegic to "walk" (Marsolais and Kobetic 1983; Petrofsky and Phillips 1983; Weber 1987).

The basic anatomical unit at each spinal level, the Sherringtonian reflex arc, belies the complex circuitry and operation of the spinal cord which is constantly being extended and refined (Ashby 1987). Continuous "signal processing" within the cord provides the substrate for motor programmes ranging from simple reflexes to the intricate patterns required, for example, in walking. No other structure within the body is so well protected physically by its membranes, the skin, the musculature of the back and the bony vertebral column. They form important defences against trauma, infection, neoplasia, autoimmune disease and iatrogenic insult but these same structures render the spinal cord inaccessible to direct clinical examination.

For years neurologists have been limited to interpretation of the results of cerebrospinal fluid (CSF) analysis obtained via a lumbar puncture needle. Myelography permitted limited visualization of the outline of the cord, marginally enhanced by CT scanning and selective angiography. By contrast, MR scanning provided a quantum leap in non-invasive cord imaging but still leaves us in ignorance of the physiological, pathological and biochemical behaviour of the cord in response to disease. Many cord lesions are not radiologically visible. In this respect motor and somatosensory-evoked potentials can be helpful (Eisen and Aminoff 1986; Eisen and Shtybel 1990). However, these neurophysiological tests do not have the localizing ability of imaging techniques. Furthermore, they are unable to discriminate between different types of pathology or disease. Although most of the advances in the physiology and neurochemistry of the spinal cord remain within the research domain, molecular genetics offers the possibility of more accurate diagnoses and the potentiality of specific treatments for degenerative disorders of the cord.

The spinal cord should be regarded as an integral and active unit of the brain, even interacting in relation to many psychological processes such as sexual libido and emotional expressiveness (Dimond 1980).The cord also possesses a controlling function over many of the physiological events occurring more peripherally; thus it may not always be easy to separate pathological changes within the cord from those directly affecting the somatic nerves or even the autonomic nervous system.

With trauma to the neck, as with a whiplash injury, we must separate the effects of cord contusion from injury to the nerve roots (Garvey and Eismont 1991; Ditunna 1994). Various neurodegenerative diseases such as Multi-System Atrophy and the Shy–Drager syndrome involve the sympathetic preganglionic neurones of the intermediolateral column which is the final site of integration of central influences on postganglionic and adrenomedullary sympathetic activity. Sexual as well as sphincter functions depend heavily on the integrity of spinal control. In spinal shock when the cord is cut off from the influence of higher centres there is a sudden diminution of sympathetic activity: muscle tone is lost, the blood pressure plummets, the bowel becomes atonic, retention of urine and faeces occurs, often followed by retention with overflow. The skin is unprotected and pressure sores can develop. Later there is a return of tone with enhanced parasympathetic outflow followed by partial restoration of sympathetic activity resulting in mass reflexes, automatic or manually stimulated bladder and bowel function; but many problems such as the postural control of blood pressure remain.

Symptomatology

The essence of history taking in suspected spinal cord disease does not differ from that for other conditions affecting the nervous system. A full description of the circumstances of the onset of symptoms can help enormously in diagnosis particularly when the onset is abrupt. Even though clinicians pride themselves that, faced with a diagnostic problem, they can correctly make the diagnosis based upon history alone in approximately 80% of patients, such clinical prowess falls far below the norm when considering disorders affecting the spinal cord. A few examples will suffice.

1. Regardless whether trauma has been sustained at work, in road traffic accidents or during sport, bony and/or neural damage involving the cervical or dorsolumbar spine is frequently overlooked. Failure to recognize the extent of such injury – or even its presence – all too often precipitates avoidable neurological deficits or death at initial handling of the patient (Rubin and Fielding 1983; Ravichandran and Silver 1984).

In sports injuries a head-on tackle, as with "spearing" in American football, may result in a fracture of the lower cervical spine. Flexion or hyperextension injuries occur in rucks (collapsed scrums) or mauls. Whiplash injury is a result of the head jolted forwards and backwards in a road traffic accident. A twisting injury during lifting, may suggest acute disc prolapse with consequent radicular pain and inability to straighten up immediately. It is useful to discover exactly how the patient was able to move from the scene of an accident or abrupt injury. What helped was required? Conversely, with certain injuries such as whiplash, symptoms may be minimal at first but develop after a few hours.

2. The history of a "crick in the neck" with burning pain across the shoulders following minor trauma, is easily misinterpreted as due to a root lesion despite unrestricted neck movement. Such patients, who are more likely to have neuralgic amyotrophy (paralytic brachial neuritis) or syringomyelia, not infrequently undergo inappropriate and unsuccessful neck traction.

3. Not every dorsal or girdle pain is the result of a prolapsed intervertebral disc or due to shingles.

4. Spinal meningitis, at the extremes of life, may escape detection unless specifically considered and sought for. Typical events heralding the acute phase of poliomyelitis and other enterovirus infections – vomiting, diarrhoea or constipation followed by a mild temperature and a meningitic reaction – are easily overlooked.

5. Any number of explanations of spastic weakness of the legs may be offered before the possibility of cord compression is finally recognized. The gradual, subacute onset of spasticity in the lower limbs should always raise the possibility of spinal cord compression.

Early symptoms include a feeling of heaviness in the legs and the complaint that walking, an automatic event, now requires conscious effort. After a set distance the feet may begin to drag, the toes may catch with a tendency to trip, and the inner aspects of the toe caps of shoes may wear excessively. Investigation to exclude neural compression should be considered before a definite sensory level is established or sphincter problems ensue.

The sudden onset of a paraparesis recognized for the first time when attempting to get out of bed can occur with spinal compression but is more usually an indication of a thrombotic lesion. Spinal multiple sclerosis may be suggested if, in addition to evidence of spasticity, the feet tend to kick out involuntarily, or unilateral symptoms are accompanied by bilateral signs.

6. Vascular accidents involving the cord often create diagnostic confusion. The symptoms of a spinal subarachnoid haemorrhage are not as readily manifest as those of an intracranial bleed. Thrombotic lesions of the cord, especially occurring in the elderly or as a consequence of blood loss, may be overlooked as may the protean symptoms ascribable to the presence of arteriovenous malformations. In fact, arteriovenous malformations of the spinal cord and dura are as often discovered by accident as by anticipation.

It may be hard to differentiate cord compression from transverse myelitis. Recurrent episodes at the same site may arise from an arteriovenous malformation. A spinal subarachnoid haemorrhage may occur with symptoms developing acutely at one level, with other symptoms such as headache and lower back pain coursing into the legs encountered several hours later.

Physical Signs

The examination provides the framework required to formulate a diagnosis, establish the level of the lesion and provide confirmatory evidence of the nature of the insult and the pathological changes found. Non-neurological physical signs provide information about the state of the overlying tissues and the likelihood of spinal cord pathology. Minor degrees of dysraphism include the presence of bifid vertebral spines, dermoids, dimpling and portwine stains. Deformities of the neck and the region of the foramen magnum such as platybasia, a short or webbed neck, torticollis, or Sprengel's deformity of the scapula, may be associated with abnormal or fused vertebrae and Arnold–Chiari malformation. If spastic paraperesis or ataxia is accompanied by the presence of kyphoscoliosis and sometimes clubbed feet, the patient is more likely to have an hereditary rather than an acquired neurological disorder. About 60%–90% of congenital and 35%–50% of acquired spinal cord disorders have associated scoliosis (Dickson 1986). A wedged vertebra may occur with a variety of inherited conditions and with Paget's disease of the spine, but acute wedging of vertebrae more commonly suggests vertebral collapse. This may cause spinal cord compression, for example in the presence of carcinomatous deposits, tuberculosis, or an epidural abscess.

Two signs, in particular, indicate acute embarrassment of the cervical spinal cord following trauma. The adoption of a cock robin posture or tilt due to post-traumatic torticollis is indicative of a Jefferson fracture and fragmentation of the ring of the atlas caused by axial compression. The actual fracture may be fairly stable but in 50% of cases it is accompanied by fractures of the odontoid or the so-called hangman's fracture separating the body of the axis from the C2–3 facet joints (Kinoshita 1994; Matsumoto 1994).

Paradoxical neurogenic ventilation is an ominous sign of a high spinal cord lesion with paralysis of the phrenic nerve (C3, 4, 5) and diaphragm. Respiratory support becomes the immediate priority. There is paradoxical distension of the abdomen during inspiration with indrawing of damaged segments of the chest wall. In this situation stimulation of the phrenic nerve and assessment of phrenic nerve conduction, as well as needle EMG of the diaphragm, is useful for documenting the presence or otherwise of nerve–muscle continuity. Lesser cervical injuries may be recognized at times by careful palpation before attempting to move the patient. Lesions affecting the anterior quadrants of the spinal cord at C2–4 may impair the autonomic control of respiration whilst leaving intact voluntary control, thus giving rise to the situation wherein respiration is unimpaired in the alert state but fails when the patient becomes drowsy (Ondine's curse). Ventilatory problems also arise with lower cervical and high dorsal lesions as these are associated with a reduced ventilatory capacity, inability to cough and the risk of atelectasis and decreased arterial Po_2 even if the CO_2 tension is maintained.

Anatomical localization within the spinal cord may be determined by piecing together, as it were on a grid, signs of vertical and horizontal dysfunction. The vertical manifestations are the less complex. Upper motor neurone signs indicate involvement of the pyramidal, or corticospinal, tracts at any level between cortex and anterior horn cells. Extrapyramidal features negate spinal disease, indicating a lesion rostral to the medulla.

Truncal ataxia and minor cerebellar signs may be mimicked by the presence of lower motor neurone weakness, loss of proprioceptive function, or damage to

Clarke's column (the nucleus dorsalis) located at the base of the posterior horns and extending from T1 to L4. Sensory signs can involve end-organ dysfunction, the peripheral nerve, or spinal tracts. Whereas peripheral nerve disease is usually associated with a graded glove and stocking distribution, a distinct upper limit is usual with spinal dysfunction. This is often accompanied, if the lesion is intrinsic, by sacral sparing or suspended sensory loss. Dissociated sensory loss may occur with predominantly spinothalamic (pain and temperature) or dorsal column (proprioception, light touch and vibration) impairment; or, as is typical in Hansen's disease, with selective involvement of the larger fibres of the posterior root ganglia.

An intriguing sign worthy of careful analysis is the presence of pseudoathetosis. Slow wandering movements of the outstretched fingers occur when the arms are extended and the eyes closed. Unlike true athetoid movements, these movements are readily suppressed when the patient is able to watch his hands. Unilateral involvement can occur with a lesion of the parietal lobe but usually pseudoathetosis is seen bilaterally with tabetic softening of the dorsal columns, or with compression of the dorsal columns as by cerebellar ectopia at the foramen magnum, carcinomatous meningitis or cervical spondylosis. It can occur, but is rare, as a result of interruption of the dorsal columns in multiple sclerosis, and here it may remit spontaneously (Bickerstaff 1980).

Another cause of pseudoathetosis is sensory neuronopathy (Asbury 1987). The lesion is of the primary afferent neurone having its cell body in the dorsal root ganglia lying within the intervertebral foramina. Sensory neuronopathies can be difficult to interpret. Degeneration of the central process occurs with lesions that are proximal to the dorsal root. In this situation electrophysiological studies are helpful. Peripheral compound sensory nerve action potentials (SNAPs) are normal, but spinal or cortical evoked potentials (SEPs) are prolonged, small or absent. Several toxic and metabolic abnormalities affecting the primary sensory neurone induce a distal axonopathy with dying back of both the peripheral and central arms of the neurone. When this happens both the peripheral SNAP and SEP are abnormal (Thomas 1982).

Sensory neuronopathies (acute or chronic) are, as a group, less common than other conditions affecting the peripheral or central components of the sensory axon. They affect the cell body directly with subsequent dying-forward of both its central and peripheral arms. Sensory neuronopathies are distinguishable from sensory neuropathies by the global, rather than distal, distribution of sensory loss, total arreflexia and absence of recordable SNAPs in the face of normal compound muscle action potentials (Asbury 1987). The chronic variety is usually associated with an underlying cancer. The rarer acute forms originally occurred in association with antibiotic therapy but more recently cases without apparent cause have been described.

Among the classical tests of sensory loss is the Romberg test. This is a test of postural instability, only apparent following closure of the eyes. Although it is used as a supportive test confirming the presence of vertigo, it is essentially dependent on the integrity of the proprioceptive pathways transmitted via the dorsal columns. Romberg's test is of little value in the assessment of ataxia as an ataxic lesion due to cerebellar dysfunction is invariably present when the eyes are open, though worsened by eye closure.

Upward extension of the spinal lesion into the medulla oblongata is usually confirmed by cranial nerve involvement. The presence of wasting and fasciculation of the tongue, an increased jaw jerk, or a spastic bulbar palsy, may obviate the need to perform a myelogram, as for example in the differential diagnosis of motor neurone disease. Abnormal visual evoked potentials may differentiate spinal multiple sclerosis from familial spastic paraparesis. Nystagmus is the only cranial nerve sign about which there is some anatomical dispute. The vestibulospinal tract, involved in the righting reflexes, descends as low as C5 where synapses are found with anterior horn cells. The tract also contains some ascending fibres and it is theoretically possible that nystagmus can arise due to a defect of afferent impulses from the cervical spine (Biemond and De Jong 1969). In clinical practice, when nystagmus is seen in conjunction with cervical cord disease, as with syringomyelia, craniovertebral anomalies or a tumour, the disorder has invariably involved structures rostral to the foramen magnum (Spillane 1968). Down beating nystagmus more prominent on lateral gaze (Ross Russell and Wiles 1985) is characteristic of lesions in the neighbourhood of the foramen magnum, especially in cases of Chiari malformation (Barnett et al. 1973). Foramen magnum lesions may also be accompanied by tingling and sensory loss confined to the finger ends. With larger lesions, such as a high cervical cyst, pin-prick and vibration sensation may be altered over the nape of the neck. Priapism may sometimes occur with high cervical lesions, e.g. following an atlanto-axial dislocation or hangman's fracture. It can occasionally prove a useful pointer in the event of sudden, unexplained collapse.

Patchy demyelination affecting the dorsal columns may result in Lhermitte's phenomenon whereby flexion or hyperextension of the neck is accompanied by a shower of electric sensations with a definite radiation: down the back, into the legs, into the arms or occasionally down the sternum or upwards to the head. These symptoms may be mentioned spontaneously or can be elicited by direct questioning. Occasionally they may present for the first time as a sign – the Barber's chair sign – with apparent discomfort when the patient is asked to flex the neck in the course of a neurological examination. The commonest cause in young people is multiple sclerosis, and in the elderly cervical spondylosis. But it may be an early sign of subacute degeneration of the cord, occur with pyridoxine excess, after intrathecal administration of vincristine, with cervical tumours or as a feature of radiation myelopathy. When Lhermitte's phenomenon follows neck trauma such as whiplash injury, there is often a latent period of about three months and the symptoms may remit spontaneously after a further three to six months.

Cervical spondylosis may present with neck stiffness, as a radiculopathy, as a myelopathy or as a combination of these. Neck movements should be examined as part of a routine neurological examination: at first as actively performed movements of flexion, extension, rotation and lateral flexion (bending the neck towards the shoulder), and then passively, gently repeating the same movement but holding the head for a moment at the extreme of each movement to check whether this elicits any particular complaint from the patient.

Myelopathies usually present with spasticity and long tract signs in the lower limbs. Thus compressive lesions of the cervical spinal cord may produce proximal leg weakness and impaired vibration in the feet. However, cases with predominant had involvement also occur. Usually sensory loss dominates. It is often global (glove distribution) and may extend proximally as far as the elbow (Voskuhl and Hinton 1990). The most probable pathophysiological mechanism is ischaemia involving the intrinsic watershed border areas of collateralization between the superficial pial network and the central arterial supply to the cervical cord. Venous stagnation may also play a role.

The presence of radiculopathy, representing the horizontal parameter of spinal cord involvement, can be recognized by means of: (a) lower motor neurone signs, (b) segmental sensory loss, and (c) altered reflex activity over the C5, 6, 7 segments. Wasting and even fasciculation may be observed proximally in the arms. Unilateral neurogenic wasting of the small muscles of the hands, if not due to a combined median/ulnar palsy usually indicates a lesion of the C8 or T1 myotome, either radiculopathy or anterior horn disease. Occasionally, lesions rostral to C8 such as anterior spinal artery thrombosis or insufficiency can cause wasting of the muscles of the hands. Rarely, mid and high cervical cord compression from cervical spondylosis may also result in hand wasting (Goodridge et al. 1987).

The power of each group of muscles is checked noting their segmental references. Likewise, segmental sensory loss to light touch, pin-prick and temperature may be examined. Loss or diminution of reflex activity accompanied by weakness or wasting suggests a lower motor neurone lesion at that segmental level. However, the reflex may also be diminished if there is sensory impairment involving afferent nerve fibres. Compression of the afferent fibres as from osteophyte formation may result in the reflex being lost.

The arm reflexes show some overlap of the segments between muscle groups. Thus percussion of the biceps tendon excites C5, 6 (chiefly 5) and at the same time evokes a slight response from the triceps muscle C6, 7 (chiefly 7), but the resulting contraction produces predominant flexion of the elbow. The spread of a reflex vibratory wave after percussion is enhanced in the presence of spasticity so that there is reflex excitation of other segments and muscle groups due to alpha motor neurone hyperexcitability affecting other muscle spindles. Thus, activating the supinator jerk C5, 6 (chiefly 6) may also elicit finger flexion C8 and contractions of the brachioradialis, biceps and triceps. In the presence of an efferent radiculopathy, where a disc or osteophyte obstructs the emergent roots at the exit foramen, spread of the reflex to unblocked segments causes other muscles to contract thus producing an inverted response.

The finding of segmental sensory loss provides an indication of root involvement but not of the site interference. However, once the afferent sensory fibres enter the spinal cord, they become dissociated: those subserving light touch and proprioception pass upwards in the ipsilateral dorsal columns, whereas those subserving pain and temperature enter the posterolateral aspect of the cord, travel upwards for two or three segments, and then cross the midline to the opposite anterolateral spinothalamic tract. An intrinsic lesion such as a cyst or solid tumour in the ventral part of the cord may have no pressure effect on the dorsal columns or on the afferent ipsilateral spinothalamic; but it will almost certainly damage the crossing spinothalamic fibres to right and left (not necessarily in a symmetrical fashion), and will encroach on the more deeply situated contralateral spinothalamic fibres in the ascending anterolateral spinothalamic tract. Within this tract there will be relative sparing of the more superficially placed anterolateral fibres, i.e. those arising from the most caudal afferents. If the intrinsic lesion is a central syrinx in the neighbourhood of the central canal the result will be bilateral impairment of spinothalamic sensation with a sharp, distinct upper level and a less distinct lower level, producing dissociated and suspended sensory loss. A suspended sensory loss is a sign of an intrinsic lesion: sacral sparing is a less definite sign of an intrinsic lesion and can occur with extrinsic lesions also.

A traumatic, infiltrative or compressive lesion affecting one half of the spinal cord will produce a Brown-Séquard syndrome. A pure hemisection is rarely seen but the concept is useful in diagnosis. Disruption of the anterolateral spinothalamic tract will produce loss of temperature and pain sensation over the opposite side of the body nearly up to the level of the lesion. Disruption of the dorsal columns will result in an ipsilateral sensory loss to light touch and joint position sensation as high as the upper level of the lesion, with an ipsilateral band of total sensory loss over a few segments just below the upper level of the lesion. The planter reflex on the ipsilateral side will be briskly extensor due to corticospinal tract involvement: that on the contralateral side will be silent because of loss of nociceptive sensation. In clinical practice it is more common to find an incomplete lesion usually with bilateral spasticity. When this is so the ipsilateral plantar reflex will be briskly extensor and the contralateral reflex less certain with a sluggish extensor response.

References

Aguayo AJ (1987) Peripheral nerve transplants used to test the regenerative capacities of central nervous system neurones. Twelfth Annual Edward H Lambert Lecture. AAEM 34th Annual Meeting. Oct 15–17 Custom Printing Inc. Rochester, Minnesota, pp 7–25

Asbury AK (1987) Sensory neuropathy Semin Neurol. 7:58–66

Ashby P (1987) Clinical neurophysiology of the spinal cord. In: Brown WF, Bolton CF (eds) Clinical electromyography. Butterworths, Boston, Toronto, pp 453–482

Barnett HJM, Foster JB, Hudgson P (1973) Syringomyelia. Saunders, London

Bickerstaff ER (1980) Neurological examination in clinical practice, 4th edn. Blackwell, Oxford

Biemond A, De Jong JMBV (1969) On cervical nystagmus and related disorders. Brain 92:437–452

Critchley EMR (1957) Sir David Ferrier. King's College Hospital Gazette 36:243–250

Dickson JH (1986) Pathogenesis and treatment of scoliosis in neuromuscular diseases. In: Dimitrijevic MR, Kakulas B, Vrbova G (eds) Recent advances in restorative neurology, Vol 2 Progressive neuromuscular disorders. Karger, Basel, pp 11–14

Dimond SJ (1989) Neuropsychology: a textbook of systems and psychological functions of the human brain. Butterworths, London, pp 518–521

Ditunna JF (1994) American spinal injury standards for neurological and functional classification of spinal cord injury: past, present and future. J Am Paraplegia Soc 17:7–11

Eisen A, Aminoff MJ (1986) Somatosensory evoked potentials in: Aminoff MJ (ed) Electrodiagnosis in clinical neurology. Churchill Livingstone, Edinburgh, pp 535–573

Eisen A, Shtybel W (1990) Clinical experience with transcranial magnetic stimulation AAEM Minimonograph. Muscle Nerve. 13:1330–1343

Garvey TA, Eismont FJ (1991) Diagnosis and treatment of cervical radiculopathy and myelopathy. Orthop Rev 20:595–603

Goodridge AE, Feasby TE, Ebers GC, Brown WF, Rice GPA (1987) Hand wasting due to mid-cervical spinal cord compression. Can J Neurol Sci 14:309–311

Guttmann L (1946) Rehabilitation after injuries to the spinal cord and cauda equina. Br J Phys Med 9: 162–180

Kinoshita H (1994) Pathology of spinal cord injuries due to fracture or fracture-dislocation of the cervical spine. paraplegia 32:642–650

Marsolais EB, Kobetic R (1983) Functional walking in paralysed patients. Clin Orthop Operations 175:30–36

Matsumoto S (1994) An unusual type of hangman's fracture with cord compression: a case report. Surg Neurol 41:322–324

Petrofsky JS, Philips CA (1983) Computer controlled walking in the paralysed individual. J Neurol Orthop Surg 4: 153–164

Ravinchandran G, Silver JR (1984) Recognition of spinal cord injury. Hosp Update 10:77–86

Ross Russell RW, Wiles CM (1985) Neurology: integrated clinical science. Heinemann, London

Rubin BD, Fielding JW (1983) Neurological sequelae of cervical cord trauma. Bull Los Angeles Neurol Sci 45:36–40

Spillane JD (1968) An atlas of clinical neurology. Oxford University Press, Oxford, p 16

Thomas PK (1982) Selective vulnerability of the centrifugal and centripedal axons of primary sensory neurons. Muscle Nerve 5(95):S117–121

Voskuhl RR, Hinton RC (1990) Sensory impairment in the hands secondary to spondylotic compression of the cervical spinal cord. Arch Neurol 47:309–311

Weber RJ (1987) Functional electric stimulation AAEM Didactic Program, 34th Annual Meeting. Custom Printing Inc, Rochester, MN, pp 29–32

Chapter 2

Anatomical Basis of Spinal Cord Function

T.J. Zwimpfer and J.D. Steeves

Despite the ability radiologically to image the spinal cord in great detail, history and physical examination remains the basis for the management of patients with disorders of the spinal cord. Knowledge of both the external and internal anatomy of the spinal cord is required for accurate interpretation of clinical findings. This chapter will review the important external features of the spinal cord as well as the main clinically relevant white matter tracts and grey matter nuclei. The reader is referred to the chapter on spinal vascular disease (Chapter 24) for details of the blood supply of the cord. In this chapter, the terms anterior and posterior will be used but they are synonymous with ventral and dorsal, respectively.

External Features

The spinal cord is covered by three meningeal layers, the inner pial layer, arachnoid and the outer layer of dura. Anteriorly, the cord has a deep midline groove, the anterior median sulcus while there is a shallow midline sulcus on its posterior surface. The lower end or conus of the spinal cord tapers into a cone. The cord is supported by three ligament-like structures that are extensions of pia and run from the pial surface of the cord to the dura. The two scalloped **denticulate ligaments**, one on either side, run from the midlateral aspect of the cord through the subarachnoid space and attach to the dura laterally. The **filum terminale** runs from the tip of the conus and inserts into the dura at the second sacral vertebra (S2).

In the fetus, the cord extends down to the S2 vertebra, which is the lower limit of the spinal dura. Due to the more rapid growth of the bony spine compared to the spinal cord, the tip of the conus lies at the level of the L3 vertebral body at birth and in the adult it is normally opposite L1 or L2. In the condition known as spinal dysraphism, the spinal cord can terminate at much lower levels, occasionally tethered by a lipoma of the conus or by a thickened and shortened filum terminale.

There are two symmetrical enlargements of the spinal cord and they contain the segments that innervate the limbs. The **cervical enlargement** (cord levels C5–T1) gives rise to the brachial plexus whereas the lumbosacral plexus originates from the **lumbar enlargement** (L2–S3). The large number of neurones associated with sensorimotor integration of the limbs account for the enlargement of the cord at these levels.

At each segmental level, the anterior and posterior roots arise from the anterolateral and posterolateral surface of the cord, respectively. Each root is formed by the union of three or four small rootlets. At each level the **anterior root** contains axons of motor neurones, while at levels T1–L2 (sympathetic) and S2–S4 (parasympathetic), these roots also carry preganglionic autonomic fibres that arise from the intermediolateral nucleus. The **posterior root** contains the central process of bipolar sensory neurones. These neurones are located in the **posterior root ganglion**, which lies in the intervertebral foramen. Some primary sensory afferents (especially visceral in origin) enter the cord through the anterior root but still terminate in the posterior horn (Coggeshall et al. 1975).

At progressively more caudal levels, the roots have a more oblique and downward course in the subarachnoid space before leaving the spinal canal. Therefore, in the lumbosacral spine, the roots of the cauda equina run almost straight down after they arise from the conus. The anterior and posterior roots leave the subarachnoid space through separate openings in the dura and then unite to form the **mixed spinal nerve**. The nerves from C1 to C7 pass above the pedicle of the corresponding numbered vertebra, C8 passes under the pedicle of C7 and below C8 each nerve passes under its corresponding pedicle. Each spinal nerve divides into a **posterior and anterior primary ramus** and each ramus contains motor, sensory and autonomic fibres. The posterior ramus innervates the paraspinal regions and the anterior ramus supplies the remainder of the trunk and the limbs.

Internal Architecture

The internal anatomy of the spinal cord can be divided into the central grey matter (Fig. 2.1) and the surrounding white matter, which contains ascending and descending fibre tracts (Fig. 2.2). Important features of the main grey matter nuclei are summarized in Table 2.1. Fibre tracts are reviewed in Table 2.2 (ascending tracts) and Table 2.3 (descending tracts).

Table 2.1.   Summary of the main grey matter columns

Nucleus	Rexed laminae	Levels	Main function
Posteromarginal nucleus	I	All	Modulate nociceptive sensory input
Substantia gelatinosa	II (III)	All	Modulate nociceptive sensory input
Principal sensory nucleus (Nucleus Proprius)	III, IV	All	Origin of main secondary sensory afferents to higher centres (e.g. spinothalamic tract)
Clarke's nucleus	VII	C8–L3	Origin of posterior spinocerebellar tract
Intermediolateral nucleus	VII	T1–L2	Origin of sympathetic preganglionic fibres
Intermediolateral nucleus	VII	S2–S4	Origin of parasympathetic preganglionic fibres
Medial motor nuclei	IX	All	Motor neurones innervating trunk musculature
Lateral motor nuclei	IX	C5–T1 and L2–S3	Motor neurones innervating upper and lower limb musculature

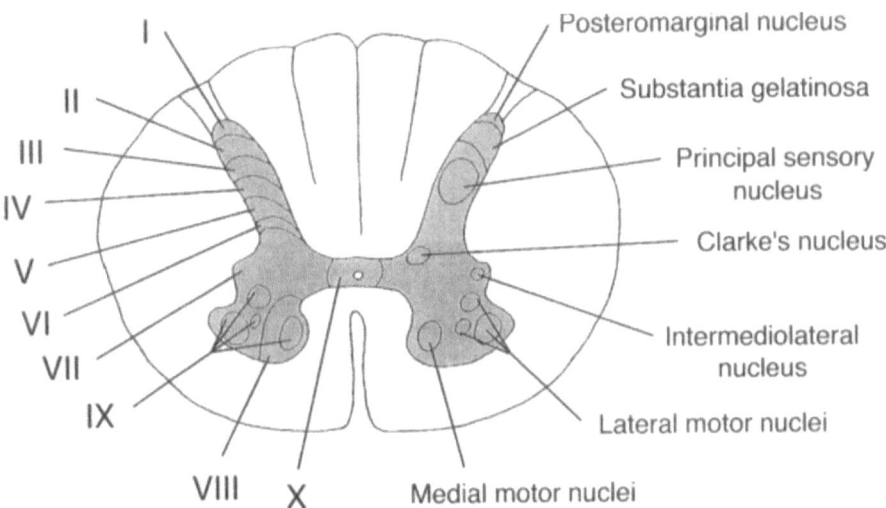

Fig. 2.1. Details of the grey matter columns in a coronal section of the spinal cord. Rexed's spinal laminae (I–X) are illustrated on the left and the major groups of nuclei are noted on the right. Not all laminae or nuclear groups are present at every level of the spinal cord (see Table 2.1).

Grey Matter

The butterfly-shaped mass of grey matter is made up of two symmetrical halves (Fig. 2.1). Each half can be divided into three parts: **posterior horn, intermediolateral horn** and **anterior horn**. The **grey commissure** is a thin strip of grey matter that crosses the midline and connects the left and right halves of the grey matter. The central canal, which is lined by ependyma, is located in the centre of this commissure.

The grey matter has been divided into 10 subdivisions or **laminae (of Rexed)** in an attempt to correlate cytoarchitecture (size, density and morphology) of neurones with information on synaptic connections and neurophysiological data from animal studies (Rexed 1954). Rexed's laminae I–VI comprise the posterior horn, laminae VII–IX constitute the anterior horn and lamina X is the central grey that surrounds the central canal within the grey commissure (Fig. 2.1).

Posterior Horn

The central process of the majority of primary sensory neurones in the posterior root ganglion terminate in and synapse with neurones in the posterior horn. Neurones in the posterior horn have several functions: (a) to modulate and process primary sensory input; (b) to relay sensory information to higher centres (i.e. thalamus and cerebellum) and (c) to participate in the segmental reflex arc.

The **posteromarginal nucleus** (Rexed lamina I) and the **substantia gelatinosa** (laminae II and part of III) are mainly involved in local modulation of pain or nociceptive sensory input and are present at all levels of the spinal cord. The **principal sensory nucleus** (nucleus proprius; laminae III and IV) relays information involving several different sensory modalities to the thalamus via the lateral and anterior spinothalamic tracts. **Clarke's nucleus** (nucleus dorsalis; lamina VII) is only present at levels C8 to L3 and provides proprioceptive input to the cerebellum via the posterior spinocerebellar tract.

Intermediolateral Horn

This column of grey matter is present in lamina VII and contains preganglionic autonomic neurones that receive input from hypothalamic and brainstem nuclei via the descending central autonomic tract. This column is present only in two regions. Levels T1–L2 contain **sympathetic preganglionic neurones** that send fibres through the anterior root to synapse with postganglionic sympathetic neurones in ganglia of the sympathetic chain. The sympathetic outflow for the entire body is through this pathway.

Parasympathetic neurones are located in the intermediolateral horn at levels S2–S4 and they give rise to the pelvic splanchnics (nervi erigentes). These nerves provide parasympathetic input to the distal colon, rectum, bladder and sexual organs and their fibres synapse with postganglionic parasympathetic neurones located in the walls of these target organs.

Anterior Horn

Large motor neurones located in lamina IX are divided into a **medial and lateral group of motor nuclei**. The medial group of motor neurones is present at all levels and supplies the axial musculature of the trunk. Lateral motor nuclei are located at the levels of the cervical (C5–T1) and lumbar (L2–S3) enlargements and innervate the musculature of the upper and lower limbs, respectively.

White Matter Tracts

The white matter is located in the periphery of the spinal cord and surrounds the grey matter. On each side, the white matter is divided into posterior, lateral and anterior columns by the posterior and anterior horns of grey matter. The proportion of white to grey matter decreases at progressively more caudal regions of the cord.

There are three different types of fibre tracts. The **ascending** and **descending** tracts are long range projections that terminate in or arise from neurones in the brainstem, diencephalon, cerebellum or cerebral hemispheres (Fig. 2.2; Tables 2.2 and 2.3). In addition, there are short range **intrasegmental** fibres that connect neurones located in the same spinal segment or **intersegmental** fibres that ascend or descend over only a few spinal segments before entering the grey matter. One group of intersegmental fibres are immediately adjacent to the grey matter, forming a thin tract called the **fasciculus proprius**. Some primary sensory fibres branch on entering the spinal cord and both ascend and descend over several segments within the **tract of Lissauer** before entering the grey matter. This tract is located between the surface of the posterolateral aspect of the cord and the tip of the posterior horn (Fig. 2.2).

ASCENDING TRACTS   DESCENDING TRACTS

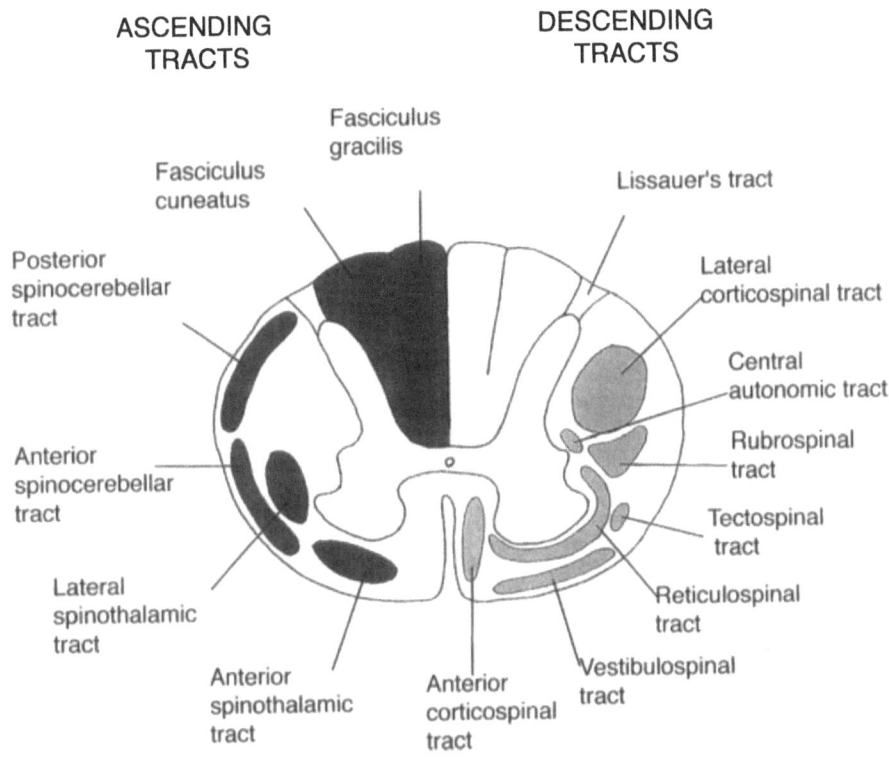

Fig. 2.2. Location of the major ascending (left) and descending (right) fibre tracts in a coronal section at a representative level of the spinal cord. Lissauer's tract contains both ascending and descending fibres.

Ascending Tracts (Fig. 2.2, Table 2.2)

Ascending tracts primarily transmit sensory information to higher relay nuclei within the main sensory pathway (e.g. thalamus) or provide sensory input (mainly proprioceptive) to the cerebellum. All ascending tracts are composed of second-order sensory afferents that arise from neurones located in grey matter, mainly the posterior horn. One exception is the posterior columns in which **fasciculi gracilis and cuneatus** are composed of primary sensory afferents from posterior root ganglia. These afferents enter the cord and ascend to the medulla without synapsing in the posterior horn. Below T6, only fasciculus gracilis is present in the posterior columns. Fasciculus cuneatus contains primary sensory afferents from posterior root ganglion above T6. At each level, these primary afferent fibres enter the most lateral aspect of the ipsilateral posterior column and take up a progressively more medial position as fibres are added at rostral levels. This results in a somatotopic organization in the posterior columns; fibres from the most caudal spinal levels (leg and lower trunk) are located most medial and fibres that arise at progressively more rostral levels are situated further lateral. Above T6, fasiculus gracilis lies medial to

Table 2.2.   Summary of the main ascending fibre tracts

Tract	Origin	Termination	Crossed/ uncrossed	Main function
Fasciculus gracilis	Posterior root ganglia below T6	Nucleus gracilis (medulla)	U	Proprioception and vibration
Fasciculus cuneatus	Posterior root ganglia above T6	Nucleus cuneatus (medulla)	U	Proprioception and and vibration
Posterior Spinocerebellar	Clarke's nucleus	Cerebellum	U	Proprioceptive, pressure and touch input to and cerebellum
Anterior Spinocerebellar	Anterior horn especially lumbosacral	Cerebellum	C	Proprioceptive, pressure and touch input to the cerebellum
Lateral Spinothalamic	Rexed laminae I, III, IV and V	Thalamus (ventral posterior nucleus)	C	Pain and temperature
Anterior Spinothalamic	Rexed laminae I, III, IV and V	Thalamus (ventral posterior nucleus)	C	Light touch and pressure

fasciculus cuneatus, separated by the dorsal intermediate septum. The main sensory modalities transmitted by these fasciculi are proprioception and vibration. Each fasciculus terminates in a nucleus (**nucleus gracilis and nucleus cuneatus**) in the posterior aspect of the lower medulla. Neurones in these nuclei give rise to second-order sensory afferents, which cross the midline at the level of the medulla, ascend in the brainstem as the medial lemniscus and terminate in the thalamus (ventral posterior nucleus).

Two spinocerebellar tracts provide sensory input to the cerebellum. The **posterior spinocerebellar tract** is an uncrossed tract that contains second-order sensory afferents that originate from Clarke's nucleus (lamina VII), which is located at levels C8 to L3. This tract lies in the posterior and peripheral aspect of the lateral column of white matter and continues into the brainstem and enters the cerebellum through the ipsilateral inferior cerebellar peduncle. The **anterior spinocerebellar tract** is a crossed tract that arises in the anterior horn, especially from neurones in the lumbar enlargement. It ascends in the anterior and peripheral aspect of the lateral column, enters the brainstem and crosses the midline again and enters the cerebellum through the superior cerebellar peduncle. Both spinocerebellar tracts transmit mainly proprioceptive information (with an additional contribution of touch and pressure) to the cerebellar vermis and paramedian aspects of the cerebellar hemispheres. This part of the cerebellum is known as the paleocerebellum or spinocerebellum and it modulates muscle tone and coordinates synergistic muscle contraction in relation to locomotion and changes in posture.

The spinothalamic tracts provide direct sensory input to the ventral posterior nucleus, the main sensory relay nucleus of the thalamus. Both the anterior and lateral spinothalamic tract are crossed tracts that originate from neurones in the principal sensory nucleus (laminae III and IV) and some neurones in laminae I and V of the posterior horn. The **lateral spinothalamic tract** is the main pathway for pain and temperature and is located in the anterior aspect of the lateral column. Neurones that give rise to this tract receive inputs from primary sensory afferents in Lissauer's tract as well as nociceptive modulatory input from the posteromarginal nucleus and substantia gelatinosa. Fibres of this tract cross the midline through the anterior grey and white commissures and at each level are added to the medial aspect of the tract. This orderly arrangement results in a somatotopic organization of fibres in this tract such that fibres from the lower extremity are lateral and the upper extremity is located medially. Considering its small surface area, the hand occupies a much larger area in the tract when compared to other regions of the body. This somatotopic arrangement underlies the loss of pain and temperature that occurs predominantly in the upper extremities (especially the hands) in central cord lesions of the cervical cord (e.g. trauma).

The **anterior spinothalamic tract** is a crossed tract and is located in the anterior column of white matter. It originates primarily from neurones in the principal sensory nucleus that receive primary afferent input of light touch and pressure. These posterior root fibres can ascend in the posterior columns over many spinal levels before they enter and synapse in the posterior horn. Therefore, the spinal cord pathway for light touch and pressure is present bilaterally and this accounts for the relative sparing of these modalities (as compared to pain and temperature) following unilateral cord lesions.

Descending Tracts (Fig. 2.2; Table 2.3)

The descending tracts can be divided into **pyramidal** and **extrapyramidal** motor pathways as well as the **central autonomic tract**. The term extrapyramidal is an inexact term but it is still frequently encountered. It is used here to describe all descending tracts that synapse on spinal neurones, excluding the lateral and anterior corticospinal tracts.

Pyramidal System Together with the corticobulbar tracts, the **lateral and anterior corticospinal tracts** comprise the pyramidal system. The corticospinal tracts contain descending fibres that originate from several different cortical areas. About 80% of the fibres originate from neurones in the primary motor cortex in the precentral gyrus (area 4 of Brodmann), primarily the large pyramidal neurones (of Betz) in cortical layer V. Other regions that contain neurones that contribute fibres to the lateral and anterior corticospinal tracts include: (a) the premotor cortex on the lateral aspect of the hemisphere (area 6); (b) the supplementary motor cortex on the medial side of the hemisphere (area 6); (c) the superior parietal lobule (area 5) and (d) the somatic sensory cortex (areas 3, 1 and 2). Fibres from these latter two sensory regions terminate in sensory nuclei in the spinal cord (e.g. the posterior horn) or brainstem, and are thought to suppress ascending sensory transmission during voluntary movements. The other descending fibres terminate in the anterior horn where they synapse, either directly or indirectly, with motor neurones. About 80% of the estimated one million fibres in the corticospinal tract cross the midline at the decussation of the pyramids in the medulla and continue on as the lateral corticospinal tract in the lateral column of white matter. Of the 20% uncrossed fibres, 5% join the lateral corticospinal tract and the remaining 15% form the uncrossed anterior corticospinal tract in the anterior column of white matter.

The lateral corticospinal tract terminates in both medial and lateral motor nuclei at all levels of the spinal cord but predominantly at the cervical and lumbar enlargements. Some fibres synapse directly on motor neurones that supply distal limb muscles and mediate the skilled movements (e.g. pincher grasp) that are unique to primates and humans. Bilateral lesions of the pyramidal tract at the level of the

Table 2.3. Summary of the main descending fibre tracts

Tract	Origin	Termination	Crossed/ uncrossed	Main function
Pyramidal system				
Lateral corticospinal	Layer V neurones in the contralateral motor cortex (major)	Medial and lateral motor nuclei at all levels	C (95%)	Skilled movements mediated by distal limb muscles
Anterior corticospinal	Layer V neurones in contralateral motor cortex	Medial and lateral motor nuclei in cervical and upper thoracic levels	U	Descending motor input to motor neurones that innervate neck musculature
Extrapyramidal system				
Rubrospinal	Contralateral Red nucleus (midbrain)	Spinal neurones primarily at cervical levels	C	Posture and locomotion primarily exor activities (small tract in man)
Reticulospinal	Bilateral reticular formation (pons and medulla)	Spinal neurones for trunk and proximal limb musculature	C and U	Posture and locomotion, respiration, modulation of pain, vasomotor tone
Tectospinal	Superior and inferior colliculi	Motor neurones for neck muscles	C	Reflex head movements toward visual and auditory stimuli
Vestibulospinal	Ipsilateral vestibular nuclei (medulla)	Spinal neurones for trunk musculature	U	Posture and locomotion primarily extensor activities
Central autonomic tract				
Sympathetic tract	Hypothalamus and brainstem nuclei	Preganglionic sympathetic neurones in intermediolateral nucleus (T1–L2)	C and U	Descending sympathetic outflow to entire body
Parasympathetic	Hypothalamus and brainstem nuclei	Preganglionic parasympathetic neurones in the intermediolateral nucleus (S2–4)	C and U	Parasympathetic supply to the distal colon, rectum, bladder and sexual organs

decussation only result in a loss of skilled hand movements, but a preservation of all gross locomotor functions (Lawrence and Kuypers 1968). Other corticospinal fibres activate axial and proximal limb muscles indirectly by synapsing with excitatory interneurons. Finally, other fibres modulate the spinal reflexes by synapsing on interneurons that are involved in the segmental reflex arc.

Fibres in the anterior corticospinal tract are uncrossed and terminate in medial and lateral motor nuclei in the cervical and upper thoracic segments. They primarily supply motor neurones that innervate neck musculature.

Extrapyramidal System Several brainstem nuclei project to the spinal cord and play prominent roles in the initiation and control of locomotion, as well as posture. Stimulation of the pontine and medullary reticular formation, indicates involvement of the reticulospinal pathways in locomotion, respiration and vasomotor phenomena. Stimulation of the lateral vestibular nucleus results in an increase in extensor muscle tone, whereas stimulation of rubrospinal neurones results in facilitation of flexor muscle tone, primarily at the cervical cord level. Tectospinal projections to the cervical cord appear to be involved in orienting responses of the head to visual and auditory stimuli. The main features of the **rubrospinal, reticulospinal, tectospinal and vestibulospinal tracts** are summarized in Table 2.3.

Central Autonomic Tract Both sympathetic and parasympathetic pathways originate in hypothalamic and brainstem nuclei (e.g. nucleus of the solitary tract) and descend to synapse on preganglionic neurones located in the brainstem and spinal cord (Loewy and Spyer 1990). This descending autonomic tract contains both crossed and uncrossed fibres and is located in the lateral column of white matter, adjacent to the intermediolateral horn. This tract supplies sympathetic outflow to the entire body and synapses with sympathetic preganglionic neurones located in the intermediolateral horn at levels T1–L2. As outlined earlier, these preganglionic fibres exit through the anterior roots and synapse on postganglionic neurones located in ganglia of the sympathetic chain.

The majority of visceral organs in the body receive preganglionic parasympathetic fibres that originate in cranial nerve nuclei in the brainstem. For example, the vagus nerve supplies all visceral organs in the chest and innervates the bowel up to the beginning of the descending colon. Preganglionic parasympathetic innervation to the distal colon, rectum, bladder and sexual organs originates from neurones in the intermediolateral horn at levels S2–S4. The central autonomic tract provides parasympathetic input to these preganglionic neurones.

References

Barr ML (1979) The human nervous system 3rd edn. Harper & Row, New York

Burt AM (1993) Textbook of neuroanatomy. WB Saunders, Toronto

Coggeshall RE, Applebaum ML, Frazen M, Stubbs TB III, Sykes MT (1975) Unmyelinated axons in human ventral roots, a possible explanation for the failure of dorsal rhizotomy to relieve pain. Brain 98:157–166

Fitzgerald MJT (1992) Neuroanatomy, basic and clinical, 2nd edn. Baillière Tindall, Toronto

Lawrence DG, Kuypers HGJ (1968) The functional organization of the motor system in the monkey. I. The effects of bilateral pyramidal lesions. Brain 91:1–14

Loewy AD, Spyer KM (eds) (1990) Central regulation of autonomic functions. Oxford University Press, New York

Rexed B (1954) A cytoarchitectonic atlas of the spinal cord in the cat. J Comp Neurol 100:297–379

Chapter 3

Prospects for Spinal Cord Repair after Injury

J.D. Steeves and T.J. Zwimpfer

Approximately 10 000 new cases of spinal cord injury (SCI) occur each year in the United States while Canada records about 1000 new cases per year (Fehlings 1994). It is estimated that there are more than 200 000 chronic SCI patients at any given time in the United States. Of these individuals, 45% are quadriplegic and 55% paraplegic. Current estimates suggest that 19% of all quadriplegic patients and 28% of all paraplegics are complete injuries (ie. no sensory or motor function below the level of the lesion). As in any traumatic central nervous system (CNS) injury, the majority of individuals who suffer SCI are male (82%) and between 16 and 30 years of age (61%) (Tator et al. 1993). In the United States, motor vehicle accidents (48%), accidental falls (21%), sports injuries (14%) and gunshot wounds (15%) constitute the major causes of SCI.

In comparison to some other neurological disorders, such as Alzheimer's disease, the total number of SCI patients is relatively small. However, the expected lifespan of many SCI patients is now comparable to that of able-bodied individuals. Consequently, over the lifetime of each SCI patient, the cost of acute and chronic medical care, as well as rehabilitation training, can easily exceed one million dollars (significantly higher after a high cervical injury). In short, the estimated annual cost for the care of all SCI patients in the United States is approximately six billion dollars. Such figures do not include the equally important personal costs of lost or reduced opportunity suffered by each SCI patient or the public expenditures necessary to make our communities more accessible for the disabled individual.

These considerations form a compelling argument for the prevention of SCI as well as the maintenance of rigorous research programmes to search for a cure for SCI. One intriguing observation is that the spinal cord is not completely severed in many clinically (i.e. functionally) complete injuries. Thus one strategy is to maximize the preservation of damaged neurones while limiting the secondary damage of uninjured neurones and axons (Dusart and Schwab 1994). Other therapies would then attempt to reform functional synaptic connections through axonal regeneration from injured neurones or sprouting from uninjured neurones. A comprehensive review of such a complex topic is not possible in one chapter. Thus, this chapter highlights (a) the overall goals of spinal cord research, (b) some of the current approaches in CNS injury and repair research, and (c) a few potential strategies that may prove fruitful in the near future.

Goal 1: To Enhance the Survival of Neurones after Injury

The primary damage in SCI is usually the result of mechanical trauma in the form of spinal cord laceration, compression or shearing of the cord due to distraction of the vertebrae. As mentioned above, most injuries have a degree of spared neural tissue at the time of injury. Thus, it is imperative to prevent cell death in injured (i.e. axotomized) neurones, as well as limit the degree of secondary damage to uninjured neurones. Examination of autopsied spinal cords from chronic SCI patients often reveals cysts within the traumatized region creating a physical gap in tissue continuity. These cavities are interlaced with scaffold-like trabeculae of connective tissue and astrocytes. Surviving axons are often associated with either these trabeculae or the pia mater around the outer rim of the spinal cord.

The essential neuronal tracts that must be either spared or repaired after SCI are: (a) the brainstem–spinal projections (e.g. reticulospinal, vestibulospinal, rubrospinal) which are critical for locomotor function and control (especially those pathways coursing through ventrolateral funiculi; Steeves and Jordan 1980); (b) the corticospinal pathways which are essential for coordinated movements (prehensile grasping) by the hand (Lawrence and Kuypers 1968); and (c) the dorsal column pathways and spinothalamic tracts which are important for somaesthetic and nociceptive function, respectively.

The known mechanisms leading to secondary neuronal damage include: (a) ischaemia resulting from reduced spinal cord blood flow; (b) inflammatory responses and attack by components of the systemic immune system due to a breakdown of the blood–brain barrier; (c) toxic effects of chemicals released from injured cells (e.g. excitatory amino acids such as glutamate); and (d) increases in intracellular free radical and calcium concentrations.

To minimize secondary damage, all SCI patients should be aggressively resuscitated to prevent or reverse hypoxia and hypotension. In addition, current standard therapy includes the intravenous administration of high dose methylprednisolone sodium succinate (MPSS or Solumedrol). When MPSS is started within the first 8 h of trauma, it appears to improve neurological outcome (when compared to placebo) in SCI patients assessed 8 months after injury using outcome measures of spared segmental sensory and motor function (Bracken et al. 1992). No benefit has been noted if MPSS is administered more than 8 h after trauma. Conclusive determination that MPSS treatment is beneficial is complicated by the observation that MPSS effects are most evident in those individuals who suffered an incomplete lesion (Young 1994). In short, there is still controversy surrounding MPSS therapy with one study even suggesting that MPSS treatment had a negative effect on the functional outcomes in patients with penetrating SCI (Prendergast et al. 1994).

Recent animal experiments (Behrmann et al. 1994) have also examined the acute administration of a 21-aminosteroid (U74006F) and a thyrotropin releasing hormone (TRH) analogue (YM-14673) after spinal cord contusion. They assessed function on an inclined plane test and with open field walking, and examined the amount of spared spinal tissue. They report that all therapeutic agents were better than controls, with the 21-aminosteroid equivalent to MPSS and the TRH analogue being slightly better than MPSS.

GM-1 ganglioside, a glycolipid (monosialoganglioside) found in most neural membranes, has also been reported to have a protective effect on spinal cord tissue after traumatic injury in a small number of patients (Geisler et al. 1991; Geisler 1993). It has been suggested that gangliosides protect neurones from the toxic effects of excess excitatory amino acids released after SCI. GM-1 may also act as a neurotrophic agent. Nevertheless, confirmation of an unequivocal therapeutic benefit awaits analysis of data from larger clinical trials.

A recent animal study suggests that the anti-inflammatory agent indomethacin (IM) has potential benefits after traumatic injury. IM uncouples cyclo-oxygenase pathways which prevents production of inflammatory mediators (prostaglandins E_2, F_2, I_2 and thromboxane A_2) from arachidonic acid, as well as reduces free radical production. Arachidonic acid is a free fatty acid liberated from phospholipids during enzymatic hydrolysis of traumatized cell membranes (Guth et al. 1994). Interestingly, corticosteroids (e.g. MPSS) are known to prevent the production of arachidonic acid by limiting lipid hydrolysis.

In addition, Guth et al. (1994) suggest that lipopolysaccharide (LPS), which is produced by the bacteria, salmonella enteritidus, may also have beneficial effects. A classical interpretation of LPS action is that it stimulates astrocytes to produce cytokines (e.g. interleukins (IL) 1,3,6, prostaglandins and tumour necrosis factor α (TNFα)) Cytokines then facilitate or maintain the local disruption of the blood–brain barrier (BBB) resulting in an infiltration of macrophages, neutrophils and lymphocytes into the CNS which have (as yet undetermined) beneficial effects. An alternative mechanism suggests that LPS may stimulate resident CNS microglia to secrete IL-1β which then stimulates astrocytes to secrete cytokines TNFα and IL-6 (Lee et al. 1993). The general cellular actions of cytokines, as well as the specific reasons they may be beneficial to traumatized CNS tissue are still poorly understood. Nevertheless, the most important finding was that the combined administration of IM, LPS and MPSS had the most beneficial effects for reducing necrosis (Guth et al. 1994).

After CNS trauma, programmed cell death (or apoptosis) is thought to be triggered in some CNS neurones, even those that were initially uninjured. Apoptosis can be described as the activation of an intrinsic genetic programme within the neurone for suicide so that it may be removed without causing damage to surrounding cells. It is characterized by shrinkage of cell size, chromatin condensation and DNA fragmentation, all within an intact cell membrane. Most experiments now focus on identifying which cellular events trigger apoptosis and how apoptotic genes might be controlled. For example, recent in vitro experiments have suggested that sympathetic neurones are dependent on the presence of nerve growth factor (NGF) for survival and undergo apoptosis when NGF is withdrawn from the culture (Allsopp et al. 1993; Greenlund et al. 1995). However, over-expression of the *bcl-2* gene will inhibit apoptosis in these cells. Other experiments have demonstrated that *bcl-2* over-expression will also rescue neurones from apoptosis induced by ischaemia (Martinou et al. 1994) or axotomy (Dubois-Dauphin et al. 1994). Alternatively, the down-regulation of the cysteine protease, ICE (interleukin 1β converting enzyme) or the human homologue gene, *CPP32*, may be another effective strategy (Gagliardini et al. 1994). Likewise, a cowpox viral gene product, *crmA*, inhibits ICE and in vitro prevents apoptosis in chick dorsal root ganglion cells. In the future, effective in vivo gene therapy will require that only specific genes be altered within selected neurones. Consequently more research is required to determine the best vector system to introduce genes into injured CNS neurones. Most current research is focused on the possible use of viral vectors to transfect the appropriate gene sequence.

Various trophic factors have been suggested to maintain the survival of developing neurones, and may also be important for the survival of injured adult neurones. They include: brain-derived neurotrophic factor (BDNF), ciliary neurotrophic factor (CNTF), epidermal growth factor (EGF), basic fibroblast growth factor (bFGF), glial derived neurotrophic factor (GDNF), platelet derived growth factor (PDGF), insulin-like growth factor (IGF), NGF, and neurotrophins (NT) 3,4/5 (e.g. Thoenen et al. 1993; Dechant et al. 1994; Oppenheim et al. 1994; Zhang et al. 1994). Administration of some of these factors has been suggested as a potential therapy to prevent neuronal death in several neurodegenerative disorders (e.g. amyotrophic lateral sclerosis, Alzheimer's, or Parkinson's disease). Similarly, there is a clear indication that axotomized neurones can be rescued from cell death by infusion of certain growth factors (Mansour-Robaey et al. 1994; Oppenheim et al. 1994). However, it is not clear whether growth factor administration only delays cell death.

As mentioned above, it is not uncommon to confirm with magnetic resonance imaging that many SCIs are anatomically incomplete. Consequently, limiting the degree of "secondary" damage to the initially spared neurones and axonal projections of the traumatized cord is imperative. It is well documented that the lysis of cell membranes can release a range of chemicals that have detrimental effects on nearby cells. For example, the exaggerated release of excitatory amino acids, such as glutamate, from injured or ischaemic cells has been implicated in functional deficits after SCI. Both the N-methyl-D-aspartate (NMDA) and non-NMDA (AMPA/kainate) subclass of glutamate receptor have been suggested to mediate the destructive events. For example, after an incomplete SCI in rats, the intraspinal infusion of a selective antagonist of the non-NMDA receptors, NBQX (2,3-dihydroxy-6-nitro-7-sulphamoyl-benzo(f)quinoxaline), reduces the subsequent loss of spinal cord tissue and improves functional recovery (Wrathall et al. 1994). The elevation of extracellular glutamate is also known to increase intracellular calcium levels within all nearby cells to toxic levels. Thus there has been a focus on strategies to preserve intracellular calcium levels within tolerable limits by increasing the buffering capacity for intracellular calcium with cell-permeant calcium chelators like BAPTA-AM (1,2-bis(2-aminophenoxy)ethane-N,N,N',N'-tetraacetic acid acetoxymethyl ester) or increasing the buffering activity of endogenous calcium binding proteins, such as calbindin and calmodulin (Tymianski et al. 1994). Finally, excess glutamate stimulation or increasing intracellular calcium levels can elevate reactive oxygen species (free radicals) which have cytotoxic properties, including stimulating apoptosis. Antioxidants such as superoxide dismutase and bcl-2 have been shown to be neuroprotective (Greenlund et al. 1995) to neurones in culture.

Goal 2: To Promote the Expression of Factors that Facilitate Axonal Regrowth and/or Replace Lost Tissue with Transplanted Cells

Considering that axonal regeneration after axotomy is dependent, at least in part, on a recapitulation of the initial developmental programme for axonal growth, it is important to characterize the known components of axonal development. Some proteins and their related genes, such as growth-associated protein 43 (GAP-43, Tetzlaff et al. 1991) and Tα1 α-tubulin (Gloster et al. 1994) are involved in axonal outgrowth during development and down-regulate their expression after axonal growth is completed. These same genes and proteins have also been observed to increase their expression in response to axonal injury. Thus, increased expression of these and other genes may be required for axonal regeneration. Elucidation of the genetic programmes necessary for axonal growth is thus an important requirement for designing future gene therapies for facilitating axonal regeneration in vivo. For example, one strategy would exploit the up-regulation of these so-called regeneration associated genes (RAGs) by coupling the promoter region of the RAG (e.g. the Tα1 gene) to another required gene (e.g. a specific neurotrophin gene) that you want expressed in an injured neurone. Since the RAG promoter should only be up-regulated in an injured neurone, expression of the coupled gene would be restricted to injured neurones (Gloster et al. 1994).

Various glycoproteins belonging to one of three structural families (immunoglobulins, cadherins and integrins) are involved as adhesion molecules and have been suggested to have various roles in cell migration, axonal fasciculation and perhaps even direct axonal growth (i.e. as a tropic factor). Neural cell adhesion molecule (NCAM, a member of the immunoglobulin superfamily) is one of the more abundant adhesion molecules found on neural cell surfaces. NCAM is expressed throughout various stages of neural development and significantly down-regulated during adult life. It is a homophilic binding protein that may play an important role in axons of similar origin associating with each other (fasciculation) during axon outgrowth to a common target (ie. it plays a role in the formation of CNS tracts and perhaps also in regeneration; Carbonetto 1991; Edelman 1994).

Transplantation of neural tissue may be used to facilitate repair after a CNS injury, in three ways: (1) replace lost neurones with fetal neurones or modified neural stem cells; (2) replenish essential depleted or down-regulated molecules with genetically modified cells that secrete the missing molecule, and (3) provide a bridge for axonal regeneration across a cyst cavity using fetal CNS or peripheral nerve tissue. The survival of transplanted fetal neurones within the CNS is well documented (Fisher and Gage 1994). Grafted fetal neurones have been observed to differentiate, integrate with host adult tissue, and even ameliorate the loss of some CNS functions (e.g. Parkinson's disease; Nikkhah et al. 1994). Since adult neurones are post-mitotic, it has been thought that the adult CNS could not generate new neurones. Recently, however, neural stem cell within the subependymal lining of the lateral ventricles of the adult brain have been identified. These cells can be removed, maintained in culture and manipulated in vitro with specific neurotrophic factors to differentiate into a number of different phenotypes. Thus, these adult neural stem cells could be the source of new neurones and glia for transplantation after CNS degeneration or trauma (Reynolds and Weiss 1992).

The transplantation into the rat spinal cord of immortalized neurotrophin-secreting cells, such as fibroblasts, has also been observed to induce axonal ingrowth into the grafted tissue (Tuszynski et al. 1994). This promises to be an interesting therapeutic avenue for the delivery of molecules important for CNS repair.

The suggestion that peripheral nerve grafts will support the outgrowth of severed axons was first made by Tello (1911) and Ramon-y-Cajal (1928). More recently, it was shown that axotomized CNS neurones will extend axons into peripheral nerve grafts inserted into the CNS of adult animals (Richardson et al. 1980; David and Aguayo 1981). These findings established that, at least some, adult CNS neurones retain the intrinsic ability to regenerate axons when provided with an environment that is conducive for growth. Schwann cells have been suggested to be the important constituent of peripheral nerve that supports axonal regeneration and Schwann cell impregnated guidance channels have been used experimentally to bridge the spinal cord cyst after SCI (Xu et al. 1995).

Finally, recent animal studies have suggested that some trophic factors may also have a role in stimulating the regeneration of axons. Neurotrophin-3 (NT-3) will facilitate increased axonal growth in axotomized corticospinal fibres when combined with an antibody (IN-1) that blocks myelin inhibitory proteins (also see below; Schnell et al. 1994).

Goal 3: To Block Expression of Factors that Inhibit Axonal Regrowth

The relatively poor capacity of the CNS for regeneration has been attributed in part to inhibitory influences intrinsic to the adult CNS. The proliferation and hypertrophy of astrocytes around the site of injury is a characteristic response in all mammals after SCI (Dusart and Schwab 1994). This reactive astrogliosis (sometimes called glial scarring) has been suggested to form a physical and/or chemical barrier to axonal regeneration. Alternatively, it may be that the astrogliosis is a CNS response to reduce the magnitude of SCI and facilitate neural repair (even if it is ultimately insufficient). Some in vitro data suggest that astrocytes can be a supportive substrate for axonal growth. Whether astrocytes are inhibitory or supportive for CNS repair has been difficult to resolve, perhaps because it has been difficult to characterize the different phenotypes or states of differentiation of astrocytes. Several molecules (e.g. tenascin, heparin sulphate proteoglycan, HSPG; chondroitin sulphate proteoglycan, CSPG; dermatan/keratan sulphate proteoglycan, KSPG) located either on the astrocyte surface or secreted by astrocytes have been shown to either inhibit or facilitate axonal growth in vitro (Riopelle and Dow 1990; Snow et al. 1990a&b; McKeon et al. 1991; Snow and Letourneau 1992.). Although there is not complete agreement, recent findings suggest that tenascin and CSPG and KSPG may be inhibitory (Taylor et al. 1993; Dow et al. 1994; Smith-Thomas et al. 1994), whereas HSPG is a supportive substrate for neuronal differentiation. Chondroitinase and keratanase enzyme pretreatment will cleave specific glycosaminoglycan side chains from CSPG or KSPG and reduce the inhibition of CSPG and KSPG as substrates for axonal growth in vitro (Dow et al. 1994; Smith-Thomas et al. 1994). Likewise, januscin (a closely related molecule to tenascin) which is primarily expressed on oligodendrocytes is also inhibitory to axonal growth by some, but not all, neurones (Schachner et al. 1994). It is likely that the different extracellular domains of these surface matrix molecules, acting via different receptors, determine whether the glial cell surface is inhibitory or supportive for axonal growth. It has also been noted that many of these extracellular matrix molecules alter their extracellular domains during development (ie. differentiate) thereby creating an inhibitory environment for axonal growth within the adult CNS (Carbonetto 1991).

As mentioned above, several lines of evidence suggest that CNS myelin or molecules associated with myelin inhibit axonal growth. Two CNS myelin proteins (NI-35 and NI-250) have been partially purified and characterized (Caroni and Schwab 1988a). A neutralizing antibody (IN-1) was then developed that blocks the inhibitory effects of myelin (Caroni and Schwab 1988b). The in vivo secretion of this IN-1 antibody from hybridoma cells placed within the adult cerebral hemispheres enhances the regeneration of some rat corticospinal axons severed at rostral spinal levels (Schnell and Schwab 1990). Independently, two groups have also observed that myelin associated glycoprotein (MAG) also inhibits or retards the rate of axonal growth in vitro (Mukhopadhyay et al. 1994; McKerracher et al. 1994). Thus there is a distinct possibility that there is more than one inhibitory myelin molecule. Does this also mean that specific therapies must be developed to overcome each inhibitory molecule or are alternative strategies needed that transiently disrupt the entire myelin structure?

In an embryonic chicken, transection of the thoracic spinal cord prior to embryonic day (E) 13 (of the 21-day developmental period) results in brainstem–spinal axonal regeneration/repair and functional locomotor recovery. Conversely repair rapidly diminishes following a transection on E13–E14 (Hasan et al. 1993). The myelination of fibre tracts within the spinal cord also begins on E13, coincident with the transition from permissive to restrictive repair periods. Interestingly, myelin never develops within any vertebrate CNS fibre tract until axonal development is complete. A immunological protocol that delays the onset of CNS myelination, extends the permissive period for axonal regeneration and functional recovery to correspondingly later stages of development (Keirstead et al. 1992). The immunological treatment involves the infusion into the cord of serum complement in combination with an oligodendrocyte/myelin-specific antibody which 'binds the complement to oligodendrocyte or myelin membranes. In adult birds, the same immunological protocol also transiently disrupts compact myelin and facilitates some axonal regeneration of axotomized brainstem–spinal neurons. The compacted form of myelin subsequently re-appears after the immunological protocol is discontinued (Steeves et al. 1994).

Goal 4: To Stimulate Appropriate Sensorimotor Capacity Necessary for Functional Recovery

There is ample clinical evidence of the need for physical and occupational therapy to maintain adequate muscle mass, and normal ranges of joint motion in patients rendered less active by a spinal cord injury. Thus, there is the need to maximize the functional capabilities of patients with incomplete lesions, including the optimization of sensorimotor coordination. If and when regeneration and reconnection within the injured spinal cord becomes possible, it will be necessary to maintain adequate function of muscle and spinal cord neuronal circuits below the lesion in order to optimize the effect of any subsequent regenerating input. In addition, in the few instances where experimental CNS regeneration has been documented, synapses have been observed to form with both appropriate and inappropriate target neurones (Zwimpfer et al. 1992). Consequently, will we have to "retrain" inopportune synaptic connections to behave in a functionally correct context? Both physical and pharmacological techniques are currently used to optimize sensorimotor potential, but they may also be important to augment or stimulate the appropriate function from any repaired pathway that has been induced to repair anatomically.

It has long been known that the spinal cord contains all the essential neuronal circuits for generating alternating limb movements characteristic of stepping (Grillner 1975; and Wallen 1985). Activation of these circuits after spinal cord injury can be achieved by altering appropriate peripheral inputs (e.g. increasing cutaneous and proprioceptive inputs during the weight support phase, in order to produce and/or improve functional stepping activity; Duysens and Pearson 1976; Barbeau et al. 1987; Lovely et al. 1990; Edgerton et al. 1992; Muir and Steeves 1995). There is evidence that the isolated spinal cord retains some degree of functional plasticity and can retain learned alterations of spinal cord reflexes (Wolpaw and Chong 1989). Training with increased weight loads has also been shown to significantly improve stepping abilities of experimental animals and humans with spinal cord injuries (Barbeau and Rossignol 1987; Barbeau et al. 1987). More recent studies have shown that the hyperactive reflexes of spinal injured patients can be conditioned, either operantly (Segal and Wolf 1995) or with appropriately timed musculocutaneous stimulation (Fung and Barbeau 1994), in order to reduce the deleterious effects of spasticity on motor function. Functional electrical stimulation (FES) has also been used to improve stepping abilities in incomplete SCI patients (Stein et al. 1993). FES employs implantable devices which provide appropriately timed stimulation to muscles during stepping. These training regimes can also be combined with pharmacological therapies to improve locomotion in spinal cord injured patients.

It is known that intravenous or intrathecal infusion of certain neurotransmitter precursors or agonists (e.g. the noradrenergic precursor L-dopa or noradrenergic agonist clonidine) will activate spinal cord neuronal networks to produce stepping activity (Barbeau and Rossignol 1990). In addition to promoting stepping activity, pharmacological agents are beneficial in reducing spasticity which is prominent after SCI in many patients and which often interferes with functional stepping abilities. In particular, cyproheptadine (a 5-HT blocker) and baclofen (a GABA agonist) have been shown in clinical trials to improve locomotor performance in significantly (Wainberg et al. 1990).

In conclusion, all SCI researchers agree it is unlikely that any single therapeutic intervention will be sufficient to promote complete functional repair of a severely traumatized cord. However, the current pace of discovery is rapidly providing many of the missing pieces to the repair puzzle. We are also quickly learning how to spatially and temporally organize the pieces to form an integrated picture for a comprehensive therapy.

Acknowledgements We would like to thank Christopher McBride, Gillian Muir and Wolfram Tetzlaff for their constructive comments and suggestions. We are grateful for the financial support of the following Canadian Agencies: The Medical Research Council, The Neuroscience Network, The Natural Sciences and Engineering Research Council and The British Columbia Health Research Foundation.

References

Allsopp TE, Wyatt SF, Davies AM (1993) The proto-oncogene bcl-2 can selectively rescue neurotrophic factor dependent neurons from apoptosis. Cell 73:295–307

Barbeau H, Rossignol S (1987) Recovery of locomotion after chronic spinalization in the adult cat. Brain Res 412:84–85

Barbeau H, Rossignol S (1990) Initiation and modulation of the locomotor pattern in the adult chronic spinal cat by noradrenergic, serotonergic and dopaminergic drugs. Brain Res 514: 55–67

Barbeau H, Wainberg M, Finch L (1987) Description and application of a system for locomotor rehabilitation. Med Biol Eng Comput 25:341–344

Behrmann DL, Bresnahan JC, Beattie MS. Modelling of acute spinal cord injury in the rat: neuroprotection and enhanced recovery with methylprednisolone, U-74006F and YM-14673. Exp Neurol 1994 Mar; 126(1):61–75

Bracken MB, Shepard MJ, Collins WF et al. (1992) Methylprednisolone or naloxone treatment after acute spinal cord injury: 1 year follow-up data. Results of the second National Acute Spinal Cord Injury Study. J Neurosurg 76:23–31

Carbonetto S (1991) Facilitatory and inhibitory effects of glial cells and extracellular matrix in axonal regeneration. Curr Opin Neurobiol 1:407–413

Caroni P, Schwab M (1998a) Two membrane protein fractions from rat central myelin with inhibitory propoerties for neurite growth and fibroblast spreading. J Cell Biol 106:1281–1288

Caroni P, Schwab M (1988b) Antibody against myelin-associated inhibitor of neurite growth neutralizes nonpermissive substrate properties of CNS white matter. Neuron 1:85–96

David S, Aguayo AJ (1981) Axonal elongation into PNS "bridges" after CNS injury in adult rats. Science 214:931–933

Dechant G, Rodriguez-Tebar A, Barde YA (1994) Neurotrophin receptors. Prog Neurobiol 42(2):347–252

Dow KE, Ethell DW, Steeves JD, Riopelle RJ (1994) Molecular correlates of spinal cord repair in the embryonic chick: heparan sulfate and condroitin sulfate proteoglycans. Exp Neurol 128:233–238

Dubois-Dauphin M, Frankowski H, Tsujimoto Y, Haurt J, Martinou J-C (1994) Neonatal motoneurons overexpressing the bcl-2 protooncogene in transgenic mice are protected from axotomy-induced cell death. Proc Natl Acad Sci 91:3309–3313

Dusart I, Schwab ME (1994) Secondary cell death and the inflammatory reaction after dorsal hemisection of the rat spinal cord. Eur J Neurosci 6:712–724

Duysens J, Pearson KG (1976) The role of cutaneous afferents from the distal hindlimb in the regulation of the step cycle of thalamic cats. Exp. Brain Res 24:245–255

Edelman GM (1994) Adhesion and counteradhesion: morphogenetic functions of the cell surface. Prog Brain Res 101:1–14

Edgerton VR, Roy RR, Hodgson JA, Proberr RJ, deGuzman CP, deLeon R (1992) Potential of adult mammalian lumbosacral spinal cord to execute and acquire improved locomotion in the absence of supraspinal input. J Neurotrauma 9:119–128

Fehlings MG (1994) Current medical management of acute spinal cord injury. Neurol Emerg Worldwide Studies 5(2):1–4

Fisher LJ, Gage FH (1994) Intracerebral transplantation: basic and clinical applications to the neostriatum. FASEB J 8:489–496

Fung J, Barbeau H (1994) Effects of conditioning cutaneomuscular stimulation on the soleus H-reflex in normal and spastic paretic subjects during walking and standing. J Neurophysiol 72:2090–2104

Gagliardini V, Fernandez PA, Lee RK, Drexler HC, Rotello RJ, Fishman MC Yuan J (1994) Prevention of vertebrate neuronal death by the crmA gene. Science 263:826–828

Geisler FH (1993) GM-1 ganglioside and motor recovery following human spinal cord injury. J Emerg Med 11(suppl 1):49–55

Geisler FH, Dorsey FC, Coleman, WP (1991) Recovery of motor function after spinal cord injury: a randomized, placebo-controlled trial with GM-1 ganglioside. N Engl J Med 324:1829–1838.

Gloster A, Wu W, Speelman A et al. (1994) The Tα1 α-tubulin promotor specifies gene expression as a function of neuronal growth and regeneration in transgenic mice. J Neurosci 14:7319–7330

Greenlund, LSJ, Deckwerth TL, Johnson EM (1995) Superoxide dismutase delays neuronal apoptosis: a role for reactive oxygen species in programmed neuronal death. Neuron 14:303–315

Grillner S (1975) Locomotion in vertebrates: central mechanisms and reflex interactions. Physiol Rev 55:247–304

Grillner S, Wallen P (1985) Central pattern generators for locomotion, with special reference to vertebrates. Ann Rev Neurosci 8:233–261

Guth L, Zhang Z, Roberts E (1994) Key role for pregnenolone in combination therapy that promotes recovery after spinal cord injury. Proc Natl Acad Sci USA 91:12308–12312

Hasan SJ, Keirstead HS, Muir GD, Steeves JD (1993) Axonal regeneration contributes to repair of injured brainstem–spinal neurons in embryonic chick. J Neurosci 13:492–507

Keirstead HS, Hasan SJ, Muir GD, Steeves JD (1992) Suppression of the onset of myelination extends the permissive period for the functional repair of embryonic spinal cord. Proc Natl Acad Sci USA 89:11664–11668

Lawrence DG Kuypers HGJM (1968) The functional organization of the motor system of the monkey. I. The effects of bilateral pyramidal lesions. Brain 91:1–14

Lee SC, Liu W, Dickson DW, Brosnan CF, Berman JW (1993) Cytokine production by human fetal microglia and astrocytes: differential induction by lipopolysaccharide and IL-1β. J Immunol 150:2659–2667

Lovely RG, Gregor RJ, Roy RR, Edgerton VR (1990) Weight-bearing hindlimb stepping in treadmill-exercised adult spinal cats. Brain Res 514:206–218

Mansour-Robaey S, Clarke DB, Wang Y-C, Bray, GM, Aguayo, AJ (1994) Effects of ocular injury and the administration of brain derived neurotrophic factor (BDNF) on the survival and regrowth of axotomized retinal ganglion cells. Proc Natl Acad Sci USA 91:1632–1636

Martinou JC, Dubois-Dauphin M, Staple JK, Rodriguez I, Frankowski H, Missotten M, Albertini P, Talabot D, Catsicas S, Pietra C, et al. Overexpression of BCL-2 in transgenic mice protects neurons from naturally occurring cell death and experimental ischemia. Neuron 1994 Oct; 13(4):1017–30

McKeon RJ, Schreiber RC, Rudge JS, Silver J (1991) Reduction of neurite outgrowth in a model of glial scarring following CNS injury is correlated with the expression of inhibitory molecules on reactive astrocytes. J Neurosci 11:3398–3411

McKerracher L, David S, Jackson DL, Kottis V, Dunn RJ, Braun PE (1994) Identification of myelin associated glycoprotein as a major myelin-dervied inhibitor of neurite growth. Neuron 13:805–811

Muir GD, Steeves JD (1995) Phasic cutaneous input facilitates locomotor recovery after incomplete spinal injury in the chick. J Neurophysiol. 74:358–368

Mukhopadhyay G, Doherty P, Walsh FS, Crocker PR, Filbin MT (1994) A novel role for myelin-associacited glycoprotein as an inhibitor of axonal regeneration. Neuron 13:757–767

Nikkhah G, Bentlage C, Cunningham MG, Bjorklund A (1994) Intranigral fetal dopamine grafts induce behavioral compensation in the rat Parkinson model. J Neurosci 14:3449–3461

Oppenheim RW, Houenou LJ, Johnson JE et al. (1995) Developing motor neurons rescued from programmed and axotomy-induced cell death by GDNF. Nature 373:344–346

Prendergast MR, Saxe JM, Ledgerwood AM, Lucas CE, Lucas WF (1994) Massive steroids do not reduce the zone of injury after penetrating spinal cord injury. J Trauma 37:576–579

Ramon y Cajal S (1928) Degeneration and regeneration of the nervous system (RM May, ed, transl). Hafner, New York

Reynolds BA, Weiss S (1992) Generation of neurons and astrocytes from isolated cells of the adult mammalian central nervous system. Science 255:1707–1710

Richardson PM, McGuinness Um, Aguayo AJ (1980) Axons from CNS neurones regenerate into PNS grafts. Nature 284:264–265

Riopelle RJ, Dow KE (1990) Functional interactions of heparan sulphate proteoglycans with laminin. Brain Res 525:92–100

Schachner M, Taylor J, Bartsch U, Pesheva P (1994) The perplexing multifunctionality of janusin, a tenascin-related molecule. Perspect Dev Neurobiol 2:33–41

Schnell L, Schwab M (1990) Axonal regeneration in the rat spinal cord produced by an antibody against myelin associated with neurite-growth inhibitors. Nature 343:269–272

Schnell L, Schneider R, Kolbeck R, Barde YA, Schwab ME. Neurotrophin-3 enhances sprouting of corticospinal tract during development and after adult spinal cord lesion {see comments] Nature 1994, 367:170–3

Schwab ME, Kapfhammer JP, Bandtlow CE (1993) Inhibitors of neurite growth. Annu Rev Neurosci 16:565–595

Segal R, Wolf S (1995) Operant conditioning of spinal stretch reflexes in patients with spinal cord injuries. Exp Neurol 130:202–213

Smith-Thomas LC, Fok-Seang J, Stevens J et al. (1994) An inhibitor of neurite outgrowth produced by astrocytes. J Cell Sci 107:1687–1695

Snow DM, Letourneau PC (1992) Neurite outgrowth on a step gradient of chondroitin sulfate proteoglycan (CS-PG). J Neurobiol 23:322–336

Snow DM, Lemmon V, Carrino DA, Caplan AI, Silver J (1990a) Sulfated proteoglycans in astroglial barriers inhibit neurite outgrowth in vtro. Exp Neurol 109:111–130

Snow DM, Steindler DA, Silver J (1990b) Molecular and cellular characterization of the glial roof plate of the spinal cord and optic tectum: a possible role for a proteoglycan in the development of an axon barrier. Dev Biol 138:359–376

Steeves JD, Jordan LM (1980) Localization of a descending pathway in the spinal cord which is necessary for controlled treadmill locomotion. Neurosci Lett 20:283–288

Steeves JD, Keirstead HS, Ethell DW et al. (1994) Permissive and restrictive periods for brainstem–spinal regeneration in the chick. Progr Brain Res 103:243–262

Stein R, Belanger M, Wheeler G et al. (1993) Assessment of electrical systems for improving locomotion after incomplete spinal cord injury. Arch Phys Med Rehabil 74:954–959

Tator CH, Duncan EG, Edmonds VE, Lapczak LI, Andrews DF (1993) Changes in epidemiology of acute spinal cord injury from 1947 to 1981. Surg Neurol 40:207–215

Taylor J, Pesheva P, Schachner M (1993) Influence of janusin and tenascin on growth cone behaviour in vitro. J Neurosci Res 35:347–362

Tello F (1911) La influencia del neurotropismo en la regeneracio de los centros nervioses. Lab Invest Biol Madred 9:123

Tetzlaff W, Alexander SW, Miller FD, Bisby MA (1991) Response of facial and rubrospinal neurons to axotomy: changes in mRNA expression for cytoskeletal proteins and GAP-43. J Neurosci 11:2528–2544

Thoenen H, Hughes RA, Sendtner M (1993) Trophic support of motoneurons: physiological, pathophysiological and therapeutic implications. Exp Neurol 124:47–55

Tuszynski MH, Peterson DA, Ray J, Baird A, Nakahara Y, Gage FH (1994) Fibroblasts genetically modified to produce nerve growth factor induce robust neuritic ingrowth after grafting to the spinal cord. Exp Neurol 126:1–14

Tymianski M, Spigelman I, Zhang L et al (1994) Mechanism of action and persistence of neuroprotection by cell-permeant Ca^{2+} chelators. J Cereb Blood Flow Metab 14:911–923

Xu XM, Guenard V, Kleitman N, Bunge MB (1995) Axonal regeneration into schwann cell-seeded guidance channels grafted into adult rat spinal cord. J Comp Neurol 351:145–160

Wainberg M, Barbeau H, Gauthier S (1990) The effects of cyproheptadine on locomotion and on spasticity in spinal cord injured patients. J Neurol Neurosurg Psychiat 53:754–763

Wolpaw JR, Chong LL (1989) Memory traces in primate spinal cord produced by opernat conditioning of H-reflex. J Neurophysiol 61:563–572

Wrathall JR, Choiniere D, Teng YD (1994) Dose-dependent reduction of tissue loss and functional impair-
    ment after spinal cord trauma with the AMPA/kainate antagonist NBQX. J Neurosci 14:6598–6607
Young W, Kume-Kick J, Constantini S (1994) Glucocorticoid therapy of spinal cord injury. Ann NY Acad
    Sci 743:241–263
Zhang L, Schmidt RE, Yan Q, Snider WD (1994) NGF and NT-3 have differing effects on the growth of
    dorsal root axons in developing mammalian spinal cord. J Neurosci 14:5187–5201
Zwimpfer TJ, Aguayo AJ, Bray GM (1992) Synapse formation and preferential distribution in the granule
    cell layer by regenerating retinal ganglion cell axons guided to the cerebellum of adult hamsters.
    J Neurosci 12:1144–1159

Chapter 4

Spinal Modulation of Noxious Stimuli

E.M.R. Critchley and M.T. Isaac

Pain is an imprecise symptom that achieves recognition as a percept within the mind. The central appreciation of pain involves the cerebral cortex, and probably also the lower end of the thalamus and upper end of the midbrain. There are both an organic component – an unpleasant experience primarily associated with physical damage and often described in terms relating to injury (Merskey and Spear 1967) – and a psychological component as interpretation takes place only in the mind, and the information recorded there is entirely personal, a private matter that cannot be shared by anyone else or described in terms that mean the same thing to another person (Mehta 1973). It is learnt from childhood onwards and the expression of that symptom is often governed by memory of previous occasions when it occurred.

At the spinal level we can refer to pain mechanisms, i.e. the processing of information whereby noxious stimuli and tissue injury at the periphery are translated centrally into awareness of pain (Fig. 4.1).

Somatic Sensibility

Normal sensibility depends on temporal and spatial summation and this fact is particularly important for the appreciation of pain (Nathan 1976). Sherrington (quoted by Denny-Brown et al. 1973) showed that any single spot on the trunk is innervated

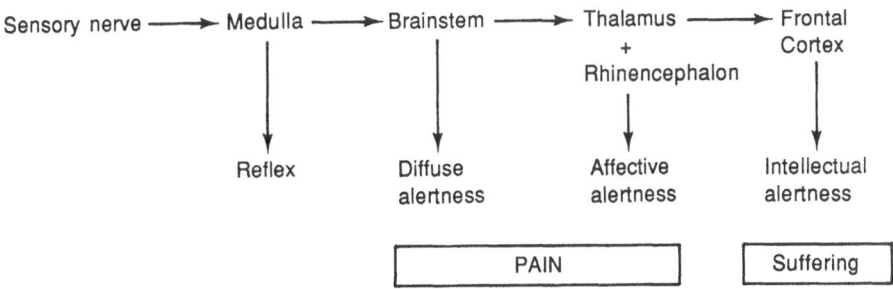

Fig. 4.1. Central regulation and integration. (From Charpentier 1968.)

33

by nerve fibres running into many neighbouring posterior roots. Thus, as part of the process of full, normal sensibility, the stimulus – response is enhanced by an overlap of fibres from neighbouring dorsal roots providing, at spinal level, a background of polysynaptic facilitation.

Historically, the many hypotheses used to explain the transmission of the various modalities of sensation from the periphery to the spinal cord can be grouped into two major theories. The stimulus-specificity theory originally depended on the finding of specific nerve endings in hairy skin. The neurones from which they arise, selectively transmit touch, cold or warmth, but if excessively stimulated give rise to nociceptive sensations. However, non-hairy skin such as that covering the human back is devoid of distinctive end-organs and the human cornea contains only one kind of nerve ending (Lele and Weddell 1956). Even so both these areas are capable of transmitting the full range of sensory modalities. The alternative, and not mutually incompatible, pattern theory is that the pattern of discharge from any given fibre could at one time contribute towards the sensation of touch, and at another towards the experience of pain, cold or warmth (Sinclair 1981). Both theories – stimulus-specificity and pattern – have had to be modified in the light of recent research. The hypothesis that all primary afferents respond to pain is questionable. Individual primary afferents are sharply tuned so that they respond well to a certain kind of stimulus and poorly to others, irrespective of the size of their fibres (Hoffert 1989).

Although the types of fibres stimulated are important, the division of afferent nerves into two groups, fast conducting medullated A fibres usually associated with specific nerve endings, and slower conducting unmyelinated C fibres, is too simplistic. C fibres also constitute a major pathway for impulses generated by various innocuous stimuli (Douglas and Ritchie 1957). Individual C fibres are sensitive to only certain stimuli; and these fibres have most amazingly different thresholds (Iggo 1965). It is now accepted that large numbers of nociceptive A delta and C fibres are present in peripheral nerves and many of these specialized fibres respond only to intense stimulation (Wall 1978).

Discrete stimulation at a single site, as for example on the skin of the trunk, will trigger impulses which are transmitted both by fast medullated fibres and by slower conducting unmyelinated fibres. If a noxious stimulus is used, additional bursts of impulses will be triggered by tissue damage with release of nociceptive chemical substances. Injury will be followed by local tenderness, primary hyperaesthesia, which is to be explained by the sensitization of previously high threshold endings to the products of tissue breakdown (Wall 1978). The kind of pain experienced depends not only on groups and sizes of afferent fibres but also on the arrangement of fibres in the tissues, on the layer that is stimulated and on the actual structure stimulated (Keele and Armstrong 1964).

It is also accepted, as was first shown by Rivers and Head (1908), that a reduction in the number of peripheral nerve fibres could cause a change in the character of a sensation, apart from a diminution in its intensity. Noordenbos (1959) found that post-herpetic neuralgia was associated with a selective loss of large fibres. This finding, since modified even for post-herpetic neuralgia, was originally incorporated into the gate control theory of Melzack and Wall (1965) (Fig. 4.2). It was assumed that the input of small fibres was inhibitory on the substantia gelatinosa and that of large fibres excitatory. Wall (1978) is more circumspect: merely stating that cells in the spinal cord, which are excited by injury signals, are also facilitated or inhibited by other peripheral nerve fibres which carry information about innocuous events. Most neuropathies manifest themselves as an irritative process followed by a

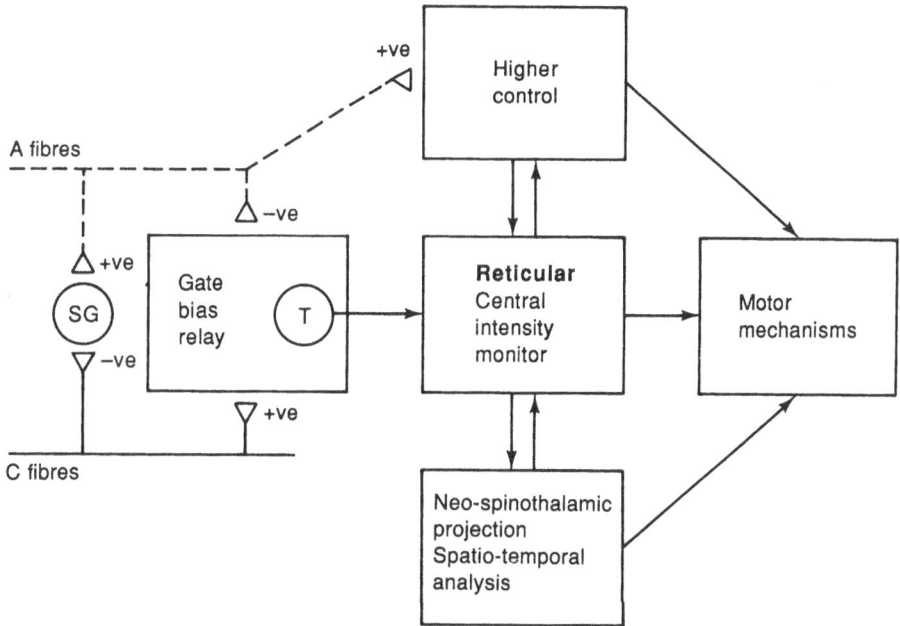

Fig. 4.2. The gate control theory. (From Melzack and Wall 1965.)

destructive one, or else are destructive from the start (Sinclair 1981). Despite the fact that some neuropathies selectively affect large fibres and others small fibres, there is no consistent relationship between the size of fibres which are lost and the painfulness or otherwise of the condition. In Friedreich's ataxia and the polyneuropathy of renal failure, there is large fibre loss without pain. Thallium neuropathy and Fabry's disease are painful conditions associated with loss of small fibres.

The Dorsal Root Entry Zone

The spinal cord has a dual role with respect to noxious stimuli: an immediate reflex avoidance response, i.e. of the trunk away from the stimulus, and the modulation and transmission of impulses to alert the sensorium (Fig. 4.3). Withdrawal of a limb probably involves more complex reflexes without requiring prior awareness of the act. The dorsal root terminals are areas of convergence of sensory information of somatic, visceral and sympathetic origin. This fact has clinical importance in the understanding of referred pain and of the role of the autonomic nervous system in pain relief.

Uncertainty exists about the exact location of modulating mechanisms within the spinal cord, the identity of the cord cells which respond to injury and transmit the impulses onward (T or transmission cells), the relative importance of presynaptic and postsynaptic inhibition in determining the input of the T cells from the periphery, and the presumed role of the substantia gelatinosa (British Medical Journal

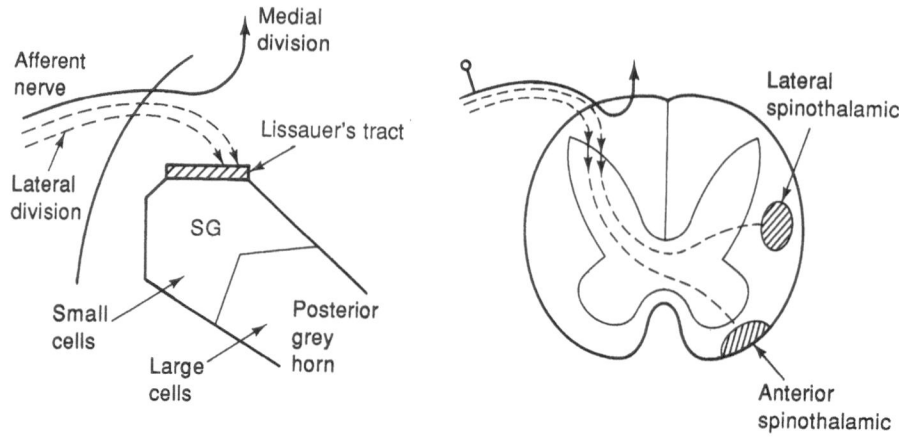

Spinothalamic tracts

Fig. 4.3.   Spinal nociceptive pathways. SG, substantia gelatinosa.

Leading Article 1978). However, certain facts are known concerning the dorsal root entry zone, the most important being that the number of impulses received from the periphery far exceeds those transmitted rostrally. It is apparent that some selection and modulation of impulses occur in this area. Such modulation would appear to be in part electrical and in part chemical.

Matthews (1934) and Barron and Matthews (1935, 1938) studied the electrical activity originating in the neurones of the posterior horns. The initial finding of a discharge conducted antidromically beyond the ganglia to the periphery in muscular and cutaneous nerves has received little subsequent attention (Nathan 1976). Of greater significance was the finding of slow potential changes spreading along the dorsal roots by a mechanism apparently identical with electrotonic spread and involving depolarization of afferent fibres near their terminals in the grey matter. The degree of depolarization had the effect of partially or intermittently blocking afferent impulses. Hongo et al. (1968) also found evidence of postsynaptic inhibition, but their work has not been widely substantiated whereas presynaptic inhibition has been extensively examined.

The dorsal root potential appears to be subject to various influences:

1. The on-going activity which precedes any new stimulus
2. Descending fibres with both facilitatory and inhibitory effects from the brain and segmental interneurones. Descending fibres from the periaqueductal grey matter have been shown to inhibit the response of lamina V cells of the substantia gelatinosa to noxious stimuli (Oliveras et al. 1974)
3. Spread of activity within the substantia gelatinosa and Lissauer's tract operative over several segments (Wall 1959, 1962)
4. The stimulus evoked activity and the relative balance of activity between different fibre systems

Although everything points to the role of the substantia gelatinosa in the modulation of nociceptive impulses the function of the various laminae is far from clear. There are two areas of particular interest.

A large number of cells in lamina V respond to both myelinated and unmyelinated nociceptive afferents, and are affected by the presence of narcotic and anaesthetic agents. Their receptive fields are complex with some cells responding to high threshold visceral afferents and also to low threshold afferents from skin (Wall 1978). Some cells project to the opposite ventral white matter and some to the thalamus.

The surface of the substantia gelatinosa contains a few cells which only respond to nociceptive afferents. Denny-Brown et al. (1973) regard these marginal cells as a region of equilibrium of neural activity in which the arrival of an impulse from any one point greatly lowers the threshold for the synapse of the axon involved and of topographically related afferents. "The mechanism provides for a combination of temporal and spatial summation."

The modulation of noxious and innocuous sensory stimuli within the substantia gelatinosa is helped by the presence of opiate receptors, including both morphine and met-enkephalin receptors. These receptors have several roles: inhibiting the release of putative nociceptive transmitters such as substance P from the primary afferent terminals, decreasing the excitability of postsynaptic cells, interfering with the activity of the excitatory nociceptive neurotransmitters, or hyperpolarizing cells and neighbouring dendrites (Haigler 1987).

Within the laminae of the substantia efferent axons run up and down the neuraxis in small closed loops or chains in contact with other gelatinosa cells. However, most of those relating to pain sensation travel for three segments or so in Lissauer's tract before crossing over and ascending in the anterolateral tract to the thalamus. It is not known how impulses that converge on cells in the substantia gelatinosa eventually reach the spinothalamic tracts which are situated deeper within the cord.

Pain transmission is best considered within the general framework of discriminative and non-discriminative sensations (Fig. 4.4). Several ascending tracts are involved. The limbic system has a role in gating or modulating the impulses. Short spinospinal interneurons may eventually reach the reticular formation. And the more rapidly ascending pain pathways are not rigidly confined within the spinothalamic tract.

Clinical Aspects of Pain Sensibility at Spinal Level

Congenital Analgesia

1. *Complete insensitivity to pain* may be a feature of congenital neuropathies, usually with a virtual absence of small primary afferent fibres in the sensory pathways. Many of these are associated with autonomic nervous system involvement which may manifest itself by disturbances in sweating and temperature control (Swanson et al. 1965).

2. *Pain asymbolia or agnosia* is a condition in which noxious stimuli are felt but the psychiatric reaction to the sensation is absent. This impairment is usually the result of an acquired lesion involving the dominant parietal lobe, but Osuntokua et al. (1968) have described two half-siblings with congenital pain asymbolia and auditory imperception.

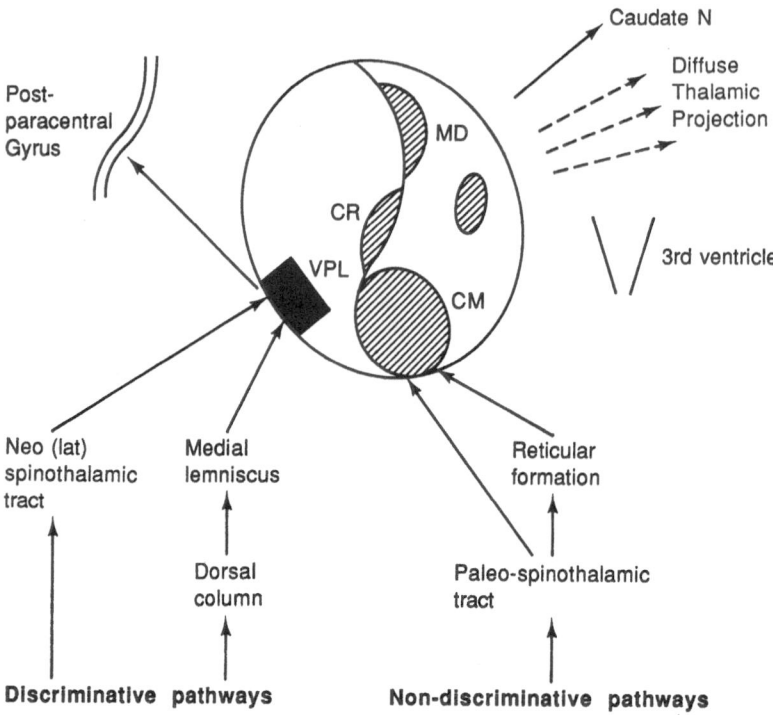

Fig. 4.4. Thalamic pain projection system. ■ ventroposterior lateral nucleus; ▨ intralammar and parafascicular nuclei.

3. *Congenital universal indifference to pain* may occur as an inherited disorder. At about the third year of life the child appears not to guard against injury. Even though deep pain is also affected, there is no demonstrable structural damage to the nervous system. Many patients show evidence of repeated self-mutilation, and about 28% are mentally retarded (Thrush 1973; McMurray 1975). Dehen et al. (1979) suggest that the condition may be a manifestation of an overactive endogenous opioid system.

Referred Pain

Disordered localization of pain occurs in three circumstances:

1. Pain derived from a hollow viscus may be experienced in a comparatively remote cutaneous area. The classical example is pain in the shoulder due to lesion under the diaphragm.

2. Pain from non-visceral structures such as muscle, bone or blood vessels is usually misinterpreted as coming from other deep tissues, but never from the skin. This is true of anginal pain which may be transmitted to the jaw and down the left arm.

3. In association with peripheral nerve or spinal injury with areas of dysaesthesia, cutaneous stimulation may be associated with an unusual area of cutaneous "refer-

ence". A good example of this phenomenon is afforded by the paraesthesiae of Tinel's sign. The word synaesthesia has a special and distinctive meaning with respect to spinal injury or amputation of limbs. Abnormal spread of sensation can occur and the term synchiria, is applied when a stimulus such as a pin-prick applied to the unaffected side produces an unpleasant sensation bilaterally. When this occurs unilaterally affecting the "mirror point" on the opposite side of the body it is known as "allochiria" (Obersteiner, 1882). Stimulation of an anaesthetic zone of a successful cordotomy may produce a sensation of pain either on the same side just above the "level" or else on the opposite side. Other terms used include allaesthesia and synaesthesialgia. A somewhat similar phenomenon was described by Bender (1945) and Henson (1949) whereby simultaneous stimulation of the "mirror point" may either enhance or extinguish the sensory response to a stimulus applied within an area of altered sensibility.

The explanation of referred pain lies in the convergence of somatic and sympathetic impulses into the same sensory pool. The localization of visceral pain is diffuse and reference is often made to a presumed body-schema based on the dermatomal site of embryonic development. Cutaneous hyperalgesia may be present at the side of the referred pain. Infiltration of this trigger area with local anaesthetic agents can bring partial relief of symptoms. Alternatively, counter-irritants may crowd out the impulses from visceral afferents.

Persistent Pathological Pain States

Spontaneous pain may arise as a result of disordered function at spinal level. Several explanations have been proposed for these central pain syndromes. Livingston (1943) postulated a multisynaptic afferent system of short spinospinal fibres capable of setting up reverberating circuits if interfered with pathologically (Fig. 4.5). Gerard (1951) proposed that a peripheral nerve lesion could bring about a temporary loss of sensory control of firing in spinal cord internuncial neurones (Fig. 4.6). These may then begin to fire in synchrony; and such synchronous firing could recruit additional units, could move along in the grey matter, and could be maintained by impulses different from and feebler than those needed to initiate it. Melzack (1972) suggested that excessive or otherwise abnormal stimulation can bring about a prolonged bias in the activity of the gate mechanism. Other properties of the "gate" – that it may be influenced by activity in spatially distant areas of the nervous system, and affected by brain mechanisms underlying psychological processes such as memory and emotion – may also serve to prolong this bias.

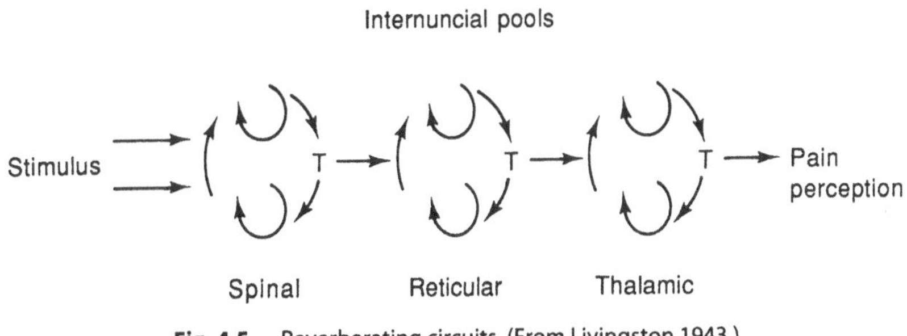

Internuncial pools

Fig. 4.5. Reverberating circuits. (From Livingston 1943.)

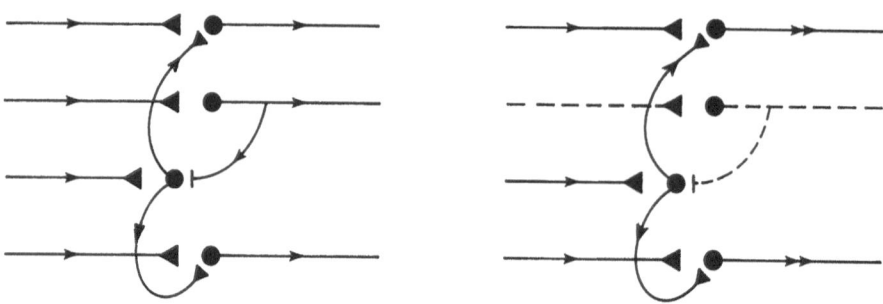

Fig. 4.6. Disruption of firing sequences. (From Gerard 1951.)

Causalgia

Causalgia originally denoted a burning quality in pain (Mitchell et al. 1864) and came to be used to describe a painful syndrome commonly found in wartime traumatic casualties. It may also arise in conjunction with fractures, sprains, crush injuries and relatively minor trauma (British Medical Journal Leading Article 1971), occurring in 2%–5% of people who sustain peripheral nerve injury. The severe and persistent unpleasant burning sensations are notoriously resistant to most forms of surgical and medical treatment.

Intense pain begins almost immediately after the accident, but occasionally is delayed for weeks or months. The pain may be spontaneous but may be aggravated or precipitated by touch, movement or psychological factors. New pains and trigger zones may spread unpredictably to other parts of the body where no pathology exists. Schott (1994) has demonstrated that visceral afferents rather than the sympathetic nerves themselves are responsible for the release of neuropeptides from C-fibres. These afferents are related to blood vessels which travel with the autonomic nerves. The limb may show typical skin changes with tightness, redness and sweating. Involuntary jerky movements may occur. If the pain is severe enough to prevent the full use of the limb, trophic changes appear in the skin and nails, and the bones become osteoporotic. Patients become demoralized by the persistence and severity of symptoms and the failure of treatment to control them (Mehta 1973).

Neuralgic Pains

Unpleasant explosive pains can occur in relation to many clinical conditions such as lesions of the thalamus, tabes dorsalis, mesencephalic tractotomy, lesions of the lemniscal system and post-herpetic neuralgia (Sinclair 1981). Some pains may be continuous but others spontaneous and paroxysmal. There may be a raised threshold for all forms of cutaneous sensibility with a painful over-reaction to such stimuli as are able to cross the threshold. The lesions are often infective or degenerative and judging from clinical observation the essential condition for the production of this syndrome at whatever level is a certain degree of incompleteness of the lesion (Symonds 1931).

Phantom Limbs

Phantom limb sensations occur in practically every patient following traumatic amputation of a limb, can occur following brachial plexus avulsion without loss of a limb, and are experienced in paraplegics following spinal injury. Phantoms are rare in those with mutilating diseases such as leprosy or gangrene (Frederiks 1980) or in children under the age of four years, but are almost invariable in adults following trauma (Simmel 1956, 1962). A phantom may last for years, and even when lost may be recovered under stress (Weddell and Sinclair 1947).

The most comprehensive studies of phantom limbs have tended to follow wartime experiences, as with the excellent study of 73 Israeli male soldiers injured in the Yom Kippur War of October 1973 (Carlen et al. 1978). All experienced an illusory awareness of the missing part. With time the phantom tended to weaken in intensity and the limb to telescope in towards the stump until the digits of the phantom merged into its substance. A painful phantom is less likely to shrink in size with the passage of time and may remain, continuing to cripple and oppress. Thus 5%–10% of patients suffered disagreeable sensations, variously described as cramp, shooting, burning and crushing. Phantom pains tend to develop in those who suffered pain in the limb for some time prior to amputation and may closely resemble in quality and localization the pain that was present before amputation. Thus burning pains generally follow irritant wounds and emergency amputation, sometimes freezing the phantom in distorted attitudes such as that occupied at the time of the accident. Pain emanates from pressure on specially sensitive areas, trigger zones which are situated initially in the injured part but gradually spread to other areas of the body which are healthy and unrelated to the injury; so much so that urination, defaecation and ejaculation may be accompanied by a burning sensation in both the phantom and the stump end.

Stump pain occurs in about 43% of amputees and is an ill-defined and painful muscle cramp occurring in the whole stump which will sometimes twitch or jerk spasmodically entirely beyond the control of the unfortunate patient. Drug-induced dyskinesias may even affect a phantom limb (Jankovic and Glass 1985). Painful neuromas may be present at the nerve ends. The overlying skin can become exquisitely tender to touch and undergo vasomotor changes of causalgic type. These symptoms occur independently or in addition to phantom limb pain.

In normal subjects, local anaesthesia of peripheral nerves, loss of sensation in a limb as in the Guillain-Barre syndrome, or avulsion of the brachial plexus may all generate phantom limb sensations, which would appear to indicate that the phantom can be generated centrally in the absence of neural impulses from affected dermatomes. This does not mean that the periphery is irrelevant to all phantoms, as electrical stimulation of the stump invariably exaggerates the phantom.

The phantom phenomena of paraplegics differ from those of amputees. Whereas the vividness of the phantom is obvious from discussion with any amputee, a similar complaint may be hard to elicit from a paraplegic. Boss (1951) cites two patients with arm and mid-thoracic amputations in whom the arm phantom was obvious while the lower body phantom required considerable concentration to describe. Paraplegics with complete cord section may feel as though their bodies caudal to the transection are missing entirely. Some paraplegics experience phantom feelings within a few days, but others note such feelings after several months have elapsed. In contrast to the detail with which a phantom limb is described, paraplegics cannot truly sense details but talk of a bizarre continuity or a vague awareness. Telescoping does not occur and painful phenomena are absent.

Phantom phenomena affecting other organs have also been described, e.g. following enucleation, tooth extraction, facial mutilation, castration or mastectomy (Frederiks 1980). In contrast to the 100% occurrence of phantom phenomena following limb amputation such phenomena – phantom pain and non-painful phantom sensations – rarely affect more than 20%–30% of those who undergo mutilation or amputation at other sites (Kroner et al. 1989).

The Origin of Phantom Phenomena

Controversy exists between those who hold Melzack's hypothesis of a central neuromatrix (1989) or a central generating mechanism for pain (Melzack and Loeser 1978) and others who suggest that phantom phenomena arise peripherally or at spinal level. Dimond (1980) sees the spinal cord (1) as a part of the brain extended longitudinally, (2) as having a localizing function at its different levels, (3) as relating to many psychological processes not usually thought to be associated with it and (4) as having an effect upon higher mental functions, including sexual libido, dreaming and emotional expressiveness. "It is clear that the cord speaks to the rest of the brain in ways we barely understand at present."

Centrally, phantom phenomena can be associated with schizophrenia (Ames 1984), parietal lesions, thalamic stimulation or epilepsy (Hecaen and de Ajurriaguerra 1952); and altered or abolished by ECT, vascular accidents, intoxication or vestibular stimulation (Frederiks 1980). Phantom limbs can arise from spinal cord lesions (Riddoch 1941; Berger and Gerstenbrand 1981), or be modified or abolished by cordotomy or section of posterior roots. That an interaction occurs between brain and spinal cord has been admirably summarized by Russell (1970): "Almost all amputees experience phantom limb sensations but these vary so widely as to indicate that the relationship between periphery and brain is variable according perhaps to personality, natural interest in giving attention to bodily sensations, previous occupation and the general threshold of the individual to pain, injury and other menacing situations. In other words, the individual's reaction to the effects of amputation partly depends on how the CNS has been trained during that person's life".

Treatment of Pain Syndromes

Two lines of treatment are of primary importance: recognition and treatment of the psychological effects of the trauma, and removal, as far as is possible, of any focus of irritation. Psychological aspects include adequate relief of pain in the acute stages, counselling, antidepressants, analgesics and the thymoleptic drugs which alter the threshold of awareness of pain. Neuralgic pains, in particular, may not respond to conventional analgesics except in doses causing drowsiness, which may be unacceptable to the patient or to a normal life-style.

Cleansing the site of trauma is best illustrated by phantom limb and stump pain. Surgical debridement of the area, removing foci of infection, removing jagged structures, ensuring that all viable tissues have an adequate blood supply, and sectioning neuromas can bring much relief. Physiotherapy is vital for the relief of symptoms in a traumatized limb. Active treatment encouraging relaxation, reducing spasticity, putting the limb through passive movements and later encouraging the full range of motion exercises can prevent joints becoming fixed and contractures developing. Traditionally, pain in the stump can be alleviated by hitting trigger areas with a blunt hammer. Ultrasound, transcutaneous electrical stimulation and vibrators can all achieve the same effect. Only rarely do phantom limbs fail to respond to apparently complete peripheral anaesthesia (Carlen et al. 1978).

With referred pain, infiltration of hyperalgesic areas is also effective. Causalgias may he helped by sympathetic nerve blockade (Loh and Nathan 1978), so much so that they have been called sympathetic-maintained pains (Portenoy 1989). Surgical sympathectomies, however, are unsatisfactory as failure to bring relief may be accompanied by further spread of the pain to previously unaffected areas. Nerve blockade is probably more useful diagnostically and prognostically than therapeutically. Peripheral nerve section is rarely of lasting help and where pain is relieved, memory of pain soon passes and the patient may find any dysesthesia of the overlying skin equally unacceptable.

Counter-irritation is a household remedy for deep pain, but nobody knows how it works (Sinclair 1981). The modern pundits have given it a new acronym, DNIC (diffuse noxious inhibitory control) for the phenomenon in which the application of a focal noxious stimulus yields analgesia in a unrelated region of the body (Portenoy 1989). Topical capsaicin is advocated for the relief of postherpetic neuralgia but the results are variable and some neurosurgeons believe that the patient should be heavily sedated before the drug is applied. Equally helpful but equally unexplained are the neuroaugmentative techniques of acupuncture, percutaneous stimulation and dorsal column stimulation (Sweet and Wepsic 1974). The assumption is that they all modify the bias of the "gate" (Melzack and Wall 1965). There is additional evidence that acupuncture and low frequency transcutaneous electrical stimulation (TENS) also stimulate the activity of endorphin systems within the substantia gelatinosa (Mayer et al. 1977). In contrast, an endorphinergic mechanism does not appear to be essential in the analgesia produced by high-frequency peripheral stimulation (Chapman and Benedetti 1977).

Rhizotomies, or section of dorsal root entry zones, have been used to bring 50% relief following spinal cord injury, but are of little value in the control of diffuse pain or predominantly sacral pain. Friedman and Nashold (1986) suggest that the best results are obtained when several roots are sectioned above a unilateral lesion. However an alternative explanation of the fact that section of the dorsal roots may not relieve pain (Coggeshall et al. 1975) may lie in the recognition that the spinal roots – and particularly the ventral root in man – contain a mixture of sensory and motor fibres. Sykes and Coggeshall (1973) found that one-third of the fibres of the ventral root are unmyelinated and presumably of sensory origin. This finding directly contradicts the early 19th century concept formulated by Bell (1811) and Magendie (1822) whereby the sensory and motor functions are discrete and localized to the dorsal and ventral roots respectively.

Chemical rhizotomy using intrathecal phenol, chlorocresol or silver nitrate is an exacting technique which can bring relief of severe pain or spasticity and can be repeated as necessary (Maher 1955). Relief of pain is unaccompanied by substantial alterations in other sensory modalities, but sphincter disturbances can arise if the patient is not skilfully positioned.

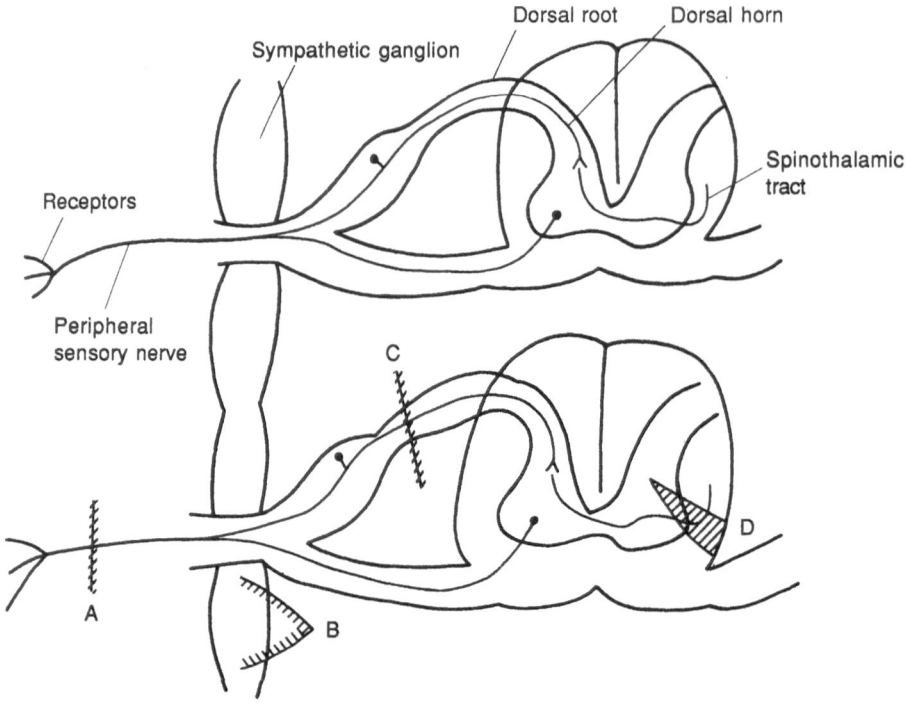

Fig. 4.7. Neurosurgical procedures for pain relief. A, neurectomy; B, sympathectomy; C, rhizotomy; D, cordotomy.

Section of the anterolateral tracts – cordotomy – can be performed percuta-neously under X-ray control but should be reserved for patients with malignant disease or a limited life expectancy (Fig. 4.7). A unilateral cordotomy performed at C2–3 will relieve pain in 70%–75% of patients, raising the threshold to pain by 40%–50%. Complications include numbness below the lesion, muscle weakness in the legs, loss of bladder and rectal control, impotence and an unstable blood pres-sure. If a bilateral cordotomy is required the second operation should be performed at C5–6 in order to avoid respiratory distress. The fact that pain perception returns despite the irreversible nature of the neurosurgical operation is of great theoretical importance, and would indicate that the relationship of pain perception to its pre-ferred spinal cord projection system is plastic (Hoffert 1989).

References

Ames D (1984) Self-shooting of a phantom head. Br J Psychiatry 145:193–194
Barron DH, Matthews BHC (1935) Intermittent conduction in the spinal cord. J Physiol (Lond) 85:73–103
Barron DH, Matthews BHC (1938) The interpretation of potential changes in the spinal cord. J Physiol (Lond) 92:272–321
Bell C (1811) Idea of a new anatomy of the brain. Strahan and Preston, London
Bender MB (1945) Extinction and precipitation of cutaneous sensation. Arch Neurol Psychiatry 54:1–9

Berger M, Gerstenbrand R (1981) Phantom illusions with spinal cord lesions. In: Siegfried I, Zimmerman M (eds) Phantom and stump pain. Springer-Verlag, Berlin, pp 66–73

Boss E (1951) Phantom limbs of patients after spinal cord injury. Arch Neurol Psychiatry 66:610–631

British Medical Journal (1971) Causalgia. Br Med J i:64 (leading article)

British Medical Journal (1978) The gate control theory of pain. Br Med J ii:586–587 (leading article)

Carlen PL, Wall PD, Nadvoma H, Steinbeck T (1978) Phantom limbs and related phenomena in recent traumatic amputations. Neurology 28:211–217

Chapman RN, Benedetti I (1977) Analgesia following transcutaneous electrical stimulation and its partial reversal by a narcotic antagonist. Life Sci 21:1645–1648

Charpentier J (1968) Analysis and measurement of pain in animals: a new conception of pain. In: Soulairac A, Cahn J, Charpentier J (eds) Pain. Proc Int Symposium on Pain, Paris, 1967. Academic Press, London and New York, pp 171–200

Coggeshall RE, Applebaum ML, Fazen M, Stubbs TB, Sykes MT (1975) A review of the Bell-Magendie hypothesis. Brain 98:157–166

Dehen H, Willer JC, Cambier J (1979) Congenital indifference to pain and endogenous morphine-like system. In: Bonica JJ, Liebeskind JC, Albe-Fessard DG (eds) Advances in pain research and therapy, vol 3. Raven Press, New York, pp 553–557

Denny-Brown D, Kirk EJ, Yanagisawa N (1973) The tract of Lissauer in relation to sensory transmission in the dorsal horn of spinal cord in the macaque monkey. J Comp Neurol 151:175–200

Dimond SJ (1980) Neuropsychology. Butterworths, London, pp 520–521

Douglas WW, Ritchie JM (1957) Non-medullated fibres in the saphenous nerve which signal touch. J Physiol (Lond) 139:385–399

Frederiks JAM (1980) Phantom limb and phantom limb pain. In: Vinken PJ, Bruyn GW, Klawans HL (eds) Handbook of clinical neurology 45. Elsevier, Amsterdam, pp 395–404

Friedman AH, Nashold BS (1986) DREZ lesions for relief of pain related to spinal cord injury. J Neurosurg 65:465–469

Gerard RW (1951) A new theory of causalgic pain. Anaesthesiology 12:1–10

Haigler HJ (1987) Neurophysiological effects of opiates in the CNS. Monogr Neurolog Soc 13:132–160

Hecaen H, de Ajurriaguerra J (1952) Méconnaissance et hallucinations corporelles. Masson et Cie, Paris

Henson RA (1949) On thalamic dysesthesia and their suppression by bilateral stimulation. Brain 72:576–598

Hoffert MJ (1989) The neurophysiology of pain. Neurolog Clin 7:183–204

Hongo T, Jankowska E, Lundberg A (1968) Postsynaptic excitation and inhibition for primary afferents in neurones of the spinocervical tract. J Physiol (Lond) 199:569–592

Iggo A (1965) The peripheral mechanisms of cutaneous sensation. In: Curtis DR, McIntyre AK (eds) Studies in physiology. Springer, Berlin, pp 92–100

Jankovic J, Glass JP (1985) Metoclopramide-induced phantom dyskinesia. Neurology 35:432–435

Keele CA, Armstrong D (1964) Substances producing pain and itch. Arnold, London

Kroner K, Krebs B, Skov J, Jorgensen HS (1989) Immediate and long-term phantom breast syndrome after mastectomy: incidence, clinical characteristics and relationship to pre-mastectomy breast pain. Pain 36:327–334

Lele PP, Weddell G (1956) The relationship between neurohistology and corneal sensibility. Brain 79:119–154

Livingston WK (1943) Pain mechanisms. Macmillan, New York

Loh L, Nathan PW (1978) Painful peripheral states and sympathetic blocks. J Neurol Neurosurg Psychiatry 41:664–671

Magendie F (1822) Experiences sur les fonctions des racines des nerfs rachidiens. J Physiol Exp 2:276–279

Maher RM (1955) Relief of pain in incurable cancer. Lancet 1:18–20

Matthews BHC (1934) Impulses leaving the spinal cord by dorsal roots. J Physiol (Lond) 81:29–31P

Mayer DJ, Price DD, Rafii A (1977) Antagonism of acupuncture analgesia in man by the narcotic antagonist naloxone. Brain Res 121:368–372

McMurray GA (1975) Theories of pain and congenital universal insensitivity to pain. Can J Psychol 29:302–315

Mehta M (1973) Intractable pain. Saunders, London

Melzack R (1972) Mechanisms of pathological pain. In: Critchley M, O'Leary JL, Jennett B (eds) Scientific foundations of neurology. Heinemann, London, pp 153–165

Melzack R (1989) Phantom limbs, the self and the brain. DO Hebb Memorial Lecture. Can Psychol 30:1–16

Melzack R, Loeser JD (1978) Phantom body pain in paraplegics: evidence for a central "pattern generating mechanism" for pain. Pain 4:195–210

Melzack R, Wall PD (1965) Pain mechanisms: a new theory. Science 150:971–979

Merskey H, Spear FG (1967) Pain: psychological and psychiatric aspects. Ballière Tindall, Cassell, London

Mitchell SW, Morehouse GR, Keen WW (1864) Gunshot wounds and other injuries of nerves. Lippincott, Philadelphia

Nathan PW (1976) The gate-control theory of pain: a critical review. Brain 99:123–158

Noordenbos W (1959) Pain. Elsevier, Amsterdam

Obersteiner H (1882) On allochiria, a peculiar sensory disorder. Brain 4:153–163

Oliveras JL, Redjemi JM, Guilbaud G, Liebeskind JC (1974) Behavioural and electrophysiological evidence of pain inhibition from midbrain stimulation in the cat. Exper Brain Res 20:32–44

Osuntokua BO, Odeku EL, Luzzato L (1968) Congenital pain asymbolia and auditory imperception. J Neurol Neurosurg Psychiatry 31:291–296

Portenoy RK (1989) Mechanisms of clinical pain: observations and speculations. Neurolog Clin 7:205–230

Riddoch G (1941) Phantom limbs and body schema. Brain 64:197–222

Rivers WHR, Head H (1908) A human experiment in nerve division. Brain 31:323–450

Russell WR (1970) Neurological sequelae of amputation. Br J Hosp Med 4:607–609

Schott GD (1994) Visceral afferents: their contribution to "sympathetic dependent" pain. Brain 117:397–413

Simmel ML (1956) On phantom limbs. Arch Neurol Psychiatry 75:637–647

Simmel ML (1962) Phantom experiences following amputation in childhood. J Neurol Neurosurg Psychiatry 25:69–78

Sinclair D (1981) Mechanisms of cutaneous sensation. Oxford University Press, Oxford

Swanson AG, Buchan GC, Alvord EC (1965) Anatomic changes in congenital insensitivity to pain. Am Med Assoc Arch Neurol 12:12–18

Sweet WH, Wepsic JG (1974) Stimulation of the posterior columns of the spinal cord for pain control: indications, technique and results. Clin Neurosurg 21:278–320

Sykes MT, Coggeshall RE (1973) Unmyelinated fibres in the human L4 and L5 ventral roots. Brain Res 63:490–495

Symonds CP (1931) The physiology of painful sensation. Lancet 2:723–726

Thrush DC (1973) Congenital insensitivity to pain – a clinical, genetic and neurophysiological study of four children from the same family. Brain 96:369–386

Wall PD (1959) Repetitive discharge of neurones. J Neurophysiol 22:305–320

Wall PD (1962) The origin of a spinal cord slow potential. J Physiol (Lond) 164:508–526

Wall PD (1978) The gate control theory of pain mechanisms – a re-examination and a re-statement. Brain 101:1–18

Weddell G, Sinclair D (1947) Pins and needles, observations on some of the sensations aroused in a limb by the application of pressure. J Neurol Neurosurg Psychiatry 10:26–46

Chapter 5

Spasticity

G.R. Critchley

Spasticity may be encountered in clinical practice as both a presenting feature and a complication of neurological disease. The patient may complain of difficulty in performing fine movements, poor coordination, difficulty walking, involuntary spasms and feelings of stiffness or rigidity. Examination may reveal a mixture of signs such as increased tone, clasp knife rigidity, loss of fine movements, brisk reflexes including spread of reflex activity, clonus and an upgoing plantar response. There may be spasms, both flexor and extensor, which may be spontaneous or precipitated by examination.

Different combinations of symptoms and signs present in different patients reflecting the heterogenous nature of pathological cause of spasticity. This translates into a plethora of management strategies based on consideration of the underlying pathophysiology.

Pathophysiology

At the simplest level, spasticity is a feature of an upper motor neurone lesion. The most widely accepted definition of spasticity is by Lance (1980): "a motor disorder characterized by a velocity dependent increase in tonic stretch reflexes (muscle tone) with exaggerated tendon jerks, resulting from hyperexcitability of the stretch reflex, as one component of the upper motor neuron syndrome." The velocity-dependent increase in tone results in the clasp knife phenomenon and distinguishes spasticity from other types of rigidity. Also to be noted is the central role of the stretch reflex in the pathophysiology of spasticity.

The stretch reflex represents the basic level of muscle control and is responsible for normal muscle tone. Gamma motor efferent fibres innervate muscle spindles and control muscle tension and length. The 1a afferent sensory nerves respond to changes in length and tension in the muscle spindles and project via the spinal cord directly to alpha motor neurones of the same muscle. They also inhibit via interneurones the alpha motor neurones of antagonist muscles. Inhibitory Renshaw cells in the anterior horn terminate the reflex. This reflex arc is under descending excitatory and inhibitory influences from upper motor neurones.

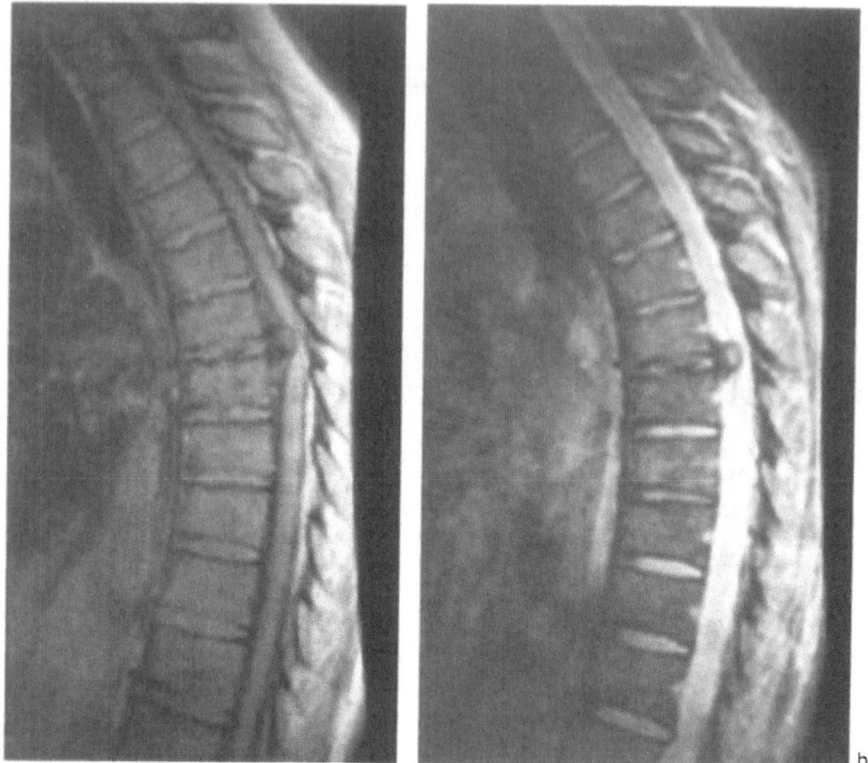

Fig. 5.1a,b   T1 and T2 weighted sagittal MR scan showing anterior spinal cord compression due to a prolapsed intervertebral disc at the level of T6/T7.

The site of a lesion along the upper motor neurone pathway from cortex to spinal cord determines the degree of excitatory or inhibitory involvement in the development of spasticity. The experimental work on this is extensively summarized by Brown (1994) who suggests that lesions at the level of the cortex or internal capsule result in loss of control of the inhibitory centre in the caudal brainstem resulting in a pattern of spasticity in which increased extensor tone and antigravity posture predominate, as in cerebral palsy. Partial cord lesions such as in multiple sclerosis result in loss of inhibitory influences from the dorsal reticulospinal tract causing severe spasticity with increased extensor tone and extensor spasms. In severe or complete cord lesions there is loss of all supraspinal influences on the cord. The result is predominantly increased flexor tone and spasms. This is shown in Figs. 5.1 and 5.2 where the underlying pathology is a T6/T7 prolapsed intervertebral disc.

Management

A description of the symptoms and signs of spasticity will also aim to elucidate the underlying pathology noting asymmetry of spasticity and involvement of upper as

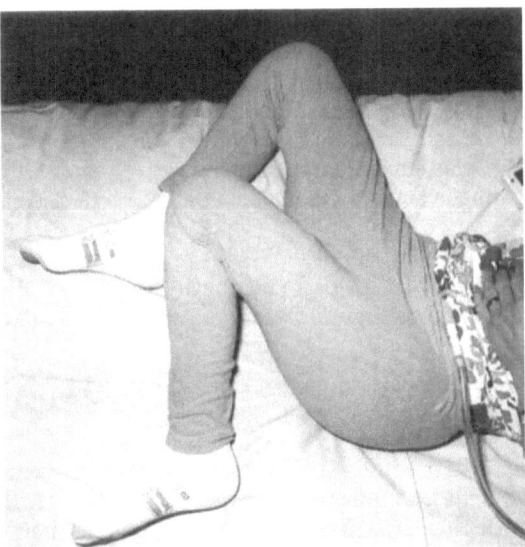

Fig. 5.2. Flexor spasm secondary to the lesion in Fig. 5.1.

well as lower limbs. Complications of spasticity and associated conditions such as contractures, pressure sores and catheter-related problems should also be noted on examination. Management plans have been aided by attempts to quantify the degree of spasticity by various systems including scales for muscle tone, reflex scores for spasms, physiotherapy scores and assessments of activities of daily living. The psychosocial consequences of spasticity for patient and family also need to be addressed.

Treatment

Prevention

Treatment of spasticity should first be aimed at preventing any deterioration. If there is a treatable cause, for example an expanding spinal tumour, then operative intervention may be necessary. In many cases, however, spasticity is the end result of neurological disease. In these patients a proper treatment strategy based on the patient's individual complaints should be devised. A reduction in extensor tone may indeed by deleterious for a patient who relies on this tone to stand. Pressure sores and bladder infections can result in an increase in spasticity due to local irritation of the reflex arc and therefore need to be treated.

Oral Drug Therapy

Oral drugs are widely used in the treatment of spasticity, baclofen and diazepam being most commonly used. Dantrolene which acts directly on muscles via inhibition of calcium release, and clonidine, an α_2 adrenergic antagonist, have also been used. Baclofen is γ-aminobutyric acid (GABA) analogue that binds to GABA-B receptors especially in the dorsal horn of the spinal cord. It causes inhibition of the stretch reflex arc by preventing release of excitatory neurotransmitters thus inhibiting both alpha and gamma efferent activity. Initial starting doses of 5 mg three times daily are used. Side effects such as confusion, drowsiness and muscle weakness may be experienced although in most cases baclofen is an effective and well-tolerated drug.

Diazepam facilitates the activity of the GABA receptor again activating inhibition of the reflex arc. It can be used in doses starting at 2 mg twice daily and is limited by side effects such as drowsiness, muscle weakness and respiratory depression.

Intrathecal Drugs

In severe cases of spasticity some patients may be unresponsive to safe doses of oral agents whereas others may become tolerant. As baclofen acts primarily on the spinal cord local delivery of this drug intrathecally has obvious theoretical attractions. Intrathecal administration of 50 μg baclofen in 1 ml saline after cessation of oral antispastic agents can be used as a therapeutic trial as well as treatment. Patients who demonstrate a good response but then require repeat doses can be considered for implantation of an intrathecal continuous delivery reservoir pump system. McLean (1993) has summarized nine recent studies involving intrathecal baclofen administration via a reservoir pump and quotes an abolition of spasticity in 164 of 168 patients. Coffey et al. (1993) also quote good results for pump use in patients with spasticity of spinal origin. Continuous intrathecal baclofen is undoubtedly useful for reduction of spasticity and improvement in function for both cerebral and spinal cord spasticity, though the enthusiasm for this method of drug delivery must be tempered by a high complication rate in inexperienced hands.

Intrathecal morphine has also been used although with less successful results than baclofen (Lazorthes et al. 1990).

Electrical Stimulation

This has been used transcutaneously, peripherally, via the cervical dorsal columns, and in the cerebellum. Although some encouraging results have been obtained, these methods remain experimental at present (Penn and Corcos 1990).

Destructive Techniques

Surgical interruption of the stretch reflex arc has been used to reduce spasticity. In principle the more destructive the technique the greater the relief but the greater the associated deficit. In patients with paraplegia and spasticity the motor deficit may not necessarily prohibit an destructive operation.

The most successful technique currently used is selective dorsal rhizotomy (e.g. Abbott et al. 1993). Peroperative electrical stimulation is used to determine which roots are involved in spasticity and the dorsal roots are cut. Other techniques such as percutaneous radiofrequency rhizotomy, chemical neurolysis, neurectomy and cordotomy have also been used.

Corrective Procedures

Orthopaedic assessment and operations such as tenotomies for severe contractures and tendon transfers for equinovarus deformities should also be considered.

Conclusions

Individualization of management strategy is important for patients with spasticity especially given the spectrum of treatment options available, from oral drugs to destructive procedures. Full assessment of the patient with a consideration of the benefits and risk of each treatment intervention should lead to selective and usually successful treatment of spasticity.

References

Abbott R, Johann-Murphy M, Shiminski-Maher T et al. (1993) Selective dorsal rhizotomy: outcome and complications in treating spastic cerebral palsy. Neurosurgery 33:851–857

Brown P (1994) Pathophysiology of spasticity. J Neurol Neurosurg Psychiatry 57:773–777

Coffey RJ, Cahill D, Steers W et al. (1993) Intrathecal baclofen for intractable spasticity of spinal origin: results of a long-term multicenter study. J Neurosurg 78:226–232

Lance JW (1980) Symposium synopsis. In: Feldman RG, Young RR, Koella WP (eds) Spasticity: disordered motor control. Chicago Year Book Medical Publications, Chicago, pp 485–494

Lazorthes Y, Sallerin-Caute B, Verdie J-C, Bastide R, Carillo J-P (1990) Chronic intrathecal baclofen administration for control of severe spasticity. J Neurosurg 72:393–402

McLean BN (1993) Intrathecal baclofen in severe spasticity. Br Hosp Med 49:262–267

Penn RD, Corcos DM (1990) Spasticity and its management. In: Youmans JR (ed) Neurological surgery, 3rd edn. W.B. Saunders, Philadelphia, pp 4371–4385

Chapter 6

Hazards of Spinal/Lumbar Puncture

J.P.R. Dick

Spinal or lumbar puncture (LP) may be used for analysis of the cerebrospinal fluid (CSF), for regional anaesthesia, for radiological investigation (e.g. myelography) or for intrathecal chemotherapy (e.g. in the management of pain, cancer or spasticity). CSF examination is an important diagnostic tool in neurological practice and this chapter is devoted to the hazards likely to be met under these circumstances. The complications of discography and chemonucleolysis are not addressed.

CSF examination can be used in diverse clinical circumstances and in some diseases it is the diagnostic test of choice (e.g. suspected purulent or carcinomatous meningitis). In many disease it provides useful diagnostic support (e.g. multiple sclerosis) and can be used as a research tool for the investigation of neuro-immunological disorders (Sharief et al. 1991) or neurotransmitter disorders (e.g. Parkinson's disease). However, it is not without its hazards and it is important to appreciate these, particularly when useful information can be obtained from other investigative modalities.

With the wider availability of computed brain tomography (CT) and magnetic resonance brain imaging (MRI) it has become unnecessary to puncture several categories of patient. Thus suspected spinal cord compression due to epidural disease (malignant or infective), previously investigated by emergency myelography, can be investigated using MR imaging (Berns et al. 1989) and the diagnosis of subarachnoid haemorrhage can usually be made in most patients with modern scanning methods. Indeed, it may be unwise to LP some patients with subarachnoid haemorrhage (SAH) as prolonged CSF drainage can be associated with an increased risk of aneurysmal rupture (Hasan et al. 1989). However, CSF examination remains essential for excluding SAH (Macdonald and Mendelow 1988; Lledo et al. 1994) and can probably be done up to 21 days after the ictus (Walton 1956; Vermeulen et al. 1983; Weir 1994).

The main contraindication to LP is the presence of a depressed level of consciousness due to raised intracranial pressure which may cause herniation of the hindbrain through the foramen magnum. In cases where there is clinical doubt concerning the level of intracranial pressure, CT can provide further information (Gower et al. 1987).Duffy (1969) reported a 40% mortality in 30 patients who underwent LP during the investigation of intracranial mass lesions. In half, the deterioration occurred immediately after the procedure and in the rest it occurred within 12 hours. Those with brain abscess did particularly badly. For intraspinal mass lesions Hollis et al. (1986) reported a 14% risk of "spinal" coning if LP was performed below a spinal block; as a result, if myelography is performed for a suspected spinal tumour a lateral cervical puncture should be performed.

Thus, although LP remains essential in the diagnosis of meningeal disease, particularly in the management of CNS infection, it may be life threatening in severe meningitis with raised intracranial pressure (Harper et al. 1985; Shapiro et al. 1986) and therapy should be started prior to CSF examination (Rennick et al. 1993). Even when necessary, certain subgroups need to be prepared carefully (haemophiliacs, neonates); thus, infants with cardiopulmonary disease may develop cardiac arrest during LP (Margolis and Cook 1973) and should be be oxygenated prior to the procedure (Fiser et al. 1993).

Complications of the Technique

Post-LP Headache Syndrome

The commonest complication of lumbar puncture is the post-LP headache syndrome (PLPHS). This is a bilateral headache coming on some time after the procedure (usually the next day) which is markedly exacerbated by standing or even by sitting. It may be accompanied by nausea, vomiting, tinnitus, stiff neck or lightheadedness and tends to last a few days. Immediate post-LP headache has a different aetiology (intracranial air, subarachnoid haemorrhage). PLPHS is thought to be due to a persistent leak of CSF through a lumbar dural tear and rarely follows cervical puncture (Frederiks 1992). It occurs less frequently in children, the aged, the demented (Blennow et al. 1993) and is perhaps more common in women of slight build (Kuntz et al. 1992), particularly if pregnant (Frederiks 1992). It is particularly common after myelography (Youl 1990). The headache is exacerbated by jugular compression and is abolished by re-injecting fluid. An identical headache occurs if sufficient CSF (25 ml) is removed initially. In neurological practice post-LP headache occurs in 13%–36% of cases (Tourtelotte et al. 1964; Hilton-Jones 1984) though lower figures are quoted in the anaesthetic literature for spinal anaesthesia (18% obstetric, 13% non-obstetric). In view of the presumed mechanism, most studies have suggested that a small diameter spinal needle should be used (22 G) to minimize dural trauma and that the bevel of the needle should be inserted in the vertical plane as the dural fibres run rostrocaudal (Hilton-Jones 1984). A prospective study in the recent obstetric literature showed no additional advantage of 24 G needles over 22 G needles (Sears et al. 1994).

Although several studies have failed to demonstrate an improvement with prolonged recumbency (e.g. Hilton-Jones 1984; Kuntz et al. 1992) most patients choose this method of management themselves. A wide variety of therapeutic agents have been advocated for symptomatic relief (indomethacin, theophylline, vasopressin, steroids) and in protracted post-LP headache syndromes epidural blood patches have been used (Frederiks 1992). However, its course is usually benign and symptomatic treatment with strong reassurance usually suffices.

Complications due to Mechanical Sequelae

Spinal anesthesia has provided useful data on the incidence of traumatic complications from LP in experienced hands. Dripps and Vandam (1951) sent questionnaires to 6147 patients who had had spinal anaesthesia over the period 1948–1951. Of the 90% who replied, 13% had had electric shock sensations radiating down one leg at the time of puncture and 1% had experienced tinnitus which resolved spontaneously. Of 637 patients who had been punctured using 16 G needles, 22% had had post-LP headaches and five of these developed horizontal diplopia which recovered spontaneously over 3 weeks to 9 months. None of their cases suffered infective complications.

Radicular Trauma

Weber and Weingarden (1979) have shown that EMG abnormalities occur in 40% of cases following myelography. They were not associated with significant symptomatology and disappeared by the fourth post-myelogram day. Although the incidence of even minor traumatic complications is low in experienced hands – 10% according to Dripps and Vandam (1951) – rarely a nerve root may be transected (Young and Burney 1971), and this has been associated with Sudeck's atrophy (Morettin and Wilson 1970), or an intervertebral disc may herniate through a stylet-induced tear (Frederiks 1992). On withdrawal of the spinal needle, the stylet should be replaced as it is possible to aspirate a nerve root and draw it through the dura (Trupp 1977). It is important to have a stylet that fits flush with its casing as there are reports of intradural epidermoid tumours resulting from the proliferation of epithelial cells originally introduced at LP (Tabaddor and Lamorgese 1975; Baba et al. 1994).

Brainstem Phenomena

Neuro-otological phenomena may occur in the context of a prolonged PLPHS (nystagmus, vertigo, vomiting, tinnitus and deafness) and this may prompt the clinical suspicion of a previously covert Arnold Chiari type I malformation (Barton and Sharpe 1993). Most patients make a complete recovery within a fortnight though rarely these phenomena take longer to resolve (Michel and Brusis 1992; Lance and Branch 1994). Occasionally an Arnold Chiari malformation can be acquired from multiple lumbar punctures (Sathi and Steig 1993).

Complications due to Associated Bleeding

Traumatic haemorrhage occurs in about 20% of LPs (Frederiks 1992) and may mimic subarachnoid haemorrhage, thereby complicating CSF analysis. In contrast to traumatic intracranial haemorrhage, traumatic haemorrhage into the spinal canal occurs in the extradural space more commonly than the subdural space. This is because the dura is attached to the inner table of the calvarium in the skull but is separated from the vertebrae by a venous plexus and loosely arranged fatty tissue in the spine. It is this venous plexus, or that surrounding a nerve root, which is most often traumatized by the LP needle. Haemorrhage is usually minimal though excessive bleeding may occur in patients who are anticoagulated or those with haematological disorders.

Haemorrhage into Epidural Space

Although this is the more common haemorrhagic complication of LP, it is rare and tends to occur in the anticoagulated patient having spinal anaesthesia. The clinical presentation is similar to that of spontaneous epidural haematoma and occurs soon after LP. Spontaneous epidural haematoma may occur after minor trauma (Dawson 1963), such as straining or turning over in bed (see elsewhere in this book). It is associated with severe local pain, may cause acute cord compression and is slightly commoner in the thoracic region (Harik et al. 1971). No structural lesion is found in many cases (presumed angiomatous malformation ablated) whereas angiomatous lesions are found in others. Extradural angiomatous malformations may be associated with vertebral or dermatologial angiomata and are less common than intradural ones. The clinical urgency is similar to that of spinal epidural abscess. Decompressive laminectomy, with adequate supplies of blood for transfusion, is urgent (Findlay 1987). Preoperative plain firms should be inspected for a vertebral angiomatous malformation, and dura, spinal cord and evacuated clot for evidence of angiomata.

Haemorrhage into Subdural Space

This is extremely rare (Edelson et al. 1974) and in those cases in which subdural blood but no subarachnoid or extradural blood has been demonstrated post mortem, it has been suggested that the haematoma resulted from blood tracking out from the subarachnoid space (Masdeu et al. 1979) and that subarachnoid blood was cleared by CSF hydrodynamics.

Haemorrhage into Subarachnoid Space

This arises as a result of trauma to radicular arteries (Masdeu et al. 1979) and may cause an acute spinal cord or cauda equina syndrome, particularly in those on anticoagulants. Brem et al. (1981) reviewed their experience in patients with stroke who were put immediately onto heparin after LP: three of 175 patients developed paraparesis, of whom two had a subarachnoid haematoma, and in one the LP had been acellular.

It is important, therefore, to consider carefully the indications for spinal puncture in patients with a coagulapathy (leukaemia, thrombocytopenia, liver disease, haemophilia), or if anticoagulated, and, if appropriate, to cover the procedure with haemostatic agents. When adequately covered LP in haemophiliacs can be safe (Silverman et al. 1993).

Infectious Complications

Rarely, infection may follow LP in an intervertebral disc (Feinbloom and Halaby 1966), in the epidural space (Rangell and Glassman 1945), in the spinal cord (Rifaat et al. 1973), in a vertebral body (Bergman et al. 1983) or in the meninges (Eng and Seligman 1981; Teele et al. 1981; Harper et al. 1985; Shapiro et al. 1986). All are uncommon (Dripps and Vandam 1951) though there remains some doubt concerning the frequency of post-LP meningitis.

Laboratory data from Petersdorf et al. (1962) demonstrated, in the dog, that dural puncture in the presence of a high-grade bacteraemia could lead to meningitis. The mechanism was uncertain though it had been known for some time that, in a spun specimen of CSF, it was not uncommon to see a cylindrical fragment of skin or incidental squamous cells with associated commensal staphylococci and occasionally, cartilage or bone marrow cells were seen (Dickson 1944). Infection could therefore be introduced directly, as above, or by causing a small haematoma which would act as a "locus minor is residentiae". Teele et al. (1981) compared the course of 277 episodes of bacteraemia in infants seen at one institution. A normal LP was seen at presentation in 46 patients (less than eight mononuclear cells, less than one polymorph and a normal sugar level); the other 231, who were not punctured, served as a control group. Seven of the 46 developed meningitis but only two of the 231 patients did. It was argued that LP had been instrumental in the development of meningitis in the seven children all of whom were under 18 months of age. However, Eng and Seligman (1981) suggested it was rare to develop LP-induced meningitis in adults and argued that previous reports of LP-induced meningitis were an expression of the high "spontaneous" potential of meningitic organisms to cause meningitis. This latter point was emphsized by Shapiro et al. (1986) who calculated an 85.6% chance of developing meningitis "spontaneously" in association with meningococcal septicaemia.

References

Baba H, Wada M, Tanaka Y, Imura S, Tomita K (1994) Intraspinal epidermoid after lumbar puncture. Int Orthop 18:116–118

Barton JJ, Sharpe JA (1993) Oscillopsia and horizontal nystagmus with accelerating slow phases following lumbar puncture in the Arnold Chairi malformation. Ann Neurol 33:418–421.

Bergman I, Wald ER, Meyer JD, painter MJ (1983) Epidural abscess and vertebral osteomyelitis following serial lumbar punctures. Pediatrics 72:476–480

Berns DH, Blaser SJ, Modic MT (1989) Magnetic resonance imaging of the spine. Clin Orthop 244:78–100

Blennow K, Wallin A, Hager O (1993) Low frequency of post lumbar puncture headache in demented patients. Acta Neurol Scand 88:221–223

Brem S, Hale A, Van Uitert RL, Ruff RL, Reichert WH (1981) A hazard of lumbar puncture resulting in reversible paraplegia. N Engl J Med 304:1020–1021

Dawson BH (1963) Paraplegia due to spinal epidural haematoma. J Neurol Neurosurg Psychiatry 26:171–173

Dickson WEC (1944) The cerebrospinal fluid in meningitis. Postgrad Med J 20:69–74

Dripps RD, Vandam LD (1951) Hazards of lumbar puncture. JAMA 147:1118–1121

Duffy GP (1969) Lumbar puncture in the presence of raised intracranial pressure. Br Med J i:407–409

Edelson RN, Chernik NL, Posner JB (1974) Spinal subdural hematoma complicating lumbar puncture: occurrence in thrombocytopenic patients. Arch Neurol 31:143–147

Eng RHK, Seligman SJ (1981) Lumbar puncture induced meningitis. JAMA 245:1456–1459

Feinbloom RI, Halaby FA (1966) Acute pyogenic spondylitis in infancy: a case report to emphasize the potential risk in lumbar puncture. Clin Pediatr 5:683–684

Findlay GFG (1987) Compression and vascular disorders of the spinal cord. In: Miller JD (ed) Northfields surgery of the central nervous system. Blackwell Scientific, Oxford, pp 707–759

Fiser DH, Gobr GA, Smith CE, Jackson DC, Walker W (1993) Prevention of hypoxaemia during lumbar puncture in infancy. Pediatr Emerg Care 9:81–83

Frederiks JAM (1992) Spinal puncture complications: complications of diagnostic lumbar puncture, myelography, spinal anaesthesia and intrathecal drug administration. In: Fankel HL (ed) Handbook of clinical neurology, vol 61, Elsevier Science Publishers Amsterdam, pp 147–189

Gower DJ, Baker AL, Bell WO, Ball MR (1987) Contraindications to lumbar puncture as defined by computed cranial tomography. J Neurol Neurosurg Psychiatry 50:1071–1074

Harik SI, Raichle ME, Reis DJ (1971) Spontaneously remitting spinal epidural hematoma in a patient on anticoagulants. N Engl J Med 284:1355–1357

Harper JR, Lorber J, Hillas Smith G (1985) Timing of lumbar puncture in severe childhood meningitis. Br Med J 291:651–652, 1123–1124

Hasan D, Vermuelen M, Wijdicks EFM, Hijdra A, Van Gijn J (1989) Management problems in acute hydrocephalus after subarachnoid haemorrhage. Stroke 20:747–753

Hilton-Jones D (1984) What is post lumbar puncture headache and is it avoidable? In: Warlow C, Garfield J (eds) Dilemmas in the management of the neurological patient. Churchill Livingstone, Edinburgh, pp 144–158

Hollis PH, Malis LI, Zappula RA (1986) Neurological deterioration after lumbar puncture block below complete spinal subarachnoid block. J Neurosurg 64:253–56

Kuntz KM, Kokmen E, Stevens JC, Miller P, Offord KP, Ho MM (1992) Post lumbar puncture headaches: experience of 501 consecutive procedures. Neurology 42:1884–1887

Lance JW, Branch GB (1994) Persistent headache after lumbar puncture (letter). Lancet 343:414

Lledo A, Calandre L, Martinez-Menendez B, Perez-Sempere A, Portera-Sanchez A (1994) Acute headache of recent onset and subarachnoid haemorrhage: a prospective study. Headache 34:172–174

Macdonald A, Mendelow AD (1988) Xanthochromia revisited: a re-evaluation of lumbar puncture and CT scanning in the diagnosis of subarachnoid haemorrhage. J Neurol Neurosurg Psychiatry 51:342–344

Margolis CZ, Cook CD (1973) The risk of lumbar puncture in pediatric patients with cardiac and/or pulmonary disease. Pediatrics 51:562–564

Masdeu JC, Breuer AC, Schoene WC (1979) Spinal subarachnoid hematoma; clue to source of bleeding in traumatic lumbar puncture. Neurology 29:872–876

Michel O, Brusis T (1992) Hearing loss as a sequel to lumbar puncture. Ann Otol Rhinol Laryngol 101:390–394

Morettin LB, Wilson M (1970) Severe reflex algodystrophy (Sudeck's atrophy) as a complication of myelography: report of two cases. AJR 110:156–158

Petersdorf RG, Swarner DR, Garcia M (1962) Studies on the pathogenesis of meningitis. II Development of meningitis during pneumococcal bacteremia. J Clin Invest 41:320–327

Rangel L, Glassman F (1945) Acute spinal epidural abscess as a complication of lumbar puncture. J Nerv Ment Dis 102:8–18

Rennick G, Shann F, de Campo J (1993) Cerebral herniation during bacterial meningitis in children Br Med J 306:953–956

Rifaat M, el Shafei I, Samra K (1973) Intramedullary spinal abscess following lumbar puncture: case report. J Neurosurg 38:366–367

Sathi S, Steig PE (1993) "Acquired" Chairi malformation after multiple lumbar punctures: case report. Neurosurgery 32:306–309

Spears DH, Leeman MI, Jassy LJ, Odonnell LA, Reisner LS (1994) The frequency of postdural puncture headache in obstetric patients: a prospective study comparing the 24G needles versus 22G Sprotte needle. J Clin Anesth 6:42–46

Shapiro D, Aaron N, Wald E (1986) Risk factors for the development of bacterial meningitis among children with occult bacteremia. J Pediatr 109:15–19

Sharief MK, Hentges R, Thomas E (1991) Significance of CSF immunoglobulins in monitoring neurological disease activity in Behcets disease. Neurology 41:1398–1401

Silverman R, Kwitatkowski T, Bernstein S et al. (1993) Safety of lumbar puncture in patients with haemophilia. Ann Emerg Med 22:1739–1742

Tabaddor K, Lamorgese JR (1975) Lumbar epidermoid cyst following single lumbar puncture. J Bone Joint Surg 57A:1168–1169

Teele DW, Dashevsky B, Rakkusan T, Klein JO (1981) Meningitis after lumbar puncture in children with bacteremia. N Engl J Med 305:1079–1081

Tourtelotte WW, Haerer AF, Heller GL, Sommers JE (1964) Post lumbar puncture headache. Thomas, Illinois

Trupp M (1977) Stylet injury syndrome. JAMA 237:2524

Vermuelen M, Van Gijn J, Blijenberg BG (1983) Spectrophotometric analysis of CSF after subarachnoid haemorrhage. Limitations in the diagnosis of rebleeding. Neurology 33:112–114

Walton JN (1956) Subarachnoid haemorrhage. Churchill Livingstone, Edinburgh

Weber RJ, Weingarden SI (1979) Electromyographic abnormalities following myelography. Arch Neurol 36:588–589

Weir B (1994) Headaches from aneurysms. Cephalalgia 14:79–87

Youl BD (1990) Les cephalees apres ponction lombaire et leur traitement. Rev Prat Paris 40:414–415

Young DA, Burney RE (1971) Complications of myelography: transection and withdrawal of a nerve filament by the needle. N Engl J Med 285:156–157

Chapter 7

Neuropathology

D.I. Graham

Introduction

The tissue of the spinal cord is similar to that of the brain and is made up of two main types consisting of the highly specialized **neurones (nerve cells)** with their processes, and the **neuroglial cells** (Lantos 1990a). Both of these are of neuroecto-dermal origin in contrast to the second main type of tissue which has an origin in mesoderm and comprises the **meninges**, the **blood vessels** and their supporting connective tissue and **microglia**. Whereas some of the diseases affecting the spinal cord are similar to those seen in other organs, e.g. inflammation, vascular disease and tumours, others are primarily diseases of spinal neurones affecting their cell body, axons and myelin sheaths. Therefore, it follows that because the constituent cells of the spinal cord are similar to those found elsewhere in the nervous system, the disease processes and the tissue reaction in response to them are similar to those found elsewhere in the brain (Hughes 1978; Esiri and Oppenheimer 1989; Lantos 1990b). However, the prevalence of the various disease processes in the spinal cord differs from that found elsewhere in the brain.

Applied Anatomy

The dura mater acts as the periosteum to the spinal canal, but it can be stripped from the vertebrae by haemorrhage or abscess formation into the potential **extradural space**. The dura and outer surface of the arachnoid are normally in contact, but the **subdural space** can more readily be distended by blood or pus than the extradural space. The arachnoid forms a continuous sheet in contact with the dura while the pia follows the contours of the spinal cord. Between the pia and arachnoid is the **subarachnoid space** traversed by delicate trabeculae of connective tissue that divide it up into a series of intercommunicating spaces filled with cerebral spinal fluid (CSF). The major spinal arteries and veins also run in the subarachnoid space, and from the arteries small blood vessels pass into the spinal cord. As an artery penetrates the spinal cord, it carries with it a potential perivascular space –

the **Virchow-Robin space** – which is separated from the substance of the spinal cord by the **blood–brain barrier**.

Microorganisms and their toxins readily spread throughout the subarachnoid space which may become filled with inflammatory exudate. Examination of lumbar CSF often provides valuable information about diseases of the nervous system. Normal CSF is clear and colourless, does not coagulate and has a specific gravity of 1006. It contains 0.15–0.45 g/l protein, 2.8–4.4 mmol/l glucose and approximately 128 mmol/l sodium and 128 mmol/l chloride. A few lymphocytes and monocytes may be seen in normal fluid but rarely more than 4/ml.

Reactions to Disease

Neurones

The neurone is one of the most complex and specialized cells in the body and since it is not capable of dividing after the first few weeks of extrauterine life any damage involving loss is structurally irreversible. A detailed understanding of the structure and function of neurones requires the application of multiple methods which show that they are made up of the **perikaryon** or cell body from which extend the **dendrites** and the **axon**. The perikarya are the main component of grey matter in which they tend to have characteristic arrangements. A conspicuous feature in the perikarya is the presence of **Nissl granules** which are rich in RNA, and are composed of stacks of rough endoplasmic reticulum and intervening groups of free ribosomes. Special staining techniques demonstrate the cytoskeleton in the cytoplasm comprising principally neurofilaments and neurotubules. Mitochondria are numerous in dendrites and in the presynaptic region. Lysosomes are also found and are a particularly characteristic feature in large neurones, such as those found in the ventral horns of the spinal cord, in their content of lipofuscin. Various substances (neurotransmitters, proteins and organelles) are relayed in fast and slow phases of **axoplasmic flow** from the cell body along the axons and dendrites to synapses. There is also a retrograde axoplasmic flow of material from the periphery towards the perikaryon.

The reactions of neurones take several forms. **Central chromatolysis** occurs in the perikaryon between 5 and 8 days after the axon has been cut. At first the cell body becomes swollen and spherical. The nucleus becomes eccentric, the Nissl granules break down into dust-like particles which may persist at the margin of the cell, and the cytoplasm becomes pale and homogeneous. This response to injury has recently been shown to be accompanied by an increase in protein synthesis. It is, therefore, considered to be a regenerative phenomenon. When it is due to damage to a spinal nerve, central chromatolysis is sometimes reversible. By contrast, effective regeneration does not occur in the central nervous system (CNS) and **retrograde degeneration** of the axon results so that following axonal transection the proximal end of the severed axon swells to form an axonal bulb: it may be found within 3–6 hours of injury, may persist for up to 60 days and is thought to be due to continuance of axoplasmic flow in both directions (Nauta and Gygax 1954; Fink and Heimer 1967; Gentleman et al. 1993; Sheriff et al. 1994).

When the cell body of a myelinated neurone is irreversibly damaged its axon and myelin sheath break down by the process of **Wallerian degeneration** (see below).

Neurones require a constant supply of oxygen and glucose and if this is inadequate, they undergo a series of changes referred to as the **ischaemic cell process** in which mitochondria become swollen, and the perikaryon shrinks and often becomes triangular in shape. Nissl granules disappear and cytoplasm becomes intensely eosinophilic and the nucleus pyknotic. A characteristic feature of recent neuronal necrosis is the presence of small dark granules known as encrustations on the surface of the perikaryon and its dendrites. Dead neurones are removed by phagocytes. Moderate neuronal loss is very difficult to recognize histologically unless there are also some reactive changes in the neuroglia. Not all neurones in the CNS are equally vulnerable to the effects of hypoxia, there being a pattern of **selective vulnerability**. Within the rank order of vulnerability the most resistant neurones to the ischaemic cell process are those found in the dorsal and ventral horns of the spinal cord.

There are many other less common changes in neurones. For example inclusion bodies may be found in certain virus infections and in many of the slowly progressive degenerative diseases such as motor neurone disease. In some of the inborn errors of metabolism the cytoplasm of neurones becomes distended with lipid-laden lysosomes.

Another form of degeneration is **trans-synaptic atrophy** which occurs in neurones, the principal afferent connections of which have been destroyed: an example is in the nucleus gracilis and nucleus cuneatus when the posterior columns of the spinal cord have undergone degeneration.

Neuroglia

These include astrocytes, oligodendrocytes and ependymal cells.

Damage to the spinal cord, whatever its cause, is invariably accompanied by hypertrophy and hyperplasia of astrocytic processes referred to as **gliosis** or **astrocytosis**. Within a day or so of tissue damage astrocytes begin to divide, this response being associated with the production of large amounts of glial fibrillary acidic protein. Characteristically, gliosed tissue is firmer than normal and tends to appear grey and translucent as in plaques of multiple sclerosis. Usually, the glial fibres are laid down in an irregular manner and in areas of long-standing gliosis **Rosenthal fibres** may be seen. These are eosinophilic structures which may be round, oval or elongated ranging in size from 10 to 40 μm. Another type of astrocytic response is seen in oedematous white matter when the cell body enlarges, becomes rounded and acquires an eosinophilic homogeneous cytoplasm and the nucleus becomes eccentric. These cells are known as **gemistocytic astrocytes** and have been found in the white matter within as little as 6 hours after the onset of acute oedema: they are also seen in relation to tumours and infarcts. Even though gliosis is the principal response of the CNS to injury in certain circumstances when there has been tissue necrosis, there is often a mixed glial and fibroblastic response referred to as a **gliomesodermal reaction**. This is most frequently seen in subacute and chronic abscesses.

Basophilic circular bodies known as **corpora amylaceae** accumulate with increasing age and in disease and they are thought to have an origin in astrocytes, and the brain tissue is firmer than normal and may have a grey translucent appearance.

Oligodendrocytes are small cells with darkly staining nuclei that resemble a lymphocyte. They are often numerous and are seen as **perineuronal satellites** in the grey matter and as rows of closely apposed nuclei between bundles of myelinated nerve fibres – the **interfascicular** oligodendroglia. Oligodendrocytes play an important role in both the formation and maintenance of myelin and loss of the interfascicular oligodendrocyte in some of the demyelinating diseases appears to precede obvious degeneration of myelin.

A single layer of ependymal cells lines the central canal of the spinal cord. They are columnar and have a ciliated free (luminal) surface immediately deep to which there is a line of small oval bodies known as blepharoplasts. Ependymal cells show few reactive changes. If the central canal becomes distended then the ependyma is stretched and then broken, but the cells do not proliferate to fill the defects.

Microglia

These respond rapidly to any noxious process, but it is not clear what proportion of reactive microglia are derived from microglia already present in the CNS and what proportion from circulating monocytes. In the process of **neuronophagia**, phagocytes engulf and eventually digest irreversibly damaged neurones. Initially microglia become elongated and their processes are more apparent; they are referred to as **rod cells**. When brain tissue is destroyed the microglia act as phagocytes; the cell becomes enlarged and rounded, the nucleus eccentric and the cytoplasm filled with ingested material, usually the breakdown products of myelin. These cells – **lipid (foamy) phagocytes** – are sudanophilic and react strongly for acid phosphatase. They are most commonly seen in relation to vascular disease and in recent plaques of demyelination. Microglia also ingest the breakdown products of haemoglobin when they are referred to as siderophages and stain positively with Perls' Prussian blue reaction.

Transverse Lesions of the Spinal Cord

Various specific disorders of the spine and spinal cord are described elsewhere, but it is appropriate at this stage to describe the events that take place when there is either partial or complete interruption of the cord. For example, acute transverse lesions may be due to **trauma** – usually a fracture dislocation of the vertebrae – **infarction** when the circulation of the anterior spinal artery is compromised, **haemorrhage** usually as a result of vascular malformation or **acute demyelination** as in neuromyelitis optica. However, transverse lesions may also develop as a result of slowly progressive pathology, such as pressure on the cord by **tumours**. Although much less common than formerly, **infections** such as tuberculosis, (Fig. 7.1), brucellosis, and *E. coli* and staphylococcal infections may cause cord compression. Compression may also occur as a result of **metabolic bone disease**.

Following partial or total interruption of the cord, in addition to the local damage, an inevitable consequence is the development of **ascending** and **descending**

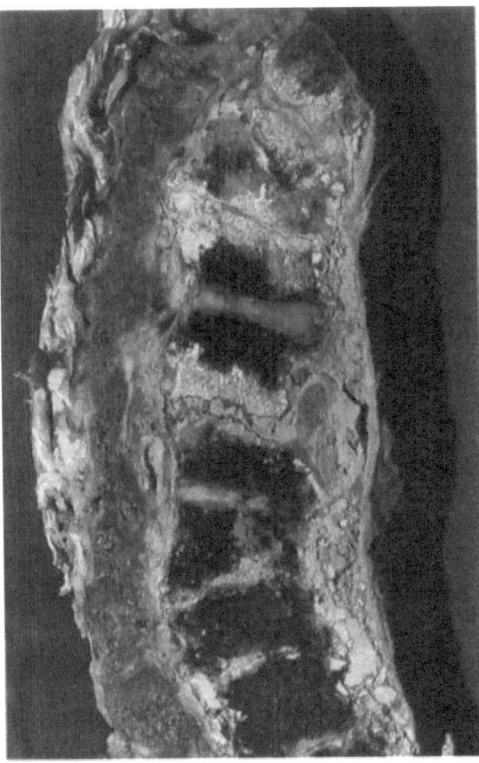

Fig. 7.1. Tuberculosis of spine. Sagittal section of the vertebral column. The "cold" abscess has led to angular curvature of the spine.

Wallerian degeneration in the interrupted tracts of the spinal cord. The distribution of the degenerative processes and its time course can be studied by one of two main staining techniques that are used to demonstrate the loss of myelin. First, there is the Marchi technique which is used to demonstrate recent breakdown of myelin within the preceding two to three months: the unsaturated fatty acids formed during this process are stained black, while normal myelin remains unstained (Smith 1951; Smith et al. 1956). Additional histological techniques that yield useful information about the state of myelin breakdown include Sudan IV, Sudan Black or Oil Red O in frozen sections. Myelin sheaths break up into ellipsoids and gradually the products of degeneration are taken up by phagocytes, a process that may be seen after 6–8 weeks. Gradually, the amount of Marchi-positive material diminishes, but it may remain in affected tracts for many months or even several years and it becomes resistant to prolonged fixation in formalin. The degenerative process is accompanied by an astrocytosis which gradually increases over several weeks and may still be evident some 6–12 months later. The second technique is one used for showing the long-term consequences of the myelin degeneration by revealing the demyelinated areas by their failure to stain with conventional stains, e.g. Luxol fast blue and by the Weigert-Pal method and its modifications.

Ascending Degeneration

The pattern following a transverse lesion in the lower thoracic spine is shown in Figs. 7.2A–D. In the section taken a few segments above the lesion (Fig. 7.2a) degeneration is seen in the posterior columns (with the exception of the small area dorsal to the grey commissure where they are chiefly commisural fibres) and the spinothalamic and spinocerebellar tracts. In the cervical region the degeneration of the posterior columns is virtually confined to the gracile tracts (Fig. 7.2b). Because the cuneate tract is composed of ascending fibres that have joined the cord above the level of the lesion, anatomical studies have shown that the degenerative process in the posterior columns ascends up to the cuneate and gracile nuclei in the medulla. On the other hand ascending degeneration in the spinocerebellar tracts extends up to the inferior cerebellar peduncle and into the cerebellum and in the anterior spinocerebellar tracts to the middle lobe of the cerebellum. The long-term consequences of this degeneration are well seen in Figs. 7.2c and d where there is a pallor of staining due to loss of myelin in the posterior columns.

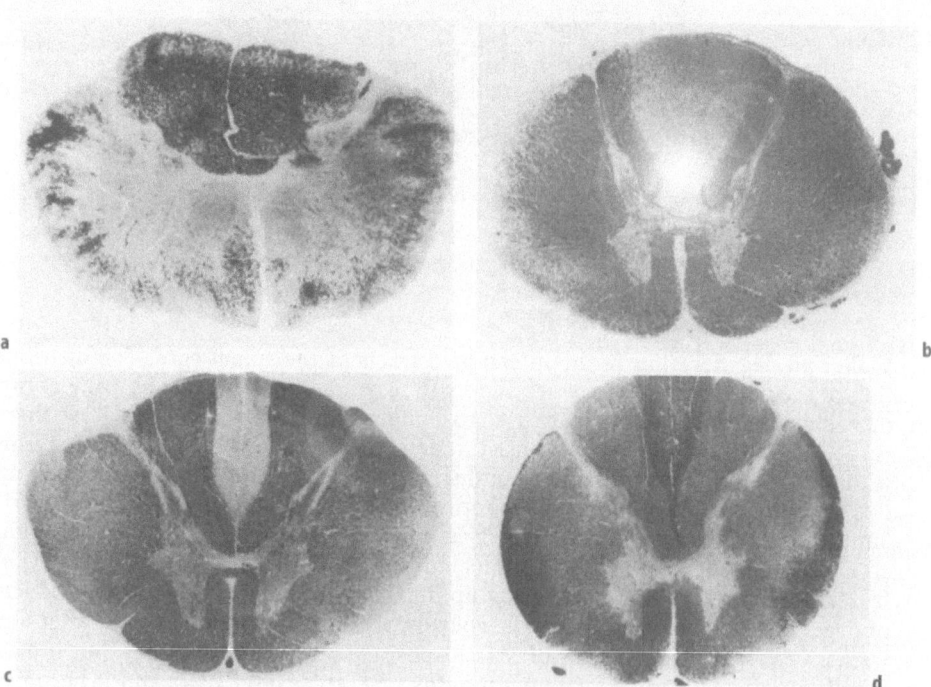

Fig. 7.2a–d. **a** Thoracic cord above lesion. The whole of the posterior columns and anterolateral ascending tracts are degenerating. Marchi. **b** Cervical region. There are fewer degenerating fibres because of the inflow of fibres above the level of the lesion. Marchi. **c** Thoracic cord above the lesion. Weigert-Pal. **d** Cervical region. Degeneration appears to be confined to the gracile tracts. Weigert-Pal. (Reproduced with permission from *Muir's textbook of pathology*, 12th edn. J.R. Anderson (ed), Edward Arnold, London, 1985.)

Descending Degeneration

In a section taken distal to a transverse lesion of the cord, marked degeneration is seen in the crossed (lateral) and uncrossed (anterior pyramidal) tracts unless the lesion is low in the cord where the uncrossed tract is no longer present (Fig. 7.3a).

A different pattern of descending degeneration is seen following a lesion, either in the brainstem or in one internal capsule, which results in retrograde degeneration of the corticospinal tract. In these situations there is degeneration of the crossed pyramidal tract on the opposite side (Fig. 7.3b) and of the uncrossed pyramidal tract on the same side. As the uncrossed pyramidal tract does not usually extend below the upper thoracic segments, its degeneration will not be seen in sections of the lower thoracic cord (Fig. 7.3c).

Spinal Injury

It has been estimated that within the United Kingdom each year between 13 and 27 per million of population suffer from serious paralysis following injury to the spinal

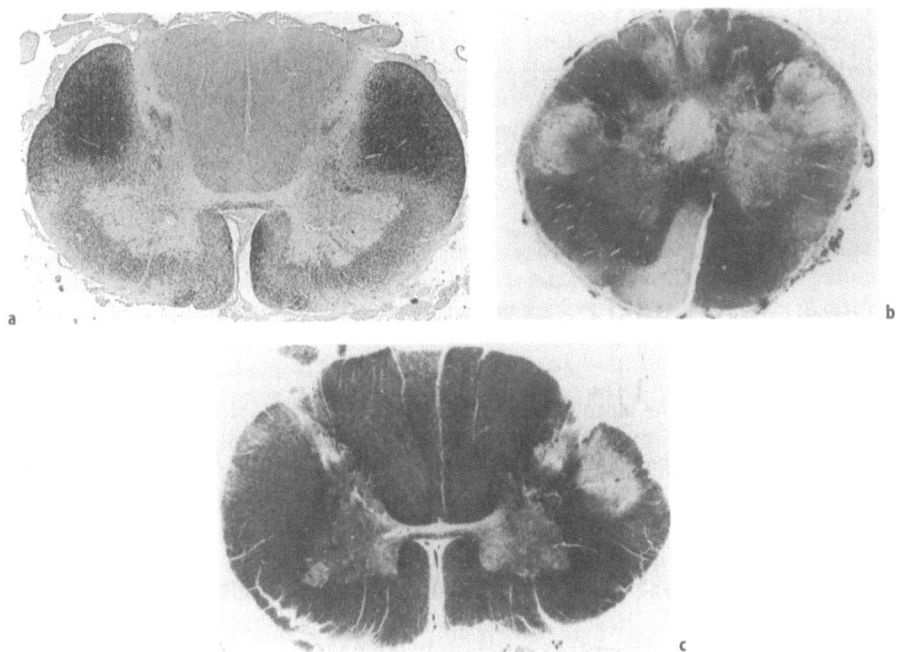

Fig. 7.3a–c. Wallerian degeneration. **a** Descending degeneration below level of lesion. There is degenerating myelin (dark area) in the lateral and anterior white columns. Marchi. **b** Medulla. The pyramid on one side is degenerated. Weigert-Pal. **c** Thoracic region. The crossed pyramidal tract on one side is degenerated. Weigert-Pal. **b** and **c** reproduced with permission from *Muir's textbook of pathology*, 12th edn. J.R. Anderson (ed), Edward Arnold, London, 1985.)

cord and an even higher prevalence if cases of sudden death after accident are included (Hughes 1984, 1992). Injuries may be classified as either **non-missile** or **missile**. The former result from subluxations and fracture dislocations of the vertebral column and in civilian practice almost half of all new cases of spinal injury result from motor car or motor cycle accidents, with 30% being due to falls and the remainder due to sporting injuries. The vertebrae may return to normal position when the fracture dislocation is said to be **stable**. If the damage to vertebrae are still capable of moving the fracture is **unstable** and any undue movement to the injured patient may intensify damage to the spinal cord. Some two-thirds of the patients are less than 40 years of age and some 90% are men.

The cervical spine at the level of C5/6 vertebrae and the thoracic spine are injured most commonly in road traffic accidents, whereas the lumbar spine is damaged most commonly in crush injuries of the type seen in mining accidents or after falls.

As with head injuries, trauma to the spinal cord may be **closed** or **open** (penetrating). There are various mechanisms which include a combination of **flexion, rotation, extension** and **compression**. An extension injury is usually due to hyperextension of the mid-cervical vertebrae which causes a separation and dislocation of intravertebral discs, local haemorrhage and possible rupture of the longitudinal ligament. If there is excessive flexion of the cervical spine, there is compression of the vertebral bodies, parts of which may be displayed posteriorly causing damage to the spinal cord. The spinal canal may be narrowed by fracture dislocation due to rotation and in patients with compressive fractures, fragments of bone may be displayed backwards into the spinal canal or if the spinal column is angulated acutely stretching and compression of the dura and cord may result. Open injuries to the cord may result from missiles such as bullets and associated bony fragments which may lodge in the cord or in the case of high velocity missiles may cause severe damage to the cord by pressure changes resulting from shock waves. In civilian practice the cord may be injured by a stab wound especially if the knife enters the spinal canal anterolaterally.

Pathology of Spinal Cord Trauma

If possible radiographs should be available to the pathologist at the time of the autopsy to allow an accurate assessment of bony lesions and location of any missile. It is essential during the post-mortem procedures to remove a block of the vertebral column extending for at least two or three vertebrae above and below the level of the injury. The specimen should then be fixed and following laminectomy the cord should be removed from the vertebral canal or the specimen be cut with a band saw in the midsagittal plane to demonstrate the damaged vertebrae and spinal cord (Fig. 7.4a).

In cases of mild injury, where there is only temporary neurological dysfunction, the term **concussion** is used as it is presumed that structural abnormalities are minimal: indeed the external surface of the cord may be normal. In more severe injuries there is **contusion** of the cord, the extent and severity of which will vary from case to case and in many there is extradural, subdural or subarachnoid haemorrhage. The lesion is characterized by **haemorrhagic necrosis** at the site of

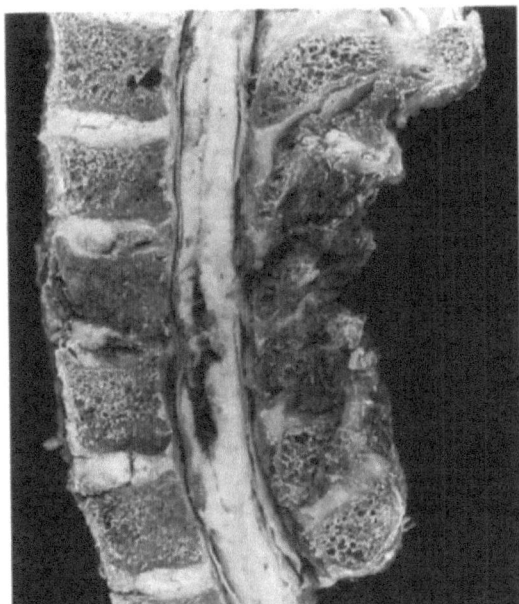
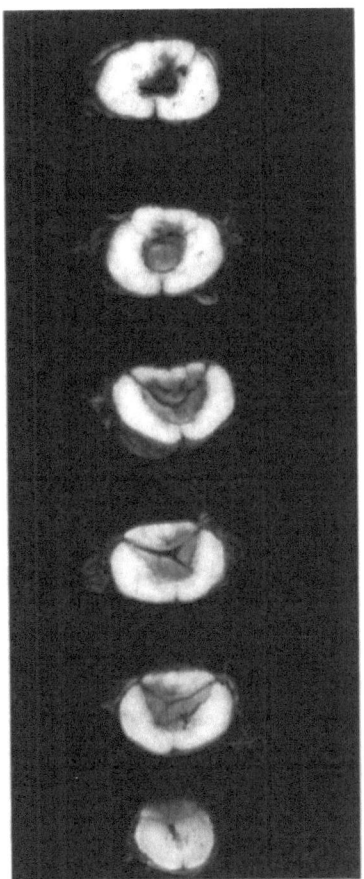

Fig. 7.4. Spinal injury. **a** There is a traumatic haematomyelia in relation to a fracture of the cervical spine. (Reproduced with permission from J.H. Adams and D.I. Graham, *An introduction to neuropathology*, Churchill Livingstone, Edinburgh, 1988.) **b** Transverse sections through traumatic haematomyelia in relation to fracture of the cervical spine.

trauma, transverse sections revealing a centrally placed fusiform mass (**traumatic haematomyelia**) which tapers to end in one or more segments above and below the site of injury (Fig. 7.4b). Histologically, there is swelling, necrosis and petechial haemorrhage formation and silver impregnation techniques reveal axonal swellings and bulb formation. Myelin sheaths become swollen and disintegrate and within a few days of injury, there is infiltration by polymorphonuclear leuco-cytes. Gradually the swelling of the cord subsides, small haemorrhages are absorbed and the necrotic tissue is gradually removed by macrophages. Eventually, a cavity is formed, the margins of which are delineated by an astro-cytosis in which iron pigment may be found. In severe cases affected segments are replaced by what is predominantly an astrocytic scar. If the injury involves root entry zones then regenerating axons in Schwann cells may invade the cord and although effective axonal regeneration does not occur, the appearances in some cases are similar to those of an **amputation neuroma**. A late consequence of injury is the development of Wallerian degeneration in both ascending and descending fibre tracts (see above). Sometimes a longitudinally disposed cavity (**post-traumatic syringomyelia**) may track upwards to the medulla or downwards from the damaged segment (Rossier et al. 1985).

Injury to the Spinal Cord and Roots Caused by Diseases of the Spine

Disease or malformation of the spine may cause local or widespread pressure either on the blood supply to the cord or the cord itself. The presentation may be acute or chronic and the histological changes in the cord depend on the duration of the compression. The clinical effects depend to a considerable extent on the rate of the development of the compressive lesion which may extend over many months or can produce paraplegia within a few days with more rapidly expanding lesions.

Many of the causes of cord compression are dealt with in more detail in the appropriate chapters. In brief, however, tumours are a common cause of compression of both the spinal cord and its nerve roots. Most commonly, these are metastatic carcinoma, lymphoma and myeloma. Primary bone tumours, meningioma, schwannomas and neurofibromas may also present in this way. Compression may also develop as a result of various inflammatory diseases. *Staphylococcus aureus* is one of the more common organisms which may cause either a localized abscess or suppuration which may track through the epidural or subdural space. Tuberculosis of the spine (**Pott's disease**) presents most frequently in the cervical and thoracic vertebrae. The disease invariably starts as tuberculous osteitis of the vertebral bodies before spreading into the paravertebral tissues and then to the adjacent epidural or subdural spaces to form a cold abscess. If kyphosis develops the cord is likely to be damaged due to compression by granulation tissue, through angulation of the spine or by interference with the vascular supply. Other inflammatory causes of cord pressure include abscess due to *Brucella abortus* and metastatic abscess due to *Escherichia coli* in association with chronic urinary tract infection.

Prolapsed Intervertebral Disc

This condition is due to herniation of the central part of the disc which consists of soft cellular fibrocartilage forming the **nucleus pulposus** through part of the **annulus fibrosus** which is a ring of much firmer fibrocartilage that is attached directly to the margin of the vertebral bodies. The nucleus pulposus develops from the notochord and forms the central portion of the disc: it often lies eccentrically because the ring of the annulus fibrosus is thicker anteriorly than posteriorly. In childhood the nucleus pulposus constitutes by far the greater part of the disc and with advancing years its bulk is reduced by an encroaching enlargement of the annulus fibrosus.

As a result of injury or of lifting a heavy weight, part of the nucleus pulposus may be forced through the annulus (Fig. 7.5) and compress a nerve root, particularly in

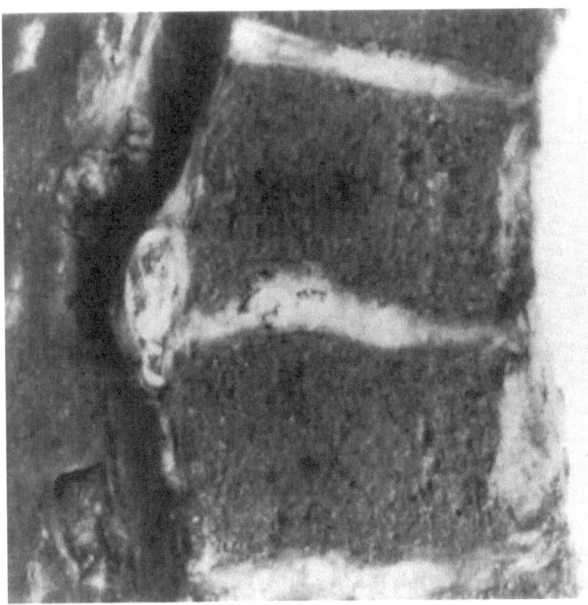

Fig. 7.5.   Prolapsed intervertebral disc. Sagittal section of vertebral column, showing ruptured disc protruding beneath the posterior longitudinal ligament. (Reproduced with permission from *Muir's textbook of pathology*, 12th edn. J.R. Anderson (ed), Edward Arnold, London, 1985.)

the lower spine between L5 and S1, and L4 and L5 and, less commonly in the neck between C5 and C6 (Hook et al. 1960). Lumbar discs are particularly common in those below the age of 40 and may be caused by a fall, or by lifting heavy weights in a stooping position. As the majority of protrusions are at the levels noted there is no damage to the spinal cord, the effects being those of compression of the roots of the cauda equina. Almost all are due to herniation of the nucleus pulposus, but spondylolisthesis with disc protrusion may occur between the lowest lumbar vertebra and the sacrum or between the two lowest lumbar vertebrae. The herniations are usually posteolateral, where they project chiefly into the intervertebral foramen to compress only one root, the most common being L4 or L5. When a disc protrudes into the canal the roots which are descending to a lower level are affected: usually only a few are involved but occasionally there is severe damage to most of the lower roots of the cauda equina. The cord, however, is also at risk in the cervical and thoracic regions, particularly if there is a centrally placed disc prolapse. Degeneration of the lumbar discs with osteophyte formation is common at the lumbar level, but prominent bony ridges on the posterior surface of the vertebral bodies are rare compared with those found in the cervical level. In severe cases osteophytes may occlude the intervertebral foramen which contains the important radicular vessels that supply the lumbosacral cord. Herniation may also occur into the bodies of the vertebrae an event which by itself is of little importance, particularly as it is seen in some 40% of normal subjects when it is referred to as **Schmorl's nodes**. However, such herniation is thought to predispose to bulging of the annulus fibrosus and to **osteophytosis**. Tissue removed at surgery should always be examined histologically where in most instances the prolapsed fragments of the disc often show mucoid degeneration, the tissue appearing devitalized with only a few normal cells remaining. Sometimes there is evidence of vascularization and macrophages containing haemosiderin may be seen. Less commonly, unexpected lesions such as granulomas and tumours may be found, both of which may simulate prolapse of the nucleus pulposus both clinically and at operation.

Spondylosis Deformans

This is a condition that affects the cervical and lumbar regions of the spine in which there is progressive degeneration of intervertebral discs. The condition is common with radiological evidence of its presence in 50% of people over the age of 50, and 75% over the age of 65 years (Frykholm 1951; Brain et al. 1952). It is characterized by ossification of the margins of the vertebral bodies in relation to thickening or lipping of the annulus fibrosus. Anterior lipping causes no neurological symptoms in many cases with minor degrees of posterior lipping also being asymptomatic. In some cases, however, bony transverse ridges on the dorsal surface of the cervical vertebrae associated with disc protrusions are the cause of paraparesis or tetraparesis. Osteophytes develop laterally where they may encroach sufficiently on the lateral recess of the spinal canal along the intervertebral foramen to compress nerve roots. The affected nerve roots become thickened and there may be interference with the blood supply of the root entry zones. There is also a risk of cord compression, but the pathogenesis of this **myelopathy** is complex and involves factors such as interference with the blood supply, trauma and protrusion of the disc material. In some cases paraplegia may develop suddenly after a minor degree of flexion or extension of the neck, and has occurred after tooth extraction or tonsillectomy. In such cases there is often radiological evidence of previous degeneration of one or more discs, so that it is doubtful whether paraplegia can follow such minor strains unless there is already degeneration of a disc. In contrast cord compression in middle-aged patients tends to be due not to disc herniation but rather to the backward protrusion of the annulus fibrosus which both at surgery and at post mortem is recognized by transverse bony ridges with which the bulging is associated. In the neck, herniation of the nucleus pulposus occurs either between the bodies of C5 and C6, or C6 and C7, which are the same sites at which chronic degenerations of the type noted above, are equally common.

The important fact in the production of the myelopathy is congenital narrowing of the cervical spinal canal: the average anteroposterior diameter of the spinal canal in controls was 17 mm and in cases with myelopathy due to **cervical spondylosis** the average measurement was 14 mm (Payne and Spillane 1957). When the neck is extended the anteroposterior diameter of the spinal canal may be reduced by 2 mm and if there is any posterior movement of one vertebra on the other the distance is even further reduced. Posteriorly in hyperextension, the ligamentum flavum may be enfolded and press on the cord. In addition there may be mechanical compression of the anterior spinal artery and tension on the ligamentum denticulatum prevents the cord from moving backwards. Under these conditions cord compression may occur and may be recognized because a segment is flatter than normal because of compression in its anteroposterior diameter. Histologically, in early lesions there are usually ill-defined areas of spongy degeneration due to distension of myelin sheaths many of which contain swollen axons. These changes are commonly found in the ventral parts of the posterior columns and in the white matter at the point of attachment of the thickened ligamentum denticulatum. The anterior third of the white matter usually remains normal. Frank necrosis may develop, and in older lesions cavitation may affect both grey and white matter.

Herniation of thoracic intervertebral discs is uncommon: some are due to trauma whereas others appear to have a more gradual onset. As with other discs they develop as a result of herniation of nucleus pulposus which later becomes fibrosed, calcified and even ossified. Such lesions are said to occur in 2%–3% of all disc protrusions occurring mainly below the level of T6, in patients of middle or later age.

Osteitis Deformans

Paget's disease of the spine is usually accompanied by a degree of kyphosis. Of greater importance, however, in patients who present with paraplegia is the general reduction in the size of the lumen of the spinal canal by prominences that develop on the posterior aspects of the vertebral bodies.

Trauma by Non-mechanical Forces

Lesions of the spinal cord are one of the more serious features of X-irradiation and acute decompression sickness (barotrauma). The cord may also be damaged by lightning, electrical damage and chemotherapy.

X-Irradiation

Radiotherapy is the mainstay of the treatment of malignant tumours of the cord, the ionizing radiation usually being given as a gamma ray beam from radioactive sources or as megavoltage X-ray beams. The dose is usually fractionated, that is the total dose is divided into equal fractions and typical conventional fractionation might be 1.8–2.0 Gy per day 5 times per week to a total dose of 60 Gy. Any complication resulting from the effects of the ionizing radiation will depend on many factors which include the total dose of radiation and the number of the fractions, the dose per fraction, the total treatment time, the volume irradiated, the elimination of "hot spots" by the use of multiple fields, and the use of other treatments such as steroids, radiosensitizers or antineoplastic chemotherapy. The main effect of irradiation on the tumour itself is to produce necrosis: this is particularly true for radiosensitive tumours where large fluid-filled cysts lined with glial scar tissue can be found following treatment, but with less radiosensitive tumours extensive central necrosis may occur although peripheral tumour may remain. Tumour irradiation may also lead to a change in tumour cytology and typically mutinucleated giant cells with irregular hyperchromatic nuclei are found: the number of mitotic figures is reduced and the affect of irradiation on the blood vessels is to induce hyalinization and thrombotic occlusion.

X-irradiation can cause injury to skin and bone and may result in impaired wound healing. Radiation myelopathy (Fogelholm et al. 1974; Godwin-Austen et al. 1975), however, is the most frequent neurological sequel of radiation therapy of which four different clinicopathological syndromes have been described. **Acute tran-**

sient myelopathy develops a few weeks after spinal irradiation, symptoms usually resolving completely over some 3–5 months. The pathogenesis is not known, but radiation-induced demyelination has been suggested. An uncommon complication is that of **acute progressive myelopathy** in which paraparesis or quadriparesis develops rapidly. It is though to be due to arterial occlusion and ischaemic necrosis of the cord. A further uncommon condition is that of **lower motor neurone syndrome** in which some months after spinal radiation the symptoms and signs of damage to the ventral horn neurones develop. The changes are usually symmetrical and are thought to be due to selective damage to the lower motor neurones.

Chronic progressive myelopathy (radionecrosis) is the commonest and most serious of the spinal syndromes caused by radiotherapy (Russell and Rubinstein 1989). The latent period may occur between 6 months and 13 years with a median of 12–15 months, the thoracic segments being the most susceptible part of the cord. Examples of this condition have been described following irradiation of extracranial tumours such as nasopharyngeal carcinoma, parotid carcinoma or basal cell carcinoma of the skull and less commonly following irradiation to tumours arising in the mediastinum. This complication is said to occur in between 1% and 2% of irradiated patients and as elsewhere in the brain the lesion is space occupying with all the features of a malignant astrocytoma (Fig. 7.6). The cord is expanded and replaced by focally cystic waxy pale yellow tissue in which there may be petechial haemorrhages. In long-standing cases the affected tissue becomes granular and is apt to crumble. Anatomical definition is blurred but in the main grey matter is spared. Histologically, the process is characterized by appearances that range from coagulative necrosis (Fig. 7.7a) around which there is no or minimal reactive change to foci of demyelination, loss of axons and infiltration by lipid-containing phagocytes, lymphocytes and plasma cells. The most important change, however, is fibrinoid necrosis and hyalinization of the walls of

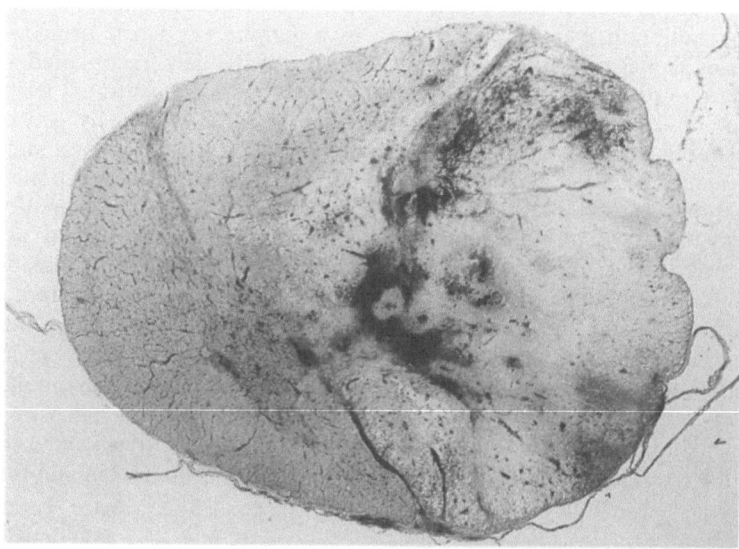

Fig. 7.6. Radionecrosis of cervical cord. The cord is swollen by a focally haemorrhagic necrotic mass of tissue. H & E × 10.

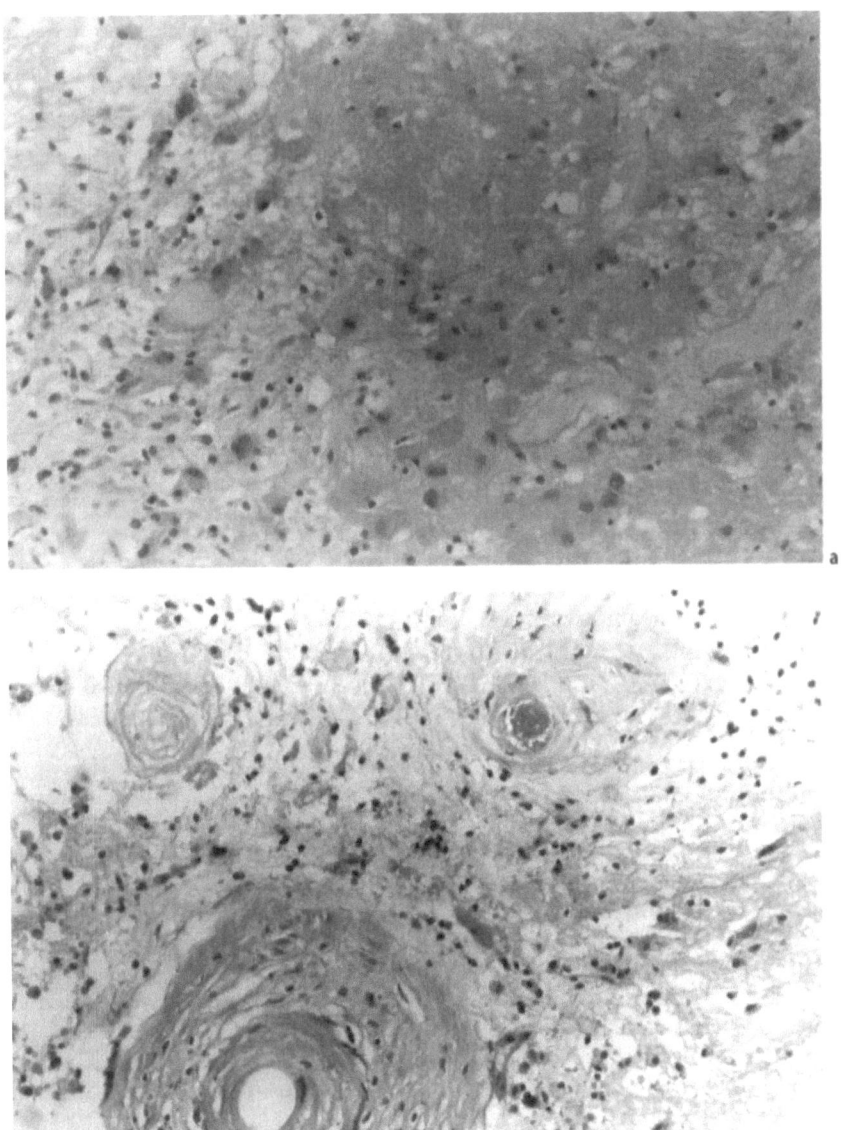

Fig. 7.7.   Radionecrosis. **a** There is coagulative necrosis with little in the way of a glial or mesodermal reaction. H & E × 9. **b** Note striking changes in small blood vessels in the form of fibrinoid necrosis and endothelial proliferation. H & E × 130.

blood vessels and the proliferation of endothelium which may be sufficient to cause an obliterative endarteritis and thrombotic occlusion of small vessels (Fig. 7.7b). Additional features include the formation of telangiectatic blood vessels, the proliferation of perivascular fibroblasts with the formation in some cases of large amounts of relatively acellular collagen and an associated astrocytosis often with bizarre multinucleated cell formation. In the later stages the segments of cord above and below the lesion are characterized by Wallerian degeneration in ascending and descending fibre tracts, respectively.

The pathogenesis of radionecrosis remains uncertain but vascular change, a direct effect of irradiation on the glia and immunological mechanisms have all been proposed. It is possible, however, that multiple mechanisms operate and that their relative importance varies with the radiation dose, and the interval between exposure and occurrence of damage. There have been many attempts to establish the tolerance level of the spinal cord to radiation. For example, a limit of 33 Gy in 42 days for field sizes less than 10 cm in length has been proposed, and generally accepted.

It is sometimes difficult to differentiate radiation from other myelopathies, especially paraneoplastic syndromes and intramedullary metastatic disease. CSF findings are non-specific and myelography is usually normal in radiation-induced myelopathy, but the cord can occasionally be swollen to such a degree that a spinal block is produced. Here CT scanning, and more recently MR imaging are helpful.

Chemotherapy

Treatment with antineoplastic agents may be given as a primary treatment or more commonly as adjunctive therapy following surgery and/or radiotherapy. The factors that limit the effectiveness of chemotherapy on malignant tumours include drug access by virtue of the blood–brain barrier for agents that are not highly lipid soluble, and low sensitivity of most tumours to single agent chemotherapy (Mena et al. 1981). Multiple agent treatments are commonly used which increase the number of potential drug-induced complications, but if a low dose of each individual agent can be used it will reduce the risk of any specific complication from arising. The cause of most CNS complications is sensitivity of the normal brain to chemotherapeutic agents. A number of syndromes have been described that include an acute and chronic myelopathy. The neurological side effects range from the insignificant acute reversible to the dose-limiting debilitating chronic and permanent. In some cases these effects are predictable varying with the dosage, duration and route of administration. However, other complications are unpredictable and are often misinterpreted because of their rarity, idiosyncratic nature or latency. The pathogenesis of these disorders is not known and may differ for each implicated drug. The differential diagnosis should include the important problem of opportunistic infection due to drug-induced immunosuppression. Myelopathies are particularly associated with the antimetabolite drugs methotrexate and cytosine arabinoside, and the alkylating agent thiopeta.

Embolism

Blood flow through the spinal cord may be arrested by emboli which according to their size become impacted in arteries, arterioles or capillaries. They may arise as a result of valvular, congenital or ischaemic heart disease and atheroma of the aorta and its large branches. They may also consist of air, nitrogen (hyperbaric and hypobaric decompression sickness) and fat.

Electricity and Lightning

When death is due to electrocution the only abnormality visible in the cord may be hyperaemia, possibly with petechial haemorrhages. If the discharge has been direct through the neuraxis as in death due to lightning, there may be charring or widespread fissuring of its surface.

System Disorders

The degenerative diseases are a diverse group, many of which are familial and hereditary, and are characterized by a progressive degeneration of neurones and their processes within anatomically and functionally defined regions or systems, but usually sparing the cerebral cortex. In many there are features of involvement of more than one system – the so-called **multiple system atrophies**. The current classification is often based on the clinical features which vary both within and between affected families and are due to differences in distribution and extent of the lesions. System disorders that affect the spinal cord include Friedreich's ataxia, hereditary spastic paraplegia (Strumpell), hereditary posterior column ataxia (Biemond) and motor neurone disease.

Friedreich's Ataxia

This rare progressive degenerative disease is the most common of the hereditary ataxias with a prevalence of 1–2 per 100 000 of the population. It is recessively inherited and presents usually before the age of 20 years and is characterized clinically by slowly progressive ataxia, loss of deep sensation, dysarthria, skeletal deformities and cardiac abnormalities. Patients often die of heart disease and there is an association with diabetes mellitus.

At autopsy the most striking macroscopic appearances are those of atrophy of the posterior roots in the lumbosacral region and cauda equina and of the spinal cord and brainstem. Histologically, this is due to atrophy of the spinal posterior roots and their associated ganglia (Oppenheimer 1979). This results in prominent degeneration of the posterior columns affecting the gracile more than the cuneate fasciculi, and of the corticospinal and spinocerebellar tracts. In typical cases the spinal cord is small, the changes in the ascending tracts being particularly affected in the upper dorsal and cervical regions whereas the changes in the descending fibre tracts are more marked in the lower spinal cord (Fig. 7.8). There is variable loss of neurones in Clarke's column. Transneuronal degeneration is seen in the gracile and cuneate nuclei and there is usually marked involvement of the dentate nuclei in the cerebellum, which in turn results in marked atrophy of the superior cerebellar peduncles. In contrast the Purkinje cell complement of the cerebellar hemispheres is usually normal. Variable loss of neurones has also been described in the motor

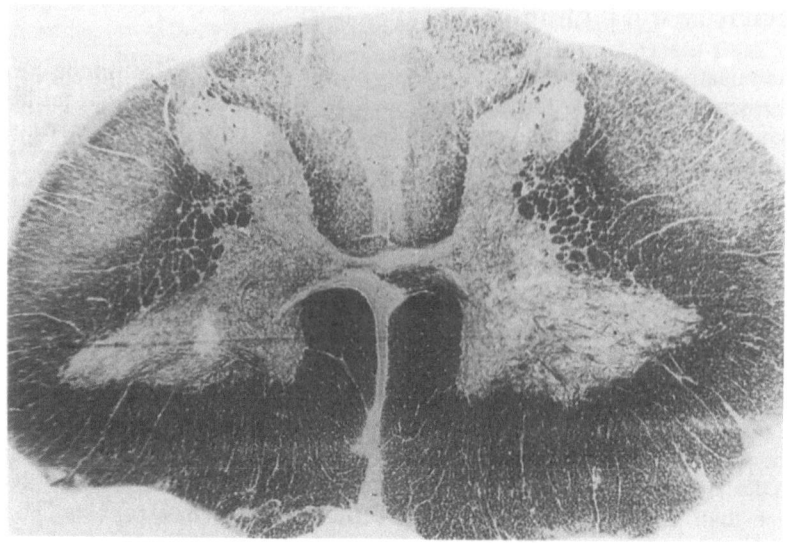

Fig. 7.8. Friedreich's ataxia. There is degeneration in posterior and lateral columns. Weigert-Pal. (Reproduced with permission from J.H. Adams and D.I. Graham, *An introduction to neuropathology*, Churchill Livingstone, Edinburgh, 1988.)

cortex and occasionally there is degeneration of the retina, the optic nerves and tracts and the lateral geniculate bodies.

There are similarities between Friedreich's ataxia and Marie's hereditary cerebellar ataxia. The two conditions sometimes overlap and there are intermediate forms. Friedreich's ataxia is frequently associated with a chronic progressive myocarditis in which focal coagulative necrosis of the muscle fibres is followed by replacement fibrosis.

Apart from impaired glucose tolerance the only other known association with Friedreich's ataxia is that of increased sensitivity to ionizing radiation.

Hereditary Spastic Paraplegia (Strumpell)

This is a slowly progressive disorder characterized by weakness of the legs that develops into a spastic paraparesis. It presents most commonly in adolescent or young adult males: in most cases inheritance is of autosomal dominant type though some also appear to be of an autosomal recessive nature.

The spinal cord may appear normal at autopsy. Histological examination shows degeneration of the lateral corticospinal tracts, particularly in the lower part of the spinal cord. There is also degeneration of the posterior columns, particularly the gracile tracts in the cervical region: and the spinocerebellar tracts may also be affected. The pathogenesis is not known, but the nature and distribution of the lesions is strongly suggestive of a distal axonopathy affecting central pathways. It has, therefore, been likened to the "dying back" process.

Hereditary Posterior Column Ataxia (Biemond)

This is a rare condition with an autosomal dominant mode of inheritance. It is characterized clinically by numbness of the hands and feet that later progresses to total absence of posterior column sensation. The spinal cord is atrophic due to degeneration of the posterior columns and partial degeneration of the posterior nerve roots.

Motor Neurone Disease

This is a progressive occasionally familial degenerative disorder of motor neurones, with a worldwide distribution, that presents clinically with wasting, weakness and eventually paralysis of muscles. It tends to occur in middle and late adult life and is more common in males than females and the disease is usually fatal in two to three years, but occasionally patients die in less than 12 months whereas others may survive for 10 years or more.

The striking feature clinically is that of loss of motor function with sparing of sensation and sphincter function and cognition. Although the name motor neurone disease highlights that the pathological features are within upper and lower motor neurones and is used as a unifying term embracing the historically defined patterns of the disease, there are nevertheless three principal clinical variants that are recognized depending on the distribution of the disease process. The commonest is **progressive muscular atrophy** when there is selectively severe involvement in the cervical region of the spinal cord as a result of which there is fibrillation and then atrophy of the small muscles of the hand. Involvement then spreads to the muscles of the arm and shoulder girdle. The term **amyotrophic lateral sclerosis** is used when upper motor neurones are affected leading to degeneration of the corticospinal tracts and a spastic paraparesis. Occasionally there is selectively severe damage to the motor nuclei in the lower brainstem, the process then being known as **progressive bulbar palsy** resulting in progressive wasting and paralysis of the muscles of the tongue, lips, jaw, larynx and pharynx.

Patients with motor neurone disease usually die as a result of respiratory insufficiency and sometimes of pneumonia. Not all muscle groups are equally affected, and the external ocular muscles are usually spared. At autopsy the ventral nerve roots of the spinal cord are shrunken and grey compared with the normal thick white posterior nerve roots (Brownell et al. 1970; Castaigne et al. 1972).

Transverse sections through the spinal cord show the ventral horns to be smaller than normal and in many instances the lateral columns of the cord are rather grey in colour, in contrast to the striking preservation of the white colour of the posterior columns (Fig. 7.9).

The principal histological change is a loss of motor neurones and associated astrocytosis seen most easily in the ventral horns of the cervical and lumbar segments of the spinal cord (Fig. 7.10a and b) and in the hypoglossal nuclei of the lower brainstem. This is in contrast to the nuclei of the oculomotor, trochlear and abducent nerves which are usually normal. Within the affected parts it is the larger motor neurones that are principally involved, the smaller and intermediate size cells tending to be preserved. Various changes are seen in the remaining neurones and include neuronophagia and ballooning (ghost cell change) and chromatolysis. Other cells show atrophy and may contain small eosinophilic inclusions (Bunina

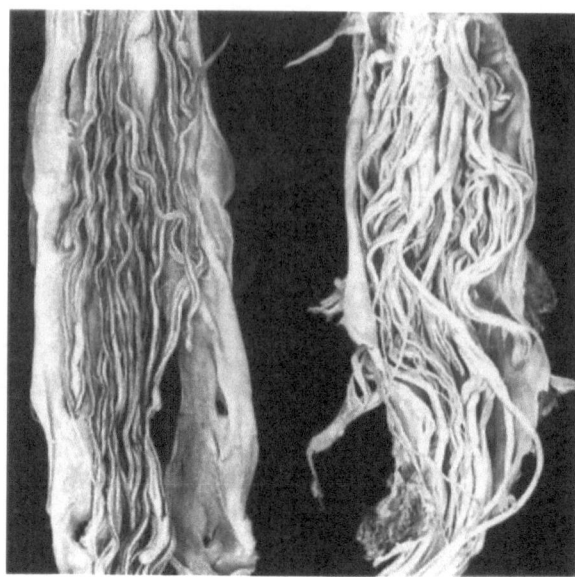

Fig. 7.9. Motor neurone disease. Compared with the normal cauda equina on the right, there is atrophy of ventral nerve roots on the left in a patient with motor neurone disease. (Reproduced with permission from J.H. Adams and D.I. Graham, *An introduction to neuropathology*, Churchill Livingstone, Edinburgh, 1988.)

bodies). Long tract degeneration is usually present (Fig 7.11) and may extend cranially beyond the cervical region into the brainstem, the cerebral peduncles, internal capsule and hemispheric white matter. All of these changes are the distal manifestation of pyramidal cell disease in the motor cortex. Detailed analysis of the motor cortex is difficult but in severe cases there is some loss of Betz cells. Sensory changes are rare in motor neurone disease and routine microscopy does not reveal obvious changes in sensory or autonomic nerves or the posterior columns. Minor changes, however, can sometimes be shown in the spinocerebellar tracts and their parent cell bodies in Clarke's column as well as in other sensory pathways.

There is increasing evidence that motor neurone disease is a heterogeneous condition due to a number of pathogenic factors that include viruses, metals, endogenous toxins, immune dysfunction and endocrine abnormalities acting upon an underlying genetic–biochemical abnormality (Tandan and Bradley 1985; Drachman and Kuncl 1989; Engelhardt et al. 1989; Siddique et al. 1991; Orell and de Belleroche 1994). The possible exogenous causes of motor neurone disease stem from observation of the Parkinsonism–dementia complex which occurs in Guam and is characterized by diffuse neuronal loss and neurofibrillary tangles in the cortex, the deep grey structures, the substantia nigra and the brainstem. The Guamanian Parkinsonism-dementia complex associated with Guamanian motor neurone disease appears to be quite different from both idiopathic Parkinsonism associated with dementia and with sporadic motor neurone disease. The principal features are that in addition to the changes in either idiopathic Parkinsonism associated with dementia or sporadic motor neurone disease there is widespread neu-

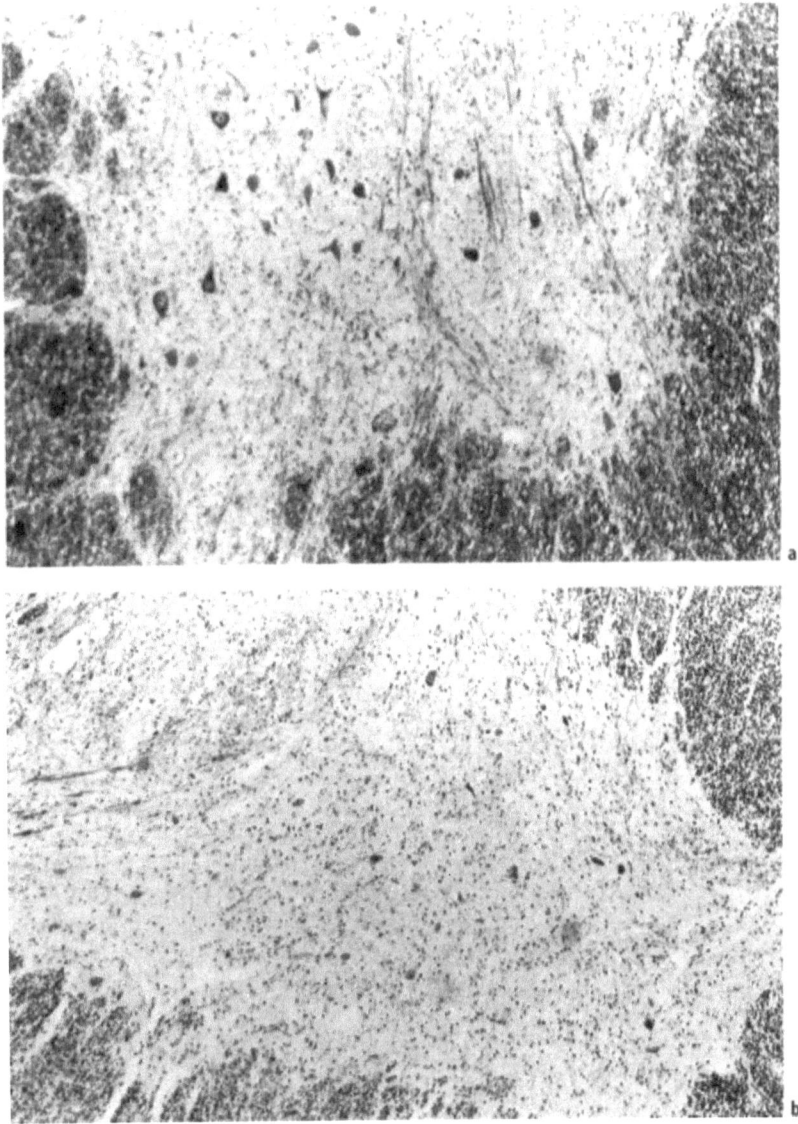

Fig. 7.10. Motor neurone disease. **a** Normal ventral horn. Luxol Fast Blue × 50. **b** Loss of ventral horn neurones in case of motor neurone disease. Luxol Fast Blue × 50. (Reproduced with permission from J.H. Adams and D.I. Graham, *An introduction to neuropathology*, Churchill Livingstone, Edinburgh, 1988.)

ronal loss and the formation of neurofibrillary tangles in the brain, brainstem and spinal cord.

The effects of denervation are well seen in muscle comprising **collateral reinnervation** from healthy subterminal axons, **fibre type grouping** and **group atrophy**. A muscle no more than moderately affected should be selected for biopsy.

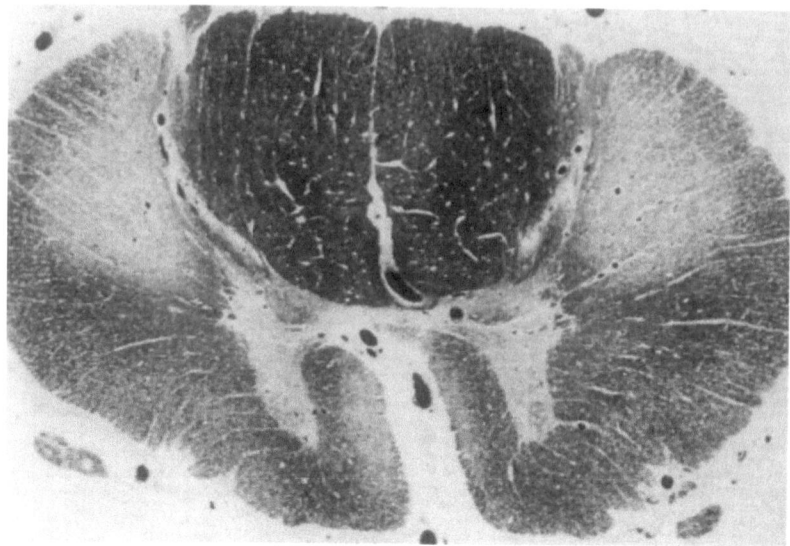

Fig. 7.11. Motor neurone disease. There is degeneration in the lateral, and to a lesser extent in the anterior, columns and preservation of the posterior columns. Heidenhain for myelin. (Reproduced with permission from J.H. Adams and D.I. Graham, *An introduction to neuropathology*, Churchill Livingstone, Edinburgh, 1988.)

Werdnig–Hoffmann Disease

This condition, also known as familial spinal muscular atrophy, is caused by degeneration of the lower motor neurone due to autosomal recessive inheritance. It is characterized by delayed motor development, weakness and hypotonia that begins at or shortly after birth. It is one of the causes of the **"floppy baby"** syndrome and is rapidly fatal. The earlier the onset, the sooner the child dies. The principal pathological features are those of loss of ventral horn neurones, atrophy of the ventral spinal nerve roots and denervation atrophy of muscles. The pyramidal and other long tracts are unaffected.

In addition to the classic and the Werdnig–Hoffmann types of motor neurone disease, there is a range of comparatively rare types with onset in later childhood or adolescence. Most are autosomal recessive in nature, and do not appear to form a continuum with classic motor neurone disease.

Demyelinating disorders

By definition these are characterized by the destruction of myelin with the relative preservation of axons (**periaxonal demyelination**). They, therefore, differ from genetic disorders of myelin formation – the leucodystrophies and from diseases causing breakdown of myelin due to destruction of neurones or their axons – Wallerian degeneration. The disorders in which demyelination is the only pathological process include a spectrum that range from acute conditions – acute dissemi-nated (perivenous) encephalomyelitis and acute haemorrhagic leucoencephalo-pathy – to chronic disorders, the most important of which is multiple (disseminated) sclerosis. Forms intermediate in both clinical and pathological fea-tures are not uncommon (Allen 1985; Weller 1985).

Acute Disseminated (Perivenous) Encephalomyelitis

This monophasic and usually self-limiting disease occurs in older children and young adults after measles, mumps, chickenpox or rubella (post-infectious encephalitis). Of rapid onset it develops some 4 to 5 days after the appearance of the rash. Recovery is generally good but the condition is associated with a 10%–20% mortality following measles or chickenpox. There is also an association with upper respiratory tract infections presumed to be viral in nature and with primary vaccina-tion against smallpox (postvaccinial) encephalitis and antirabies inoculation.

At autopsy the CNS may either appear normal or merely show congestion and oedema. This contrasts with histological changes in the white matter in which there is widespread cuffing of small blood vessels (probably venules by inflammatory cells (Fig. 7.12a). Initially, the inflammatory infiltrate comprises neutrophil polymorphs but these are replaced by lymphocytes and macrophages. The inflammatory process may extend into the meninges. The most distinctive histological change, however, is that of perivascular demyelination (Fig. 7.12b) within which axon cylinders are pre-served in contrast to a total loss and disintegration of myelin sheaths. In the spinal cord, especially, these lesions may coalesce, and with recovery there is an astrocytosis.

The available evidence is that acute disseminated perivenous encephalomyelitis is not infectious in nature, but represents a **delayed hypersensitivity reaction**. For example, the clinical course of the disease, the inability to isolate any virus and the onset of the illness, and the similarity between the lesion to those seen in **experimen-tal allergic encephalomyelitis**, all suggest that autoimmune mechanisms may be involved. The exact cause of the immunological reaction has not been established, but it would seem that a humoral reaction to constituents of myelin and a T-lymphocyte reaction to myelin basic protein combine to cause myelin as the target of the immunological attack. Other possibilities include shared antigens between viruses and oligodendrocytes or that the demyelination is simply a consequence of a bystander effect in which myelin becomes damaged as a result of an immunologi-cally mediated attack on viral particles.

Acute Haemorrhagic Leucoencephalitis

This is a relatively uncommon disorder which may occur as a sequel to any one of a number of several viral infections that may also complicate septic shock, treatment with various drugs, and other diseases assumed to be hypersensitive reactions, e.g. asthma and acute glomerular nephritis. It has a rapid course and is usually fatal within a few days of onset.

The principal finding at autopsy is that of swelling and multiple petechial haemor-rhages, particularly in the white matter. The grey matter of both the cerebral cortex and basal ganglia are often spared, but there may be involvement of the brainstem,

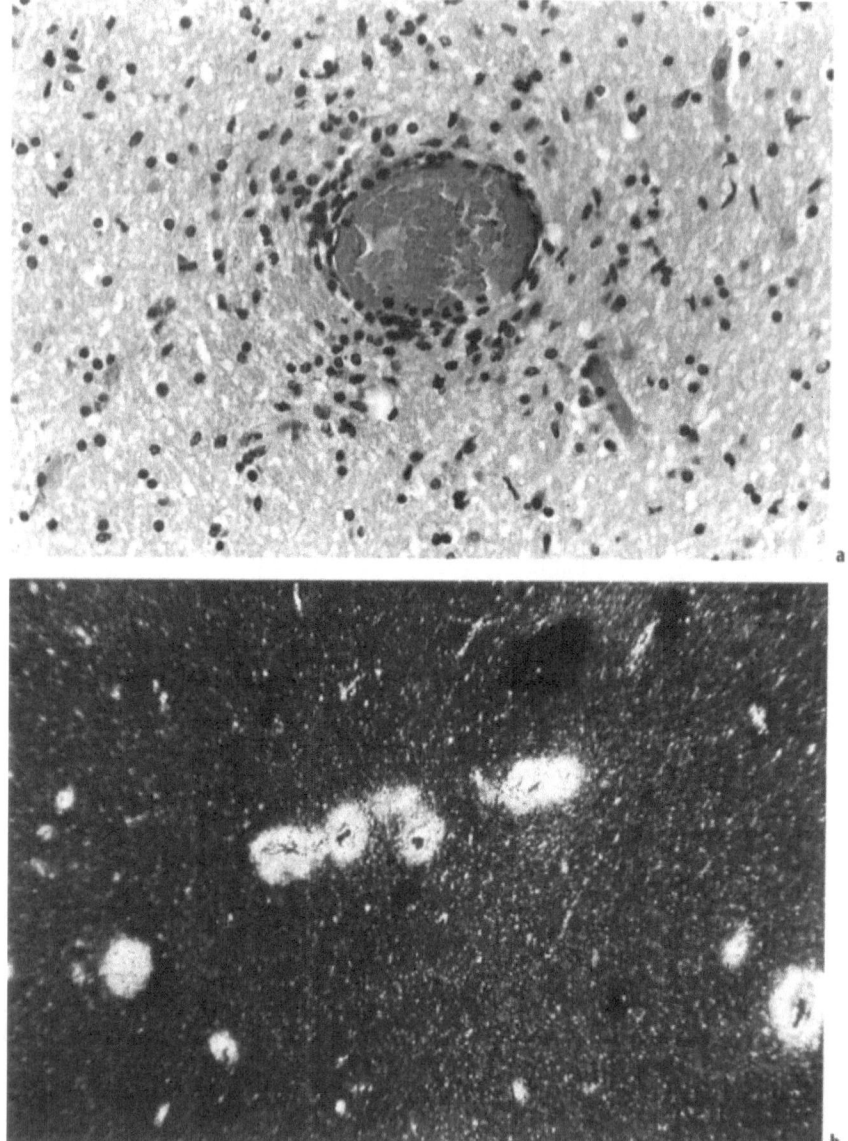

Fig. 7.12 Acute disseminated (perivenous) encephalomyelitis. **a** There is a diffuse inflammatory process in which lymphocytes and some monocytes are seen around a small blood vessel and in white matter. H & E × 330. **b** There is perivascular demyelination. Heidenhain for myelin × 50. (Reproduced with permission from J.H. Adams and D.I. Graham, *An introduction to neuropathology*, Churchill Livingstone, Edinburgh, 1988.)

cerebellum and spinal cord. The haemorrhagic lesions are often symmetrical and if severe the haemorrhages may become confluent. Histologically the principal abnormalities are in the walls of small blood vessels in which there is necrosis and exudation of fibrin into and through the blood vessel walls into the perivascular spaces.

Some of the blood vessels may be occluded by thrombus. In cases of short survival there is perivascular infiltration by neutrophil polymorphs and later by monocytes and lymphocytes. The disease is characterized by perivascular demyelination with associated microglia and macrophages. In some cases because of the intensity of the vascular reaction, small infarcts develop.

Aetiology is unknown but is thought to be a hyperacute variant of acute disseminated encephalomyelitis, and to be caused by the deposition of immune complexes and the activation of complement.

Multiple (Disseminated) Sclerosis

This is the most common of the demyelinating disorders with an incidence that varies with latitude ranging from 30 per 100 000 with a band of high frequency that lies between the 40th and the 60th parallels to less than 10 per 100 000 in lower latitudes. The disease virtually disappears at the equator. It is more common in women than men, and its incidence increases from early adolescence with a peak at the third and fourth decade. The disease in its classic form is characterized by relapses and remissions and some two-thirds of patients ultimately show continuous deterioration. Although this is true for the majority there are a small number, however, who have an acute unremitting form of the disease. The initial symptoms and signs vary but include paraesthesiae, limb weakness, ataxia, bladder dysfunction, nystagmus, optic neuritis and very rarely psychiatric symptoms.

The pathological features at autopsy vary with the rapidity with which the disease is progressing. For example naked eye examination in cases of **acute active multiple sclerosis** may reveal few abnormalities, though, when the brain is sliced lesions may appear as areas of yellow granular discolouration in white matter. Histologically, there are sharply defined areas of demyelination within which there are many surviving axons. Stains for lipid show large amounts of the breakdown products of myelin within phagocytes and there is widespread cuffing of blood vessels by lymphocytes, plasma cells and macrophages. Most of the lymphocytes are T-cells and the plasma cells contain IgG. Such cells also define the margins of the plaques. A further feature of the acute lesions is that of considerable hypertrophy and hyperplasia of astrocytes. This is in contrast to the oligodendrocytes in the centre of the lesions which are greatly reduced in number: at the margins, however, attempts at remyelination may be seen giving rise to an appearance that has been referred to as **shadow plaques**. Finally, using silver impregnation techniques and immunochemistry for neurofilament proteins, the integrity of the majority of axons can be, readily, identified.

In **chronic multiple sclerosis** there may be little abnormality post mortem, although on the ventral aspects of the pons and medulla, it may be possible to see irregular shrunken grey plaques on stripping the meninges. Plaques of multiple sclerosis may occur anywhere within the CNS, although the optic nerves and chiasm, the periventricular white matter, the brainstem and spinal cord are sites of predilection. Indeed in some patients the optic nerve, brainstem and spinal cord (Fig. 7.13) are severely affected and the brain may contain only a few plaques. Multiple sectioning of the spinal cord reveals plaques to be rather shrunken grey areas of demyelination which are commonly present in the cervical region with a high proportion involving the lateral columns (Oppenheimer 1978). As a result of the plaques, secondary changes may be seen in the form of long tract degeneration.

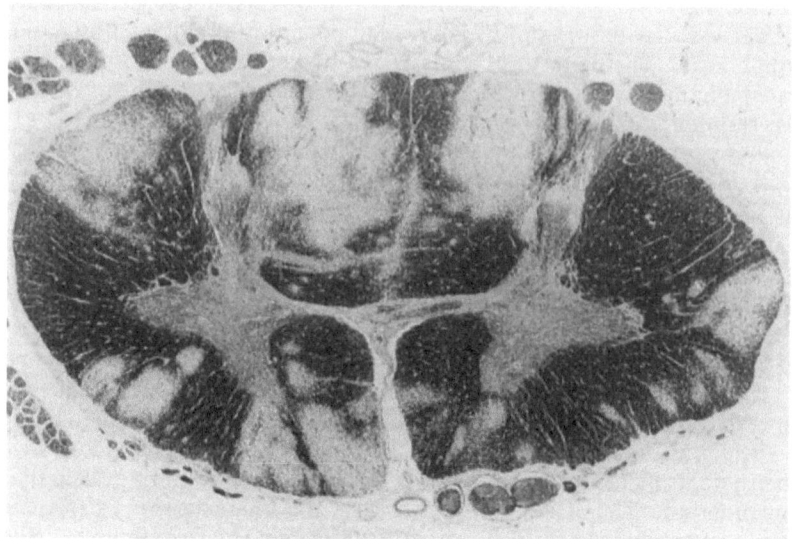

Fig. 7.13. Chronic multiple sclerosis. There are multiple plaques in the spinal cord. Luxol fast blue/cresyl violet. (Reproduced with permission from J.H. Adams and D.I. Graham, *An introduction to neuropathology*, Churchill Livingstone, Edinburgh, 1988.)

Histologically, the disease is characterized by sharply defined areas of demyelination (Fig. 7.14a) many of which are centred on small venules. If the plaque involves grey matter within the demyelinated area the neurones are preserved, a feature that distinguishes the lesion from infarction. Oligodendrocytes are reduced in number and there is an astrocytosis which in all plaques takes the form of a dense network of

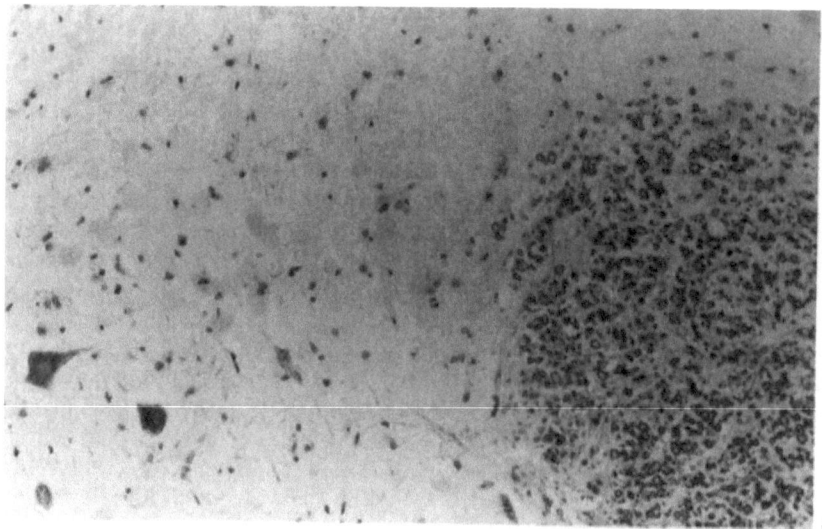

Fig. 7.14. Multiple sclerosis. **a** The edges of the plaque are usually well demarcated because of the complete demyelination. Luxol fast blue/cresyl violet × 130. **b** There is mild perivascular cuffing of blood vessels by lymphocytes. H & E × 330. **c** There is preservation of axons within the plaques. Palmgren × 130

astrocytic processes. In chronic active plaques, a few of the associated blood vessels are cuffed by lymphocytes and macrophages (Fig. 7.14b) and at the margins of the lesion signs of active myelin breakdown are seen in the form of lipid-containing macrophages. Similar cells may be seen in the related meninges and there is preservation of the majority of axons (Fig. 7. 14c). In chronic multiple sclerosis the histo-

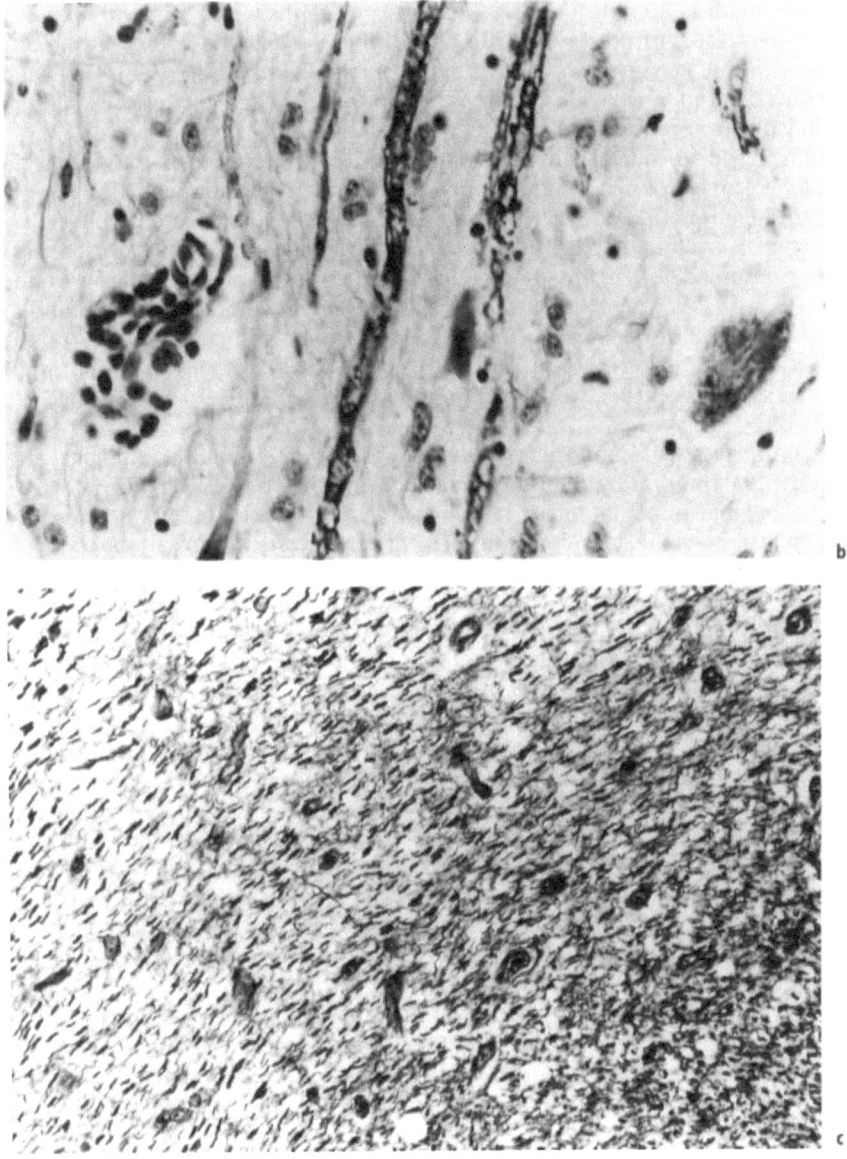

Fig. 7.14. *(Continued)*

logical appearances differ in that there are very few inflammatory cells. Astrocytes are less prominent although there is a marked gliosis and there are very few macrophages. Again the number of oligodendrocytes is greatly reduced and although many axons are preserved their numbers become reduced over time. The histological appearance in chronic multiple sclerosis, therefore, will vary depending on the activity of the process ranging from chronic active to chronic burnt out plaque formation. Commonly, in long-standing cases there is ultimately Wallerian degeneration in ascending and descending tracts within the spinal cord.

There is a variant of multiple sclerosis – **Devic's disease** or **neuromyelitis optica** – in which there is a clinical association of visual failure and signs of spinal cord involvement. Apart from the distribution of the plaques, the pathological features are those of the classic form of multiple sclerosis. Fulminating examples have also been described in which there is necrosis over several segments of the spinal cord, possibly due to secondary vascular damage.

Following an episode of exacerbation in multiple sclerosis, there may be partial or complete recovery of neurological function. This may in part be explained by subsidence of inflammation and swelling in and around the plaque and by physiological adaptation. Certainly there is little evidence of effective remyelination probably due to the widespread destruction of oligodendrocytes. Post mortem studies have shown that in some cases of clinically mild multiple sclerosis, there are large numbers of plaques whereas devastating clinical disease may be associated with a relatively small number. Furthermore, in as many as 10%–20% of cases in which multiple sclerosis is observed post mortem, there may be no clinical signs of the disease during life.

The pathogenesis of multiple sclerosis is not known, but epidemiological studies on individuals migrating from areas of high incidence to areas of low incidence suggest an environmental factor inter-reacting with genetic factors may be important. Thus, patients born in low latitudes appear to carry the lower attack rate with them if they move to higher latitudes after the age of 15 years. Conversely, patients migrating after the age of 15 from Northern Europe to, for example, South Africa and to Israel retain the high risk of their country of origin as those leaving at a young age seem to be relatively protected. There is also an increased incidence of multiple sclerosis in the families of patients with the disease but it is not known whether this is attributable to genetic or environmental factors or to a combination of both. Although these studies might suggest an infective aetiology, there is no convincing evidence yet for this theory. Multiple sclerosis has not been transmitted to experimental animals and no viral agent has been consistently isolated from brain tissue, though many studies have demonstrated an increased titre of antibodies – particularly to measles and less consistently to vaccinia, rubella and herpes simplex. The meaning of these increased titres is not clear, as it has not been possible to relate the specific antibodies to the oligoclonal bands of immunoglobulin that are so commonly found in CSF. It is also pertinent to note that the disease does not resemble any known persistent or slow virus infection of the CNS in humans or animals. There is considerable evidence for an immune reaction in the pathology of multiple sclerosis. Certainly, the presence of lymphocytes and plasma cells in acute plaques is in keeping with such a theory, and recent work has shown that in patients with acute attacks of multiple sclerosis there is a marked decline in the activity of suppresser T-cells in the peripheral blood, the activity rising again after an attack. So multiple sclerosis may, therefore, be a disorder of immune regulation. In support of an autoimmune aetiology, antibodies which together with complement cause demyelination of cultured brain tissue have been detected in the serum of patients with multiple sclerosis. Such antibodies have also been found in various non-demyelinating diseases. In spite of considerable effort the antigens under immune attack are not known. One suggestion is that some patients with multiple sclerosis have an increased cell mediated immunity against myelin basic protein. However, even in diseases such as acute post-infectious encephalomyelitis in which antibodies to myelin basic protein are present in the serum it is uncertain whether this indicates a primary aetiological factor or a secondary effect of the disease. As with acute disseminated encephalomyelitis, it has been suggested that demyelination in multiple sclerosis may be the result of a "bystander" effect. In this way myelin damage would result from the immune attack on a non-myelin antigen.

Metabolic Disorders

It is not intended in this section to cover the primary metabolic diseases which make a considerable contribution to morbidity and mortality in children, many of which are inherited as autosomal recessive diseases. Although the onset of clinical symptoms may not become apparent until adult life, the majority appear during childhood and frequently in the first few days of life.

For the brain to function normally, it requires that other systems in the body are also functioning normally. In view of this dependence it is perhaps not surprising that secondary metabolic affects on the CNS are an early manifestation of systemic disease. In many instances the clinical features are reversible and there are minimal morphological changes, both occurrences supporting the belief that many of the disorders are attributable to biochemical derangement rather than a structural abnormality. It is only when the metabolic disorder has been profound and prolonged that structural changes occur, thus accounting for the permanent clinical neurological deficits that some of these patients manifest. Such secondary acquired CNS manifestations of systemic disease occur at all ages. However, only a few that affect the spinal cord will be highlighted.

Subacute Combined Degeneration

Since highly effective purified preparations of vitamin B_{12} have become available for the treatment of **pernicious anaemia**, this complication is now uncommon. Similar lesions have been found even more rarely in some other chronic diseases, e.g. malabsorption syndromes, leukaemia, diabetes and carcinoma. The administration of vitamin B_{12} in adequate doses is completely effective in preventing the development of CNS lesions.

Signs and symptoms referable to the spinal cord are usually marked in early features of the disorder. The cord may appear entirely normal externally and on section, at autopsy. Histologically, however, the disease is characterized by the multifocal development of vacuoles in the white matter of the dorsal and lateral columns (Fig. 7.15), particularly of the lower thoracic region before extending both upwards and downwards. As the vacuolation increases in amount and severity it is

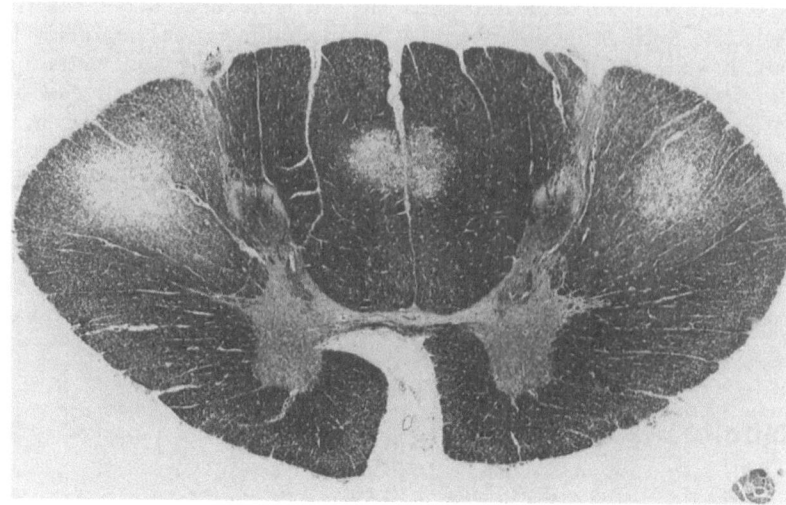

Fig. 7.15. Subacute combined degeneration of the cord. There is focal pallor of myelin staining in the posterior and lateral columns. Luxol fast blue/cresyl violet. (Reproduced with permission from J.H. Adams and D.I. Graham, *An introduction to neuropathology*, Churchill Livingstone, Edinburgh, 1988.)

accompanied by the breakdown of myelin and some evidence of axonal degeneration. Lipid-containing macrophages are present around small blood vessels. In untreated cases there is a remarkable absence of astrocytic reaction but with long survival and appropriate treatment, gliosis eventually develops. The symptoms depend on the degree and extent of tract involvement.

Vitamin B_{12} is required for the normal growth and maintenance of the nervous system. With the exception of vegans, dietary deficiency of the vitamin is uncommon. Other conditions, however, may be associated with the reduced absorption of vitamin B_{12} and include the absence of the "intrinsic factor" from gastric mucosa that is required for its absorption, infestation by tapeworms and severe gastritis or gastric surgery which removes the region secreting the intrinsic factor. Biochemistry has identified that within the nervous system of mammals there are two vitamin B_{12}-requiring enzymes, namely methionine synthetase and methylmalonyl CoA (coenzyme A) mutase. There is evidence that methyl donation is the underlying biochemical defect, the peculiar sensitivity of humans compared to other species in the development of myelin lesions, being their higher requirement of myelin basic protein for labile methyl groups. Evidence in support of such a mechanism has been found from various experimental studies that include the study of cage paralysis in non-human and experimental primates, intoxication by nitrous oxide and cycloleucine.

Acquired Hepatocerebral Encephalopathy

A metabolic encephalopathy invariably accompanies severe liver failure. Cases of massive hepatic necrosis are accompanied by an acute hepatic encephalopathy characterized by rapidly developing coma. On the other hand in cases of liver disease with cirrhosis, particularly when there is portosystemic shunting, **chronic hepatic encephalopathy** develops. Both types are potentially reversible so the patients often present an episodic and relapsing course: it may, however, become chronic and progressive. One such manifestation of hepatic disease is the occasional development of **myelopathy** in which there is symmetrical demyelination of lateral corticospinal tracts, of the cervical cord. There may in addition be some loss of fibres in the gracile tracts of the dorsal columns. The pattern of the pathology is suggestive of the "dying back" type of neuronal degeneration.

Myelopathy of Diabetes Mellitus

Complications of diabetes in the CNS are usually attributable to cerebrovascular disease. An exception to this generalization is the not uncommon finding of partial demyelination of the posterior columns of the spinal cord. The changes may be so marked that the cord acquires a distinctive shape referred to as "**pseudotabes**". **Demyelination of the lateral columns has been reported as diabetic amyotrophic lateral sclerosis.** The pathogenesis of the demyelination is not known: possibilities include primary demyelination, toxic metabolic factors or a microangiopathy due to thickening of the basement membrane and changes in the blood–brain barrier. The loss in the posterior columns is invariably associated with a **chronic peripheral neuropathy**.

Non-Metastatic (Remote) Effects of Carcinoma

Many patients present with deposits of metastatic carcinoma within the brain and fewer with signs of cord compression as a result of deposits in the extradural tissues. Other tumours, particularly carcinoma of the bronchus and lymphoma may have indirect (remote) effects on the central or peripheral nervous systems, either singly or in combination. Indeed up to 6% of patients with carcinoma are said to present neurological syndromes as a manifestation of the non-metastatic effects of carcinoma (Henson and Urich 1982). There is no constant relationship between the course of the neurological disorder and that of the carcinoma, in that they may develop concurrently or the neurological disorder may antedate objective evidence of tumour by several years. Furthermore, the severity of the neurological disease is not related to the size of the tumour.

There are five main categories of disorder that include **neuromuscular, metabolic** and **vascular** syndromes and those secondary to **infections** and **therapy**. Included within the neuromuscular syndromes are a group of conditions that closely simulate motor neurone disease, and an amyotrophic lateral sclerosis-like syndrome. Within the encephalomyelitic syndromes, is the uncommon condition of subacute necrotizing myelopathy, the principal features of which are the presence of lymphocytes and some plasma cells around small blood vessels within the spinal cord, and small aggregates of microglia (Fig. 7.16). Grey matter is affected more than white matter and inflammatory changes are associated with loss of neurones and Wallerian degeneration. Many suggestions have been put forward about the pathogenesis of these neurological syndromes that include toxins, infection, autoimmune processes, and both metabolic and endocrine disorders. The presence of inflammatory lesions

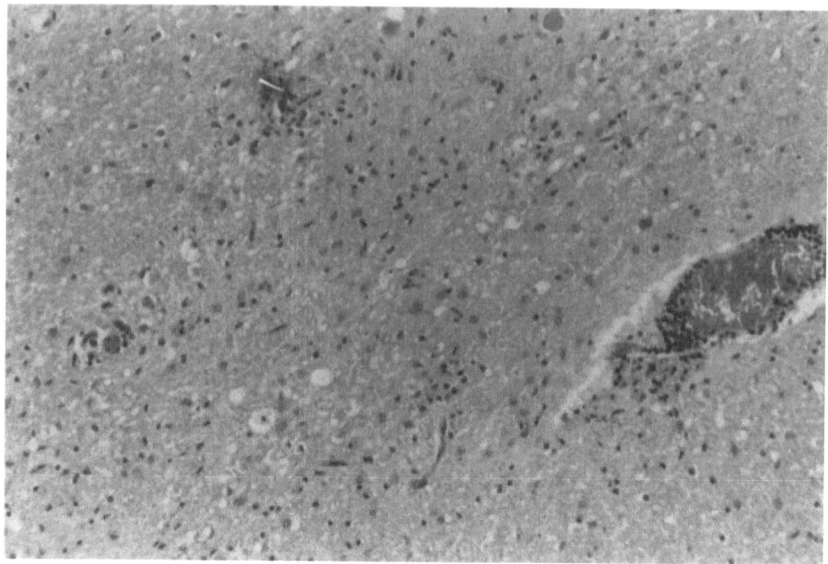

Fig. 7.16. Non-metastatic effects of carcinoma: spinal cord. There is slight perivascular cuffing by lymphocytes, clusters of microglia and an astrocytosis. H & E × 130.

similar to those seen in virus infections, certainly suggests the possibility that a neurotropic virus is the causal agent. An alternative explanation is that of an antigen–antibody reaction following the discovery of specific circulating antibodies against brain tissue.

Malformations of the Spinal Cord

To be discussed here is syringomyelia. The dyraphic abnormalities of the cord, that include diastematomyelia and spina bifida are considered elsewhere.

Syringomyelia

This is an uncommon condition in which a cyst-like space (**syrinx**) or spaces develop within the spinal cord and contain clear fluid enclosed by neuroglia. The lesion may extend over several centimetres usually lying immediately dorsal to the central canal, though it may extend eccentrically into one or both dorsal horns of the grey matter (Fig. 7.17). Occasionally the cyst communicates with either the fourth ventricle or the central canal. As it enlarges the cord becomes swollen and not infre-quently there is an associated Chiari Type 1 malformation. Occasionally, syringomyelia occurs in association with intradural spinal tumours and vascular malformation (Williams 1992).

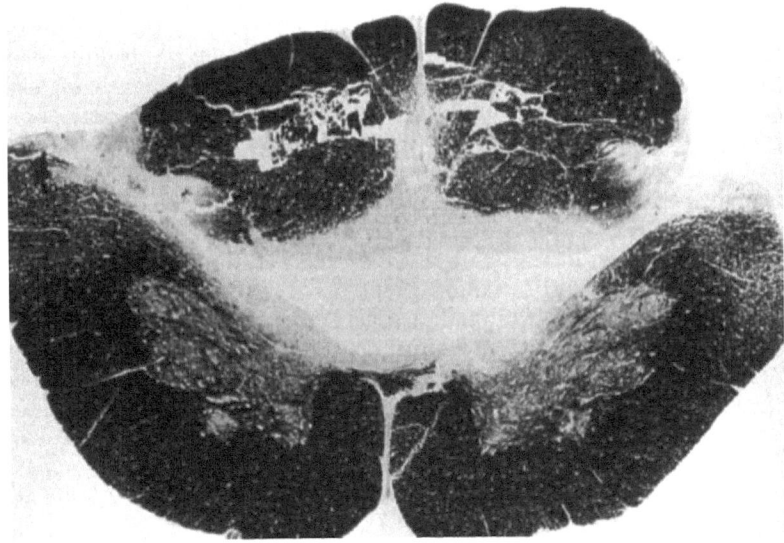

Fig. 7.17. Syringomyelia. There is a cavity extending into both columns in the cervical cord. Weigert-Pal for myelin. (Reproduced with permission from J.H. Adams and D.I. Graham, *An Introduction to neuropathology*, Churchill Livingstone, Edinburgh, 1988.).

The clinical effects are due principally to destruction of the cord by the enlarging cavity. The first fibres to be affected are those that decussate conveying the sensations of heat and pain. This results in **dissociated anaesthesia** which is a selective insensibility to heat and pain in the region corresponding to the involved segments of the cord. A **neuropathic arthritis** similar to that seen in tabes is common, and as syringomyelia usually occurs in the cervical region, the joints of the upper limbs are chiefly involved. Trophic lesions also occur in the skin. If the cavity enlarges it ultimately affects the lateral white columns leading to spastic paraparesis, the ventral grey horns leading to neurogenic atrophy of muscles and the posterior white columns leading to even greater disturbances of sensation.

The nature and pathogenesis of syringomyelia remain controversial. However, is now well accepted that in at least some cases it is caused by CSF being propelled through a valve-like opening between the caudal extremity of the fourth ventricle and the central canal. An alternative view is that syringomyelia is a form of disraphism in which there has been instability in the lines of junction of the alar and basal laminae with each other. In other words the cavity is a greatly distended central canal.

Inflammatory Diseases of the Spinal Cord and Dorsal Root Ganglia

Included amongst these are **tropical spastic paraparesis** which is a form of neuromyelopathy recognized in some tropical countries in which inflammatory changes are present in the spinal cord, nerve roots and sensory ganglia. Initially, the changes are those of a mononuclear infiltrate but with long-standing survival the amount of inflammation is greatly reduced, the most prominent feature then being extensive fibrosis of the meninges and around the small blood vessels at the sites of previous inflammation. There is neuronal loss in the ventral horn neurones and sensory ganglia. Raised antibody titres to the retrovirus HTLV-1 in serum and CSF have been described (Rogers-Johnson et al. 1985).

Involvement of dorsal spinal roots is particularly characteristic of neurosyphilis and gives rise to **tabes dorsalis** as a result of degeneration of the posterior spinal nerve roots immediately proximal to the dorsal root ganglia with selective involvement of the fibres responsible for pain, temperature and proprioception. The posterior nerve roots become grey and shrunken and the spinal cord also becomes reduced in size particularly in its anteroposterior diameter because of demyelination and shrinkage of the posterior columns. Tabes dorsalis most frequently affects the lumbosacral nerve roots but occasionally cervical nerve roots are the most severely affected, this being referred to as cervical tabes.

Since the initial description of neurological diseases associated with AIDS an extensive nomenclature has evolved about which there is now some consensus (Budka et al. 1991). Among the various HIV-associated diseases is **vacuolar myelopathy** in which there are multiples areas of vacuolated myelin with macrophages in the dorsolateral columns of the spinal cord. The appearances are very similar to those described in subacute combined degeneration of the cord (see above) and in the opinion of some, it is not specific for AIDS and may occur in the absence of HIV infection. Vacuolar myelopathy may or may not occur in association with HIV-positive multinucleated giant cells usually as part of multifocal giant cell leucoencephalitis or HIV encephalitis. However, a few cases have now been described in which there is a spinal equivalent of HIV encephalitis, the multinucleated giant cells being restricted to the spinal cord (Geny et al. 1991).

Involvement of the CNS as a complication of varicella-zoster virus infection is not common in immunocompetent individuals. The virus becomes latent in dorsal root ganglia to reactivate in later life when immunity, both humerol and cellular has declined. Following reactivation in the ganglia virus may spread centripetally to dorsal nerve roots and to the ventral horns to produce myelitis. Histologically, there is a marked mononuclear cell infiltrate that is almost exclusively lymphocytic within the affected ganglia: there may be associated necrosis. The sensory nerve cells of the affected ganglia undergo degenerative changes and neuronophagia may be seen. In patients who die during or soon after the acute stages of the disease any histological abnormalities will be seen within the segment of the spinal cord appropriate for the affected ganglion. Under circumstances of immunodeficiency, such as that associated with AIDS, with involvement of the CNS, myelitis is much more common (Devinski et al. 1991; Gray et al. 1992).

Acknowledgements My thanks to Mrs H. Boyd for having typed this manuscript.

References

Allen IV (1985) Demyelinating diseases. In: Adam JH, Corsellis JAN, Duchen LW (eds) Greenfield's neuropathology, 4th edn. Edward Arnold, London, pp 338–384

Brain WR, Northfield D, Wilkinson M (1952) The neurological manifestations of cervical spondylosis. Brain 75:187–225

Brownell B, Oppenheimer DR, Hughes JT (1970) The central nervous system in motor neurone disease. J Neurol Neurosurg Psychiatry 33:338–357

Budka H, Wiley CA, Kleihues P et al. (1991) HIV-associated disease of the nervous system: review of nomenclature and proposal for neuropathology-based terminology. Brain Pathol 1:143–152

Castaigne P, Lhermitte F, Cambier J, Escourolle R, Le Bigot P (1972) Etude neuropathologique de 61 observations de sclérose latérale amyotrophique: discussions nosologique. Rev Neurol 127:401–414

Devinski O, Cho E-S, Petito CK et al. (1991). Herpes Zoster Myelitis. Brain 114:1181–1196

Drachman DB, Kuncl RW (1989) Amyotrophic lateral sclerosis: an unconventional autoimmune disease? Ann Neurol 26:269–274

Engelhardt JI, Appez SH, Killian JM (1989) Experimental autoimmune motoneuron disease. Ann Neurol 26:368–376

Esiri MM, Oppenheimer DR (1989) Histology. In: Diagnostic neuropathology, Blackwell Scientific Publishers, Oxford, pp 46–66

Fink RP, Heimer L (1967) Two methods for selective impregnation of degenerating axons and their synaptic endings in the central nervous system. Brain Res 4:369–374

Fogelholm R, Haltia M, Andersson LC (1974) Radiation myelopathy of cervical spinal cord simulating intramedullary neoplasm. J Neurol Neurosurg Psychiatry 37:1177–1180

Frykholm R (1951) Lower cervical vertebrae and intervertebral discs. Surgical anatomy and pathology. Acta Chir Scand 101:345–359

Gentleman SM, Nash MJ, Sweeting CJ, Graham DI, Roberts GW (1993) ß-amyloid precursor protein (β-APP) as a marker for axonal injury after head injury. Neurosci Lett 160:139–144

Geny C, Gherard R, Boudes P et al. (1991) Multifocal multinucleated giant cell myelitis in an AIDS patient. Neuropathol Appl Neurobiol 17:157–162

Godwin-Austen RB, Howel DA, Worthington B (1975) Observations in radiation myelopathy. Brain 98:557–568

Gray F, Mohr R, Rozenberg F et al (1992) Varicella-zoster virus encephalitis in acquired immunodeficiency syndrome: report of four cases. Neuropathol Appl Neurobiol 18:502–514

Henson RA, Urich H (1982) Cancer and the nervous system. The neurological manifestations of systemic malignant diseases. Blackwell Scientific, Oxford

Hook O, Lidvall H, Astrom KE (1960) Cervical disk protrusions with compression of the spinal cord. Neurology 10:834–841

Hughes JT (1978) Introduction. In: Pathology of the spinal cord, Lloyd-Luke, London, pp 1–16

Hughes JT (1984) Regeneration in the human spinal cord: a review of the response to injury of the various constituents of the human spinal cord. Paraplegia 22:131–137

Hughes JT (1992) Disorders of the spine and spinal cord. In: Adams JH, Duchen LW (eds) Greenfield's neuropathology, 5th edn. London, Edward Arnold, pp 1083–1115

Lantos PL (1990a) Cytology of the normal central nervous system. In: Weller RO (ed) Nervous system, muscle and eyes. Systemic Pathology, 3rd edn, vol. 4, Churchill Livingstone, Edinburgh, pp 3–35

Lantos PL (1990b) Histological and cytology reactions. In: Weller RO (ed) Nervous system, muscle and eyes. Systemic Pathology, 3rd edn, vol. 4, Churchill Livingstone, Edinburgh, pp 36–63

Mena H, Garcia JH, Velandia F (1981) Central and peripheral myelinopathy associated with systemic neoplasia and chemotherapy. Cancer 48:1724–1728

Nauta WJH, Gygax PA (1954) Silver impregnation of degenerating axons in the central nervous system. A modified technic: Stain Technol 29:91–93

Oppenheimer DR (1978) The cervical cord in multiple sclerosis. Neuropathol Appl Neurobiol 4:151–162

Oppenheimer DR (1979) Brain lesions in Friedreich's ataxia. Can J Neurol Sci 6:173–176

Orrell RW, de Belleroche JS (1994) Superoxide dismutase and Als. Lancet 344:1651–1652

Payne EE, Spillane JD (1957) The cervical spine. An anatomo-pathological study of 70 specimens (using a special technique) with particular reference to the problem of cervical spondylosis. Brain 80:571–596

Rogers-Johnson P, Gajdusek DC, Morgan OSEC et al. (1985) HTLV1 and HTLV111 antibodies and tropical spastic paraparisis. Lancet ii:1248–1249

Rossier AB, Foo D, Shilito J, Dyro FR (1985) Post-traumatic cervical syringomyelia. Brain 108:439–461

Russell DS, Rubinstein LJ (1989) Effects of radiation and other forms of energy on intracranial and intraspinal tumours and their surrounding tissues. In: Pathology of tumours of the nervous system, 5th edn. Edward Arnold, London, pp 871–879

Sheriff FE, Bridges LR, Sivaloganathan S (1994) Early detection of axonal injury after human head trauma using immunocytochemistry for ß-amyloid precursor protein. Acta Neuropathol 87:55–62

Siddique T, Figlewicz DA, Pericak-Vance MA et al. (1991) Linkage of a gene causing familial amyotrophic lateral sclerosis to chromosome 21 and evidence of genetic-locus heterogeneity. N Engl J Med 324:1381–1384

Smith MC (1951) The use of Marchi staining in the later stages of human tract degeneration. J Neurol
    Neurosurg Psychiatry 14:222–225
Smith MC, Strich SJ, Sharp P (1956) The value of the Marchi method for staining tissue stored in formalin
    for prolonged periods. J Neurol Neurosurg Psychiatry 19:62–64
Tandan R, Bradley WG (1985) Amyotrophic lateral sclerosis: part 2. Etiopathogenesis. Ann Neurol
    18:419–431
Weller RO (1985) Pathology of multiple sclerosis. In: Mathews WB, Acheson ED, Batchelor JR, Weller RO
    (eds) McAlpine's multiple sclerosis. Churchill Livingstone, Edinburgh, pp 301–343
Williams B (1992) Syringomyelia. In: Findlay G, Owen R (eds) Surgery of the spine, vol 2. Blackwell
    Scientific Publications, Oxford, pp 891–906.

Chapter 8

Embryology and Paediatric Aspects of Spinal Cord Disorders

A. Hill

This chapter reviews normal embryonic development of the spinal cord and related structures, e.g. vertebral column, to provide a basis for understanding of major congenital anomalies of these structures, which may be considered as errors in the normal developmental sequence. In addition, there are reviews of spinal cord trauma and degenerative diseases of the spinal cord which present during childhood to provide an overview of paediatric aspects of spinal cord disorders.

Embryology of Spinal Cord and Related Structures

During the second week of embryonic development, there is implantation of the trophoblast into the endometrium of the uterus followed, during the third week of gestation, by formation of a trilaminar embryonic disc which contains three germ layers, i.e. mesoderm, ectoderm and endoderm. The embryonic period (four to eight weeks gestation), involves folding of the embryonic disc as a result of a process of relatively rapid elongation and growth of midline structures (notochord, neural tube) into a cylindrical embryo. During the first months of gestation, one germ layer has the potential of acting on another such that the second group of cells differentiate or otherwise after their behaviour in a process termed "induction" (Moore 1988; Sadler 1990).

"Primary neurulation" (also termed "dorsal induction") refers to transformation of ectoderm, under the inductive influence of the mesoderm on the dorsal aspect of the embryo, which results in formation of the brain and segments of spinal cord above the sacral region. The subsequent formation of lower sacral segments of the spinal cord is termed "caudal neural tube formation" or "secondary neurulation" (Volpe 1995). An understanding of these two processes forms the basis for later discussion of major developmental abnormalities of the spinal cord.

Primary Neurulation (Dorsal Induction)

Primary neurulation occurs during the third and fourth weeks of gestation. The nervous system begins as a thickening of tissue in the midline of the dorsal aspect of the ectoderm which differentiates into the neural plate at approximately 16–18 days of gestation under the inductive influence of the underlying notochordal and chordal mesoderm (Lemire et al. 1975). The cuboidal ectoderm is transformed into columnar neural epithelium and there is longitudinal elongation of the cells of the neural plate guided by a cytoskeletal network of microtubules and microfilaments as well as perhaps neurotransmitters and local messengers (Nagele et al. 1989; Copp et al. 1990). As the neural plate becomes attached and anchored by the prechordal plate mesoderm anteriorly and the notochord posteriorly, a groove develops in the midline of the neural plate. Under the continuing inductive influence of the epidermis and mesoderm, the lateral margins of the neural plate invaginate to form neural folds which fuse dorsally to form the neural tube. The first fusion of the neural folds occurs in the region of the lower medulla at approximately 22 days. Midline fusion of the neural folds proceeds both rostrally and caudally with closure of the anterior neuropore at 24–26 days of gestation and closure of the posterior neuropore in the lumbosacral region at 26–28 days (O'Rahilly and Mueller 1989). The mechanism of this fusion is not understood completely. However, it appears to involve the adhesion of nerve cell molecules (N-CAM) or other components within the extracellular matrix (Bally-Cuif et al. 1993).

Spinal cord occlusion occurs at the same time as neural fold fusion and is considered an essential pre-requisite for distension of the ventricular system of the brain by intraluminal fluid accumulation (Norman et al. 1995).

As the neural folds are fusing to form the neural tube, the "neuromeres", a series of lateral bulges, develop and then disappear in sequence from rostral to caudal. It appears that the neuromeres represent areas of proliferation of germinal cells. A longitudinal band, the "sulcus limitans" develops on each side of the ventricular surface of the neuromeres which divides the neural tube into alar and basal plates, which give rise to the motor and sensory systems, respectively. In the embryo, neurones proliferate in the ventricular zone and migrate into the alar and basal plates which consequently enlarge in size. Primary motor axons develop during the fourth week of embryonic development followed by formation of the first synapses in the marginal layer of the basal plate after the seventh week of gestation. There is migration of cells to form the visceral motor (intermediolateral) cell column. All definitive cell groups in the central grey matter are recognizable by the 14th week of gestation.

During the process of neuronal proliferation, axons extend up and down within the periphery of the cord around the central grey matter. Axons of the corticospinal tracts reach the lower medulla by 10–14 weeks of gestation and subsequently decussate at this level at approximately 14 weeks. They reach the mid-thoracic level at 17 weeks and the lower spinal cord by the 29th week (Norman et al. 1995). The length of the spinal cord increases approximately tenfold between 16 weeks and term (Friede 1989). This growth of neurones and axonal processes results in thickening of the walls of the spinal cord with gradual obliteration of the central canal.

Specific cells at the edge of the neural folds are not incorporated into the neural tube and form the "neural crest cells" which migrate to become dorsal root ganglia, sensory ganglia of cranial nerves, autonomic ganglia, Schwann cells, cells of the pia and arachnoid and certain skeletal elements. Processes from primary sensory neurones grown into the spinal cord to synapse with neurones in the alar plate and then ascend to the cerebellum, thalamus and other locations. Interaction of the neural tube with the surrounding mesoderm gives rise to the dura and axial skeleton, i.e. skull and vertebral column. The neural tube detaches from the ectoderm and the overlying surface ectoderm forms the epidermis (Norman et al. 1995).

Initially, the spinal cord extends along the full length of the embryo to the coccygeal region. Subsequently, the vertebral column, which has been developing in the surrounding mesoderm, begins to grow more rapidly than the spinal cord, such that by term, the lower end of the spinal cord lies at the level of the third lumbar vertebrae and in the adult at the lower border of the first lumbar vertebrae, with individual variations ranging from the twelfth thoracic to third lumbar levels (Barson 1970). Postnatal growth of the spinal cord amounts to approximately 2.7 times its length at birth. The disproportionate rate of growth of the vertebral column and spinal cord results in downward angulation of spinal nerve roots below the upper cervical level with increasing degrees of obliquity. The lower end of the vertebral column contains the cauda equina and the filum terminale which remains as a remnant of the spinal cord. The subarachnoid space extends to the mid sacral level, below which the nerves and filum terminale are surrounded by dura mater (Norman et al. 1995).

Secondary Neurulation (Caudal Neural Tube Formation)

Formation of the caudal neural tube, i.e. the lower sacral and coccygeal segments, occurs later than primary neurulation and involves serial processes of canalization and retrogressive differentiation which varies from individual to individual. Between 28 and 38 days of gestation, undifferentiated cells at the caudal end of the neural tube (caudal cell mass) develop small vacuoles which gradually coalesce, enlarge and make contact with the posterior lumen of the central canal of the neural tube by 30 days of gestation. Occasionally, accessory lumens remain and give rise to congenital anomalies. The process of canalization continues until approximately seven weeks of gestation. Subsequently from seven weeks of gestation until after birth, retrogressive differentiation results in regression and resorption of much of the caudal cell mass except certain residual structures, e.g. the ventriculus terminalis in the conus medullaris and the filum terminale (Lemire et al. 1975; Volpe 1995).

Developmental Abnormalities of the Spinal Cord and Vertebral Column

Based on the previous discussion of the embryology of spinal cord formation, developmental abnormalities of the spinal cord may be classified as disorders of primary neurulation, i.e. failure of neural tube closure (Table 8.1) or disorders of secondary neurulation or caudal neural tube formation, i.e. occult dysraphic states (Table 8.2).

Table 8.1. Spinal cord disorders resulting from abnormal primary neurulation

Craniorachischisis totalis
Myeloschisis
Meningomyelocele

Table 8.2.   Spinal cord disorders resulting from abnormal secondary neurulation

Myelocystocele
Diastematomyelia
(Lipo) Meningocele
Lipoma, tumours, arteriovenous malformations
Dermal sinus (may be associated with dermoid, epidermoid)
Tethered cord

Adapted from Volpe (1995).

Disorders of Primary Neurulation: Neural Tube Defects

Errors in neural tube closure include failures of anterior neural tube closure, e.g. anencephaly, encephalocele. However, this discussion will be restricted to disorders of primary neurulation that result in developmental abnormalities of the spinal cord. Disorders of primary neurulation are among the most severe congenital anomalies and often result in a shortened life span. They are associated with abnormalities of the axial skeleton, meningovascular and dermal coverings.

Craniorachischisis Totalis

This severe disorder, which originates prior to 22 days of gestation, involves total failure of neurulation and results in an open, neural-plate-like structure with absence of overlying skin and axial skeleton. Most affected embryos are aborted spontaneously (Lemire et al. 1975; Lemire and Siebert 1990; Volpe 1995).

Myeloschisis

Failure of posterior neural tube closure, which occurs before 26 days of gestation, presents with extensive portions of the spinal cord appearing as a raw neural plate-like structure without overlying vertebrae of skin. Most affected fetuses are stillborn (Lemire et al. 1975).

Myelomeningocele

This condition which results from restricted failure of posterior neural tube closure may be considered the most important variant of abnormal primary neurulation in that most affected infants survive. There are large variations in incidence between different geographic locations, with highest incidences reported from Ireland, Scotland and Wales. A decreasing incidence has been reported in Great Britain and North America during the last two decades (Leech and Payne 1991; Stone 1987).

In 80% of cases, myelomeningoceles are located at or below the thoracolumbar and the lesion presents as plate-like neural tissue which is displaced dorsally and is associated with invariably with defects of the spinal column, e.g. lack of fusion or absence of vertebral arches, and variable, incomplete skin covering. The meninges are thin and rupture easily resulting in a high risk of infection. Neurological abnormalities include motor, sensory and sphincter dysfunction and depend primarily on the level of the lesion. Determination of the functional level of the lesion may permit reasonable prediction of long-term outcome, although there is considerable variability between the apparent segmental neurological level (especially in the mid-lumbar region) and long-term ambulatory status (McDonald et al. 1991). In general, children with sacral lesions are ultimately able to walk unaided and those with lesions above the L2 level are predominantly wheelchair dependent (McDonald et al. 1991).

Cranial abnormalities are often associated with myelomeningocele, especially the Chiari II malformation which occurs in a majority of cases and consists of partial displacement of the medulla and cerebellum (especially the vermis) through the foramen magnum inferiorly into the upper cervical canal, overriding the spinal cord. The fourth ventricle is usually elongated and partially herniated and there are associated bony abnormalities of the foramen magnum, posterior fossa and upper cervical vertebrae. Hydrocephalus occurs in more than 90% of cases of Chiari II malformation and most commonly relates to aqueduct stenosis (Gilbert et al. 1986). In children with myelomeningocele the hydrocephalus develops usually before six weeks of age and a significant number (approximately 30%) exhibit lower brainstem dysfunction, e.g. feeding disturbances, vocal cord paralysis and central apnoea, which may be the cause of death in approximately 50% of cases (Hesz and Wolraich 1985; Hays et al. 1989; Swaminathan et al. 1989). In addition to Chiari II malformation, 92% of brains of children with myelomeningocele demonstrate evidence of cortical dysplasia, especially neuronal migration abnormalities (Gilbert et al. 1986), which accounts for the occurrence of seizures in 25% of children with myelomeningocele (Noetzel and Blake 1991).

The diagnosis of myelomeningocele is based primarily on clinical observation. Although CT or MRI may delineate the precise relationship between skin and spinal lesion (Lee et al. 1985), complete neuroimaging is often not necessary prior to primary surgical repair of the back lesion. MRI permits visualization of the extent of abnormalities associated with the Chiari II malformation (Altman and Altman 1987).

The management of infants with myelomeningocele raises difficult ethical issues. Important advances have been made in the primary goal of prevention. Thus, there are compelling data which suggest that a daily periconceptional intake of folic acid may reduce the risk of neural tube defect by approximately 60% (Czeizel and Dudans 1992; Oakley 1993; Werler et al. 1993). This has led some authorities to advocate that daily dietary supplementation with folic acid should be considered for all females of child-bearing potential. To date, prenatal diagnosis of open neural tube defect is based principally on elevated levels of alphafetoprotein in amniotic fluid at 14–16 weeks of gestation (Kimball et al. 1977). More recent data suggest that a rapid immunoassay of acetylcholinesterase may be a superior diagnostic test compared with alphafetoprotein for detection of open neural tube defect and may approach 100% sensitivity (Loft et al. 1993). Determination of maternal serum alphafetoprotein levels have been proposed as a useful screening procedure (Milunsky et al. 1980). However, screening is considered uneconomical in geographic areas which have a low incidence of spina bifida. The other diagnostic technique which plays a major role in prenatal diagnosis is real-time ultrasonography (Morrow et al. 1991).

The initial decision in the management of an infant with myelomeningocele is determination of the optimal means of delivery. Data suggest that exposure of the open neural tube to mechanical stresses associated with labour and vaginal delivery may further injure the spinal cord and worsen outcome sufficiently to make the difference between a child being ambulatory or wheelchair bound. Thus, scheduled caesarian section prior to onset of labour should be considered for all fetuses with myelomeningocele without other major anomalies (Luthy et al. 1991). Subsequent decision to proceed with surgical intervention must be based on a clear understanding of the prognosis of the lesion. If surgery is undertaken, early closure of the back lesion within 24–48 h is usually considered optimal to minimize risk of infection (Sharrard et al. 1963), preferably with prophylactic antibiotic coverage (Charney et al. 1985). Following primary closure of the back lesion , subsequent surgery may be required to shunt progressive hydrocephalus. Posterior fossa decompression may be undertaken in cases with lower cranial nerve paralysis. The numerous problems that confront patients with myelomeningocele during later childhood are managed most successfully by a multidisciplinary team of specialists including a paediatrician, neurosurgeron, urologist, physiotherapist and psychologist.

Disorders of Neural Crest-Derived Cells

Recognized anomalies of cells derived from neural crest are uncommon. Congenital aplasia or hypoplasia of spinal and autonomic ganglia have been recognized in certain conditions, e.g. congenital insensitivity to pain, familial dysautonomia (Friede 1989). Congenital aganglionosis of the colon (Hirschsprung's disease), which involves a congenital lack of neurones in the enteric plexus of the rectum and colon, due to either failure of migration or differentiation of neural crest cells, is the most common cause of neonatal colonic obstruction (Touloukian 1979).

Disorders of Secondary Neurulation: Caudal Neural Tube Abnormalities

Disorders of secondary neurulation (Table 2) are distinguished from abnormalities of primary neurulation by their caudal location, i.e., lower sacral and coccygeal segments. The presence of intact skin over the lesions combined with the observation that the neural abnormality may be subtle and often remains undetected for many years has led to the term "occult dysraphic state". A relationship between disorders of primary and secondary neurulation is suggested by the fact that defects of primary neurulation have been documented in 4.1% of siblings in patients with occult dysraphic states (Carter et al. 1976).

Clinical Features Approximately 80% of disorders of secondary neurulation have dermal lesions, e.g. abnormal collections of hair (Fig. 8.1), cutaneous dimples or sinus tracts, superficial haemangiomas or subcutaneous masses (lipomas) (Fig. 8.2a, b). In addition, vertebral defects, most commonly vertebral laminar defects or a widened spinal canal, occur in 85%–90% of cases (Scatliff et al. 1989). Elongation of the conus medullaris and a thickened filum terminale are often associated with "tethering" or fixation of the caudal end of these structures by a fibrous band, lipoma or related lesion which may impair the normal mobility of the lower spinal cord and result in "traction injury" associated with growth and flexion/extension movements of the trunk (Yamada et al. 1981). In addition to the presence of visible skin lesions, clinical neurological dysfunction may develop, e.g. primary or secondary abnormality of sphincter control, asymmetry of size or function of lower limbs, progressive foot deformalaities (pes cavus, pes equinovarus), scoliosis. Pain in the back or lower extremities may develop. Most commonly, neurological deterioration is gradually progressive, although sudden deterioration may occur and may not resolve despite prompt surgery (Dubowitz et al. 1965; Pasternak and Volpe 1980). Recurrent meningitis is an unusual presentation but may occur when there is communication between skin and spinal subarachnoid space. Hydrocephalus is not associated with occult dysraphic states.

Diagnosis and Management Suspicion of the presence of an occult dysraphic abnormality, based usually on skin abnormalities in the region of the lower spine, should lead to more detailed investigation to enable definitive diagnosis. Before one year of age, incomplete ossification of the posterior spinal elements permit initial non-invasive evaluation of the spinal cord, subarachnoid space, conus and filum terminale using real-time ultrasonography (Fig. 8.3) (Scheible et al. 1983; Naidich et al. 1984). In the absence of abnormality on both spine radiographs and ultrasonography during the newborn period, further neuroimaging may not be required and clinical follow-up is appropriate. It is important to emphasize that spine radiographs are normal in 10%–15% of patients with occult dysraphic states. In other children, MRI

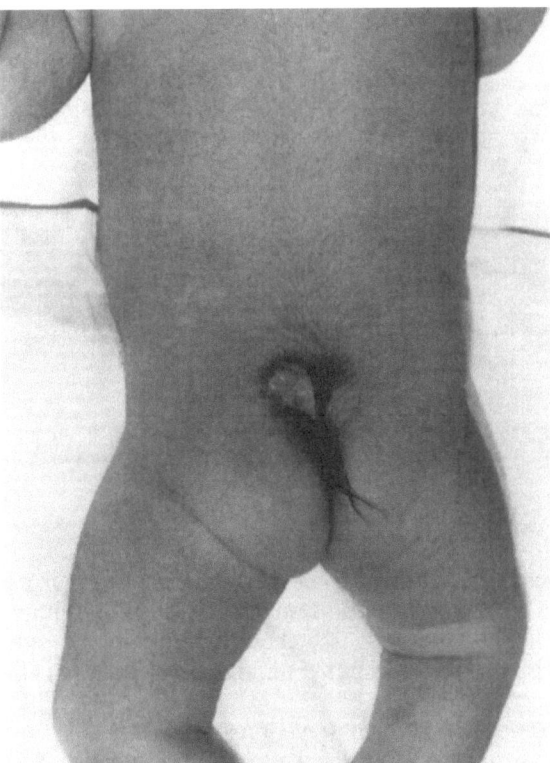

Fig. 8.1. Occult spinal dysraphism: note abnormal collection of tissue and hair in lumbosacral region. (Courtesy of Dr Paul Steinbok.)

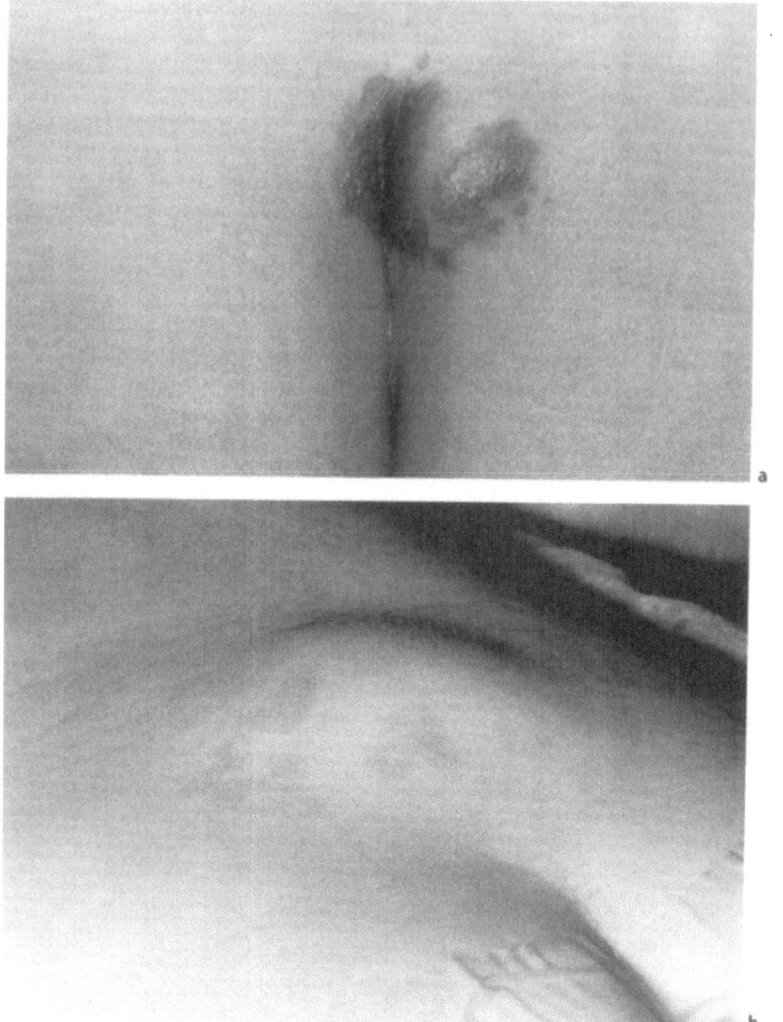

Fig. 8.2. Occult spinal dysraphism: **a** superficial haemangioma in midline in sacral region; **b** subcutaneous lipoma and haemangioma in lumbosacral region. (Courtesy of Dr Paul Steinbok.)

or CT myelography permit delineation of spinal cord lesions (Fig. 8.4) (Naidich et al. 1983; Packer et al. 1986; Peacock and Murovic 1989; Scatliff et al. 1989; Harwood-Nash and McHugh 1990) whereas associated bony lesions, e.g. diastematomyelia spurs, are better visualized by computed tomography (Scatliff et al. 1989; Pang et al. 1992).

Surgery is performed primarily to prevent neurological deficits or further deterioration and it may partially reverse deficits of recent onset (Fig. 8.5). At the present time, the optimal timing of surgery is controversial in a young infant without neurological deficits (Naidich et al. 1983; Hoffman et al. 1985; Scatliff et al. 1989).

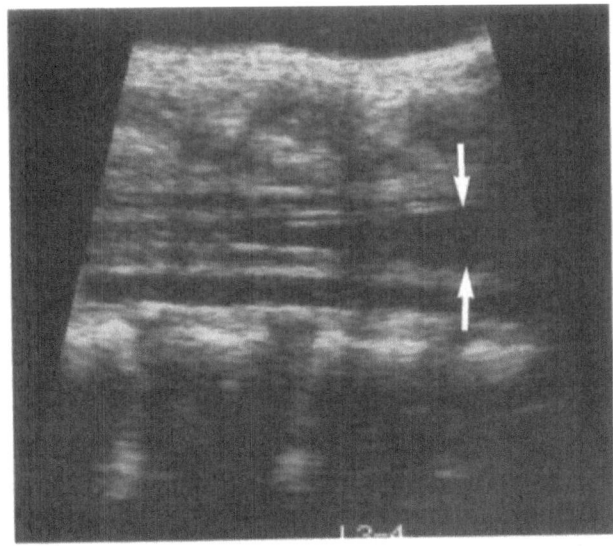

Fig. 8.3. Ultrasound of back in newborn with occult spinal dysraphism: Note widened spinal canal (*arrows*).

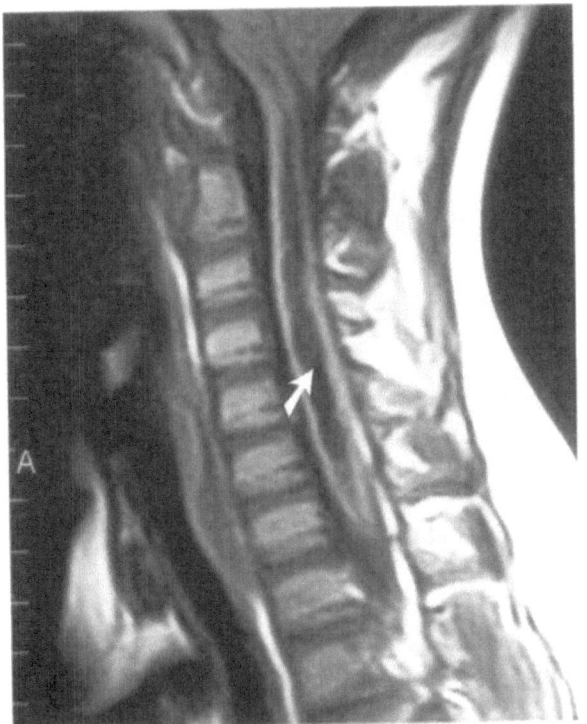

Fig. 8.4. MRI scan of syringobulbia and cervical syringomyelia (*arrow*).

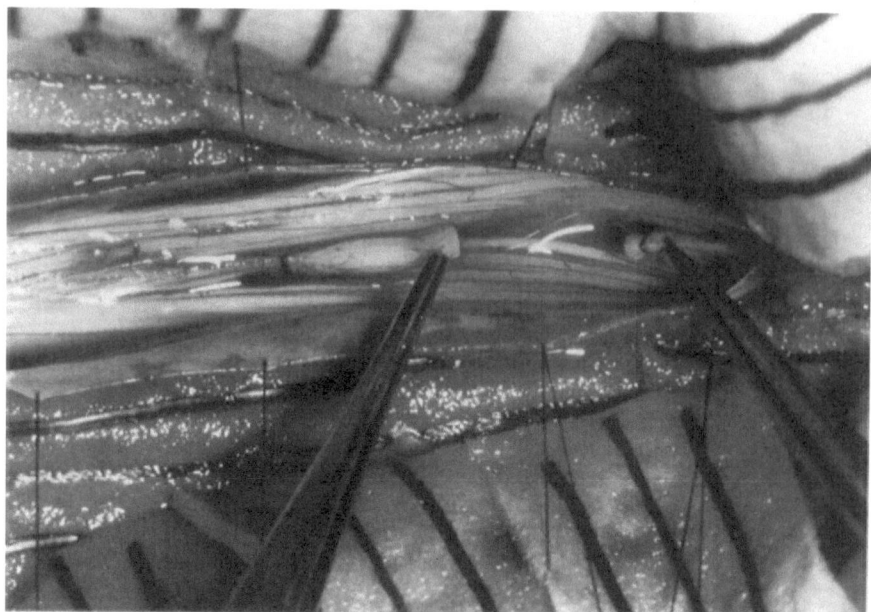

Fig. 8.5. Surgical release of tethered and thickened filum terminale. Note edges of cut filum (held by forceps) have separated by approximately 2 cm. (Courtesy Dr Paul Steinbok.)

Myelocystocele

This anomaly, which originates at approximately 28 days of gestation, involves localized excessive dilatation of the central canal of the caudal spinal cord and is often associated with cloacal exstrophy, omphalocele, imperforate anus and vertebral anomalies (Lemire et al. 1975; Peacock and Murovic 1989).

Diastematomyelia, Diplomyelia

This condition involves division of the caudal cord by a bony, cartilaginous or fibrous septum arising from the dorsal aspect of the vertebral body into two "half-cords" each surrounded by individual pia mater. Diplomyelia is a term which may be used to describe a divided or duplicated spinal cord without the presence of a septum (Lemire et al. 1975; Gower et al. 1988; Scatliff et al. 1989; Pang et al. 1992).

Meningocele, Lipomeningocele

Meningocele which refers to herniation of meninges posteriorly through a bony defect in the lumbar region, covered by skin and not associated with gross abnormality of brain or spinal cord. The term "lipomeningocele" is used when there is an associated infiltration by fibrous and fatty tissue (Seeds and Jones 1986; Hirsch and Pierre-Kahn 1988, Seeds and Powers 1988).

Lipoma, Congenital Tumours

Subcutaneous lipomas with intradural extension are more common than lipomeningoceles. Congenital tumours, e.g. teratoma, neuroblastoma, ganglioneuroma, haemangioblastoma, presumably originating from germinal tissue in the caudal cell mass or arteriovenous malformations may extend into the dural space (Lemire and Beckwith 1982; Michaud et al. 1988; Baraitser and Shieff 1990).

Dermal Sinus, Dermoid, Epidermoid Cyst

A cutaneous dimple in the lumbosacral region may extend inwardly and rostrally in a sinus tract which may connect with the vertebral canal. Such tracts may enlarge into subcutaneous cysts that contain dermal structures ("dermoid") or epidermal structures ("epidermoid") (Wright 1971).

Isolated Tethered Cord

This anomaly involves elongation of the conus, thickening of the filum terminale and fixation of the caudal end of the spinal cord by fibrous bands (Lemire et al. 1975; Hoffman et al. 1976).

Congenial Abnormalities of the Vertebral Column

In addition to abnormalities of the spinal cord discussed previously, congenital or familial osseous abnormalities of the vertebral column may result in significant neurological complications in children.

Narrow Foramen Magnum

In some of the skull dysplasias, e.g. achondroplasia, there is significant decrease in the transverse diameter of the foramen magnum which may indent the posterior aspect of the spinal cord (Reid et al. 1987; Nelson et al. 1988). Compression myelopathy may develop insidiously, with subtle neurological signs rather than acute quadriplegia or paraplegia. Apnoea, which may lead to sudden death, may be the only manifestation of myelopathy (Fremion et al. 1984; Nelson et al. 1988). Syringomyelia occurs rarely and may be prevented by posterior fossa and cervical decompression surgery (Hecht et al. 1984).

Abnormal Odontoid Process

This condition may occur as a congenital anomaly or as a result of trauma (Hukuda et al. 1980). Hypoplasia of the odontoid process occurs in approximately 6% of children with Down's syndrome (Davidson 1988).

Vertebral Stenosis

Cervical vertebral block may occur in certain syndromes, e.g. Klippel–Feil syndrome, acondroplasia. Stenosis of the lumbar vertebral canal may be a complication of achondroplasia, which may result in root or spinal cord compression manifested by motor or sensory disturbances or deterioration in bowel or bladder function (Nelson et al. 1988).

Atlantoaxial Dislocation

Atlantoaxial dislocation occurs in conditions which are associated with excessive ligamentous laxity or abnormalities of the dens, e.g. Down's syndrome, Morquio syndrome, or it may develop as a complication of cervical or pharyngeal infection, trauma or rheumatoid arthritis. Atlantoaxial dislocation is often associated with acute onset of quadriplegia but may be preceded by clinical features such as head tilt, staggering gait and hemiplegia (Corio et al. 1983). Children at high risk for developing atlantoaxial dislocation, e.g. children with Down's syndrome who have radiological evidence of wide atlanto-dens space separation (> 7 mm) should be advised to refrain from activities such as somersaulting or trampolining (Pueschel 1988). Diagnosis of atlantoaxial dislocation is based on the presence of greater than 5 mm distance between the anterior aspect of the odontoid and atlas on X-ray and rotation and lateral displacement of the dens on CT or MRI (Chaudry et al. 1987). Surgical vertebral fusion is recommended for symptomatic cases.

Lumbosacral Agenesis

Although the pathogenesis of this entity is unclear, a large percentage of affected children are offspring of mothers who are diabetic or who have a strong family history of diabetes (Passarge and Lenz 1966). In fact, this abnormality has been reported in 1% of infants of diabetic mothers. The degree of disability relates directly to the level of the vertebral lesion (Sarnat et al. 1976). Thus, infants with lumbar or complete sacral agenesis have severe deformities whereas those with partial sacral or coccygeal agenesis may be asymptomatic. In severe cases, paralysis usually corresponds anatomically to the level of the vertebral lesion whereas sensation (including perineal sensation) is often much better preserved. Club-foot deformity may be present. Bladder incontinence is a constant feature even with relatively mild hemisacral defects. In fact, many mild cases remain unrecognized until problems with toilet-training arise.

Spinal Cord Injury in Childhood

Neonatal Spinal Cord Injury

Neuropathology and Pathogenesis

In contrast to spinal cord injury in adults, which involves primarily compression injury, neonatal spinal cord injury sustained during delivery results principally from excessive traction or rotation (Volpe 1995). The true incidence of neonatal spinal cord injury is unknown. Although spinal cord lesions have been documented in approximately 10% of neonatal autopsies (Towbin 1969), some abnormalities, e.g. perivascular petechiae, are probably of limited clinical significance. However, the incidence of occult cervical trauma in newborns who present with hypoxic-ischaemic or traumatic cerebral injury may be considerable. Most acute spinal cord lesions involve epidural or intraspinal haemorrhage, especially within dorsal or central grey matter and are associated with varying degrees of oedema, laceration or disruption of the spinal cord. These lesions subsequently evolve into chronic changes, i.e. focal gliosis, syringomyelia, or even total separation of transected cord segments (Friede 1989). Although dural tears occur frequently in association with cord injury, complete cord transection with intact dura has been documented (Byers 1932).

In the newborn, the vertebral column is almost entirely cartilaginous and very elastic. In fact, the newborn spine can stretch up to 5 cm without bony disruption, whereas the spinal cord can only stretch to a maximum of 6–8 mm (Towbin 1969). Thus, vertebral lesions, e.g. fractures, dislocations or separation of the vertebral epiphysis (Couvelaire 1903), are uncommon and complete transection of the spinal cord can occur without radiological evidence of bony disruption.

Most spinal cord lesions in the newborn involve the cervical or upper thoracic region, reflecting sites of particular mobility and anchoring of the spinal cord. The two principal sites of injury relate to the type of delivery, i.e. in cephalic delivery, torsion may result in upper and midcervical injury (Shulman et al. 1971; MacKinnon et al. 1993) whereas excessive longitudinal or lateral traction in breech delivery is associated with lower cervical and upper thoracic lesions (Bresnan and Abroms 1974, Friede 1989; MacKinnon et al. 1993). The pathogenesis of neonatal spinal cord injury at a cellular and molecular level has not been studied in detail. Based on studies of experimental animals and adult humans, injured neurones may release excitotoxic amino acids and arachidonic acid, associated with increased cytosolic calcium, vasoactive prostanoids and free radicals which result in cell membrane injury and cell death (Faden and Simon 1988; Volpe 1995).

Clinical Features In the majority of cases, the affected infant is born by difficult midforceps or breech delivery often associated with maternal drugs or anaesthesia or intrauterine asphyxia which may contribute to fetal hypotonia and depression (DeSouza and Davis 1974; Volpe 1995). Hyperextension of the fetal head (which occurs in approximately 5% of breech presentations) may be an important factor. Vaginal breech delivery of a fetus with hyperextended head results in death or severe spinal cord injury in 20%–25% of cases. Thus, in one series, of 73 infants with hyperextension of the neck and who were born by vaginal breech delivery, 15 died or had severe cord injury, whereas none of the 35 infants delivered by caesarean section developed such problems (Caterini et al. 1975). Rarely, infants with hyperextended fetal head in utero may sustain major cord injury prior to delivery (MaeKawa et al. 1976), presumably due to subluxation/dislocation of upper cervical vertebrae with compromise of vertebral arteries which supply the upper cervical cord via the anterior spinal artery (Sladky and Rorke 1986; Clancy et al. 1989).

Clinical manifestations range from stillbirth or rapid death secondary to respiratory failure to prolonged survival. During the first days of life, there is usually flaccid weakness with areflexia of lower extremities, variable involvement of upper extremities, paradoxical respiration and respiratory insufficiency, a sensory level, atonic anal sphincter and distended bladder which may be emptied by means of suprapubic pressure. There may be evidence of Horner's syndrome. Hypotonia may persist or evolve into spasticity (Byers 1975; Bucher et al. 1979; MacKinnon et al. 1993; Volpe 1995).

In infants with cervical lesions who require mechanical ventilation there may be clinical evidence of hypoxic-ischaemic encephalopathy which may mask the signs of spinal cord injury (Volpe 1995). In one series of 14 cases of neonatal spinal cord injury, nine infants had concomitant encephalopathy. Furthermore, cognitive deficits have been documented in approximately 40% of survivors (MacKinnon et al. 1993).

The long-term prognosis of neonatal spinal cord injury is poor with persistence of neurological deficits and occurrence of respiratory or urinary complications. Disturbances of autonomic function, e.g. sweating, may produce wide fluctuations in body temperature in young infants. Trophic disturbances of muscle and bone may lead to orthopaedic complications (Volpe 1995).

Diagnosis and Management In addition to careful neurological examination, ultrasonography may be considered as the initial imaging technique of choice. It may demonstrate cord disruption and echogenic blood without requiring that the infant be moved. Serial examinations may be performed easily at the bedside. Subsequently, MRI appears to be the imaging technique of choice in subacute or chronic situations (Lanska et al. 1990; Minami et al. 1994).

In the absence of effective, specific therapy for neonatal spinal cord injury, emphasis must be directed towards prevention including cautious management of breech delivery and dysfunctional labour with avoidance of fetal depression. In infants who have evidence of spinal cord injury, it is important to rule out a surgically correctable lesion. In the absence of a large epidural haemorrhage, there is little evidence that laminectomy or surgical decompression are beneficial (Volpe 1995). Supportive therapy includes ventilation, maintenance of body temperature, prevention of urinary tract infection and joint contractures. In infants who require mechanical ventilation, there are major ethical issues concerning continuation of life support. Available data which may assist in the prediction of outcome during the neonatal period is limited. In one series of nine infants with cervical spinal cord injury, only two infants who survived had good outcome (independent daytime breathing and good motor function) and they had spontaneous breathing movements on the first day of life. In contrast, all four survivors who were completely apnoeic beyond 30 days of age required long-term mechanical ventilation and developed sever motor disability (MacKinnon et al. 1993). Clearly, only limited conclusions can be drawn from such a small study population.

Neonatal Spinal Cord Infarction

Spinal cord infarction occurs rarely following catheterization of the umbilical artery, or accidental injection of air into a peripheral vein related presumably to progressive thrombosis or spasm of the anterior spinal artery or artery of Adamkiewicz (Dulac and Aicardi 1975). Rarely, non-traumatic intramedullary spinal haemorrhage has been reported (Mutoh et al. 1989).

Table 8.3. Metabolic disorders which present as spinocerebellar degeneration

Adrenomyeloneuropathy
GM1 gangliosidosis
GM2 gangliosidosis
Abetalipoproteinemia
Vitamin E deficiency
Mitochondrial disorders

Metabolic and Heredodegenerative Spinal Cord Disorders in Childhood

Hereditary degenerative disorders which involve the spinal cord during childhood are heterogeneous. Generally, they involve premature failure or degeneration of specific neuronal systems or pathways in the spinal cord which may also involve cerebellum and brainstem (e.g. spinocerebellar degeneration). In most instances, the specific underlying metabolic derangements are not known and there are no known identifiable biochemical markers. Table 8.3 lists the major known metabolic disorders which may present as spinocerebellar degeneration in childhood. Furthermore, neoropathological abnormalities may be variable even in several affected individuals within the same family.

Friedreich's Ataxia

This is the most common and best delineated of the spinocerebellar degenerations. Usually, the mode of inheritance is autosomal recessive (some autosomal dominant cases have been documented) and there is a mutation at the centromeric region of chromosome 9 (Harding 1981; Chamberlain et al. 1988). Pathological abnormalities include degeneration of long ascending and descending spinal cord tracts (cerebellar tracts, pyramidal tracts, posterior columns), posterior root ganglia and large sensory fibres of peripheral and optic nerves with relative sparing of the cerebellum itself (Ouvrier et al. 1982). In addition to neuronal degeneration, most cases also have a hypertrophic cardiomyopathy with fibre necrosis and fibrosis affecting the left ventricle predominantly. Diagnosis of Friedreich's ataxia is based principally on the recognition of the stereotypical constellation of clinical abnormalities which are summarized in Table 8.4 (based on data from Harding 1981). Motor and sensory nerve conduction velocities are normal or mildly delayed although the sensory evoked potential is absent or greatly reduced in amplitude (Ouvrier et al. 1982). Visual evoked responses are abnormal in two thirds of patients (Pinto et al. 1988). Abnormal electrocardiogram (T-wave and ST segment abnormalities) and echocardiogram occur in two thirds of cases. There is progressive deterioration of neurological function: most affected individuals are wheelchair bound by age 25 years. More than 50% of patients die of cardiac failure (Leone et al. 1988).

At the present time, spinocerebellar degenerations in children are best regarded as a large number of heterogeneous, unrelated conditions that are grouped together

Table 8.4.   Clinical features of Friedreich's ataxia

Clinical feature	Frequency (%)
Onset before 20 years	100
Progressive ataxia	100
Absent tendon reflexes	100
Extensor plantar respons	>90
Sensory disturbance	>90
Cardiomyopathy	60–90
Weakness, muscle wasting	50–80
Scoliosis and/or pes cavus	90
Optic atrophy	<30
Nystagmus	20–50
Axonal neuropathy	Most
Diabetes	10–25
Dementia	0

Based on data from Harding (1981).

merely for convenience and have different modes of inheritance. In most instances, it is impossible to determine whether a disorder represents a single condition with variable clinical presentations or are distinct and separate diseases that share common clinical and pathological features. Accurate diagnosis and classification must be based on molecular genetic data and awaits identification of specific metabolic defects which should permit accurate diagnosis, genetic counselling and ideally, prenatal diagnosis.

References

Altman NR, Altman DH (1987) MR imaging of spinal dysraphism. AJNR 8:533–538

Bally-Cuif L, Goridis C, Santoni M-J (1993) The mouse NCAM gene displays a biphasic expression pattern during neural tube development: Development 117:543–551

Baraitser P, Shieff C (1990) Cutaneomeningo-spinal angiomatosis: the syndrome of Cobb. A case report. Neuropediatrics 21:160–161

Barson AH (1970) The vertebral level of termination of the spinal cord during normal and abnormal development. J Anat 106:489–497

Brabyn PS, Chuang SH, Daneman A et al. (1988) Sonographic evaluation of spinal cord birth trauma with pathologic correlation. AJR 9:765–768

Bresnan MJ, Abroms IF (1974) Neonatal spinal cord transection secondary to intrauterine hyperextension of the neck in breech presentation. J Pediatr 84:734–773

Bucher HU, Boltshauser E, Friedreich J et al. (1979) Birth injury to the spinal cord. Helv Pediatr Acta 34:517–527

Byers RK (1932) Transection of the spinal cord in the newborn. Case with autopsy and comparison with normal cord at the same age. Arch Neurol Psychiatr 27:585

Byers RK (1975) Spinal cord injuries during birth. Dev Med Child Neurol 17:103–110

Carter CO, Evans KA, Till K (1976) Spinal dysraphism: genetic relation to neural tube malformations. J Med Genet 13:343–350

Caterini H, Langer A, Sama JC et al. (1975) Fetal risk in hyperextension of the fetal head in breech presentation. Am J Obstet Gynecol 123:632

Chamberlain S, Shaw J, Rowland A et al. (1988) Mapping of mutation causing Friedreich's ataxia to human chromosome 9. Nature 334:248–250

Charney EB, Weller SC, Sutton LN et al. (1985) Management of the newborn with myelomeningocele: time for a decision-making process. Pediatrics 75:58–64

Chaudry V, Sturgeon C, Gates et al. (1987) Symptomatic atlanto-axial dislocation in Down's syndrome. Ann Neurol 21:606–609

Clancy RR, Sladky JT, Rorke LB (1989) Hypoxic-ischemic spinal cord injury following perinatal asphyxia. Ann Neurol 25:185–189

Copp AJ, Brook FA, Estibeiro AS et al. (1990) The embryonic development of mammalian neural tube defects. Prog Neurobiol 35:363–403

Corio F, Quintana F, Villalba M et al. (1983) Craniocervical abnormalities in Down's syndrome. Dev Med Child Neurol 25:252–255

Couvelaire A (1903) Hemorragies du systeme nerveux central des noveau-nes dans leurs rapports avec la naissance prematuree et l'accouchement laborieux. Ann Gynecol Obstet (Paris) 59:253–268

Czeizel AE, Dudas I (1992) Prevention of the first occurrence of neural tube defects by periconceptional vitamin supplementation. N Engl J Med 327:1832–1835

Davidson RG (1988) Atlanto-axial instability in individuals with Down's syndrome: a fresh look at the evidence. Pediatrics 81:857–865

DeSouza SW, Davis J (1974) Spinal cord damage in the newborn infant. Arch Dis Child 49:70

Dubowitz V, Lorber J, Zachary RB (1965) Lipoma of the cauda equina. Arch Dis Child 40:207

Dulac O, Aircardi J. (1975) Paraplegic compliquant le catheterisme arterial ambilical. Arch Fr Pediatr 32:659–664

Faden Al, Simon RP (1988) A potential role for excitotoxins in the pathophysiology of spinal cord injury. Ann Neurol 23:623–626

Fremion AS, Garg BP, Kalsbeck J (1984) Apnea as the sole manifestation of cord compression in achondroplasia. J Pediatr 104:398–401

·Friede RL (1989) Developmental neuropathology (2nd edn). Springer Verlag, New York

Gilbert JN, Jones KL, Rorke LB et al. (1986) Central nervous system anomalies associated with meningomyelocele, hydrocephalus and the Arnold–Chiari malformation: reappraisal of theories regarding the pathogenesis of posterior neural tube closure defects. Neurosurgery 18:559–564

Gower DJ, Del Curling O, Kelly DL et al. (1988). Diastematomyelia – a 40 year experience. Pediatr Neurosurg 14:90–96

Harding AE (1981) Friedreich's ataxia: a clinical and genetic study of 90 families with an analysis of early diagnostic criteria and intrafamilial clustering of clinical features. Brain 104:589–620

Harwood-Nash DC, McHugh K (1990) Diastematomyelia in 172 children: the impact of modern neuroradiology. Pediatr Neurosurg 16:247–251

Hays RM, Jordan RA, McLaughlin JF et al. (1989). Central ventilatory dysfunction in myelodysplasia: an independent determinant of survival. Dev Med Child Neurol 31:366–370

Hecht JT, Butler IJ (1990) Neurologic morbidity associated with achondroplasia. J Child Neurol 5:84–97

Hecht JT, Butler IJ, Scott CI (1984) Long-term neurologic sequelae in achondroplasia. Eur J Pediatr 143: 58–60

Hesz N, Wolraich M (1985) Vocal-cord paralysis and brain stem dysfunction in children with spina bifida. Dev Med Child Neurol 27:528–531

Hirsch JF, Pierre-Kahn A (1988) Lumbosacral lipomas with spina bifida. Childs Nerv Syst 4:354–360

Hoffman HJ, Hendrick EB, Humphreys RP (1976) The tethered spinal cord: its protean manifestations, diagnosis and surgical correction. Childs Brain 2:145–155

Hoffman HJ, Taecholarn C, Hendrick EB et al. (1985) Management of lipomyelomeningoceles. Experience at the Hospital for Sick Children, Toronto. J Neurosurg 62:1–8

Hukuda S, Ota H, Okabe N et al. (1980) Traumatic atlanto-axial dislocation causing OS odontoideum in infants. Spine 5:207–210

Kimball ME, Milunsky A, Alpert E (1977) Prenatal diagnosis of neural tube defects. III. A re-evaluation of the alphafeto-protein assay. Obstet Gynecol 49:532–536

Lanska MJ, Roessman U, Wiznitzer M (1990) Magnetic resonance imaging in cervical cord birth injury. Pediatrics 85:760–764

Lee BCP, Zimmerman RD, Manning JJ et al. (1985) MR imaging of syringomyelia and hydromyelia. AJNR 6:221–228

Leech RW, Payne GG Jr (1991) Neural tube defects: epidemiology. J Child Neurol 6:286–287

Lemire RJ, Beckwith JB (1982) Pathogenesis of congenital tumors and malformations of the sacrococcygeal regions. Teratology 25:201–213

Lemire RJ, Siebert JR (1990) Anencephaly: its spectrum and relationship to neural tube defects. J Craniofac Genet Dev Biol 10:163–174

Lemire RJ, Loeser JD, Leech RW et al. (1975) Normal and abnormal development of the human nervous system. Harper & Row, Hagerstown

Leone M, Rocca WA, Rosso MG et al. (1988) Friedreich's disease: survival analysis in an Italian population. Neurology 38:1433–1438

Loft AGR, Hogdall E, Larsen OS et al. (1993) A comparison of amniotic fluid alphafeta-protein and acetylcholinesterase in the prenatal diagnosis of open neural tube defects and anterior abdominal wall defects. Prenat Diag 13:93–109

Luthy DA, Wardinsky T, Shurtleff DB et al. (1991) Cesarian section before the onset of labor and subsequent motor function in infants with meningomyelocele diagnosed antenatally. N Engl J Med 324:662–666

MacKinnon JA, Perlman M, Kirpalani H et al. (1993) Spinal cord injury at birth: Diagnostic and prognostic data in twenty-two patients. J Pediatr 122:431–437

Maekawa K, Masaki T, Kokubun Y (1976) Fetal spinal-cord injury secondary to hyperextension of the neck: no effect of caesarian section. Dev Med Child Neurol 18:229–232

McDonald CM, Jaffe KM, Mosca VS et al. (1991) Ambulatory outcome of children with myelomeningocele: effect of lower-extremity muscle strength. Dev Med Child Neurol 33:482–490

Michaud LJ, Jaffe KM, Benjamin DR et al. (1988) Hemangioblastoma of the conus medullaris associated with cutaneous hemangioma. Pediatr Neurol 4:309–312

Milunsky A, Alpert E, Neff RF et al. (1980) Prenatal diagnosis of neural tube defects. IV. Maternal serum alphafeta-protein screening. Obstet Gynecol 55:60–66

Minami T, Ise K, Kukita J et al. (1994) A case of neonatal spinal cord injury: magnetic resonance imaging and somatosensory evoked potentials. Brain Dev 16:57–60

Moore KL (1988) The developing human. Clinically oriented embryology 4th edn. WB Saunders, Philadelphia

Morrow RJ, McNay MB, Whittle MJ (1991) Ultrasound detection of neural tube defects in patients with elevated maternal serum alphafeta-protein. Obstet Gynecol 78:1055–1057

Mutoh K, Ito M, Okuno T et al. (1989) Non-traumatic spinal intramedullary hemorrhage in an infant. Pediatr Neurol 5:53–56

Nagele RG, Bush KT, Kosciuk MC et al. (1989) Intrinsic and extrinsic factors collaborate to generate driving forces for neural tube formation in the chick: a study using morphometry and computerized three-dimensional reconstruction. Dev Brain Res 50:101–111

Naidich TP, McLone DG, Mutluer S (1983) A new understanding of dorsal dysraphism with lipoma (lipomyeloschisis): radiologic evaluation and surgical correction AJR 140:1065–1078

Naidich TP, Fernbach SK, McLone DG et al. (1984) Sonography of the caudal spine and back: congenital anomalies in children AJR 142:1229–1242

Nelson FW, Hecht JT, Horton WA et al. (1988) Neurological basis of respiratory complications in achondroplasia. Ann Neurol 24:89–93

Noetzel MJ, Blake JN (1991) Prognosis of seizure control and remission in children with myelomeningocele. Dev Med Child Neurol 33:803–810

Norman MG, McGillivray BC, Kalousek DK, Hill A, Poskitt KJ (1995) Congenital malformations of the brain: pathological, embryological, clinical, radiological and genetic aspects. Oxford University Press, New York, pp. 105–179

Oakley GP (1993) Folic acid preventable spina bifida and anencephaly. JAMA 269:1291–1293

O'Rahilly R, Mueller F (1989) Bidirectional closure of the rostral neuropere in the human embryo. Am J Anat 184:259–268

Ouvrier RA, McLeod JG, Conchin TE (1982) Friedreich's ataxia – early detection and progression of peripheral nerve abnormalities. J Neurol Sci 55:137–145

Packer RJ, Zimmerman RA, Sutton LN et al. (1986) Magnetic resonance imaging of spinal cord disease of childhood. Pediatrics 78:251–256

Pang DL, Hoffman HJ, Rekate HL (1992) Split cord malformation: Part II: Clinical syndrome. Neurosurgery 31:481–500

Passarge E, Lenz W (1966) Syndrome of caudal regression in infants of diabetic mothers. Pediatrics 37:672–675

Pasternak JF, Volpe JJ (1980) Lumbosacral lipoma with acute deterioration during infancy. Pediatrics 66:125–128

Peacock WJ, Murovic JA (1989) Magnetic resonance imaging in myelocystoceles. Report of two cases. J Neurosurg 70:804–807

Pinto F, Amantini A, DeScisciolo G et al. (1988) Visual involvement in Friedreich's ataxia: PERG and VEP study. Eur Neurol 28:246–251

Pueschel SM (1988) Atlanto-axial instability and Down syndrome. Pediatrics 81:879–880

Rehan VK, Seshia MMK (1993) Spinal cord birth injury – diagnostic difficulties. Arch Dis Child 69:92–94

Reid CS, Pyeritz RE, Koptis SE et al. (1987) Cervicomedullary compression in young patients with achondroplasia: value of comprehensive neurologic and respiratory evaluation. J Pediatr 110: 522–530

Sadler TW (1990) Langnon's medical embryology, 6th edn. Williams & Wilkins, Baltimore

Sarnat HB, Case ME, Graviss R (1976) Sacral agenesis: neurologic and neuropathologic features. Neurology 26:1124–1129

Scatliff JH, Kendall BE, Kingley DP et al. (1989) Closed spinal dysraphism: analysis of clinical radiological and surgical findings in 104 consecutive patients. AJNR 10:269–277

Scheible W, James HE, Leopold GR et al. (1983) Occult spinal dysraphism in infants: screening with high-resolution real-time ultrasound. Radiology 146:743–746

Seeds JW, Jones FD (1986) Lipomyelomeningocele. Prenatal diagnosis and management. Obstet Gynecol 67:534–537

Seeds JW, Powers SK (1988) Early prenatal diagnosis of familial lipomyelomeningocele. Obstet Gynecol 72:469–471

Sharrard WJW, Zachary RB, Lorber J et al. (1963) A controlled trial of immediate and delayed closure of spina bifida cystica. Arch Dis Child 38:18

Shulman ST, Madden JD, Shaklin DR et al. (1971) Transection of the spinal cord: a rare obstetrical complication of cephalic delivery. Arch Dis Child 46:291–294

Sladky JT, Rorke LB (1986) Perinatal hypoxic-ischemic spinal cord injury. Pediatr Pathol 6:87–101

Stone DH (1987) The declining prevalence of anencephalus and spina bifida: its nature, causes and implications. Dev Med Child Neurol 29:541–546

Swaminathan S, Paton JY, Davidson-Ward SL et al. (1989) Abnormal control of ventilation in adolescents with myelodysplasia. J Pediatr 115:898–903

Touloukian RJ (1979) Colon aganglionosis. In: Bergsma D (ed) Birth defects compendium. Alan Liss, New York, p 240

Towbin A (1969) Latent spinal cord and brain stem injury in newborn infants. Dev Med Child Neurol 11:54

Volpe JJ (1995) Neurology of the newborn, 3rd edn. WB Saunders, Philadelphia

Werler MM, Shapiro S, Mitchell AA (1993). Periconceptional folic acid exposure and risk of occurrent neural tube defects. JAMA 269:1257–1261

Wright RL (1971) Congenital dermal sinuses. Progr Neurol Surg 4:175–191

Yamada S, Zinke DE, Sanders D (1981) Pathophysiology of "tethered cord syndrome". J Neurosurg 54:494–503

Chapter 9

Imaging of the Spine and Spinal Cord

J. S. Lapointe

Introduction

Between 1896, when Roentgen discovered X-rays and 1975, when spinal computed tomography (CT) became available thanks to improvements to Hounsfield's 1971 invention, the spinal cord had to be studied by indirect means. Plain film radiography, and linear and complex motion tomography were used to image the bony spine. The outline of the spinal cord was first seen with pneumomyelography, after Dandy outlined the medulla with air in 1919 but a safe opaque contrast medium for myelography was only introduced in 1940. This iophendylate (Pantopaque) was replaced by non-ionic water-soluble metrizamide (Amipaque) in 1973. Spinal angiography, since its introduction by Djindjian in 1963, has had a limited role in the investigation of vascular lesions of the spinal cord.

After 1975, perfected CT body scanners made axial images of the spinal cord possible. With the aid of intrathecal contrast, better visualization of the contour of the cord and its position within the spinal canal was achieved. Following improved resolution of the CT scans in the 1980s, cysts, haemorrhages, and tumours within the substance of the cord could be detected without intrathecal contrast and without or with intravenous contrast enhancement (Ruggiero et al. 1981). At the same time, rapid progress in the image quality of magnetic resonance studies was being made and the first clinical units became available at the beginning of the 1980s. This new and expensive technology, whose first images were produced by Lauterbur in 1973, will be the imaging modality of choice in the 1990s for diseases affecting the spinal cord, as it is the first method which consistently outlines the substance of the cord in any plane and the effect of the surrounding tissues on it. Recent advances have increased the resolution in MRI of the cord to the point that grey and white matter differentiation is possible.

Imaging Tools

In this period of concern over health care costs, it is important for the physician ordering examinations to understand what information each type of examination is likely to yield, and to tailor these requests to the patient's neurological status. The availability of the technology should not be the only determining factor in the choice of examination. The degree of radiological expertise available and the familiarity with the conditions being studied are also very important. If the patient is to be transferred to a more specialized centre for management, it is often advisable to have that centre's neuroradiologists perform the examinations, to reduce unnecessary duplication and to increase diagnostic yield. While the following is not all-inclusive, its aim is to elucidate what place these examinations have in the overall investigation.

Plain Films

Plain film radiography (Banna 1985) is available in all radiology departments and is the first radiographic examination performed when trauma to the spine has been sustained. Obtained supine, often on a trauma board, with the neck in a brace or collar, the examination consists mainly of AP and cross-table lateral films. In an uncooperative patient, it may be difficult to obtain a good open-mouth view to see the base of the odontoid. When the patient has a short neck or wide shoulders, a swimmer's view will delineate the cervicothoracic junction. Oblique views of the cervical spine may not be routinely obtained in trauma. Satisfactory information may be gained by angling the X-ray tube without moving the patient, resulting in a somewhat distorted view of the oblique cervical spine. Another method is to obtain oblique views of the cervical spine by doing oblique scout views (digital radiograph) by CT. These add only a few seconds to a CT examination of the head. Alignment of pedicles and shingling or imbrication of the laminae can be easily ascertained by either method, attesting to the normal alignment of the vertebral bodies and obviating the need for spinal precautions in the multi-traumatized patient (Fig. 9.1a and b).

The size of the intervertebral foramina and the integrity of the pedicles and laminae are assessed on routine oblique views of the cervical spine, while oblique views of the lumbar spine help to assess the pars interarticularis and the apophyseal joints. Flexion and extension views are performed if abnormal mobility of the spine, usually at the cervical level but occasionally at the lumbar level, is suspected. Ligamentous injury of the cervical spine can easily be missed on the initial supine study. These flexion and extension views should always be performed with the patient's cooperation and in a sitting or standing position when the patient's condition permits. Supine flexion and extension films done passively may give the physician a false sense of security and not demonstrate the presence of ligamentous injury. Spinal precautions should be maintained as long as instability is still suspected.

Tomography

Tomography is of two types, linear and complex motion, and is equipment dependent. The second type better delineates bony detail and is used to study complex congenital anomalies of the spine such as segmentation anomalies and scoliosis. It is also used to study fractures f the spine, where CT scanning is not available. As many cases of trauma occur in young people, CT scanning is preferred because the dose of radiation is much less with CT scanning than with tomography, and the examination

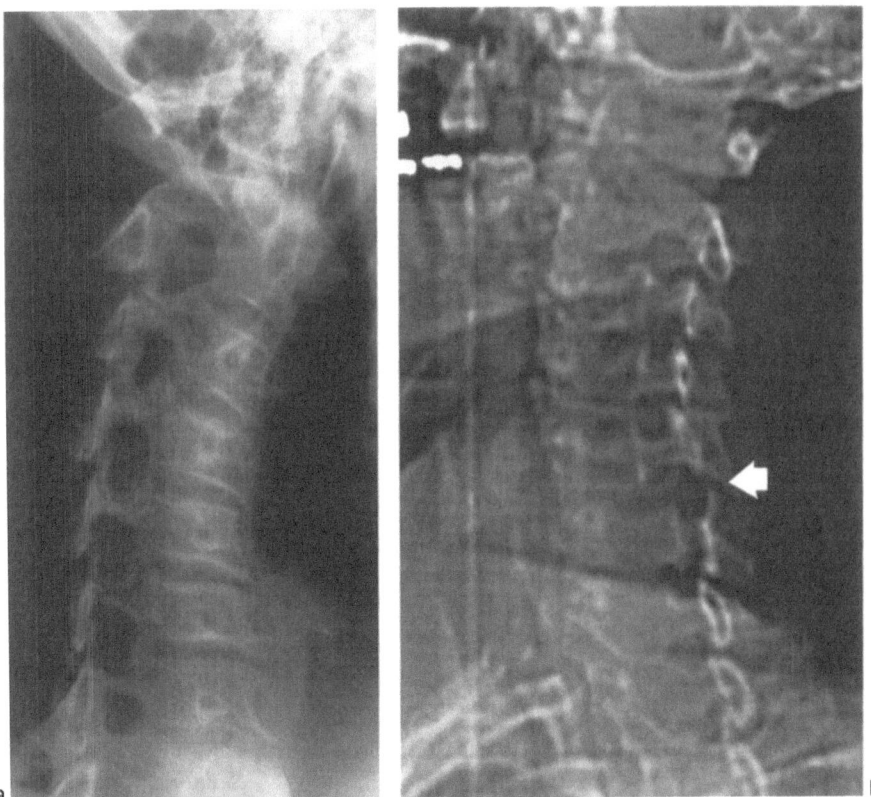

Fig. 9.1. **a** Oblique view of the cervical spine showing normal imbrication (shingling) of the cervical laminae. **b** Oblique digital radiography (scout view) showing a facet look at C5–6: loss of shingling of the laminae, disrupted alignment of the round pedicles and of the posterior margin of the vertebral bodies.

can be performed more quickly and with better resolution, and with less manipulation of the injured spine (Donovan-Post 1984).

Myelography

This consists of injection of a iodinated contrast medium into the subarachnoid space and gravitation of this contrast to various segments of the spinal canal under fluoroscopic control. Myelography helps to determine the presence of blocks due to intradural, extradural, and intramedullary lesions, as well as to outline the position, size and shape of the spinal cord and nerve roots. While it was the investigation of choice for 40 years to determine the presence of disc herniation and tumour, it has largely been replaced by CT scanning and MR imaging. It is still used in many centres that do not have ready access to these two latter technologies, and the introduction of improved non-ionic, water-soluble contrast media such as iohexol (Omnipaque) and iopamidol (Isovue) has greatly decreased the amount of side effects of this procedure. The incidence of post lumbar puncture headache in many centres has been further decreased by the use of 25 and 26 gauge spinal needles (Vezina et al. 1989). Myelography is currently used in conjunction with computed tomography when CT scanning or MRI (either non-enhanced or intravenously enhanced) have not resolved the clinical dilemma. It is particularly useful in delineating subtle mass effect on root sleeves due to disc herniation, as well as subtle epidural spread of tumour, and also for demonstrating cord atrophy due to spondylosis presenting as cervical myelopathy (Shapiro 1984) (Fig. 9.2a and b).

CT Scanning

This has been widely used since the early 1980s to study the disc herniations and spinal stenosis. CT scanning of the virgin lumbar spine requires no intravenous contrast as the presence of fat in and around the spinal canal helps define disc margins, root sleeves, thecal sac, and epidural veins and outlines the relationship of these soft tissue structures to the bony canal, intervertebral foramina, and apophyseal joints.

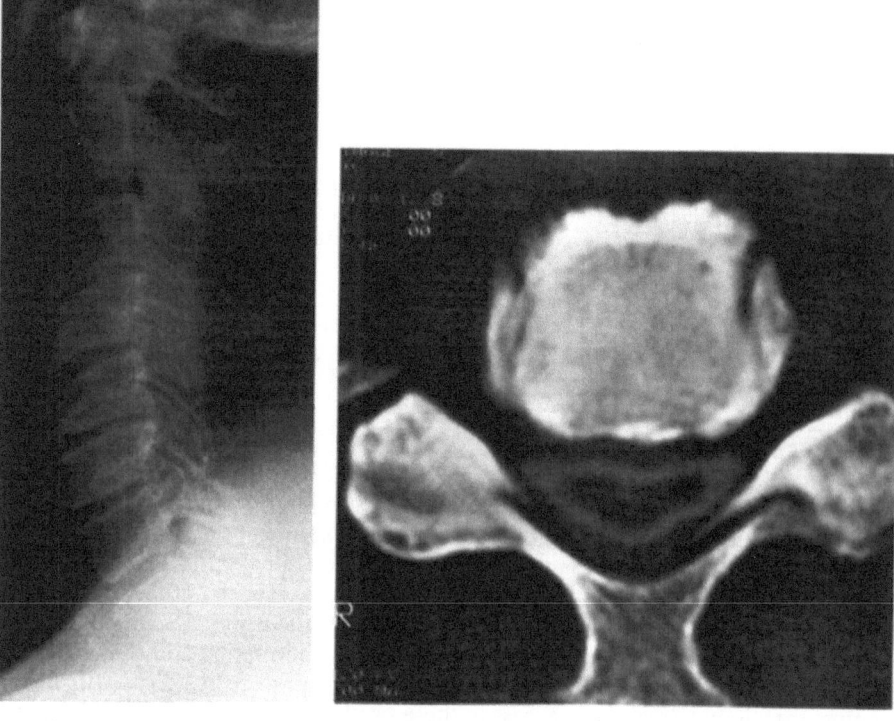

Fig. 9.2. **a** Lateral cervical spine shows severe spondylosis and spinal stenosis. **b** Postmyelogram axial CT scan at C3–4 shows a flattened spinal cord consistent with atrophy in a 48-year-old man complaining of neck pain and weakness in the right arm.

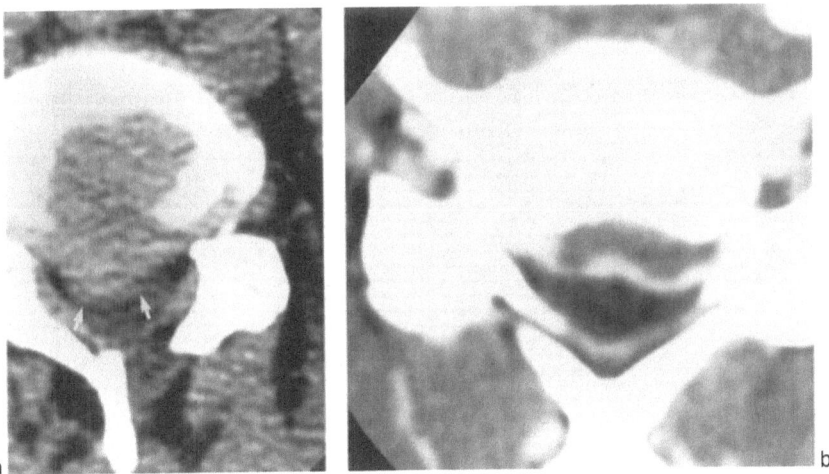

Fig. 9.3. **a** Axial CT scan showing a large central lumbar disc herniation at L5–S1 in a 40-year-old woman with back pain. **b** Axial CT scan with intravenous contrast enhancement showing a large central and left sided C4–5 disc herniation in a 36-year-old man with left arm weakness.

Intravenous contrast is used to outline the epidural venous plexus and in some instances to help differentiate between recurrent disc herniation and post surgical scarring (Figs. 9.3a and b, 9.4a and b). In the cervical spine, the convex configuration of the end plate makes visualization of the margin of the disc more difficult; intravenous contrast, by highlighting the vertebral venous plexus, which is closely apposed to the posterior margin of the vertebral body and disc, is used routinely to detect subtle indentation on the dural sac and nerve roots. Neoplasms such as neurofibromas, meningiomas, and intramedullary tumours may also be enhanced with intravenous contrast, improving their delineation (Fig. 9.5) (Newton and Potts 1983).

MR Imaging

This is the newest addition to imaging techniques. The lack of radiation is viewed as an advantage over CT scanning by both physicians and patients. Contraindications to its use are many and include the presence of ferromagnetic metals such as certain cerebral aneurysm clips and metallic orbital foreign bodies, which may be displaced by the pull of the magnet, and the presence of pacemakers which may malfunction. The current configuration of the scanner and its relatively small aperture makes scanning large patients, claustrophobic patients, and certain severely ill patients difficult or impossible. Patient cooperation is important as motion degrades the quality of the images. Sagittal and coronal imaging of the spinal canal is easily obtained, contrary to CT. While the cord can be seen on one image from the foramen magnum to the conus, surface coils over areas of interest have improved resolution and focus attention on specific areas of the cord. Paramagnetic contrast agents such as gadolinium DTPA enhance lesions in a similar fashion as CT intravenous contrast, increasing lesion conspicuity. MRI is rapidly replacing

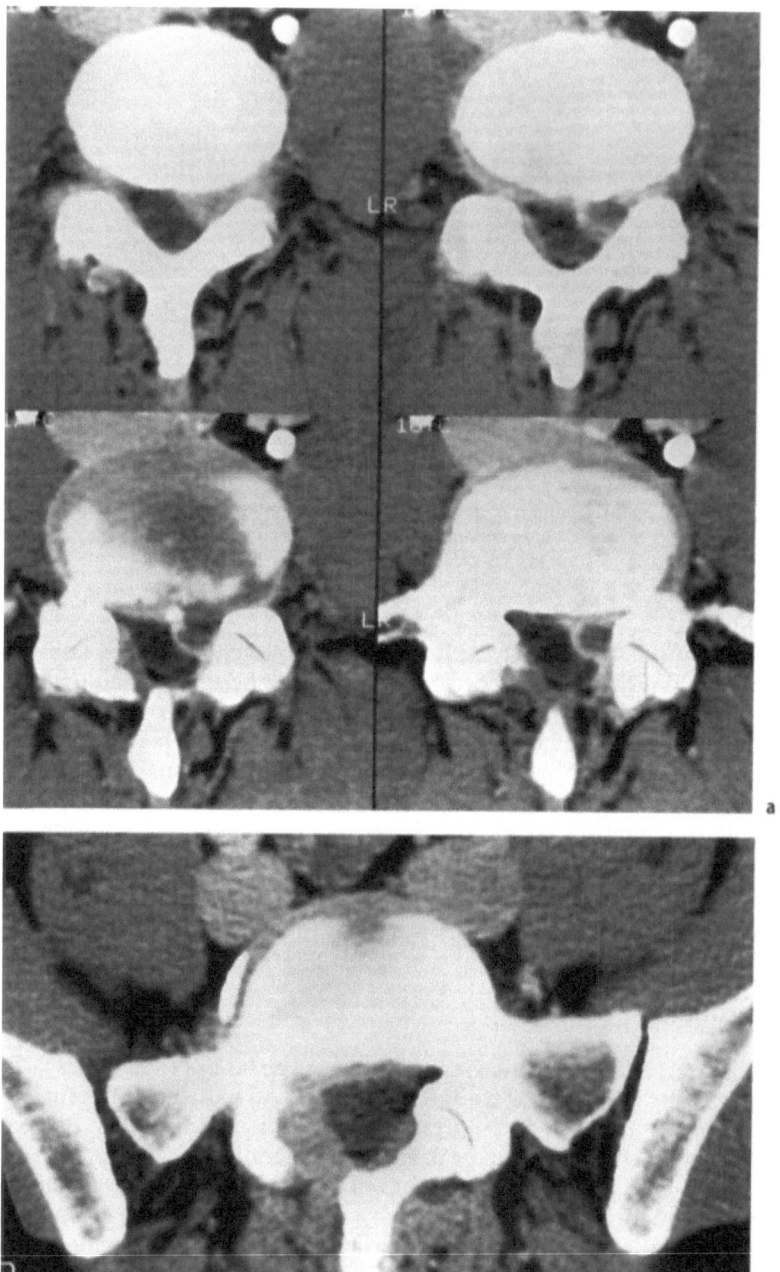

9.4. **a** Axial CT scan with intravenous contrast enhancement showing a recurrent left sided L4–5 disc herniation in a 45-year-old man with left L5 root symptoms. **b** Axial CT scan with intravenous contrast showing enhancing scar along the right side of the dural sac, at the site of previous L5–S1 laminectomy in a 46-year-old man complaining of recurrent right leg pain.

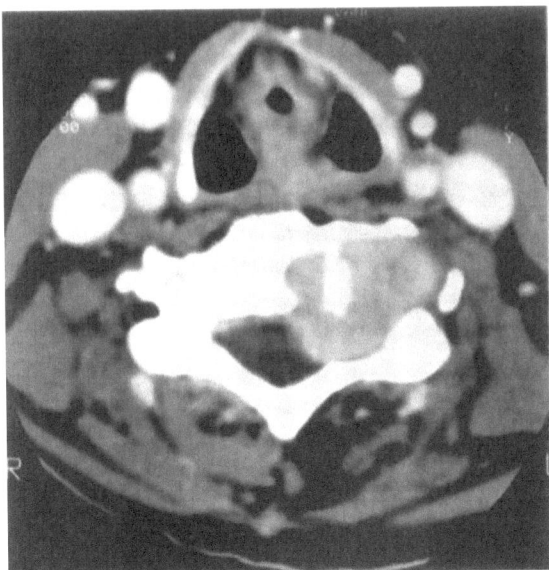

Fig. 9.5.   Axial CT scan of the cervical spine, with intravenous contrast, showing an enhancing dumb-bell schwannoma of the left C2–3 foramen in a 69-year-old woman with left shoulder pain and weakness for six months and a prior history of breast carcinoma.

myelography, especially when an intramedullary lesion is suspected. Cysts, syrinxes, and intramedullary masses and cerebellar tonsillar herniation are readily demonstrated (Figs. 9.6 and 9.7) and physiological processes such as myelination and CSF flow can be studied (Norman 1987).

Spinal Angiography

This examination is used when myelography, CT scan, or MRI have suggested the presence of an arteriovenous malformation, a dural fistula or a vascular tumour. It is time-consuming and tedious and results in a large amount of radiation to the patient. To outline the vascular supply of the spinal cord, selective injections in all the intercostal and lumbar arteries are necessary, with additional injections of vertebral arteries, thyrocervical trunks, costocervical trunks, and internal iliac arteries sometimes necessary. This often means 25 to 50 separate vessels must be studied at one or more sittings. Digital subtraction angiography, when available, speeds the examination as well as decreases the radiation dose and the volume of iodinated contrast material. Embolization, surgery, or a combination of both can then be planned. This type of examination should be limited to specialized centres (Thron 1988) (Fig. 9.8a and b).

Nuclear Medicine Bone Scans

These are useful to pinpoint early metastatic disease not evident on plain film, and may help localize benign bone lesions such as osteoid osteoma which is a common

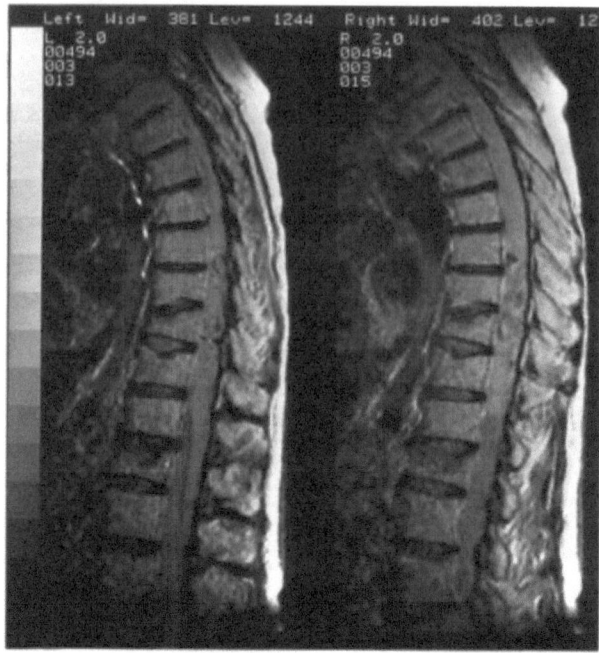

Fig. 9.6. Sagittal MRI of the thoracic cord showing mixed density changes of an astrocytoma in a 73 year-old woman with multiple compression fractures.

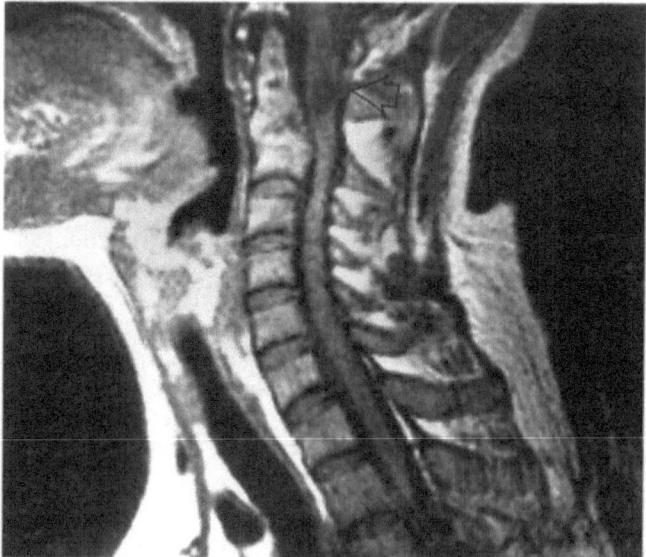

Fig. 9.7. Sagittal MRI of the cervical spine showing a high cervical cord syrinx in a 31-year-old man who suffered an injury to C2 and C3 ten years ago with persistent mild quadriparesis and recent increasing left limb weakness.

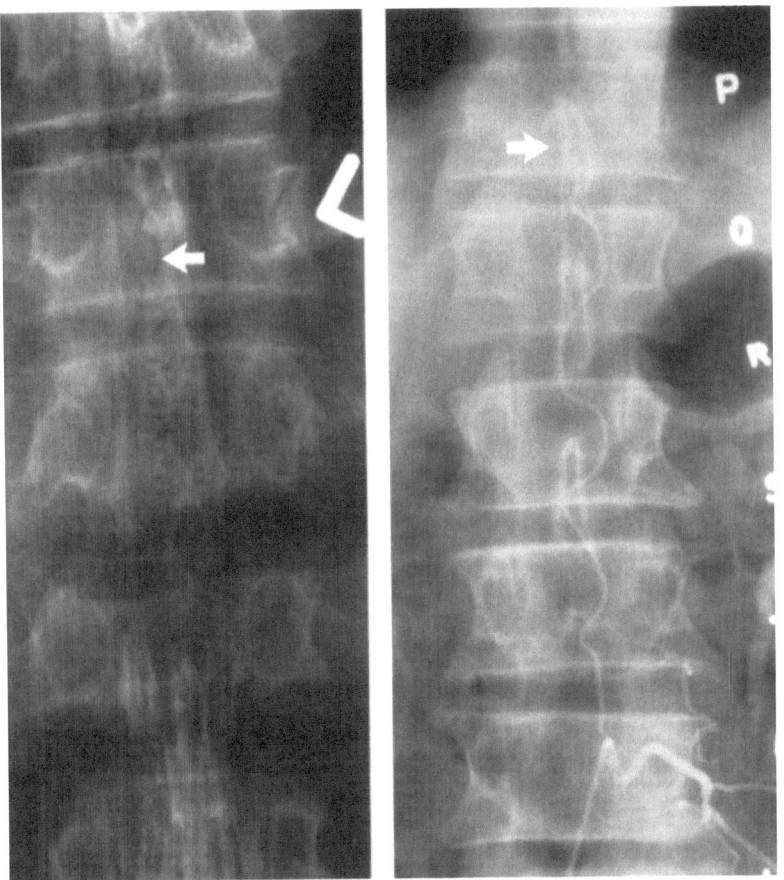

Fig. 9.8. **a** Myelogram and **b** spinal angiogram showing the abnormal vessels of a dural fistula of the conus medullaris in a 52-year-old man complaining of progressive lower limb weakness with sphincter difficulties.

source of bone pain in young people and which occasionally presents in the spine. Gallium scans and tagged leucocyte scans may pinpoint vertebral infection in the absence of plain film bony changes. Further studies by CT or MRI may then be warranted.

Ultrasound

This can be used as readily in the neonatal spine as it is in the neonatal brain. It is particularly useful in patients with dysraphic states of the lower lumbar spine suspected because of a skin covered lumbosacral mass and can be performed without radiation or sedation. Lipomyelomeningocele, teratoma, and status post repair of myelomeningocele can be evaluated. Absence of cord motion on real-time scanning indicates cord tethering and the need for further evaluation. In the adult, ultrasound of the spine is an intraoperative tool used to localize intramedullary cysts for shunting, intramedullary masses for removal, and to minimize the myelotomy and thus reduce postoperative sensory changes, to assess the spinal canal for adequate decompression of spinal stenosis, and to rule out the presence of subarachnoid cysts (Pasto et al. 1984). It is also used to determine the adequacy of decompression of spinal fractures and normal realignment of structures and to localize foreign bodies such as bone fragments or bullet fragments intraoperatively (Naidich and Quencer 1987).

Current Concepts

A review of the entire spectrum of conditions studied with these available tools is outside the scope of this monograph. The enclosed references will yield more specific detail to the interested reader. A summary of current practices and new knowledge of common conditions follows. It is hoped that the reader will be able to extrapolate from these examples useful and practical information concerning the investigations of conditions affecting the spine and spinal cord.

Anatomy – Normal vs. Abnormal

Evaluation of the alignment of the vertebral bodies, the pedicles, the spinous processes, the apophyseal joints and the laminae, symmetry of the soft tissues including the discs and ligaments and the integrity of the bone and its density can and should be determined.

The appearance of the various bony structures evolves during growth, but following closure of the epiphyses, a fairly uniform configuration is attained. Familiarity with the spine in childhood helps to recognize developmental abnormalities, such as limbus vertebra, hypoplastic disc, transitional vertebra, tropism of the apophyseal joints, and prevents erroneous diagnoses.

Plain films depict the bones well, but CT scan with its greater sensitivity to calcium illustrates subtle bony alterations to better advantage. Cross-sectional imaging may make it easier to understand the compressive or obstructive effects of certain types of lesions on the dural sac and the exiting nerve roots, for example, nerve roots exiting through a narrowed intervertebral foramen or the extraspinal extension of tumour or infection.

MRI, because of its ability to image more subtle changes in tissue density than CT, has improved our understanding of the changes affecting the ageing spine in health and disease. Alterations in vertebral bone marrow and in the intervertebral disc are now better understood and can be distinguished from disease. Distinction of grey and white matter columns in the cord has been achieved (Czervionke et al. 1988; Carvlin et al. 1989; Curtin et al. 1989).

Until the advent of MRI, the spinal cord, intrathecal nerves, and the cerebellar tonsils could only be accurately depicted with intrathecal contrast during myelography of CT. Concurrently, improved real-time ultrasound scanning led to visualization of the lumbar spine and its contents in the neonate, but abnormalities were usually confirmed by invasive studies prior to surgery.

The cerebellar tonsils and the conus medullaris are now easily visible on MRI and their normal position has been determined in vivo. Tonsillar ectopia (Chiari I) takes many forms and is deemed to be present when the tip of the rounded or pointed tonsils are found 5 mm below the level of the foramen magnum, measured by a line drawn from the caudal cortex of the basion to the opisthion (Barkovich et al. 1986). Similarly, the position of the normal conus is at the adult level in the first few months of life. The normal range of the tip of the conus extends from T12 to L3 (Wilson and Prince 1989).

Tethering of the conus is no longer a condition found mainly in childhood and adolescence, but is being increasingly recognized in middle-aged adults. In children with lumbosacral dimples or hair patches, without or with a subcutaneous lipoma, cord tethering can be easily diagnosed on CT scan and MRI or by ultrasound in neonates. Adults often have no cutaneous abnormality and present with an abnormal gait or difficulty in urination, which in males can mimic prostatic hypertrophy. Myelography, intrathecally enhanced CT or MRI will show the thickened filum terminale, usually associated with a lipoma (72%) and a conus below L2 (84%). An associated cavitary lesion or myelomalacia was recognized in 9 of 20 patients on MRI in one series (Merx et al. 1989; Raghavan et al. 1989).

A better understanding of complex anomalies of the spine including segmentation anomalies, tethering, diastematomyelia and syringomyelia associated with meningomyelocele usually require combined investigations to elucidate all facets of the process so that adequate treatment may be instituted.

Trauma

Plain films are the mainstay of the investigation of spinal trauma as they are readily obtained and measures to stabilize the spine may be instituted rapidly. Spinal trauma is often associated with multiple head, chest, or abdomen injuries which require more immediate attention. It is rarely necessary to obtain detailed information on the spine once the level of injury has been recognized, on an emergency basis, as experience has shown that immediate decompression of spinal fractures does not alter the prognosis for recovery, the maximum deficit having been caused at the time of injury. It is necessary to determine the extent of the injury before the patient is mobilized, especially in those patients who have suffered fractures with little or no neurological deficit to prevent the occurrence of second injury. In many instances, the plain film findings underestimate the extent of the bony injuries. CT scanning in particular and, where not available, tomography should be used (Figs. 9.9a and b, 9.10a and b).

Spinal Stability vs. Instability

One of the main questions regarding a spinal fracture is determining its stability (Dunsker et al. 1986) i.e., will motion with resulting change in position of the various elements of the spine further compromise the spinal cord? Fractures affecting both the vertebral body and neural arch are always unstable. When in doubt, a useful system is to divide the spine into three columns, the first centred on the interlaminar line, the second on the posterior margin of the vertebral body, and the third on its anterior margin. The integrity of the bones and ligaments is considered along each

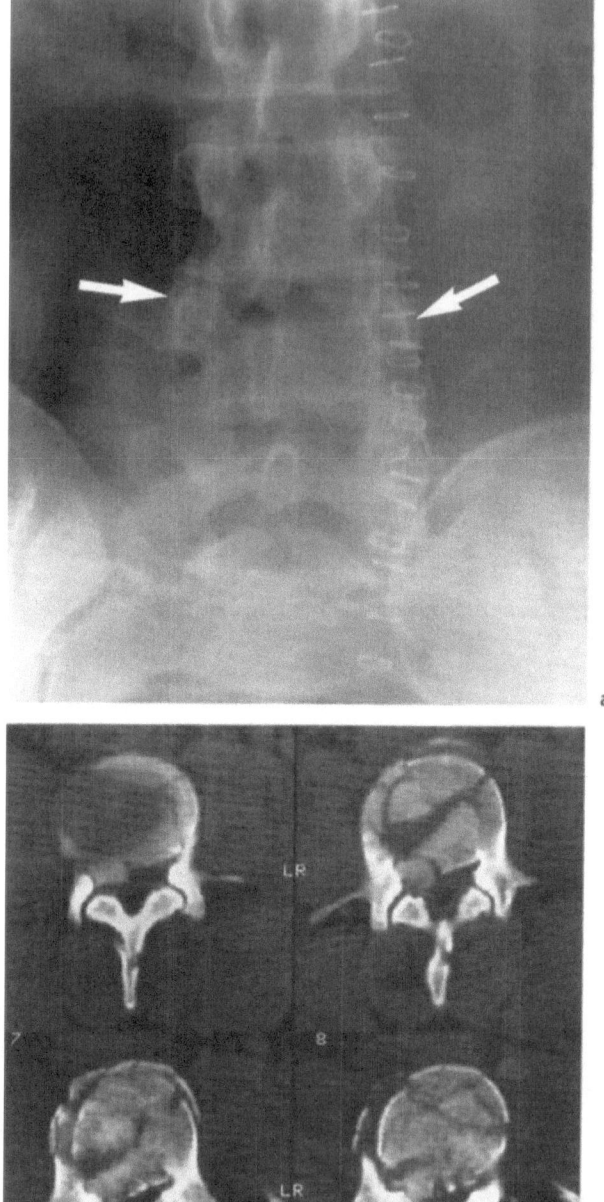

Fig. 9.9. **a** Plain film of the lumbar spine obtained portably after an emergency laparotomy on a 20-year-old man who sustained multiple injuries in a motor vehicle accident. The left L3 and L4 transverse processes are avulsed, the pedicles of L4 are splayed, and the body of L4 is decreased in height. **b** The axial CT scan shows a burst fracture of L4 with marked narrowing of the spinal canal by retropulsed bone fragments.

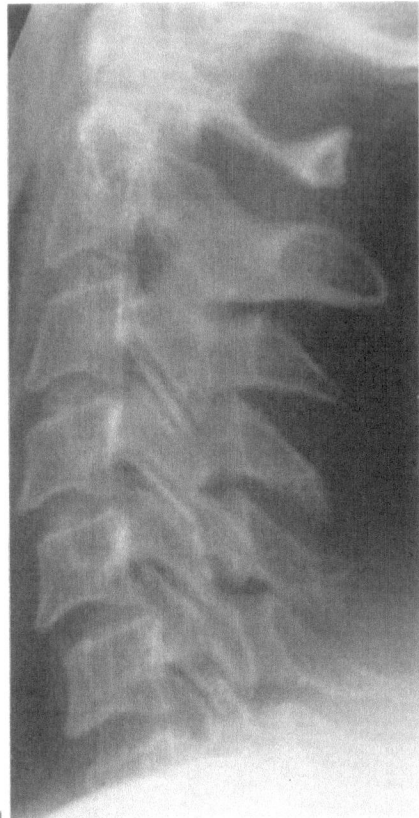
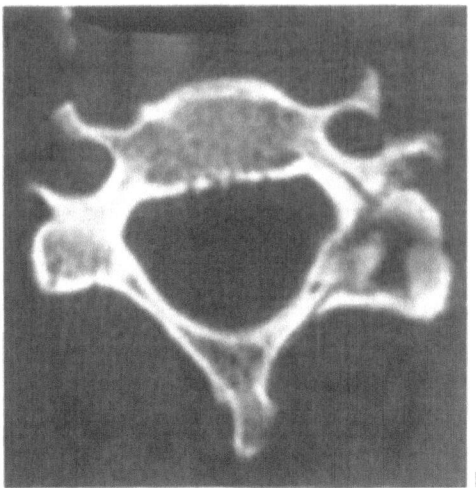

Fig. 9.10. **a** The lateral cervical spine shows subluxation of C5 on C6 without distortion of the inter-laminar line. **b** The axial CT scan shows a unilateral fracture involving the left C5 pedicle, lamina and articular pillar in a 40-year-old woman who sustained a fall.

of these lines. If the injury has disrupted ligaments and/or bones of two of the three columns, the spine is considered acutely unstable and appropriate management precautions should be taken (Denis 1983). A more chronic instability may occur if only one column, usually the posterior one, is damaged.

Intraspinal Haemorrhage

Haemorrhage has to be sizable before it can be detected on non-contrast spinal CT in an epidural, subdural, subarachnoid or intramedullary location. MRI has rarely been used in acute spinal trauma because of the difficulties in obtaining an adequate examination. Once the patient is stabilized, however, it may prove quite useful for prognosis and management. Any deterioration of spinal function following spinal trauma warrants thorough investigation. Early diagnosis and treatment may reverse the deterioration and maintain function. Early MRI results suggest that recovery is insignificant with intramedullary haematoma and good with contusion or oedema (Naseem et al. 1986; Kadoya et al. 1987; Kulkarni et al. 1987).

Post-traumatic Syrinx (Fig. 9.7)

A progressive neurological deficit whether subacute or chronic warrants detailed investigation. The most common lesion is the development of post-traumatic syringomyelia which can progress in a cranial or caudal direction (Aubin et al. 1987). Cranial extension of the syrinx results in an ascending neurological deficit. MRI is particularly useful in delineating the extent of these cysts, believed by some authors to represent dilatation of the central canal secondary to obstruction or compression of the cord and subarachnoid space. The absence of haemosiderin as a marker of previous haemorrhage does not support the theory of a syrinx starting from a cord haematoma (Norman 1987).

Water-soluble intrathecal contrast medium, followed by a 6 to 24 hour or 48 hour delayed CT scan of the spine, was used in the past to delineate these syrinxes. While it was useful prior to the advent of MRI, it is no longer the study of choice because the timing of contrast accumulation within the cord varies from patient to patient, making diagnosis more difficult, and the extent of the cyst is not accurately shown.

CSF flow dynamics is currently an area of intense MRI study. Shunting of the syrinx into the subarachnoid space or into the peritoneum is used to arrest progression of the deficit. Syrinxes exhibiting flow are thought more likely to be undergoing active expansion (water-hammer effect) and the patient should benefit from shunting, while cysts with non-pulsatile fluid are believed to be at little risk of expansion (Sherman et al. 1986; Castillo et al. 1987). The most caudal position possible for the shunt is preferred to assist in decompression and to minimize new deficits.

Fractures (Figs. 9.9a and b, 9.10a and b)

The types of spinal fractures are too numerous to detail here and the reader is referred to the works of Rogers (1982) or Banna (1985) for easy reading. The following points warrant special attention:

1. Patients can survive craniovertebral dislocation; alignment of the tip of the clivus with the tip of the odontoid should always be ascertained on the lateral view of the skull or cervical spine to avoid missing this injury (Woodring et al. 1981; Lee et al. 1987).

2. Fractures of the base of the odontoid can be missed if undisplaced. Its cortical outline should be easily followed on the lateral and open-mouth view. In an uncooperative patient with an inadequate open-mouth view, a Caldwell view of the skull often shows the C2 vertebra well.

3. To view the cervicothoracic junction, a frequent site of fracture dislocation, it may be necessary to obtain the oblique views discussed previously before resorting to tomography (Fig. 9.1).

4. Burst fractures frequently result in serious neurological injury. They can mimic a simple compression fractures on the lateral view if the integrity of the posterior margin of the vertebral body is not properly assessed and if the intraspinal position of the fragment of bone originating from the posterior superior aspect of the vertebral body is not recognized. CT scan frequently shows more extensive fractures than originally demonstrated on plain films (Atlas et al. 1986; Kim et al. 1988).

5. Injuries in a purely axial plane, such as the so-called seat belt fracture and ligamentous disruption without or with subluxation, are difficult or impossible to see on axial images alone. Reformatted sagittal or coronal images will give adequate information provided the patient has not moved between slices which have been obtained at small intervals, usually 3 or 5 mm. This technique is useful when a short segment of spine is being studied. Not only the level of injury but also usually at least one-half of the vertebral body above and below the fracture should be imaged.

6. It is not uncommon for the patient to suffer injury at more than one vertebral level, sometimes quite distant from the first. Only a high index of suspicion will lead to its early recognition and investigation (Gehweiler et al. 1980).

Degenerative Disc Disease and Spinal Stenosis

Back and neck pain are very common complaints. Pain radiating to an extremity, especially when localized in a neuroanatomical distribution, helps to pinpoint the source of the symptom. A neurological deficit need not be present

In the past, investigation by myelography was reserved for presumed surgical candidates. When the myelogram was normal the patient was sometimes sent to a psychiatrist for treatment of functional pain. Even after apparently successful surgery, a large number of patients suffered from persistent or recurrent symptoms. This has been termed the "failed back syndrome".

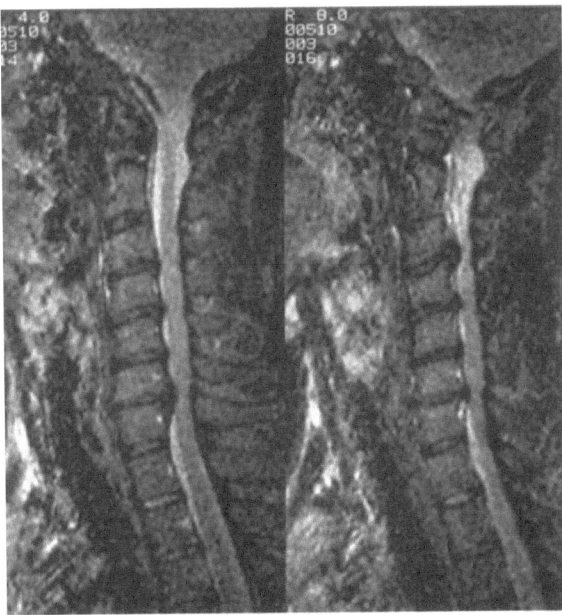

Fig. 9.11. Sagittal MRI of the cervical spine showing spondylosis maximum at C6–7, with cord compression in a 40-year-old man with hyper-reflexia.

Degenerative Disc Disease

CT and MRI have shown that degenerative disc disease is very prevalent, especially after age 45. In one series, asymptomatic cervical cord impingement (by disc) was found in 26% of patients over 64 years of age on MRI (Teresi et al. 1987). The progressive changes in the intervertebral disc with ageing have been documented with MRI and pathological correlation obtained, from the neonatal period to adulthood (Pech and Haughton 1985; Ho et al. 1988; Yu et al. 1988a,b,c; Yu et al. 1989). Types of tears of the annulus fibrosis have been characterized on MR (Yu et al. 1988b) and the radial tear may be responsible for the bulging annulus. Transverse tears, resulting in rupture of Sharpey's fibres at the periphery of the annulus near the ring apophysis, may account for the focal herniation (Yu et al. 1988a,b,c; Bonneville et al. 1989).

Not all disc bulges (defined as a concentric extension of disc material with an intact but often thin annulus), or disc herniations (diagnosed when a disruption of the annulus is associated with focal disc extrusion), are symptomatic (Norman 1987). Free fragments, often called sequestered discs, herniate through the lateral part of the posterior longitudinal ligament because its midportion is much thicker than its lateral aspects. This lateral herniation is more likely to result in symptoms because the exiting nerve roots are impinged upon by the free fragment. Myelography is not always capable of distinguishing herniation from bulge, especially when the defect is central. MRI and CT are of similar sensitivity and specificity in the diagnosis of herniation (Brown et al. 1988; Hedberg et al. 1988; Masaryk et al. 1988) (Fig. 9.3).

CT and MRI both demonstrate types of disc herniation not visible on myelography. The far lateral or extreme disc herniation is the type that compresses the existing nerve root in the intervertebral foramen and slightly lateral to it, distal to the nerve root sleeve. Often an overlooked entity and a cause for failed back syndrome, it is more commonly found at higher disc levels than routine disc herniations, with about one-half seen at L2–3 and L3–4 and only one-third or so at L4–5. Migratory (free) fragments are found in half the cases and typically there is no intraspinal herniation (Osborn et al. 1988). A routine laminectomy will not disclose this type of herniation and a facetectomy of foraminotomy may be necessary to remove the fragments.

Institutions with large volumes of spinal MRI are noticing an apparent increased incidence of thoracic disc herniations (Ross et al. 1987a). As in other parts of the spine, not all are symptomatic, but the small diameter of the subarachnoid space surrounding the cord increases the potential for harm. Some of these herniations have mimicked spinal multiple sclerosis. Prior to MRI, thoracic disc herniation was diagnosed with myelography. In the absence of a block, supine AP and cross-table lateral films of the thoracic region were obtained and subtle indentations on the dural sac sought. A postmyelogram CT scan of the suspicious area may be obtained to determine whether the herniation is central or lateral. If the patient has symptoms localized to a specific dermatome, an intravenously enhanced CT scan with thin slices (1.5–3mm) may disclose the herniation, in a similar fashion to herniated cervical discs.

The above types of disc have been termed neurogenic and represent the well-known disc herniations. Recently, vertebrogenic symptoms, consisting of local and referred pain and autonomic reflex dysfunction, mainly sympathetic, have been ascribed to lumbar disc extrusion anterior to the pedicles. Twenty-nine per cent of patients in one series had this anterior type of disc herniation (Jinkins et al. 1989). Further studies will determine the place of this type of herniation in the diagnosis of back pain.

Spondylosis and Diffuse Idiopathic Skeletal Hyperostosis

Spinal pathology causing pain or neurological dysfunction is not limited to disc disease. Spondylosis, the formation of osteophytes at the margins of the vertebral bodies due to loss of resilience of the discs and increased stress on Sharpey's fibres, can impinge on the dural sac or nerve roots. Extensive ossification of the anterior longitudinal ligament, with preservation of the disc height, has been termed diffuse idiopathic skeletal hyperostosis (DISH). While this entity was thought benign, affecting only the mobility of the spine, a 50% incidence of associated ossification of the posterior longitudinal ligament (OPLL) has been documented (Resnick et al. 1978). OPPL can contribute to spinal stenosis and lead to severe myelopathy. Its current treatment consists of unroofing of the spinal canal, either anteriorly or posteriorly, to relieve the stenosis.

Spinal Stenosis

Spinal stenosis, or narrowing of the spinal canal, can be congenital (due to short pedicles and/or laminae) (Fig. 9.2). acquired (due to overgrowth of the articular facets without or with arthrosis, thickening of the laminae or ligamentum flavum), or a combination of these factors (Rosa et al. 1986; Postacchini 1988). It is commonly focal, affecting only short segments of the spinal canal, and is recognized on axial images (on CT or MRI) as distortion of the dural sac from its rounded shape to a triangular shape. Normally the dural sac tapers gradually the more caudally the scans progress, maintaining its rounded shape. Assessment of adequate surgical decompression is aided in some centres by intraoperative ultrasound; lateral decompression has been achieved when the dural sac has a normal configuration. Effects of chronic cervical cord compression seen as increased intensity on MRI are thought to be proportional to the severity of the myelopathy and the degree of spinal stenosis. The presence of these changes suggests a less favourable response to medical or surgical therapy (Takahashi et al. 1989).

Post Surgical Scarring

(See Fig. 9.4b.) The formation of excessive scar following surgery is a cause of recurrent symptoms. Re-exploration is difficult or impossible and can exacerbate symptoms. It has always been a difficult diagnostic problem, because retained or recurrent disc herniation can coexist with scar.

On intravenously enhanced CT, scar enhances while herniated disc rarely does (Teplick and Haskin 1984; Braun et al. 1985; Yang et al. 1986; Sotiropoulos et al. 1989). The degree of enhancement is variable however and is dependent on the amount of iodine (total grams) used and the timing of the scans. The amount of scar present will also vary and the evolution of scar enhancement on CT is still being determined. A large amount of contrast, such as 300 ml of Conray 60%, representing

84 g of iodine, infused rapidly while scans are being obtained yields the best results. The use of a similar amount of iodine with the safer non-ionic materials remains costly.

On MRI, epidural scar is of variable intensity. Its irregular configuration and extension is an important feature in differentiating it from recurrent disc herniation (Bundschuh et al. 1988a; Hochhauser et al. 1988). The mechanism and time course of enhancement of epidural fibrosis with gadolinium-DTPA has been studied. As in CT, herniated disc does not enhance, whereas epidural fibrosis surrounding herniated disc does. In the unoperated spine, epidural fibrosis occurs as an attempt at healing around a herniation, and it must be distinguished from the epidural venous plexus (Ross et al. 1989a,b).

Infection and Inflammation

Infection (Figs. 9.12a and b, 9.13a and b)

Discitis and vertebral osteomyelitis, whether bacterial or tuberculous, though infrequent in developed countries, may be insidious in onset and difficult to recognize and to treat (Burke and Brant-Zawadzki 1985; Kopecky et al. 1985). Disc space narrowing, irregularity and sclerosis of vertebral end plates followed by more pronounced bone destruction and demineralization are its signs on plain films, tomography, CT and MRI. Paravertebral spread of infection and epidural or subdural extension may be recognized with intravenously enhanced CT scan, intrathecally enhanced CT scan, and MRI without or with gadolinium-DTPA. Myelography is rarely needed. The examination most likely to produce the best information in the cooperative patient is MRI; intravenously enhanced CT is the next choice. Subtle changes in the disc and bone marrow on MRI may pinpoint the infection before it is visible by other imaging modalities. Tuberculous spondylitis may spare the discs and mimic metastatic disease (Smith et al. 1989; Thrush and Enzmann 1989).

Arachnoiditis

This inflammatory process results in adhesion of the pia-arachnoid to the cord or, more commonly, lumbar nerve roots and it may be associated with spinal cord atrophy (Donaldson and Gibson 1982). In the late stages, fibrosis involves the dura, leptomeninges, and nerve roots. On myelography, CT, or MRI, the nerve roots are clumped together and move poorly in the decreased subarachnoid space. The margins of the dural sac are irregular, with amputation of he nerve root sleeves. Complete obstruction may occur (Ross et al. 1987b). Iophendylate (Pantopaque, Ethiodan, Myodil), used for myelography until the late 1970s when safe water-soluble compounds became widely available, is known to have caused arachnoiditis, especially if blood was present in the CSF. It is absorbed at the rate of 1 ml per year and evidence of previous oil myelography is still present in many patients. This retained oily contrast has the MRI characteristics of fat (Braun et al. 1986). It is often loculated and may have caused small arachnoid cysts at the points of adhesion, which may further compromise root sleeves.

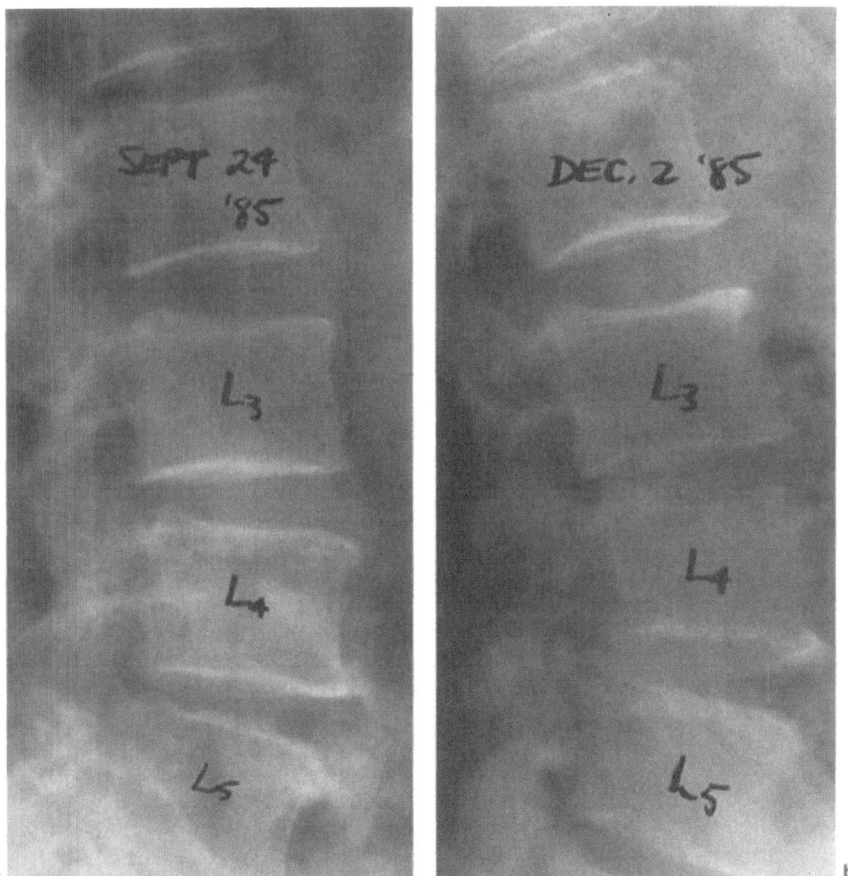

Fig. 9.12. **a** and **b** Lateral lumbar spine views showing discitis as progressive disc space narrowing of L3–4, with demineralization of the adjoining end plates, following L3 to L5 laminectomy for spinal stenosis in a 65-year-old man.

Rheumatoid Arthritis

Rheumatoid arthritis is another condition which has greatly benefited from the advent of MRI as pannus can now be readily discerned and its effect on the thecal sac observed. Abnormal mobility due to ligamentous laxity or disruption is best assessed with flexion and extension views. Plain films, tomography, and CT scans show the bone changes to best advantage.

Synovial hypertrophy, joint effusion, and cartilage thinning are better appreciated on MRI (Beltran et al. 1987). Sagittal MRI of the cervicomedullary junction in one group of 15 patients showed that those with a cervicomedullary angle of less than 135 degrees had brain stem compression, cervical myelopathy or C2 radicular pain, and all were neurologically abnormal. Purely bone changes such as apophyseal joint disease, cystic changes of the C1–2 facets, erosion of the spinous processes and the basiodental interval were better studied by other methods than MRI (Bundschuh et al. 1988a,b; Petterson et al. 1988)

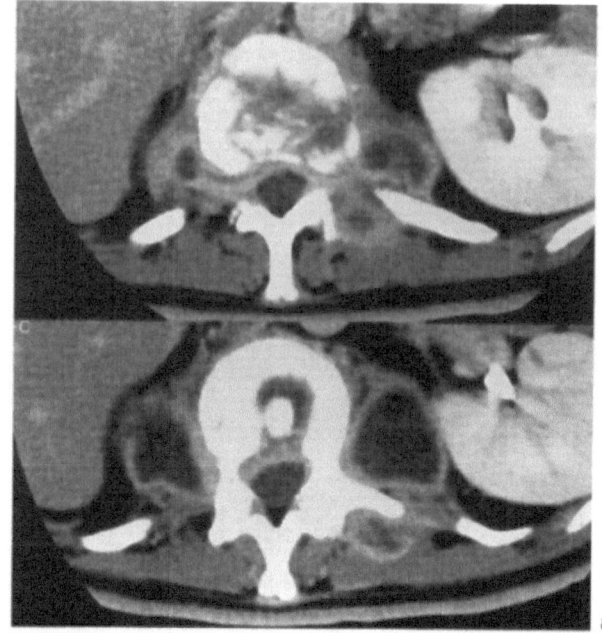

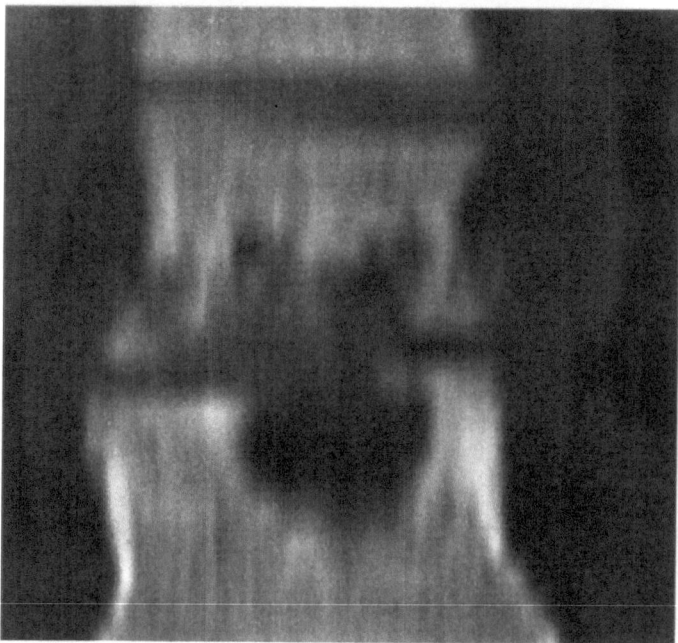

Fig. 9.13. **a** Axial CT scans with intravenous contrast enhancement, showing bilateral psoas abscesses with T12–L1 tuberculous discitis in a 37-year-old man presenting with low back pain, gradual weight loss, and recent fevers and chills. **b** Coronal reformatted image showing the bone destruction of the end plates.

Stainless steel fixation wires used to reduce C1–2 instability may result in poor MR images. For this reason, surgeons are urged to use titanium wires or alloys which do not interfere with the MRI signals. Fixation will not only immobilize the spine and reduce cord compression, but pannus may regress as a consequence, further reducing cord impingement (Mirvis et al. 1988; Larsson et al. 1989a).

Neoplasms

The management of spinal tumours has been altered as a result of improved imaging and surgical techniques (Jeanmart 1986) (Figs. 9.5, 9.6, 9.14a and b, 9.15). Removal of many of these tumours is feasible, the effect of radiation therapy and the follow-up of the consequence of longstanding compressive lesions is now possible. Myelomalacia, atrophy and small intramedullary cysts may be found at the site of compression. Some believe that syringomyelia, which develops months to years after

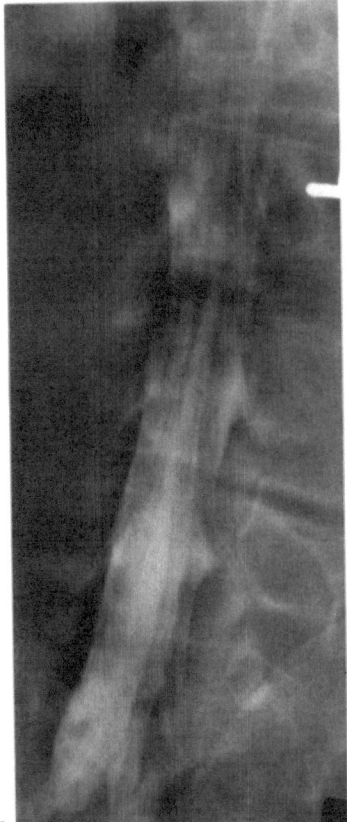
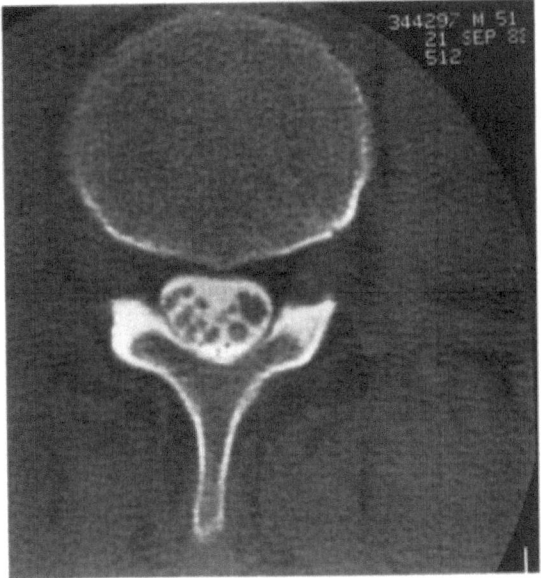

Fig. 9.14. a Oblique view of a lumbar myelogram. **b** axial image of the postmyelogram CT scan showing thickened nodular nerve roots consistent with metastatic subarachnoid seeding in a 51-year-old man presenting with weakness and pain in his legs, who had an adenoid cystic carcinoma of his larynx removed one year ago.

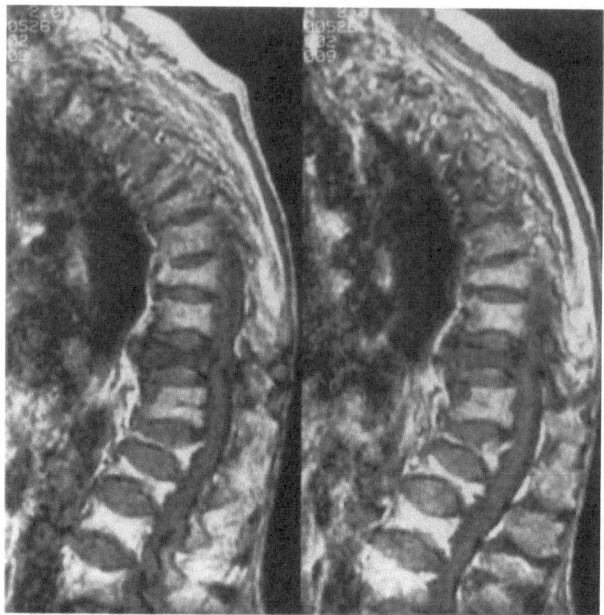

Fig. 9.15. Sagittal MRI of the thoracic spine showing breast carcinoma metastasis in T10 and T11 replacing normal bone marrow, with cord compression at T10 and severe compression fractures of T12 and L1, with normal marrow, in a 78-year-old woman with urinary symptoms.

removal of the mass, has its origin in these areas of abnormal tissue (Castillo et al. 1987). Early detection of such syrinxes and their treatment may prevent progression and result in maintenance of neurological function. Clinical deterioration can also be due to tumour recurrence which can be detected and in some cases removed, with preservation or restoration of function.

Myelography is traditionally used to confirm the level of spinal block often caused by epidural spread of metastatic tumour, the most common type of spinal neoplasm. Intradural masses can be sharply demarcated and the extent of intramedullary expansion visualized. Contrast administered via a lumbar puncture can be supplemented by further water-soluble contrast injected at the C1–2 level. The entire length of the subarachnoid space is thus evaluated and the level and number of spinal segments involved determined, to limit the number of decompressive laminectomies or to define radiation portals.

CT scanning following a myelogram sometimes discloses an incomplete block where the myelogram suggested it was complete. This is because very small amounts of contrast passing beyond the block can be detected by CT. A C1–2 puncture can be averted in these patients when the limits and the character of the mass have been satisfactorily shown on CT.

Intravenously enhanced CT can be used to localize the solid component of an intramedullary mass, or extraspinal extension of an intradural extramedullary tumour. Epidural and paravertebral masses, especially when associated with bone destruction, are also well shown (Lapointe et al. 1986; Shapiro et al. 1986).

Spinal angiography is performed when the presence of a haemangioblastoma is suspected in isolation or associated with von Hippel–Lindau disease. Single or multiple tumours may be intramedullary or extramedullary. A cyst may be associated with the tumours nodule, as in cerebellar haemangioblastoma, and be responsible for most of the symptoms including an ascending deficit due to cephalad progression of the "syrinx" (Rebner and Gebarski 1985).

MRI delineates intramedullary masses very well and provides more information than other imaging modalities (DiChiro et al. 1985; Carsin et al. 1987). Ependymomas and astrocytomas comprise 90% of all intramedullary tumours. Of these, 30%–50% have one or more cysts adjacent to the solid portion. These cysts, of variable size, can be proximal and/or distal to the solid component. Enhancement with gadolinium DTPA demarcates the tumour nodule to best advantage (Sze et al. 1988a,b; Valk 1988; Parizel et al. 1989). Evidence of prior haemorrhage within a tumour is seen on MRI as well as peritumoural oedema. Calcification, rare in spinal tumours and found most commonly in schwannoma and meningioma, is not easily detected on MRI. CT scan is the most sensitive method for the detection of calcium.

Leptomeningeal metastatic disease may be subtle. On myelography or on intrathecally enhanced CT, small tumour nodules along the margins of the dural sac, irregularity and/or nodularity of cord or nerve roots, are considered diagnostic (Fig. 9.14a and b). Early experience with MRI was discouraging, but new imaging sequences and the use of gadolinium DTPA have greatly increased the diagnostic yield (Smoker et al. 1987; Krol et al. 1988; Sze et al. 1988a,b; Carmody et al. 1989).

Ultrasound of spinal tumours is utilized intraoperatively to localize the solid component within an expanded cord. Small cysts may be detected which were not apparent on MRI (Goy et al. 1986).

Multiple Sclerosis

Multiple Sclerosis (MS) remains a diagnostic dilemma. While only 15%–20% of patients present with purely spinal symptoms, investigation of the patient for silent cerebral plaques has proved useful and an aid to diagnosis (Edwards et al. 1986). Spinal plaques are only very rarely visible on CT scan obtained with a double dose delay technique (scan obtained 45 minutes after injection of 84 g of iodine), the technique most commonly used to demonstrate cerebral plaques. MRI consistently shows intracranial plaques better than CT. In the event of a normal cerebral MRI study, a spinal study should be performed, as plaques may be demonstrated in the cord. The MS plaques are seen as high signal intensity and with the improved resolution of grey and white matter of the cord, it may be possible to correlate the clinical findings with the actual spinal tracts involved, similar to what is possible in the brain, bearing in mind that the appearance of cerebral lesions wax and wane with time and that the location of cerebral plaques does not always correlate with symptoms and/or signs. Gadolinium DTPA may prove useful to study the activity of the plaques (Larsson 1989b). These MRI studies have disclosed the presence of unrecognized herniated thoracic discs in some patients presumed to have MS. No doubt a large number of asymptomatic disc herniations will also be discovered.

Myelography was traditionally used in suspected spinal MS to rule out compressive lesions such as disc herniation or foramen magnum meningioma. Dural arteriovenous fistulas (Fig. 9.8) are another mimic of spinal MS, increasingly diagnosed since the use of water-soluble contrast for myelography became widespread in the late 1970s. Presenting as paraparesis, paraesthesias, sphincter disturbance, sensory deficits or muscle atrophy, usually in middle age, the effects of these arteriovenous shunts can be arrested or reversed with surgery and/or embolization. Congestion of the spinal cord and resulting hypoxia caused by interference with normal venous drainage by the arteriovenous shunt is believed responsible for the symptoms. Myelography, and in some cases MRI, discloses the presence of tortuous draining veins, usually on the dorsal aspect of the cord. Only spinal angiography will accurately outline the vascular supply of the dural nidus, originating from one or more radicular branches of a segmental artery. Spinal angiography should not be carried out when tortuous and moderately dilated vessels on the dorsal aspect of the thoracolumbar enlargement are found incidentally, and in the absence of suggestive symptoms or signs of a fistula, as these "varices" may be a normal finding (N'Diaye et al. 1984; Thron 1988).

Conclusion

Development of CT in the 1970s resulted in the first cross-sectional images of the brain. Development of MRI in the 1980s has furthered the evaluation of the spinal cord and its adjoining structures. Resolution of spinal cord cross-sectional anatomy is approaching that of brain. MRI has improved our understanding of CSF flow dynamics. By revealing the temporal alterations in multiple sclerosis, it is helping to elucidate the pathophysiology of this disorder and to discern the effects of various therapies.

Improved knowledge of spinal anatomy, pathology, and physiology is largely responsible for the favourable outcome of many of these patients who are now treated more aggressively than in the past.

References

Atlas SW, Regenbogen V, Rogers LF, Kim KS (1986) Radiographic characteristics of burst fractures of the spine. AJNR 7:675–682; AJR 147:575–582

Aubin ML, Balériaux D, Cosnard G, et al. (1987) MRI in syringomyelia of congenital, infectious traumatic or idiopathic origin. A study of 142 cases. J Neuroradiol 14:313–336

Banna M (1985) Clinical radiology of the spine and spinal cord. Aspen Systems Corp, Rockville, Maryland

Barkovich AJ, Wippold FJ, Sherman JL, Citrin CM (1986) Significance of cerebellar tonsillar position on MRI. AJNR 7:795–799

Beltran J, Caudill JL, Herman LA, et al. (1987) Rheumatoid arthritis: MR imaging manifestations. Radiology 165:153–157

Bonneville JF, Runge M, Cattin F, Potelon P, Tang Y-S (1989) Extraforaminal lumbar disc herniations: CT demonstration of Sharpey's fibers avulsion. Neuroradiology 31:71–74

Braun IF, Hoffman Jr JC, David PC, Landman JA, Tindall GT (1985) Contrast enhancement in CT differentiation between recurrent risk herniation and postoperative scar: prospective study. AJNR 6:607–612; AJR 145:785–790

Braun IF, Malko JA, Davis PC, Hoffman Jr JF, Jacobs LH (1986) The behavior of pantopaque on MR: in vivo and in vitro analyses. AJNR 7:997–1001

Brown BM, Schwartz RH, Frank E, Blank NK (1988) Preoperative evaluation of cervical radiculopathy and myelopathy by surface-coil MR imaging. AJNR 9:859–866; AJR 151:1205–1212

Bundschuh CV, Modic MT, Ross JS, Masaryk TJ, Bohlman H (1988a) Epidural fibrosis and recurrent disc herniation in the lumbar spine. MR imaging assessment. AJNR 9:169–178; AJR 150:923–932

Bundschuh C, Modic MT, Kearney F, Morris R, Deal C (1988b) Rheumatoid arthritis of the cervical spine: surface coil MR imaging. AJNR 9:565–571; AJR 151:181–187

Burke DR, Brant-Zawadzki M (1985) CT of pyogenic spine infection. Neuroradiology 27:131–137

Carmody RF, Yang PJ, Seeley GW, Seeger JF, Unger EC, Johnson JE (1989) Spinal cord compression due to metastatic disease: diagnosis with MR imaging versus myelography. Radiology 173:225–229

Carsin M, Gandon Y, Rolland Y, Simon J (1987) MRI of the spinal cord: intramedullary tumors. J Neuroradiol 14:337–349

Carvlin MJ, Asato R, Hackney DB, Kassab E, Joseph PM (1989) High-resolution MR of the spinal cord in humans and rats. AJNR 10:13–17

Castillo M, Quencer RM, Green BA, Montalvo BM (1987) Syringomyelia as a consequence of compressive extramedullary lesions: postoperative clinical and radiological manifestations. AJNR 8:973–978; AJR 150:391–396

Curtin AJ, Chakeres DW, Bulas R, Boesel CP, Finneran M, Flint E (1989) MR imaging artifacts of the axial internal anatomy of the cervical spinal cord. AJNR 10:19–26

Czervionke LF, Daniels DL, Ho PSP, et al. (1988) The MR appearance of gray and white matter in the cervical spinal cord. AJNR 9:557–562

Denis F (1983) The three column spine and its significance in the classification of acute thoracolumbar injuries. Spine 8:817–831

DiChiro G, Doppman JL, Dwyer AJ, et al. (1985) Tumors and arteriovenous malformations of the spinal cord: assessment using MR. Radiology 156:689–697

Donaldson I, Gibson R (1982) Spinal cord atrophy associated with arachnoiditis as demonstrated by computed tomography. Neuroradiology 24:101–105

Donovan-Post JM (1984) Computed tomography of spinal trauma. In: Donovan-Post JM (ed) Computed tomography of the spine. Williams and Wilkins, Baltimore, London, pp 765–808

Dunsker SB, Schmidek HH, Frymoyer J, Kahn E (eds) (1986) The unstable spine (thoracic, lumbar and sacral regions). Grune and Stratton, Orlando, New York

Edwards MK, Farlow MR, Stevens JC (1986) Cranial MR in spinal cord MS: diagnosing patients with isolated spinal cord symptoms. AJNR 7:1003–1005

Gehweiler Jr JA, Osborne RL, Becker RF (1980) The radiology of vertebral trauma. Sauders, Philadephia

Goy AM, Pinto RS, Raghavendra BN, Epstein FJ, Kricheff II (1986) Intramedullary spinal cord tumors: MR imaging, with emphasis on associated cysts. Radiology 161:381–386

Hedberg MC, Drayer BP, Flom RA, Hodak JA, Bird CR (1988) Gradient echo (GRASS) MR imaging in cervical radiculopathy. AJNR 9:145–151; AJR 150:683–689

Ho PSP, Yu S, Sether LA, Wagner M, Ho K-C, Haughton VM (1988) Progressive and regressive changes in the nucleus pulposus. Part I. The neonate. Radiology 169:87–92

Hochhauser L, Kieffer SA, Cacayorin ED, Petro GR, Teller WF (1988) Recurrent postdiskectomy low back pain. MR-surgical correlation. AJNR 9:769–774; AJR 151:755–760

Jeanmart L (ed) (1986) Radiology of the spine. Tumors. Springer-Verlag, Berlin, Heidelberg, New York, Tokyo

Jinkins JR, Whittemore AR, Bradley WG (1989) The anatomic basis of vertebrogenic pain and the autonomic syndrome associated with lumbar disk extrusion. AJNR 10:219–231; AJR 152:1277–1289

Kadoya S, Nakumura T, Kobayashi S, Yamamoto I (1987) Magnetic resonance imaging of acute spinal cord injury. Neuroradiology 29:252–255

Kim KS, Chen HH, Russell EJ, Rogers LF (1988–89) Flexion teardrop fracture of the cervical spine: radiographic characteristics. AJNR 9:1221–1228; AJR 152:319–326

Kopecky KK, Gilmor RL, Scot JA, Edwards MK (1985) Pitfalls of computed tomography in diagnosis of discitis.Neuroradiology 27:57–66

Krol G, Sze G, Malkin M, Walker R (1988) MR of cranial and spinal meningeal carcinomatosis. Comparison with CT and myelography. AJNR 9:709–714; AJR 151:583–588

Kulkarni MV, McArdle CB, Kopanicky D, et al. (1987) Acute spinal cord injury: MR imaging at 1.5T. Radiology 164:837–843

Lapointe JS, Graeb DA, Nugent RA, Robertson WD (1986) Value of intravenous contrast enhancement in CT evaluation of intraspinal tumors. AJR 146(1):103–107

Larsson EM, Holtås S, Zygumunt S (1989a) Pre and postoperative MR imaging of the craniocervical junction in rheumatoid arthritis. AJNR 10:89–94

Larsson EM, Holtås S, Nilsson O (1989b) GD-DTPA-enhanced MR of suspected spinal multiple sclerosis. AJNR 10:1071–1076

Lee C, Woodring JH, Goldstein SJ, Daniel TL, Young AB, Tibbs PA (1987) Evaluation of traumatic atlanto-occipital dislocation. AJNR 8:19–26

Masaryk TJ, Ross JS, Modic MT, Boumphrey F, Bohlman H, Wilber G (1988) High resolution MR imaging of sequestered lumbar intervertebral disks. AJNR 9:351–358; AJR 150:1155–1162

Merx JL, Bakker-Niezen SH, Thijssen HOM, Walder HAD (1989) The tethered spinal cord syndrome: a correlation of radiological features and preoperative findings in 30 patients. Neuroradiology 31:63–70

Mirvis SE, Geisler F, Joslyn JN, Zrebeet H (1988) Use of titanium wire in cervical spine fixation as a means to reduce MR artifacts. AJNR 9:1229–1231

Naidich TP, Quencer RM (eds) (1987) Clinical neurosonography: ultrasound of the central nervous system. Springer-Verlag, Berlin, Heidelberg, New York, London, Paris, Tokyo

Naseem M, Zachariah SB, Stone J, Russell E (1986) Cervicomedullary hematoma: diagnosis by MR. AJNR 7:1096–1098

N'Diaye M, Chrias J, Meder JF, Barth MO, Koussa A, Bories J (1984) Water soluble myelography for the study of dural arteriovenous fistulae of the spine draining into the spinal venous system. J Neuroradiol 11:327–339

Newton TH, Potts DG (1983) Computed tomography of the spine and spinal cord. Modern neuroradiology vol 1. Clavadel Press, San Anselmo, CA

Norman D (1987) The spine. In: Brant-Zawadzki M, Norman D (eds) Magnetic resonance imaging of the central nervous system. Raven Press, New York, pp 289–328

Osborn AG, Hood RS, Sherry RG, Smoker WRK, Harnsberger HR (1988) CT/MR spectrum of far lateral and anterior lumbosacral disk herniations. AJNR 9:775–778

Parizel PM, Balleriaux D, Rodesch G, et al. (1989) GD-DTPA-enhanced MR imaging of spinal tumors. AJNR 10:249–258; AJR 152:1087–2096

Pasto ME, Rifkin MD, Rubenstein JB, Northrup BE, Colter JM, Goldberg BB (1984) Real-time-ultrasonography of the spinal cord: intraoperative and postoperative imaging. Neuroradiology 26:183–187

Pech P, Haughton VM (1985) Lumbar intervertebral disk: correlative MR and anatomic study. Radiology 156:699–701

Petterson H, Larsson EM, Holtås S, et al. (1988) MR imaging of the cervical spine in rheumatoid arthritis. AJNR 9:573–577

Postacchini F (1988) Lumbar spinal stenosis. Springer-Verlag, Wien, New York

Raghavan N, Barkovich AJ, Edwards M, Norman D (1989) MR imaging in the tethered spinal cord syndrome. AJNR 10:27–36

Rebner M, Gebarski SS (1985) Magnetic resonance imaging of spinal cord hemangioblastoma. AJNR 6:287–289

Resnick D, Guerra J, Robinson C, Vint V (1978) Association of diffuse idiopathic skeletal hyperostosis (DISH) and calcification and ossification of the posterior longitudinal ligament. AJR 131(6):1049–1053

Rogers LF (1982) Radiology of skeletal trauma, vol 1. Churchill Livingstone, New York, pp 273–338

Rosa M, Capellini C, Canevari MA, Prosetti D, Schiavoni S (1986) CT in low back and sciatic pain due to lumbar canal osseous changes. Neuroradiology 28:237–240

Ross JS, Perez-Reyes N, Marsaryk TJ, Bohlman H, Modic MT (1987a) Thoracic disk herniation: MR imaging. Radiology 165:511–515

Ross JS, Marsaryk TJ, Modic MT, et al. (1987a) MR imaging of lumbar arachnoiditis. AJNR 8:885–892; AJR 149:1025–1032

Ross JS, Delamarter R, Hueftle MG, et al. (1989a) Gadolinium-DTPA-enhanced MR imaging of postoperative lumbar spine: time course and mechanism of enhancement. AJNR 10:37–46; AJR 152:825–834

Ross JS, Modic MT, Marsaryk TJ, Carter J, Marcus RE, Bohlman H (1989b) Assessment of extradural degenerative disease with Gd-DTPA-enhanced MR imaging: correlation with surgical and pathologic findings. AJNR 10:1243–1249; AJR 154:151–158

Ruggiero R, Capece W, Del Vecchio E, Palmieri A, Ambrosio A, Calabro A (1981) High resolution CT spinal scanning with ACTA 0200 FS. Neuroradiology 22:23–25

Shapiro M, Kier EL, Reed D, et al. (1986) Intravenous contrast enhanced CT alternative to myelography in neoplasms involving spinal canal (ASNR abstract). AJNR 7:549

Shapiro R (1984) Myelography, 4th edn. Year Book Medical Publishers, Chicago

Sherman JL, Barkovich AJ, Citrin CM (1986) The MR appearance of syringomyelia; new observations. AJNR 7:985–995

Smith AS, Weinstein MA, Mizushima A, et al. (1989) MR imaging characteristics of tuberculous spondylitis vs. vertebral osteomyelitis. AJNR 10:619–625; AJR 153:399–405

Smoker WR, Godersky JC, Knutzon RK, Keyes WD, Norman D, Bergman W (1987) The role of MR imaging in evaluation metastatic spinal disease. AJNR 8:901–908; AJR 149:1241–1248

Sotiropoulos S, Chafetz NI, Lang P, et al. (1989) Differentiation between postoperative scar and recurrent disk herniation: prospective comparison of MR, CT and contrast enhanced CT. AJNR 10:639–643

Sze G, Krol G, Zimmerman RD, Deck MDF (1988a) Intramedullary disease of the spine: diagnosis using gadolinium DTPA-enhanced MR imaging. AJNR 9:847–858; AJR 151:1193–1204

Sze G, Abramson A, Krol G, et al. (1988b) Gadolinium-DTPA in the evaluation of intradural extramedullary disease. AJNR 9:153–163; AJR 150:911–921

Takahashi M, Yamashita Y, Sakamoto Y, Kojima R (1989) Chronic cervical cord compression: clinical significance of increased signal intensity of MR images. Radiology 173:219–224

Teplick JG, Haskin ME (1984) Intravenous contrast enhanced CT of postop lumbar spine: improved identification of recurrent disk herniation, scar, arachnoiditis and diskitis. AJNR 5:373–383; AJR 143:845–856

Teresi LM, Lufkin RB, Reicher MA, et al. (1987) Asymptomatic degenerative disk disease and spondylosis of the cervical spine: MR imaging. Radiology 164:83–88

Thron AK (1988) Vascular anatomy of the spinal cord. Springer-Verlag, Wien

Thrush A, Enzmann DR (1989) MR of infectious spondylitis (ASNR abstract). AJNR 10:880

Valk J (1988) GD-DTPA in MR of spinal lesions. AJNR 9:345–350; AJR 150:1163–1168

Vlezina JL, Fontaine S, Laperriere J (1989) Outpatient myelography with fine needle technique: an appraisal. AJNR 10:615–617; AJR 153:383–385

Wilson DA, Prince JR (1989) MR imaging of the location of the normal conus medullaris throughout childhood. AJNR 10:259–262

Woodring JH, Selke AC, Duff DE (1981) Traumatic atlantooccipital dislocation: two cases with survival. AJNR 2:251–254

Yang PJ, Seeger JF, Dzioba RB, et al. (1986) High dose IV contrast in CT scanning of the postoperative lumbar spine. AJNR 7:703–707

Yu S, Haughton VM, Ho PSP, Sether LA, Wagner M, Ho K-C (1988a) Progressive and regressive changes in the nucleus pulposus. Part II. The adult. Radiology 169:93–98

Yu S, Sether LA, Ho PSP, Wagner M, Haughton V (1988b) Tears of the annulus fibrosus: correlation between MR and pathologic findings in cadavers. AJNR :367–370

Yu S, Haughton VM, Sether LA, Wagner M (1988c) Annulus fibrosus in bulging intervertebral disks. Radiology 169:761–763

Yu S, Haughton VM, Lynch KL, Ho KC, Sether LA (1989) Fibrous structure in the intervertebral disk: correlation of MR appearance with anatomic sections. AJNR 10:1105–1110

Chapter 10

Clinical Features of Spinal Compression

N.T. Gurusinghe

The term "spinal cord compression" is widely used in clinical practice to indicate the pathological and clinical entity caused by an expanding lesion within the spinal canal. There are a great number of causes of compression (Table 10.1). The pressure effect could be on the spinal cord and/or the nerve roots emerging from the cord. A rapidly expanding lesion will cause an "acute" clinical presentation whereas the symptoms of a slow-growing benign tumour will evolve over a much longer period. Occasionally, "chronic" compression can lead to an acute course usually due to sudden rapid expansion or ischaemia from vascular occlusion. The neurological features are determined by the rate of expansion of the lesion and the spinal level involved. Careful neurological assessment will localize the anatomical site of compression. There are well recognized patterns or "syndromes" of clinical presentation. Certain diseases display symptoms and signs due to involvement of other systems. Early diagnosis results in a better prognosis and functional outcome. This can be achieved by combining good clinical knowledge with careful assessment of patients followed by appropriate investigations.

Surgical Anatomy

A sound knowledge of anatomy is important in achieving a clinical diagnosis and to perform a successful surgical procedure. Modern microsurgical methods have enlightened surgeons regarding the finer anatomical details of healthy and diseased tissue.

Spinal Column and Cord

The spinal canal extends from the foramen magnum to the coccyx. It comprises 33 vertebral segments named cervical (7), dorsal (12), lumbar (5), sacral (5) and coccygeal (4) vertebrae. The intradural and subarachnoid compartments containing the neural elements end at the level of the second sacral segment. The cord lies within these meningeal sleeves and in a normal adult, the conus medullaris tapers to an end at about the L1/L2 intervertebral disc level (Fig. 10.1). Below this the subarachnoid space is

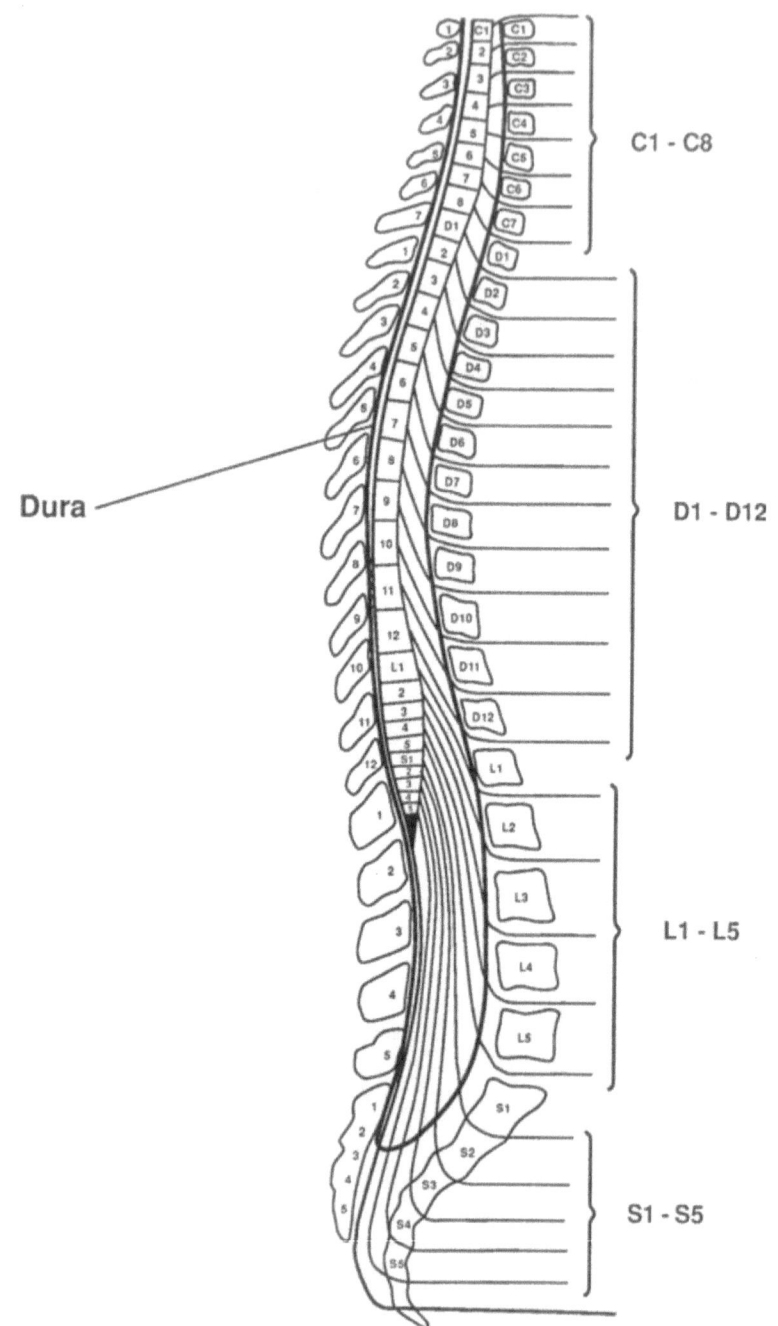

Fig. 10.1. Relationship of signal segments to vertebral bodies. (Reproduced with permission from Duus P., *Topical diagnosis in Neurology*. Translation by R. Luidenberg, drawing by G. Spitzer. Georg Thieme Verlag, 1989.)

occupied by the filum terminale and the lumbar–sacral roots forming the cauda equina (Fig. 10.2). At birth the cord terminates at L3 level, but due to differential growth rates of the cord and the vertebral column, the cord ascends to the adult position.

The cord measures 42–45 cm in men and is slightly shorter in women. It is divided into 31 functional units, but the segmentation is not externally recognizable except by the pairs of spinal roots emerging from each segment. There are eight cervical,

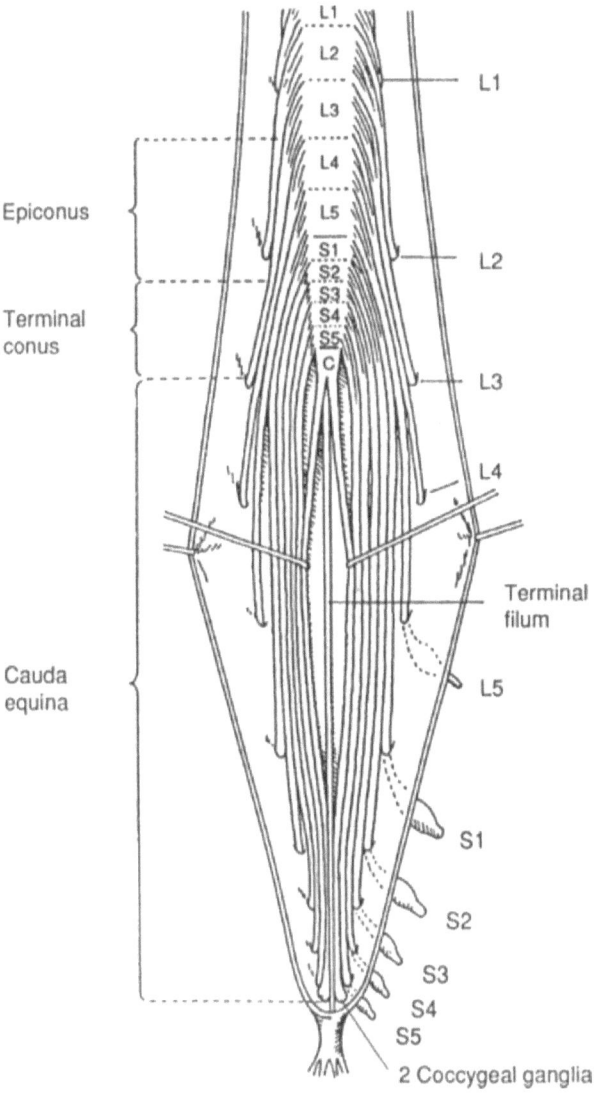

Fig. 10.2. Anatomy of epiconus, conus and cauda equina. Reproduced with permission from Duus P, *Topical diagnosis in Neurology*. Translation by R. Luidenberg, drawing by G. Spitzer. Georg Thieme Verlag, 1989.)

twelve thoracic, five lumbar, five sacral and one coccygeal segments in the cord. The spinal canal has a finite volume akin to the cranial cavity. The longitudinal and axial dimensions of the canal change with movements of the spine and may adversely affect the cord within if an intraspinal mass is also present. The cord occupies less than half the transverse area of the canal. The diameter of the cord averages 12 mm in the transverse plane and increases between C4 to T1 and L2 to S3 segments forming the cervical and lumbar enlargements owing to the abundance of neurones required to innervate the upper and lower extremities respectively. The internal structure of the cord relevant to basic clinical assessment is described later.

As the spinal cord is shorter than the extent of the spinal canal, the cord segments are not situated opposite their corresponding vertebrae (Fig. 10.1). This discrepancy is most prominent in the dorsal region. The dorsal spinous processes slope down-wards and their tips, as palpated by the surgeon externally are situated lower than the corresponding vertebral body. The clinical examination will indicate the level of the tumour according to the spinal segment(s) involved ("clinical level") but the radiologist will indicate the level of the lesion according to the vertebral body oppo-site the tumour ("radiological level"). The neurosurgeon attempting spinal tumour excision must be mindful of this discrepancy of anatomical terminology but tradi-tionally uses the radiological level to plan the surgical approach. It is sound practice to identify the appropriate vertebral level during the operation by a lateral X-ray with a needle marking the relevant spinous process. This will ensure that the bone removal is performed only at the required level/s.

Nerve Roots

A spinal nerve is formed by the union of an anterior (motor) and posterior (sensory) root within each intervertebral foramen. The roots are attached to the cord by a series of rootlets. The ganglion of the sensory root lies within the intervertebral foramen. The roots corresponding to spinal segments C1–C7 leave the vertebral canal rostral to their corresponding vertebrae. The C8 and D1 roots exit rostral and caudal to the D1 vertebra respectively. From D1 downwards the roots exit on the caudal side of the same vertebral unit (Fig. 10.1). The roots are named according to the corresponding spinal segment. Each root is attached to the cord by 6–8 rootlets. The cervical roots lie horizontal in their course to the intervertebral foramen. A pro-gressively caudal course is observed in the dorsal and lumbar–sacral roots because the cord is shorter than the spinal canal.

Extradural Space

The spinal canal is lined with a layer of extradural fat. Benign, slow-growing intradural neoplasms invariably cause pressure necrosis and atrophy of the extradural fat. This is a useful sign to the surgeon in recognizing the level of the lesion at operation. Malignant extradural tumours will change the normal yellow–brown appearance of the fat. The internal vertebral plexus is a system of longitudinal, valveless venous channels in the extradural fat. They communicate with the basivertebral plexus which drain the vertebral bodies and act as an additional system of venous flow to supple-ment the inferior vena cava when this vessel may be impeded due to increased intra-abdominal pressure. Therefore, it is important that the abdomen is kept free of direct pressure during spinal surgery in the prone position to achieve a safe and relatively bloodless field for the surgeon. Spinal frames used by surgeons achieve this in most instances and a 20 degree "head down" tilt of the operating table facilitates this end even further. The internal vertebral plexus communicates with the superior vena cava which drains the breast, thyroid as well as the pelvic veins which serve the prostate gland. This was thought to be significant in the dissemination of secondary cancer deposits from these sites to the vertebrae but it is now believed that arterial spread is responsible. The extradural veins may be engorged due to impairment of flow caused by a space-occupying lesion within the spinal canal.

Meninges

The dura of the spinal canal is an extension of the membrane covering the cerebellum. It extends to the S2 vertebral level and is pierced by pairs of spinal roots at each vertebral level. A dural sleeve surrounds the nerve roots into the intervertebral foramen and blends with the epineurium. It is a tough membrane which acts as a firm anatomical barrier to confine neoplastic infiltration and infection. Yet, it is a pain-sensitive structure supplied segmentally by meningeal branches of the spinal nerves. In disease, dural irritation is a potent cause of spinal pain.

The arachnoid membrane is a much more flimsy but as important to the surgeon treating spinal disease. It also extends into the dural root sleeves. The cerebrospinal fluid is contained within the arachnoid membrane. Its chief function is to contain the cerebrospinal fluid (CSF). This compartment is invaluable in diagnostic radiology including magnetic resonance imaging (MRI). The subarachnoid space allows the surgeon a well-lubricated milieu to handle the delicate vessels and nerves attached to the cord. It also forms an investment around tumours which provides a convenient tissue plane for dissection.

The spinal subarachnoid space extends from C1 to S2 and communicates with the cranial subarachnoid compartment. The space is narrow at the cervical and lumbar enlargements of the cord, but is capacious in the region of the cauda equina. Here, intradural tumours can enlarge as elongated sausages and grow to a large size before becoming symptomatic. In the cervical and dorsal regions however, a tumour will cause symptoms much earlier due to the reduced space available for tumour expansion. The resultant impediment to CSF flow will create a high concentration of protein below the level of the tumour, (i.e. Froin's CSF loculation syndrome). The block will also result in a negative Queckenstedt's test in which compression of the abdomen or jugular vein fails to cause a rise of lumbar CSF pressure. A "dry tap" may result when a lumbar puncture is attempted to perform a myelogram because CSF is scanty below the tumour. Alternatively, a tumour at the cauda equina may be traumatized by the unsuspecting radiologist who attempts the examination. Severe back pain or sciatic pain when CSF is withdrawn or contrast is injected, is almost pathognomonic of an intradural tumour occupying the lumbar spine compartment. Fortunately, MRI has virtually obviated the need for these invasive procedures to diagnose spinal compression.

The pia mater envelops the cord closely and blends with the epineurium of nerve roots. At the conus it extends downwards as the filum terminale. A continuous lateral pial extension stretches between the cord and the dura at each spinal level. The intermittent dural attachment of this membrane on either side produces a scalloped edge and the tooth-like points of adhesion explain the term "ligamentum denticulatum".

The anterior and posterior spinal roots pass on either side of the ligament to reach their intervertebral foramina. Since most neurinomas arise from the posterior spinal roots, these tumours are usually situated posterior to the dentate ligament. The ligament can be safely divided at its attachment to the dura during surgery and used as a means of gentle manipulation of the cord to gain access to the anterior spinal canal. The last dentate ligament is at the L1 level. The roots, dentate ligaments and filum suspend the spinal cord in the subarachnoid space, but allow a degree of movement of the cord within the canal during spinal flexion and extension.

Vascular Anatomy

The spinal cord derives blood from the single anterior spinal artery and the pair of posterior spinal arteries (Fig. 10.3). Their rostral origin is from the vertebral arteries, but the three vessels have several communications with each other via circumferential branches around the cord and at their termination near the conus medullaris. The arterial input to these vessels is boosted at several points along their course by radicular arteries which arise from the vertebral artery and the thyrocervical trunk (subclavian origin) as well as intercostal and lumbar arteries (from the aorta). These vessels will enter the spinal canal via the intervertebral foraminae. Of the 31 such pairs of arteries only seven or eight participate significantly in supplying blood to the cord. The other vessels supply only the roots and meninges. The large radicular vessel usually entering the canal from the left between T12 and L2 is the artery of Adamkiewicz (arteria radicularis magna). This is an important vessel which boosts the blood supply even up to the upper dorsal region. The vascular dynamics of this arrangement creates watershed areas of relatively precarious blood supply. The most important of these is the area between C8 and D4 level which is shared by the rostral subclavian supply and the caudal aortic contribution.

The three main spinal arteries give off deep medullary branches which supply the grey and white matter of the cord. The anterior spinal arteries supply the anterior two thirds of the cord while the posterior vessels provide blood to the posterior columns and the posterior horn of grey matter. A spinal tumour may endanger the blood supply of the cord by compressing the anterior spinal artery. The wasting of the hand muscles (neurones at D1 level) seen in tumours of the foramen magnum may be due to ischaemia from a disturbance of the anterior spinal artery.

The venous drainage accompanies the arterial organization akin to elsewhere in the body. The anterior three fourths drain into channels which converage on a large vein in the anterior median fissure. The dorsal horns as well as the posterior and lateral columns drain into paired posterior spinal veins situated near the entry of the dorsal roots. The coronal plexus of veins surrounding the cord connects these two systems. This plexus drains via vessels which exit through the intervertebral foraminae at several levels.

Pathology and Pathophysiology

Until recently the importance of the spinal cord was overshadowed by the complexity and mysteries of the brain. It is now recognized that the cord is a metabolically

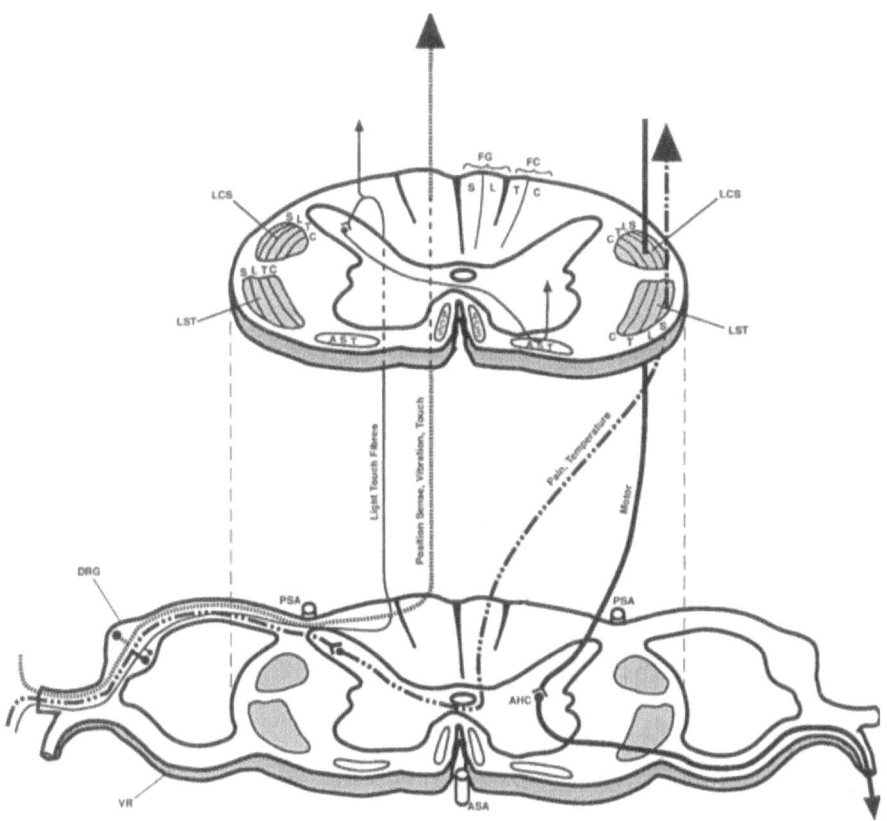

Fig. 10.3 Diagram showing main ascending and descending tracts within the spinal cord and the somatotopic arrangement of fibres in each tract. ——, light touch fibres; ....., position sense, vibration, touch; .-..-, pain, temperature; ▬▬ , motor. ACS, anterior corticospinal tract; AHC, anterior horn cell; ASA, anterior spinal artery; AST, anterior spinothalamic tract; DRG, dorsal root ganglion; FC, fasciculus cuneatus; FG, fasciculus gracilis; LCS, lateral corticospinal tract; LST, lateral spinothalamic tract; PSA, posterior spinal artery; VR, ventral root; S, L, T, C, sacral, lumbar, thoracic, cervical fibres (i.e. somatotopic organization within main tracts).

active structure which is vulnerable to damage due to inadvertent handling or vascular insufficiency. The blood flow to the cord is similar to brain tissue. Grey matter receives a greater flow than the axons of the white matter because of the higher metabolic activity of the cell. Oxidative metabolism of glucose and an abundant oxygen supply is required to maintain normal function of the neurones (Hayashi et al. 1983). The flow is protected against fluctuations of perfusion pressure by an inherent "autoregulation" mechanism as long as the mean arterial pressure remains between 40 and 135 mm Hg (Kobrine et al. 1976).

The lesions causing spinal compression are numerous. Each is described in greater detail in the respective chapters in this book. It is customary to classify them according to the anatomical compartments in which the lesion is situated (Table 10.1). The mechanisms by which an expanding lesion causes a neurological disturbance are complex accounting for the variety of known clinical presentations.

Table 10.1.   Causes of spinal compression

Extradural	Extradural and intradural	Intradural) (extramedullary)	Intradural (intramedullary)
Disc prolapse	Neurofibroma	Neurofibroma	Astrocytoma
Secondary tumours of axial skeleton	Meningioma	Meningioma	Ependymoma
Primary tumours of axial skeleton		Haemangioblastoma	Haemangioblastoma
Abscess including Tuberculosis		Ependymoma	Dermoid and epidermoid cysts
Haematoma		Secondary carcinoma	Lipoma

A more detailed classification is shown in Chapter 30.

Mechanical Compression

The spinal canal is a closed compartment of finite volume akin to the cranial cavity. It contains nerve tissue, meninges, CSF and vessels filled with blood. A lesion which occupies the canal will cause compression of these components. The size and rate of expansion of the lesion will determine the physical force imparted.

Many extradural lesions can present with an "acute" clinical course due to rapid expansion of the lesion. Moreover, these lesions cause earlier symptoms due to the involvement of pain sensitive structures, e.g. dura, nerve roots. An acute lumbar disc prolapse presents with pain due to stretching of the dura (back pain) and compression of the nerve root (sciatica). A rapidly expanding lesion will cause early mechanical compression of all the spinal contents and manifest as an acutely evolving neurological disturbance.

The time course of "chronic" compression allows more time for compensatory adjustment and thereby preserves neurological function for a longer period. The neurosurgeon is often impressed by the degree of retained function despite severe compression of the spinal cord by a benign slow growing tumour (Fig. 10.4). Mechanical compression will impair conduction in nerve tissue. Large diameter nerve fibres such as in the corticospinal tract are more vulnerable to the effects of compression. This will explain the early occurrence of spastic limb weakness in extramedullary cord compression. In this situation, the rarity of lower motor neurone paralysis may be explained by the fact that grey matter is less susceptible to compression than white matter. On the other hand, this is found early in the course of the clinical evolution of an intramedullary tumour which directly involves the grey matter of the cord containing anterior horn cells.

Ischaemia Due to Vascular Occlusion

The lesion could displace and distort arteries and veins which supply nutrients to the spinal cord. This may affect the main arteries around the cord, the penetrating branches or even the microcirculation at the neuronal level. Occlusion of a major vessel will cause rapid neurological deterioration. This is a probable explanation for the acute presentation of spinal compression sometimes caused by extradural metastatic disease.

The microscopic changes observed in compressed spinal cord tissue are compatible with nutritional deficiency due to arterial ischaemia or venous congestion.

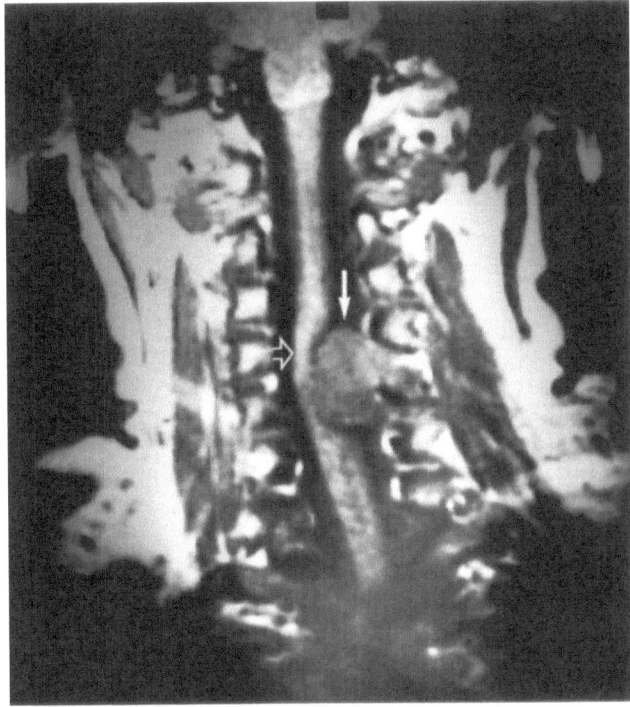

Fig. 10.4.   MR scan (coronal T1 image of cervical cord) showing intradural extramedullary Schwannoma (*solid arrow*) causing severe compression of the cord (*open arrow*). The tumour extends into the intervertebral foramen. The patient was a 55-year-old woman presenting with progressive walking difficulty due to a spastic paraparesis.

Unlike mechanical compression, anoxia is more harmful to grey matter than the axons of the white matter due to the greater metabolic demands of the nerve cells.

All the above factors will contribute in producing the neurological disturbance. Mechanical compression is by far the most potent factor concerned and the relative contribution of each factor varies with different lesions. The compression can involve the cord and/or nerve roots. Therefore, the term "spinal neural compromise" which embraces the above pathophysiological and anatomical concepts is suggested as an alternative to "spinal cord compression".

Clinical Presentation

Strictly, spinal cord compression can only be caused by a lesion situated between C1 and L1/2. Below this level neural compression only involves the roots of the cauda equina. A lesion which impinges on the cord can also disturb the nerve roots attached to the cord at that level. This is most common at the conus medullaris where the cord is surrounded by the roots of the cauda equina. Lesions between C1

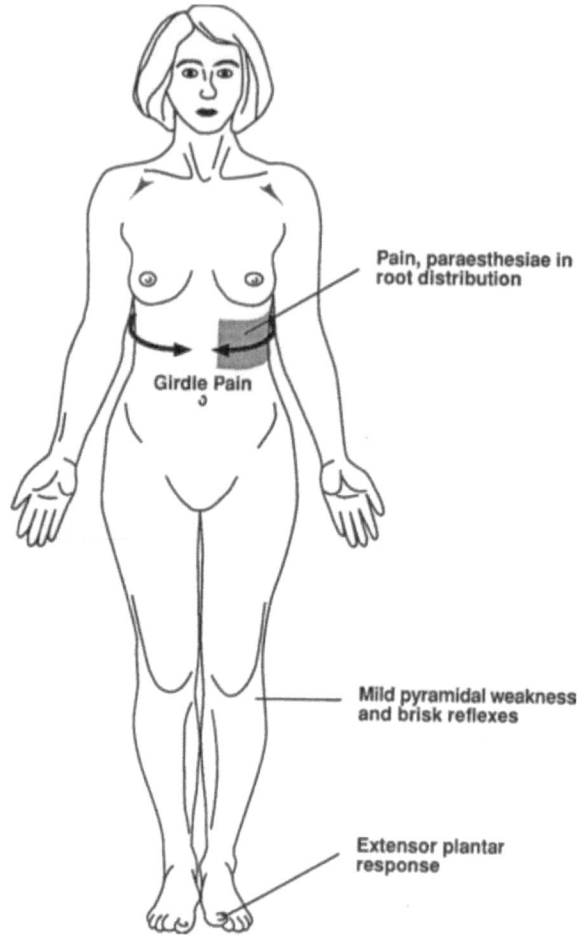

Pain, paraesthesiae in
root distribution

Girdle Pain

Mild pyramidal weakness
and brisk reflexes

Extensor plantar
response

Fig. 10.5. Clinical features of neuralgic stage of cord compression.

and L1/2 sited in or near the intervertebral foramen may initially involve the nerve root only and compress the cord when the lesion encroaches into the spinal canal. Radicular (i.e. root) symptoms are an early feature of most causes of spinal compression. This was recognized by Oppenheim (1923) who described three stages of "cord compression".

1. Neuralgic stage (Fig. 10.5) characterized by root pain in the distribution of the spinal nerve involved. This is a distinct feature of disc prolapse, intradural tumour, e.g. neurofibroma, and extradural metastatic tumours. There may be subtle signs of cord disturbance which can be detected only by careful examination. For the best outcome to be achieved the diagnosis of spinal compression should be made at this early stage.

2. Stage of incomplete cord transection is the commonest encountered in clinical practice. There is a wide spectrum of neurological disturbance involving motor, sensory and autonomic function.

3. Stage of complete cord transection is characterized by the absence of neurological function below the level of the lesion. Despite the wide availability of medical facilities and sophisticated imaging methods a small number of patients have severely disturbed neurological function before the diagnosis is reached.

A high index of clinical suspicion is the key to the early diagnosis of spinal compression. The main feature of the clinical history is the gradual progression of the neurological disturbance invariably heralded by pain. In contrast, primary vascular disease affecting the cord is usually characterized by the sudden onset of a profound neurological syndrome with gradual improvement. Multiple sclerosis causes episodic disturbances especially in the early stages.

The recognition of spinal compression is achieved by applying the art of neurological diagnosis. A careful history of the onset and progress of symptoms will lead the astute clinician to suspect the diagnosis of spinal compression. The neurological examination will reveal the site of the lesion. This process of localization of the lesion begins during the history and is consolidated on the findings of the clinical examination. A knowledge of the anatomy of the spinal cord and its main neural pathways and the peripheral innervation of muscles and dermatomes is essential to enable this task of localization to be completed. Radiological imaging methods to confirm the diagnosis should concentrate on the area of the spine indicated by the clinical assessment. The decision regarding surgical treatment can be merited only when the clinical findings correlate well with the radiological features.

The clinical manifestations of spinal compression can be grouped into four categories:

1. Pain (midline spinal and radicular and central types)
2. Motor (paralysis)
3. Sensory (pain and temperature, position sense)
4. Autonomic (bladder, bowel and sexual function)

The neurological findings will differ to some degree depending on whether the lesion responsible is extradural, extramedullary or intramedullary indicating the transverse (axial) localization. The spinal level of compression will be determined by the longitudinal extent of the neurological disturbance.

Midline Spinal Pain

This is localized to the area of disease in the spine and arises from pain-sensitive structures in the dura and tissues of the axial skeleton. Careful enquiry as to the exact site of the pain is important in the process of localization. Midline pain is particularly common and severe in extradural lesions when it is accompanied by localized tenderness over the related spinous processes. Collapse of a vertebra afflicted with extradural metastatic disease is a potent cause of pain. Careful palpation along the spines may reveal a "step" when vertebral collapse is present. In contrast, a benign intradural tumour, e.g. neurofibroma may be present for several years without causing midline pain. Nocturnal pain or recumbent exacerbation of pain which is relieved by walking should alert the clinician to the likelihood of a spinal neoplasm because this pattern is unusual with degenerative disease.

Radicular Pain (Radiculopathy)

Compression of a root causes pain in the peripheral distribution of the nerve over the myotome or dermatome supplied by the root. This pattern is extremely useful in localizing the spinal level affected by the disease. Therefore, an essential part of the process of localization is to identify the distribution of root pain during the clinical assessment. Such pain is usually aggravated by coughing, sneezing or movement of the spinal segment involved. Upper limb radicular pain (i.e. brachialgia) arises from compression of the C5, 6, 7, 8 or D1 root. Dorsal root pain radiates around the trunk in the area supplied by the corresponding intercostal nerve. Bilateral dorsal root pain may be described by the patient as a tight belt or girdle around the trunk. Unilateral trunk pain may be mistaken as arising from an abdominal viscus, e.g. gall bladder. Lower limb root pain is usually in the distribution of the sciatic nerve (sciatica) or the femoral nerve (i.e. anterior thigh). The commonest cause of radicular pain is root compression caused by disc disease. It is also a classical symptom of a benign intradural extramedullary neurofibroma because the tumour usually arises from a sensory nerve root. Atypical radicular pain in a limb should always raise clinical suspicion of an intradural spinal neoplasm. Incessant dorsal radicular discomfort may be due to extradural malignant disease of the vertebra with collapse of the pedicle resulting in compression of the exiting nerve root.

Radicular compromise also produces sensory symptoms and signs in the area supplied. The commonest is hypoaesthesia (numbness) or paraesthesiae (tingling or pins and needles) but even hyperaesthesia is seen in clinical practice. Objective impairment of superficial sensation in the dermatomal area of the root is to be expected but often absent in the early stages because of dermatomal overlap from adjacent roots. Awareness of the dermatomal map enables good clinical localization of the lesion (Fig. 10.6).

The motor features of radicular compression are of a lower motor neurone disturbance. The muscles supplied display wasting, fasciculation, weakness and a reduced or absent stretch reflex. The limb muscles are supplied by a group of consecutive roots but one root has a dominant innervation (Tables 10.2 and 10.3). On this basis,

Table 10.2. Upper limb muscle assessment indicating root supply

	Flexion	Extension	Abduction	Adduction
Shoulder			Deltoid C5 Supraspinatus C5	Pectoralis major Latissimus dorsi C6, 7, 8
Elbow	Biceps **C5 (reflex)** Brachio-radialis) **C6 (reflex)**	Triceps **C7** **(reflex)**		
Wrist	Flexor carpi radialis and ulnaris C7	Extensor carpi radialis longus and brevis and EC ulnaris C6, 7		
Thumb	Flexor pollicis along us and brevis D1 (C8) Opponens pollicis D1	Extensor pollicis longus and brevis C7 (C8)	Abductor pollicis longus C7 and Abductor pollicis brevis D1	Adductor pollici D1
Fingers	Flexor digitorum profundus C8	Extensor digitorum communis C7	Dorsal interosseii D1	Palmar interossei D1

The blank spaces indicate movements which are absent or can be ignored in routine clinical examination. The root values in parentheses are supplementary.

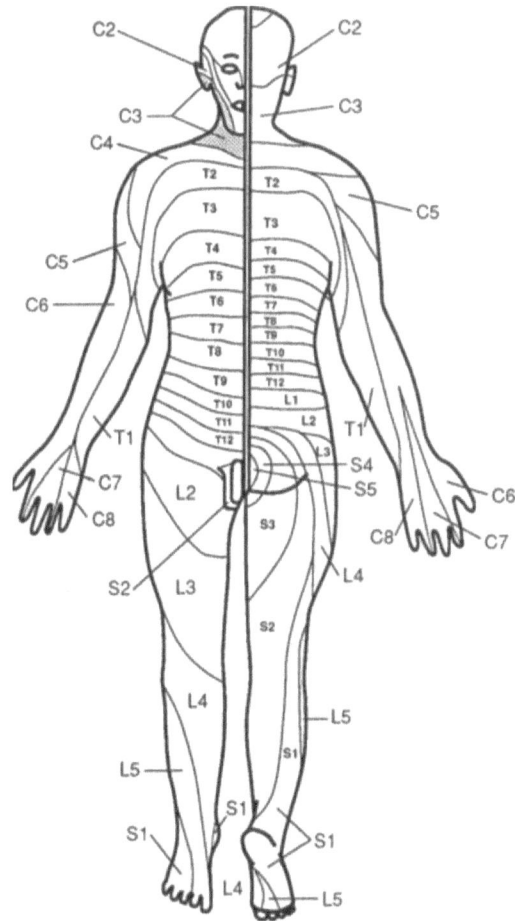

Fig. 10.6. Dermatomal map indicating spinal segmental supply.

Table 10.3. Lower limb muscle assessment indicating root supply

	Flexion	Extension	Abduction	Adduction
Hip	Ilio-psoas L1, 2	Gluteus maximus L5, S1	Gluteus medius and Tensor fascia latae L5	Adductor group L2, L3
Knee	Hamstring L5, S1	Quadriceps **L3, 4 (Reflex)**		
Ankle	Tibialis anterior L4	Gastrocnemius and Soleus **S1** **(Reflex)**	Peroneii L5, S1 (eversion)	Tibialis posterior L4, L5 (inversion)
Hallux		Extensor Hallucis longus L5		
Toes		Extensor digitorum brevis L5		

The blank spaces indicate movements which are absent or can be ignored in routine clinical examination. The root values in parentheses are supplementary.

each tendon reflex has a designated root of major supply. Again, these clinical features provide evidence to localise the spinal lesion.

The clinical features of root compression constitute a "radiculopathy".

Central Pain

Some patients complain of a peculiar discomfort often of an uncomfortable burning quality (dysaesthesia) distributed over a wide area of the trunk or occasionally in a limb. This is usually indicative of disease involving the spinothalamic tracts of the cord and seen most commonly in intramedullary lesions. A tight band like sensation around a limb or trunk results from compression of the posterior columns. They are usually distributed over several spinal segments. Pain of unusual quality and distribution should raise the suspicion of a neoplasm.

Despite the complex neural connections and tracts within the spinal cord beside clinical assessment can be confined to the evaluation of the corticospinal tracts, posterior columns (position sense) and spinothalamic tracts (pain and temperature).

Motor Disturbances (Myelopathy)

The motor manifestations of root compression are those of a lower motor neurone (LMN) lesion as described already. Weakness resulting from root compression is usually a late feature. An intramedullary tumour will disturb anterior horn cells of the cord and also produce LMN weakness. The distribution of this weakness will identify the segmental extent of the cord lesion.

Examination of the limbs to detect muscle weakness should be systematic and performed with a knowledge of the "root value" of each muscle. The upper limb is innervated by C5 to D1 and the lower limb by L1 to S2 roots. Movements are achieved by contraction of groups of muscles but there is a dominant muscle (prime mover) in each action. A spinal motor root invariably supplies more than one muscle. Most muscles are supplied by more than one root but there is a dominant root of motor innervation. This fact is invaluable in localization of the compressive lesion when the muscles affected are identified by clinical examination. It is impractical and time consuming to attempt examination of all the muscles. I have found it sufficient to confine the primary motor examination to a selection of movements which encompass muscles supplied by all the roots innervating the limb (Tables 10.2 and 10.3).

Cord compression causes interruption of the corticospinal (pyramidal) tract/s and results in an upper motor neurone paralysis (myelopathy). Cervical lesions cause quadriparesis and dorsal compression leads to paraparesis. The limbs display spasticity (hypertonia) with hyperreflexia, clonus and extensor plantar responses. In the acute stage the tone is flaccid and the reflexes absent or subdued (spinal shock). Motor symptoms may be the initial complaint. The legs feel heavy and stiff and walking becomes difficult due to easy fatigability. Difficulty in managing stairs and tripping over carpet edges and kerbs occurs due to weakness of foot dorsiflexion. Hurrying or running exaggerates the difficulty and causes falls. The recognition of a spastic gait is an invaluable sign of a cord disturbance. Spasticity involving the upper limbs manifests usually as clumsiness of the hands with inability to perform fine and repetitive movements. A mild weakness of the arm affects fine distal movements prior to the more proximal muscles.

The corticospinal tracts contains about a million axons of neurones arising from the motor, premotor and sensory cortex. The majority (90%) fibres decussate in the medulla and descend in the lateral corticospinal tract of the cord (the axons destined to anterior horn cells serving the upper limbs cross more rostrally than those of the lower limbs). The other 10% mainly innervating muscles of the neck descend ipsilaterally in the uncrossed (anterior) corticospinal tract and cross at a lower level to reach their anterior horn cells. This tract separation is not important for ordinary clinical purposes. In the lateral corticospinal tract the axons are arranged so that cervical fibres are medial and lumbar and sacral fibres are lateral (Fig. 10.3). Therefore, the axons destined to the lower limbs may be more vulnerable to extradural and extramedullary compression explaining the earlier occurrence of spasticity of the legs. The pyramidal weakness affects the extensors more than the flexors in the upper limbs. In the legs, the flexors of the hip, knee, ankle and toes are more affected. The stronger muscles display a greater degree of hypertonia. Therefore, the chronic quadriplegic acquires a posture with elbow flexion and knee extension.

The tendon reflexes each have a cord segment (and root) value. A lesion above C5 will cause all the reflexes to be exaggerated. A lesion below C7 will cause hyperreflexia in the legs only. Cord compression at C6 causes an inverted supinator (brachioradialis) reflex and is of excellent localizing value. The biceps, triceps and knee reflexes can also be inverted with cord lesions at C5, C7 and L4, respectively. Moderate hyperreflexia can be quite normal particularly in an anxious patient. The presence of Hoffmann and Wartenberg reflexes usually indicate pathological hyperreflexia in the upper limbs.

A lesion of the pyramidal tract above D9 abolishes the ipsilateral abdominal, cremasteric and plantar responses. The last is replaced by the Babinski (extensor plantar) response.

Sensory Disturbances (Myelopathy)

This part of the examination needs patience on the part of the examiner and complete cooperation from the patient. Subjective sensory complaints are often not accompanied by concrete objective sensory abnormalities. The sensory modalities useful in clinical practice are proprioception, stereognosis (posterior columns) and pain and temperature (lateral spinothalamic tracts). Assessment of light touch sensation (posterior columns and anterior spinothalamic tracts) is less important in the process of localization sufficient to warrant special attention.

Sensory symptoms are often the first to appear in neural compression. It is difficult to correlate particular symptoms to disease affecting a definite anatomical site but certain patterns are recognized in clinical practice. Spontaneous abnormal sensations experienced are termed paraesthesiae. The common symptoms indicating root compression are tingling or pins and needles. Fine tingling in the hands and feet, tight bands around a limb or trunk, the feeling of being covered with gravel, sand, gloves, stocking or a tight cast and swelling (without visible increase) usually denote involvement of the posterior columns. Hypersensitivity to touch (hyperaesthesia) or pain (hyperalgesia) may be due to root or cord disturbance. Dysaesthesiae are sensations of a burning quality, coldness or of an uncomfortable painful nature implying origin from disease of the spinothalamic tracts. Numbness means impairment of normal sensation (touch, pain or temperature) but is often used by patients to convey the idea of weakness. Lhermitte's sign ("Barber's chair" sign) is an electric shock like sensation traversing along the spine and/or into the limbs on flexion or extension of the neck and is caused by a lesion compressing the posterior columns in the cervical region or demyelination in this area.

Posterior Columns (Fig. 10.3): Proprioception

These contain large myelinated central fibres of the pseudo-unipolar calls situated in the ipsilateral dorsal root ganglia. They convey joint position sense, vibration, discriminatory touch (including stereognosis), pressure and some light touch impulses. The medially situated *fasciculus gracilis* contains fibres from the sacral, lumbar and lower six dorsal segments. The lateral *fasciculus cuneatus* contains the cervical and upper six dorsal fibres. This somatotopic arrangement occurs because the fibres which enter the cord at a higher level displace those which entered below. Both tracts terminate in their respective nuclei in the ipsilateral medulla. The second order neurones decussate in the medulla (rostral to the decussation of the pyramidal tracts) and traverse as the medial lemniscus to the thalamus whence the third order neurones project to the parietal cortex.

These tracts are especially vulnerable to lesions which compress the cord from the dorsal aspect when bilateral involvement is common. Lateral compression causes a disturbance of the ipsilateral tract first.

Disease of the lower limb fibres causes "sensory gait ataxia" because of the loss of position sense. The feet are lifted high above the ground and brought down heavily onto the ground ("steppage gait") The patient is unsteady with the eyes shut (Romberg's sign). The ataxia is enhanced when in a dark room or when washing the face ("sink" sign). If the hands are involved they become clumsy and unable to perform fine tasks such as buttoning, knitting, sewing or tying shoe laces. It becomes difficult to identify an object given to the hand by feeling its shape (astereognosis) or to recognize a letter or number written on the palm of the hand by the examiner (graphaesthesia).

Lateral Spinothalamic Tracts (Fig. 10.3): Pain and Temperature Sensation

These contain unmyelinated and fine myelinated fibres serving pain and temperature sensation. On entering the cord via the dorsal root they ascend in the posterior columns (Lissauer's tract) but soon terminate in laminae III, IV and V of the ipsilateral dorsal horn. The second order neurones ascend gradually crossing the midline within 2-3 spinal segments traversing anterior to the central canal to reach the lateral spinothalamic tract. The fibres are arranged in somatotopic order with the sacral fibres outermost as they reached the tract first. There is evidence that the pain and temperature fibres are also separated within the tract (Friehs et al. 1995). In the brainstem the fibres form the lateral lemniscus and reach the thalamus where the third order neurones project to the parietal cortex.

There are two definite sites at which these fibres are disturbed in cord compression. The decussating fibres are affected by a lesion such as an expanding syrinx or tumour situated around the central canal. This causes pain and temperature loss bilaterally over the dermatomes served by those fibres. The cervical region is often the site of these lesions. The patients present with an inability to feel the temperature of a cup, bath water or radiator. Some especially smokers present with painless burns in the hands. Sensation is impaired over selective adjacent dermatomes with normal sensation above and below. The shape of the sensory loss resembles a "cape" draped over the shoulders and arms. The highest dermatome affected indicates the lowermost cord segment occupied by the lesion because the fibres cross over two or three segments. When the lesion extends to the upper cervical segments and lower brainstem the trigeminal nucleus is also affected. The sensory loss increases to involve the back of the head and the face ("cape with a hood" distribution). The other sensory modalities are not disturbed at this stage and this pattern of "dissociated sensory loss" is typical of an intrinsic cord lesion. When the lesion expands transversely the lateral spinothalamic tracts are disturbed. The medially situated cervical and dorsal fibres are affected first. The sensory symptoms and impairment extend further gradually spreading to the lower dermatomes. This descending sensory disturbance is characteristic. The sacral dermatomes are affected in the late stages only. "Sacral sparing" is a typical feature of intrinsic cord compression.

With extramedullary cord compression the lateral spinothalamic tracts are affected before the decussating fibres. This results in a "sensory level" initially contralateral to the side of the lesion because the fibres affected have already crossed the midline. The sacral fibres are outermost and disturbed early in the disease. Paraesthesiae and dysaesthesiae are the typical symptoms. They ascend on the limbs and trunk as the lesion expands and the pattern is characteristic of extramedullary compression. There is a band of hyperaesthesia just above the sensory level probably due to the associated radiculopathy. The lesion is located at the cord segment corresponding to the area of hyperaesthesia. With severe compression the opposite spinothalamic tract is affected and the sensory level becomes bilateral. The posterior columns are also disturbed by the compression. Therefore, joint position and light touch are disturbed initially ipsilateral to the lesion and then bilaterally. On occasion, the sensory level is well below the level of compression ("suspended sensory level"). This occurs most often with cervical cord lesions when the sensory level may be detected on the trunk.

Anterior Spinothalamic Tract (Fig. 10.3): Light Touch

The fibres serving light touch enter the cord via the dorsal root. Their central processes ascend in the posterior columns for a short distance. During this course they synapse with second order neurones in the dorsal horn which cross the midline in the anterior commissure and ascend in the anterior spinothalamic tracts. A lesion of this tract in the lower part of the cord may not result in loss of light touch because the fibres travel along two pathways. A lesion in the cervical cord is more likely to cause a disturbance which can be detected clinically as most light touch fibres have reached these tracts at that level. Light touch is not a useful sensory modality for neurological localization.

Disturbance of Sphincter and Sexual Function

Disorders of sphincter (bladder and bowel) control and sexual function are common accompaniments of spinal compression. Their onset invariably signifies decompensation and impending rapid deterioration of cord function. The symptoms are a result of disruption of spinal autonomic reflex pathways and/or their central connections with the higher centres situated in the brainstem, frontal lobes and hypothalmus. These systems are complex and the suggested pathophysiology in disease conditions is often tentative. Only bilateral lesions cause significant disturbance of these autonomic functions.

Micturition

This is a reflex function coexisting with voluntary control so that the individual can respect accepted social behavior relating to this natural act. Therefore, loss of continence is not only a personal nuisance but a social embarrassment. Emptying of the bladder is predominantly controlled by the parasympathetic system which on stimulation induces contraction of the detrusor and relaxation of the internal sphincter. These detrusor impulses originate from cell bodies in the intermediolateral grey matter within the sacral segments S2, 3, 4 ("sacral bladder centre") on receiving afferent input indicating that the bladder is full. They traverse along the sacral parasympathetic plexus (nervi erigentes) to the bladder. The sensation of bladder fullness is conveyed to the higher centres situated in the pons, cerebellar vermis, basal ganglia and the medial frontal lobes by fibres closely associated with the pyramidal tracts.

There are two systems which assist in maintaining continence. The sympathetic innervation of the bladder originates in the intermediolateral grey matter of cord segments D12, L1 and L2 and efferent impulses reach the bladder via the hypogastric plexus. Stimulation causes contraction of the internal sphincter at the bladder neck and relaxation of the detrusor. The striated muscle of the external sphincter situated in the pelvic diaphragm is supplied by anterior horn cells in the S2, 3, 4 segments. These impulses traverse along the pudendal nerves and contract the sphincter. This mechanism maintains continence during coughing and straining and can withhold micturition temporarily even with detrusor contraction.

The common symptoms of disturbed control are urgency, incontinence, acute retention, hesitancy and frequency. The symptoms cannot be used to definitely localize the site of the lesion but certain generalizations can be made based on clinical experience. It is important to remember that through embarrassment patients are often reluctant to divulge symptoms such as incontinence and dribbling. Tactful probing often reveals a worse situation than obtained with a cursory inquiry.

Severe cord compression above S2, 3, 4 will obliterate the normal inhibitory action of the higher centres causing hesitancy or urgency, the latter resulting in incontinence because of reflex bladder contraction. This is called the "reflex neurogenic bladder". The associated impairment of walking ability caused by the lesion often enhances the predicament of the sufferer. This is typically seen in patients with cervical spondylotic myelopathy or dorsal intradural tumour. Compression of the conus medullaris (extradural or extramedullary tumour) will affect the reflex pathway within the cord. Similarly, if the roots of the cauda equina are disturbed (e.g. acute lumbar disc prolapse), the spinal reflex is abolished. Both usually result in acute retention or dribbling (overflow) incontinence ("autonomous neurogenic bladder"). The symptoms become worse when infection is superimposed on chronic retention. Early catheterization is recommended in the acute phase of the illness to avoid infection and changes in bladder capacity. Bladder training including intermittent self-catheterization must be commenced early in the rehabilitation programme.

Defaecation

This is very similar to the bladder mechanism and mediated by the parasympathetic innervation of the rectum and internal sphincter originating in the S2, 3, 4 spinal segments. Fortunately, most patients with spinal compression tend to become constipated rather than incontinent of faeces. The former is far easier to treat and less distressing to the individual concerned. Faecal impaction causes mucosal irritation with the formation of liquid faeces which leads to incontinence especially with concomitant loss of the anal reflex due to the tumour.

Erection and Ejaculation

Erection and ejaculation are mediated by complex autonomic pathways. Parasympathetic impulses originating from the S2, 3, 4 segments of the cord produce erection and sympathetic messages originating from the L1, 2 segments achieve ejaculation with erection. These spinal centres are connected to higher function control by pathways in the central grey matter of the cord. Disorders of potency affect males only. However, lesions affecting the S2 roots will cause diminished genital sensation and thus impair sexual enjoyment in either sex. Cord lesions above L1 can lead to impotence or reflex priapism and lesions involving S2, 3, 4 may produce loss of erection and ejaculation ability. Lesions of the cauda equina can have similar effects but may also cause priapism or spontaneous ejaculation. Careful inquiry into these aspects of bodily function is required in establishing the nature of sexual inability. It must be remembered that psychological and endocrine disease are the commonest causes of male impotence.

Recognized Clinical Syndromes

The lesion causing compression may be situated anywhere in the axial plane in relation to the cord. Also, it may occupy the extradural, extramedullary or intramedullary compartments. Nevertheless, the consistent anatomical organization of cord segments, tracts and nerve roots yield certain easily recognizable patterns of clinical presentation. In practice, it is common to encounter partial syndromes which are variations of the typical clinical picture. It is often difficult to differentiate between extradural and intradural extramedullary compression purely on clinical evidence. On the other hand, intramedullary compression due to tumour, syrinx or haematoma results in a distinctive clinical presentation.

The neurological features caused by an intradural neurofibroma sited posterolaterally on the left at D6, provides an ideal model to describe Oppenheim's three stages of compression. These features could also be present in cord compression caused by a centrolateral disc prolapse at D6/7 causing extradural compression.

Neuralgic Syndrome (Fig. 10.5)

The initial stage of compression will involve the left D6 posterior root with mild effects on the left hemicord. The clinical features can be summarized as follows.

1. Root pain and paraesthesiae around trunk in the left inframammary (D6) region. This dermatomal area may be hypersensitive to touch and pin stimulus.
2. Tight band-like sensations around the trunk affecting the lower costal area (girdle pain)
3. Subtle weakness of left hip flexion (early pyramidal weakness), exaggeration of lower limb reflexes (more on the left), a left Babinski response.
4. Usually no sensory loss can be demonstrated.
5. Urinary hesitancy or urgency will be uncommon.

This is the stage when diagnosis is difficult because the physical signs are not obvious without a careful examination.

Hemicord Syndrome (Incomplete Transection at D6 Cord Level)

With further expansion of tumour the cord becomes more compromised. The left hemicord is more affected but the signs are usually bilateral. The clinical picture is similar but not typical of hemisection syndrome of the cord as described by Brown-Séquard (1850).

1. Left D6 root pain.
2. Pain and temperature sensation lost over left D6 dermatome and right (contralateral) lower limb and trunk up to D8 (the sensory level is below the level of the lesion).
3. Posterior column function impaired in left (ipsilateral) lower limb.
4. Spastic weakness in left (ipsilateral) lower limb with brisk reflexes and Babinski response. The right lower limb is affected similarly but to a lesser extent
5. Urgency of micturition with occasional incontinence.

   Hemicord compression due to an extradural tumour will have a very similar clinical picture. A lesion situated posterior to the cord will predominantly affect the posterior columns in the initial stages. Anterior compression (e.g. extramedullary meningioma) will disturb the spinothalamic and pyramidal tracts before producing an impairment of position sense.

Complete Transection Syndrome (at D6 level)

The transition from the first to the final stage occurs slowly with benign extramedullary compression and more rapidly with extradural malignant tumours. All motor and sensory function is lost below the level of the lesion.

1. Bilateral sensory level at D6 below which all modalities are either severely impaired or absent. A zone of hyperaesthesia may be present at the upper part of the area of sensory loss. The upper margin of this represents the true sensory

level and the level of the tumour. In extradural cord compression, sensation is often preserved over the lower sacral segments (sacral sparing)

2. Spastic paraplegia (flaccidity and areflexia in the stage of spinal shock)
3. Urgency with incontinence or acute retention of urine

Cervical Cord Compression

Cord compression between C5 to D1 (cervical enlargement) produces a clinical picture which is different from that due to a lesion in the high cervical or foramen magnum area. Therefore, the features of the latter will be considered separately. The neurological picture is characterized by the mixed upper and lower motor neurone disturbance of the upper limbs associated with a spastic paraparesis. This radiculomyelopathy occurs with an intradural extramedullary neurofibroma or extradural compression due to cervical spondylosis. Spondylosis can produce a pure myelopathy without radicular features.

1. The radicular pain is situated along the radial (C5, 6) medial (C8, D1) or posterior (C6, 7) border of an upper limb (Fig. 10.6). Root pain from C6 and C7 can also be felt at the ipsilateral medial scapular border. The root area may be anaesthetic or hyperaesthetic. The muscles supplied by each root affected may be painful and even tender in addition to being weak and wasted. The corresponding tendon reflex is depressed or absent (Table 10.2). These effects are ipsilateral and at the level of the lesion.
2. Spastic quadriparesis/plegia (with lower motor features in those upper limb muscles affected by root involvement). The reflexes are brisk below the level of the lesion ("reflex level"). With compression at C5, 6 the supinator jerk may be inverted. Hyperreflexia in the upper limbs is manifested by finger jerks, positive Hoffman reflexes and Wartenberg's sign. The plantar responses are extensor.
3. The sensory level is usually at the level of compression. It may be on the trunk in some cases ("suspended sensory level"). Also, sacral sparing is possible because these fibres are outermost in the lateral spinothalamic tract. Loss of position sense occurs initially in the lower limbs.
4. A Horner's syndrome can be observed in lesions between C8 and D2 due to interruption of the cervical sympathetic pathway within the cord or from extraspinal involvement of the stellate ganglion.
5. Urinary urgency and/or incontinence.
6. Lesions at C3, 4, 5 will cause abdominal breathing due to paralysis of the diaphragm.
7. Lhermitte's sign

Extramedullary Foramen Magnum and High Cervical Cord Compression

This region is clinically very important because the main causes of cord compression are (a) benign neoplasms, (b) spondylotic(disc) compression at C3/4, (c) rheumatoid pannus at C1/2 associated with atlantoaxial instability and

(d) cerebellar ectopia associated with Arnold–Chiari malformation. The typical clinical picture is well described but easily overlooked without careful clinical assessment. The region of the foramen magnum is difficult to visualize by routine radiological methods. Therefore, once clinical suspicion has been alerted the process of investigations must be pursued diligently to conclude or exclude the diagnosis. It is possible to be distracted by an incidental midcervical disc prolapse seen on radiographs. Accepting this diagnosis and missing the tumour will have disastrous consequences to the patient. MRI is essential in investigating this region of the spine (Fig. 10.7).

The clinical picture is as expected by the anatomical structures being compressed. In essence foramen magnum lesions involve the lower brainstem, cerebellum and cranial nerves (IX, X, XI, XII), in addition to the upper part of the spinal cord. High cord lesions rostral to the upper limb outflow inevitably causes a spastic quadriparesis and pathologically brisk tendon reflexes in all limbs. The cranial nerves affected are V (trigeminal nucleus in upper cervical cord) and XI because the spinal accessory nerve arises from C2, 3, 4. Although lower motor type weakness is not expected, wasting of the small hand muscles is well described, probably occurring due to

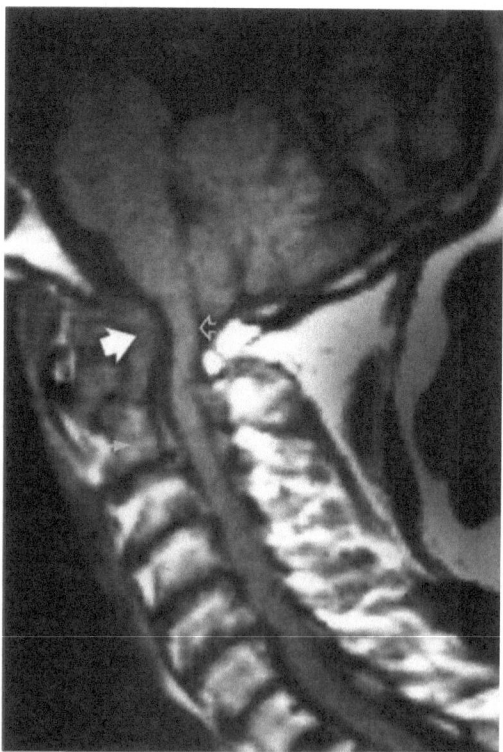

Fig. 10.7.   MR scan (T1 image) of craniocervical junction showing rheumatoid pannus (*large solid arrow*) situated anterior to the spinal cord (*open arrow*) at the foramen magnum. The C2 vertebra is indicated by the *small solid arrow*.

remote ischaemia caused by compression of the anterior spinal arteries. Any combination of the following list of clinical features is possible:

1. Suboccipital pain often radiating towards the vertex (C2 root pain), commonly associated with neck stiffness due to spasm of paraspinal muscles. It is important to localize the pain to the high cervical region.
2. Wasting of suboccipital, paraspinal neck muscles, sternomastoid and trapezius muscles noticeable especially if it occurs unilaterally. Also weakness of the sternomastoid and trapezius muscles often causing a head tilt (torticollis) and weakness of head turning movements and elevation of the shoulder. These features are due to involvement of the motor roots of C2, 3, 4 and the XI cranial nerve.
3. Wasting and paralysis of the tongue, hoarse voice and swallowing difficulty (bulbar paresis).
4. Spastic quadriparesis with brisk reflexes in all four limbs with Babinski responses.
5. Wasting of the small hand muscles (with mild weakness).
6. Downbeat nystagmus on horizontal gaze.
7. Acroparaesthesiae (tingling) in the fingertips is common. Impairment of position sense worse in the hands than in the feet. Stereoanaesthesia is present in the hands.
8. Spinothalamic sensory level at C2 or C3 but since the trigeminal sensory nucleus occupies the upper cervical cord, facial sensation can also be disturbed. Accurate knowledge of the dermatomal map and careful testing are essential to detect sensory levels over the neck and scalp.
9. Mild cerebellar ataxia.
11. Pseudo-tremor of the hands.

Dorsal Cord Compression

The following clinical features are possible in addition to those described at the beginning of this section.

1. Radicular pain is of intercostal nerve distribution (intercostal neuralgia). Unilateral pain can be mistaken for being of visceral origin. Bilateral pain is felt like a tight belt or girdle discomfort. The motor disturbance of root compression is difficult to detect.
2. Spastic paraparesis with brisk reflexes and Babinski responses. The ipsilateral abdominal reflexes are lost in cord lesions above D9 or if the D8 to D12 roots are involved with tumour.
3. Sensory level to pain on the trunk about two segments below the level of the lesion, or a suspended level below groin (D12) level. Physiological sensory levels exist because the supraclavicular (C4) inframammary (D5, 6) and groin (D12) regions are more sensitive to pain in most individuals. The patterns of involvement of posterior columns and spinothalamic tracts have already been described.
4. The abdominal reflexes are lost in cord lesions above D6 and those involving the D8 to D12 cord segments or roots. The reflexes are normal with lesions below D12.

5. Paralytic ileus especially in rapid compression due to involvement of splanchnic nerves.
6. Urgency/incontinence, hesitancy or frequency of micturition.
7. Lesions above D5 cause autonomic disturbances, e.g. syncope due to orthostatic hypotension or excessive sweating, flushing and bradycardia when the bladder or rectum are distended.

Central Cord Syndrome (Intramedullary Tumour)

Intrinsic cord compression has a unique clinical presentation virtually unknown in extramedullary spinal compression. The common causes are syringomyelia, astrocytoma and ependymoma. They may be confined to one region or extend to involve the entire length of the cord. The lesions originate in the area around the central canal of the cord. Therefore, the decussating fibres of the spinothalamic system are disturbed very early. Initially, the zone of pain and temperature loss which is usually bilateral, is confined to the dermatomes of the spinal segments two or three segments caudal to the lesion because the fibres cross over gradually. As the tumour expands longitudinally within the cord more segments are affected and the sensory loss becomes more widespread, still adhering to a dermatomal pattern. The distribution of the sensory loss is an index of the longitudinal extent of the tumour. No other sensory modality is affected in the early stages whilst the tumour is confined to the central cord. This "dissociated" sensory loss is typical of the early central cord syndrome. An intrinsic tumour of the cervical cord will eventually produce a cape-like pattern of dissociated sensory loss over the face, arms and upper trunk.

Transverse growth of tumour affects the anterior horn cells in the ventral grey matter causing wasting and weakness in the myotomes corresponding to the cord segments involved by the tumour. As the tumour expands longitudinally the lower motor paralysis will spread to adjacent muscles. Further expansion in the transverse plan disturbs the crossed pyramidal tracts producing a bilateral, probably asymmetric spastic paralysis below the level of the lesion. Similarly, the lateral spinothalamic tracts will be affected and the sensory loss will spread caudally following the somatotopic representation of fibres in the cord. Eventually all except perhaps the lower sacral segments will be involved and a sensory level with "sacral sparing" is detected. Even the sacral areas can be anaesthetic in the final stages. By this time the posterior columns are also affected by the transverse expansion and all modalities of sensation are involved so that the sensory loss is no longer "dissociated".

Radicular pain is absent in intramedullary disease. Midline spinal pain sometimes occurs with tumours occupying many cord segments. Central pain is experienced in the late stages probably arising from the disturbance to the ascending tracts.

Cervical Intramedullary Tumour

The cervical enlargement from C5 to D1 is a common site of intramedullary tumours. The clinical features can be summarized:

1. Deep aching or burning pain over the trunk, shoulders or arms involving many dermatomes.
2. Painless burns or injuries in the hands.
3. Lower motor neurone paralysis of the upper limbs.
4. Cape (with or without hood) distribution of dissociated sensory loss followed by sensory level (with sacral sparing). Position sense and light touch affected in the late stages only.
5. Spastic paralysis of the lower limbs with brisk reflexes and Babinski responses (late stage).
6. Unilateral or bilateral Horner's syndrome.
7. Urgency or incontinence of urine/faeces.

When the tumour extends into the dorsal cord the spinothalamic sensory loss will descend over the trunk. The spread of the lower motor paralysis is more difficult to detect as it involves intercostal and abdominal wall muscles. The abdominal reflexes will disappear when D6 to D12 are affected. Weakness of the paraspinal muscles causes scoliosis.

Lumbar and Sacral Compression Syndromes

The anatomy of this region is complex (Fig. 10.2) and the motor and sensory features of compression are dependent on the extent and pattern of cord and nerve root disturbance. The D12 cord segment lies behind the D10/D11 intervertebral disc. Therefore, a lesion between D11 and L1/2 vertebral level can cause compression of the lumbosacral cord (conus medullaris) and the associated roots. Below L1/2 only the roots of the cauda equina are disturbed. The root syndromes arising from this area can be identified by the distribution of the pain and the associated motor and sensory deficits (Table 10.3 and Fig. 10.6). The radicular pain is experienced in the myotome distribution. Therefore pain from L1, 2 roots is felt in the hip/groin (hip flexor); from the L2, 3 roots in the medial aspect of thigh(adductor compartment); from the L3, 4 roots in the anterior thigh (quadriceps compartment). L5 root pain is projected to the lateral thigh and leg and dorsum of foot and S1 pain to the posterior thigh and leg and lateral foot. However, often, L5 pain can also be in the latter distribution because the hamstrings are innervated by both roots. Paraesthesiae or hypalgesia can occur in the appropriate root distribution. The radicular pain of root compression due to tumour is often atypical and different from the sciatica of disc disease and yet increased with coughing, sneezing and certain postures.

The pattern of muscle paralysis is also determined by the level of compression. Cord and root involvement will give rise to a mixed upper and lower neurone paralysis the latter determined by the roots affected (Table 10.3). Compression at the L1 cord level will result in a spastic paraparesis with a sensory level at the groin. Compression at L4 segment will result in a paraparesis which spares the hip and knee flexors. The knee jerks are depressed but the ankle reflexes are brisk and the plantar responses extensor. Cauda equina compression results in a lower motor neurone paralysis.

The midline spinal pain in contrast is worse when lying flat and often wakes the patient at night who then finds relief by walking about. Sensory impairment can occur over the appropriate areas and pain is more reduced than any other modality. Autonomic functions such as sweating and piloerection are absent and the skin may be blotchy and cold. Pain from the lower sacral segments localizes to the perineum, rectum and genitalia.

Several well-recognized syndromes occur in this region. The terminal part of the spinal cord is surrounded by a sheath of nerve roots. Pure intramedullary tumours usually do not disturb nerve roots but an ependymoma involving the lower sacral cord often sprouts through and intermingles with the corresponding roots. The commonest compressive lesions are disc prolapse and neoplasms.

Disc Prolapse Syndromes (Fig. 10.8)

Low back pain is invariably present especially with disc degeneration. Disc prolapse is commonest at L5/S1 and then in descending order of frequency at each higher disc level up to L1/2. The herniation can be central, lateral, centrolateral or extralateral. A lateral prolapse at L5/S1 will compress the S1 root which crosses the disc level traversing to the sacral exit foramen below. The radicular pain (sciatica) will be experienced in the ipsilateral posterior thigh and leg and the lateral sole of the foot. Likewise, a lateral prolapse at L4/5 will cause a radiculopathy of L5. The pain of a lateral prolapse at L3/4 will be in the anterior thigh (L4 root). Thus, the root affected relates to the lower vertebral level. A centrally situated prolapse at either level will occupy the spinal canal more medially and disturb the S 2, 3, 4 nerve roots of both sides and the L5 roots depending on the lateral extent of the lesion (cauda equina syndrome). A combined central and lateral herniation will result in a mixed unilateral root syndrome. An extralateral disc prolapse compresses the root after its exit from the spinal canal. Such a lesion at L5/S1 will cause a L5 radiculopathy. The rule is that in an extralateral prolapse the root involved is the same as the upper vertebra identifying the disc level (Fig. 10.8). A disc prolapse at D12/L1 or L1/2 will give rise to a mixed cord and root syndrome as outlined below.

The clinical syndromes of lumbar-sacral compression can be classified as follows:

1. Intramedullary lesions
    a) Cord between L1–L4
    b) Epiconus (L4–S2)
    c) Conus (S3–S5)
2. Mixed cord and root lesions (extramedullary)
    a) High – involving cord or epiconus
    b) Low – involving conus
    c) Midline – intrinsic conus lesion involving lower sacral roots
3. Cauda equina lesion

Intramedullary Lesion (Lower Cord or Epiconus)

The clinical picture evolves in a similar pattern to that described for cervical and dorsal tumours. An intramedullary tumour can cause lower motor type weakness in

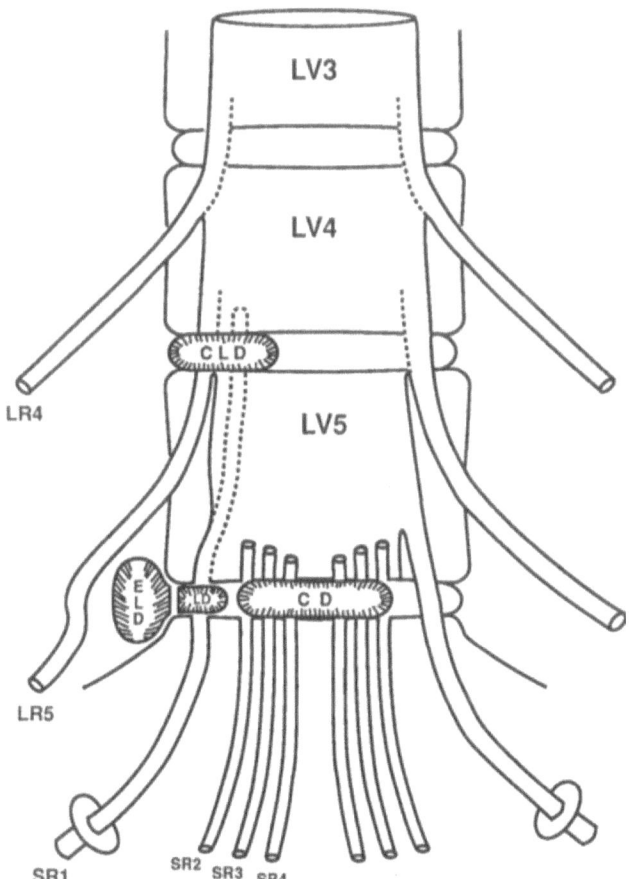

Fig. 10.8. Root syndromes caused by lumbar-sacral disc prolapse. At L5/S1 a central prolapse (CD) causes compression of sacral roots, a lateral prolapse (LD) affects the S1 root and an extralateral prolapse (ELD) compresses the L5 root. At L4 a centrolateral prolapse (CLD) will compress the L5 and S1 roots. LV, lumbar vertebra; SR, sacral root; LR, lumbar root. See text for description of root syndrome.

all the muscles of the lower limbs. The knee (L3, 4) and ankle (S1) reflexes are affected dependent on the extent of the tumour. The spinothalamic loss can spread from L1 to S4 segments and sacral sparing is not common only in the early stages. Bladder and rectal sphincter disturbance is inevitable and impotence is common. The common causes are astrocytoma, ependymoma and syringomyelia.

Intramedullary Lesion (Terminal Conus Medullaris)

The cord segments affected are S3, 4 and 5. The main features of a pure (intramedullary) conus syndrome centre around the innervation of the bladder and rectum by S2, 3, 4 and the sensory supply to the "saddle" area. These are:

1. Saddle anaesthesia
2. Acute urinary retention, incontinence or overflow with retention

3. Faecal incontinence
4. Impotence
5. Absent anal reflexes

An intrinsic tumour of the conus can extend into the extramedullary space and then compress sacral nerve roots. Usually, the root involvement will be bilateral and in descending order of root value. In addition to the features of a conus tumour described above the following can be noted in the clinical picture:

1. Rectal, genital or perineal pain
2. Loss of ankle reflexes
3. Weakness of muscles supplied by L5 and S1 roots
4. The sensory loss may extend beyond the "saddle" area

It is important to note that there is no paralysis of the lower limbs and the ankle reflexes are preserved if the lesion remains confined to the conus.

Mixed Cord and Root Compression Syndromes

The clinical features of this variety of compression are best described by illustrating an intradural neurofibroma arising from the root of L4 on the left side (Fig. 10.9). The root syndrome will comprise the following:

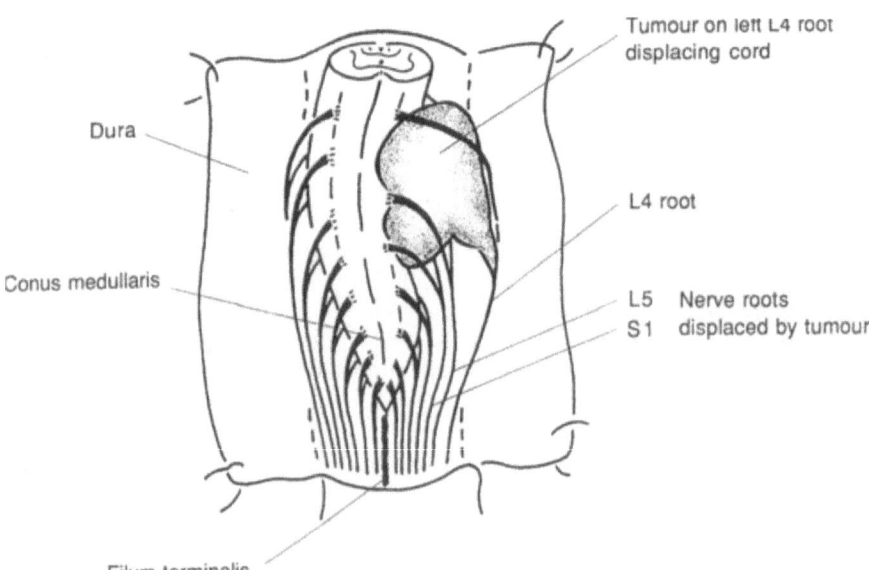

Fig. 10.9. Intradural extramedullary schwannoma arising from left L4 dorsal root causing cord and root compression.

1. Root pain over the left anterior thigh
2. Wasting of the left quadriceps muscle
3. Weakness of left knee extension and ankle inversion (L4 root)
4. Reduced left knee reflex

If cord compression occurs, additional physical signs will appear. These will vary in severity depending on the degree of compression. In the extreme situation complete motor and sensory loss will occur below L5 (cord level) associated with loss of autonomic function. In the early stages however the signs are:

5. Brisk ankle reflexes with clonus
6. Extensor plantar responses

Cauda Equina Syndrome

This syndrome occurs with lesions sited below the L1/2 disc level which can only cause a disturbance of the spinal roots. The L1, 2 and 3 roots exit from the canal above the level of the lesion. The L4, L5 and all the sacral roots have a longer course within the canal and therefore can be affected by compression situated anywhere in that path. The commonest lesion encountered is an acute disc prolapse the clinical features of which have been described above. The capacious intradural subarachnoid space of the canal in this region will accommodate growth of a tumour. The nerve roots become draped around its outer surface. They are capable of accepting some displacement before neurological disturbance occurs. On the other hand, extradural metastases, myeloma and lymphoma occur commonly in this area often associated with vertebral collapse which adds to the mass effect of the lesion. Vascular channels accompanying the roots and the filum terminale may also become compromised and cause further neurological dysfunction. The usual clinical features of a cauda equina tumour are:

1. Radicular pain in the anterior (L4) lateral (L5) or posterior (S1) thigh with paraesthesiae in the corresponding dermatomes. The pain is bilateral in large lesions.
2. Lumbar-sacral back pain especially if vertebral collapse is present. Nocturnal pain is common and in the case of a tumour the pain may be relieved by walking!
3. Wasting and weakness of the muscles supplied by L4, L5, S1 and S2 roots. Absent ankle reflexes and plantar responses.
4. Saddle anaesthesia (S 2, 3, 4) extending into the L4, L5 and S1 segments with large lesions.
5. Urinary urgency, incontinence or acute retention. Faecal incontinence or constipation.
6. Loss of anal and bulbocavernosus reflexes.
7. Impotence.

It is often impossible clinically to distinguish between a tumour of the conus from one arising within the cauda equina.

General Clinical Features

In addition to the detailed neurological examination described above a careful examination of the other systems must be made including the breasts and pelvic structures when appropriate. Shortness of breath associated with signs of pleural effusion or pulmonary consolidation should lead to suspicion of malignancy. Diabetics are particularly prone to spinal extradural abscess. A cutaneous septic focus may be present in these patients. Cafe-au-lait patches and iris hamartomas (Lisch nodules) signify neurofibromatosis. Papilloedema can occur due to associated hydrocephalus caused by the high protein content of the CSF (Raynor 1969). The phenomenon of reverse spinal coning can occur in this situation if the hydrocephalus is treated with ventricular drainage (Jooma and Hayward 1984).

Deformities of the spine such as kyphosis, scoliosis and torticollis can be associated with spinal neoplasms due to the imbalance of muscular activity. The presence of a tuft of hair, pigmented naevus, skin dimple or sinus in the lumbosacral area indicates the presence of spina dysraphism which in turn can be associated with tumours such as lipomas, dermoid and epidermoid cysts. The extraspinal portion of a neurofibroma may be palpable in the neck and occasionally the paravertebral extension of a metastatic deposit in the spine is palpable as a mass. Anterior wedge collapse of the vertebral body due to a metastatic tumour, myeloma or lymphoma may be recognized posteriorly by tenderness over the corresponding spinous process which is often more prominent or sunken giving the impression of a "step" when the palpating finger is run gently along the spines.

References

Brown-Séquard CE (1850) De la transmission crosse des impressions sensitives par la moelle epiniere. CR Biol 2:33

Friehs GM, Schrottner O, Pendl G (1995) Evidence for segregated pain and temperature conduction within the spinothalamic tract. J Neurosurg 83:8–12

Hayashi N, Green BA, Gonzales-Carvajal M et al. (1983) Local blood flow, oxygen tension and oxygen consumption in the rat spinal cord. Part 2. J Neurosurg 58:526–530

Jooma R, Hayward RD (1984) Upward spinal coning: impaction of occult spinal tumours after relief of hydrocephalus. J Neurol Neurosurg Psychiatry 47:386–390

Kobrine AI, Doyle TF, Rizzoli HV (1976) Spinal cord blood flow as affected by changes in systemic arterial blood pressure. J Neurosurg 44:12–15

Lhermitte J, Bollack, Nicholas M (1924) Les douleurs a type de decharge electrique consecutives a la flexion cephalique dans la sclerose en placques; sclerose multiple Rev Neurol 31:56–62

Raynor RB (1969) Papilloedema associated with tumours of the spinal cord. Neurology Minneapolis 19:700

Chapter 11

Electrophysiological Investigation of Disorders of the Spinal Cord

A.A. Eisen

Introduction

This chapter explores the value, and limitations, of clinical neurophysiology in the investigation of spinal cord disease. In an age of gigantic advances in visualization of the spinal cord – made possible by CT scanning and, more so, by magnetic resonance imaging (MRI) – one may reasonably ask what is the role of clinical neurophysiology? The disease specificity of neurophysiology is poor and localization to a single segmental level is seldom possible. However, such techniques can be cost-effective, yielding important information concerning function. For example, after spinal cord trauma it is possible to gauge the extent to which function has been impaired and to comment on prognosis. Many diseases affecting the spinal cord have no radiological correlates. This statement is relevant to: most of the motor neurone diseases, non-structural diseases of the dorsal root ganglion better termed the ganglioneuronopathies, diseases of the dorsal columns such as vitamin B_{12} deficiency and Friedreich's ataxia, diseases of the motor tracts such as latharysm and Konzo and autonomic dysfunction secondary to spinal cord disease.

Subsequent sections consider in turn each of the spinal tracts, the anterior horn cells and spinal interneurones and discuss which electrophysiological tests are most appropriate to examine the various disease states.

Aside from these pragmatic issues much remains to be learnt about the physiological and pathophysiological functioning of the human spinal cord. This is most readily achieved through neuro- (and particularly electro-)physiological methods and the chapter concludes with a short commentary on current research trends in spinal cord physiology. For a digest of the numerous, excellent, past and recent writings on spinal cord physiology and electrophysiological assessment of disorders of the spinal cord, the reader is encouraged to consult the following references: Brown (1981), Davidoff (1984), Ashby (1987), Davidoff and Hackman (1991), Schoenen (1991), Schwartz and Swash (1992).

The Descending Motor Pathways

Motor control is complex perhaps reaching its phylogenetic acme in humans. There are several interdependent (and interconnected) parts of the motor system. They include the primary motor cortex and its surrounds, the pre-motor areas and supplementary motor cortex, basal ganglia, thalamus, cerebellum, brainstem and the reticular formation. The motor neurones of the spinal cord are the "final common pathway" to which these higher centres make direct or more commonly indirect connections. In non-human primates and other mammals several descending tracts converge on the spinal motoneurone (SMN). In humans some of these have been largely sacrificed at the expense of the corticomotoneuronal system. This system arises from cells in the primary motor cortex and is the only descending motor pathway that makes monosynaptic connection with the SMNs. (See Porter and Lemon (1993) for a comprehensive review of corticospinal function in humans.)

The corticomotoneuronal (C-M) system is highly developed in humans and to some extent in the great apes (chimpanzees, gorillas and orangutans). In lower mammals it is largely absent. Their descending motor connections synapse with the SMNs through one or more intervening neurones. In humans the C-M system synapses with the motor neurone pools of all SMNs excepting those innervating the external ocular muscles and Onuf's nucleus supplying the bladder wall. It is noteworthy that these are the only motor nuclei spared in amyotrophic lateral sclerosis (ALS), for which, among other reasons, it has been suggested that ALS, which is primarily a disorder of the C-M system, starts in the motor cortex (Eisen et al. 1992).

The C-M system, which has its origin in the primary motor cortex, is not synonymous with the corticospinal tract which arises from several neocortical areas including the motor cortex, pre-motor areas and primary sensory cortex. Elegant physiological studies performed over the last decade have demonstrated that each corticomotoneurone synapses with many SMNs and each SMN receives input from many different C-M cells. This arrangement of convergence and divergence, which is most abundant for the distal muscles especially of those responsible for hand and facial innervated musculature, accounts for the amazing degree of fractionated movement that humans are capable of. In turn it allows for a large repertoire of different movements involving the same muscle. Corticomotoneuronal control is largely responsible for delicate control of force, precision grip, angulation, rate of change of movement and muscle tension. It is likely that the C-M system is vital in the acquisition of new motor skills, which, once learnt, are relegated to more caudal parts of the nervous system, including the spinal cord. Glutamate is probably the sole (excitatory) neurotransmitter of the C-M system.

It was originally believed that C-M SMN connections were all fast conducting and that the originating pyramidal neurones were all of large diameter including the Betz cells. This would mean that very few pyramidal neurones (< 2%) in the motor cortex participate in a system that has become very important in humans. However, recent evidence indicates that slow conducting, monosynaptic, connections, arising from small diameter pyramidal cells also exist so that it is likely that a large complement of the motor cortical pyramidal cells, in humans, make up the C-M system.

The spinal cord is also responsible for much automated (learnt) movement including walking, running, stepping, hopping and stereotyped responses to a variety of stimuli. Even if it is disconnected from supraspinal input its circuitry is sufficient to generate a variety of automatic behaviour through the implementation of "spinal generators". However, these are much more obvious in lower mammals and other animal species. "A chicken can walk without its head."

In Vivo Investigation of the Corticomotoneuronal System in Humans

The remarkable discovery by Merton and Morton (1980) that it was possible to stimulate the awake and intact human motor cortex opened a new era of human neurophysiological investigation. These initial experiments were performed using high voltage, short duration electrical stimuli making the procedure tolerable but uncomfortable. It has been largely replaced by transcranial magnetic stimulation (TMS). This method is virtually free of any discomfort. It also appears very safe in both the short and long term. Over the last decade many thousands of individuals throughout the world have had TMS. (For recent reviews of all aspects of TMS see: Rossini and Marsden 1988; Lissens 1992; Eisen 1992; Murray 1993; Beric 1993.)

TMS activates the C-M system presynaptically through the apical dendrites of the corticomotoneurone. It is not possible to stimulate descending motor tracts in the spinal cord directly; the current density induced by the magnetic coil is insufficient. Also, most general anaesthetic agents, which act presynaptically preclude using TMS in the operating room.

Nonetheless, Merton and Morton's method originally described for cortical stimulation can be directly applied to the spinal cord. Direct stimulation is readily performed and increasingly used to monitor spinal cord integrity intraoperatively under anaesthesia. In this situation pain induced by high voltage electrical stimulation is no longer relevant. Intraoperative monitoring of spinal cord function is especially important in scoliosis corrective surgery and obliteration of abdominal aortic aneurysms. In the past both procedures were monitored using somatosensory evoked potentials (SEPs) which record the integrity of afferent sensory function. However, SEPs do not provide information concerning the motor spinal tracts which are more vulnerable in these situations.

In the awake subject, many laboratories use TMS routinely to provide indirect estimation of the fast conducting (primarily) direct corticomotoneuronal tract passing through the spinal cord. Motor cortex and spinal roots (to account for the peripheral component) are stimulated in turn whilst recording from the same target muscle (see Fig. 11.1). When the responses are recorded from an arm or hand muscle the latency difference between cortical and radicular stimulation reflects central motor conduction through the cervical cord. Motor conduction through the whole spinal cord can be measured if responses are recorded from a leg muscle. Recording is possible from almost any limb muscle.

It is equally valid to use the F-wave latency to determine the peripheral component of the motor pathway, using subtraction to calculate the central motor conduction through the spinal cord. However, F-waves are not easily recorded from proximal muscles, their latency is inconsistent, and they can only be evoked by electrical stimulation. For these reasons the author prefers to use root stimulation with the magnetic coil to determine the peripheral contribution to the overall conduction time.

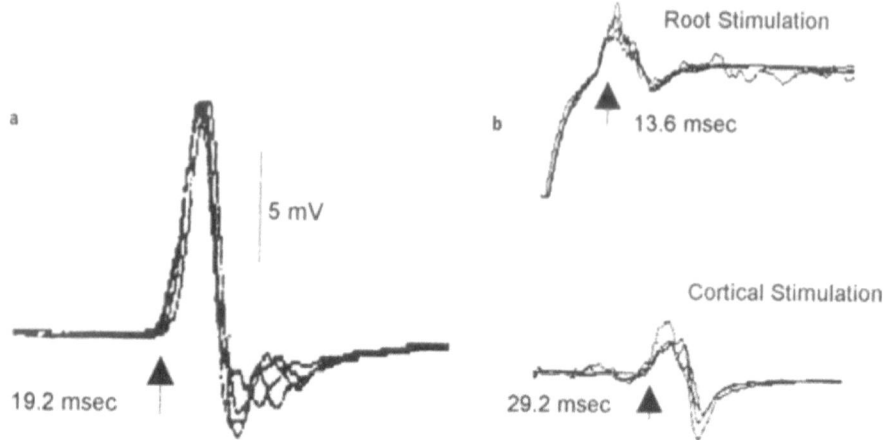

Fig. 11.1. **a** Normal motor evoked potential evoked by stimulation of the left cortical hand area and recorded from the slightly contracting contralateral thenar muscle. **b** Same normal subject. Stimulation of the fifth spinal root (top traces) and left cortical leg area (lower traces). The motor evoked potentials were recorded from the right tibialis anterior. Amplitude calibration as for the thenar recording. Central motor conduction from cortex to the L5 spinal segment is 15.6 ms (normal value < 18.5 ms).

The normal limits given in Table 11.1 were derived from over 500 normal studies. The subjects mean age was 42.7 years (range 17–81 years) and the values are the upper (for latency, threshold and central conduction time, CCT) and the lower (for MEP amplitude and MEP/CMAP ratio) normal limits (±3 standard deviations). Latency correlates with arm length ($r = 0.655$) and to some extent with height ($r=0.420$). Central conduction times also increase by 1–2 ms with age. Age is also a factor in MEP amplitude causing a decrease of about 10% per decade. Side to side differences for latency for a given target muscle should not exceed 3 ms for upper limb muscles and 5 ms for lower limb muscles. The values were measured with the target muscle contracting at about 15% maximum. When measured from a relaxed target muscle latency (and CCT) are longer and amplitude of the MEP is lower. Cortical threshold, which is the lowest stimulus needed to evoke a motor response in

Table 11.1. Normal evoked potential values for selected muscles

Target muscle	Latency (< ms)	MEP AMP (> mV)	MEP/CMAP (> %)	Threshold (> %)	CCT (< ms)
Thenar	25	2	20	65	9
Hypothenar	25	2	20	65	9
EDC	20	2	20	65	8.5
Biceps	15.5	1.5	15	70	8.5
TA	35	1.5	15	70	18.5

Abbreviations: AMP, amplitude; CCT, central conduction time; CMAP, compound muscle action potential; MEP, motor evoked potential; EDC, extensor digitorum communis; TA, three out of five trials of amplitude greater than 50 μV, is always measured with the target muscles relaxed.

Clinical Application of TMS to Spinal Cord Disease

TMS has a particular role in cord diseases that cannot be visualized radiologically. In these conditions, which include, among many others, multiple sclerosis, vitamin B_{12} deficiency, ischaemic cord disease, amyotrophic lateral sclerosis (especially initial primary lateral sclerosis), lathyrism and Konzo, it is often reassuring to both physician and patient to have objective documentation of disease.

Amyotrophic Lateral Sclerosis (ALS) and Other Motor Neurone Diseases

Early studies in ALS employed electrical cortical stimulation. (Hugon et al. 1987) They showed, an anticipated attenuation or in some cases absence of the MEP and prolongation of central motor conduction time in some patients, especially in the lower limbs (Ingram and Swash 1987) (Fig. 11.2). Schriefer et al. (1989) studied 22 ALS patients using transcranial magnetic stimulation and correlated hypothenar MEP abnormalities with clinical deficit. There was only a weak correlation between central motor conduction prolongation and hyperreflexia of the limb including brisk finger flexion. No correlation was apparent between central motor conduction and impairment of fine finger movement or hypthenar muscle weakness. Abnormal MEPs were also recorded in some patients with a normal clinical examination of the limb studied and normal MEPs were recorded in five cases without neurological deficit involving the hand.

Subsequently, Eisen et al. (1990) studied 40 patients with ALS recording from the thenar, extensor digitorum communis and biceps muscles. No responses were elicited in 12 patients with severe bulbar palsy, usually associated with generalized hyperreflexia. In others the main abnormality was a marked reduction in the MEP amplitude (Fig. 11.2) and MEP/CMAP ratio. Latency to all three muscles was only modestly, but significantly prolonged, as was central motor conduction time.

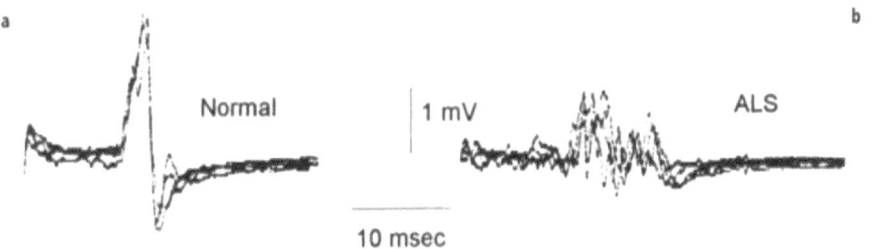

Fig. 11.2. Motor evoked potentials recorded from the thenar muscle. Stimulation contralateral cortical hand area. **a** Normal potential. **b** Small dispersed and slightly prolonged potential often seen in ALS. This is particularly true in patients with bulbar palsy and marked upper motor neurone features.

Recent studies have explored other aspects of the MEP in ALS, particularly threshold measurements, cortical inhibitory mechanisms and the size of the compound excitatory post synaptic potential (EPSP) facilitating a single spinal motor neurone using peristimulus time histograms (PSTHs). Early in ALS cortical threshold is frequently normal or paradoxically even lower than normal for the patient's age (Caramia et al. 1991; Eisen et al. 1993). Threshold, which is a reflection of motor cortical excitability, increases with disease progression and eventually no response can be obtained. It has been suggested that the increased cortical excitability (reduced stimulus threshold) in early ALS might result from glutamate excitotoxicity. Another measure of cortical excitability is the duration of the inhibitory period induced by a single cortical stimulus applied during voluntary contraction of the target muscle. This is shortened in ALS compared to aged-matched controls. Most of the cortical silent period is due to cortical (as opposed to spinal) inhibitory mechanisms and its shortening in ALS may be due to glutamate toxicity.

Postpoliomyelitis Syndrome

This syndrome has been reviewed by Dalakas and Illa (1991). The majority of patients with postpolio syndrome have a history of prior paralytic disease. Some, however, do not (paralytic poliomyelitis develops in only 1%–2% of individuals infected by the virus). In these, a postpoliomyelitis syndrome is most easily explained on the basis of motor neurones being scarred and only later in life succumbing to the interaction of ageing and previous subclinical insult (Calne et al. 1986).

The spinal cord of patients known to have had prior poliomyelitis (with and without postpolio syndrome) shows evidence of perivascular inflammation and gliosis which is disproportional to the neuronal loss. However, there is no evidence of retrograde involvement of the corticospinal tracts even years later (Pezeshkpour and Dalakas, 1988). This makes postpoliomyelitis a good model to compare with ALS since only the anterior horn cell and not the corticomotoneurone is involved. In keeping with the reported pathological findings it has always been possible to elicit a MEP in patients with postpolio syndrome. In 14 patients with postpolio syndrome studied using transcranial magnetic stimulation the amplitude of the MEP was reduced proportionally to the degree of muscle wasting, but MEP/CMAP ratio was normal (Fig. 11.3). Central motor conduction time was normal in all patients. Threshold to cortical stimulation was measured in six patients seen more recently and was also normal (< 65%).

Toxic Myelopathies

Lathyrism is due to toxicity from the consumption of *Lathyrus sativus* (the chickling pea). The responsible ingredient is N-oxalylamino-L-alanine (BOAA) is an excitotoxic amino acid. Lathyrism is endemic in geographic areas subject to famine and drought such as Bangladesh, China, Ethiopia and India. The chickling pea, is a drought-resistant crop, and at times of famine and drought it becomes a cheap and often the only source of nutrition. For unknown reasons the disease affects men more frequently than women and characteristically induces pyramidal leg weakness. The arms are typically much less involved (Spencer et al. 1991). Use of transcranial

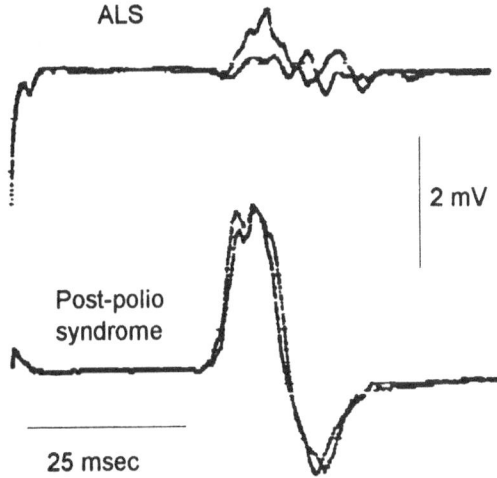

Fig. 11.3. Comparison of motor evoked potentials in ALS (top traces) and postpoliomyelitis syndrome (lower traces). Both sets were recorded from the tibialis anterior stimulating the cortical leg area. Despite having had severe poliomyelitis about 30 years prior to the study the potential recorded from the patient with postpoliomyelitis is normal, That from the patient with ALS is reduced in amplitude and slightly prolonged in latency.

magnetic stimulation in lathyrism has demonstrated prolonged central conduction to the lumbar spine in patients in whom a leg MEP could be recorded. However, in many no response can be elicited. MEPs recorded from hand muscles are usually normal.

Konzo has many similarities to lathyrism. It too causes an acute-onset spastic paraparesis, particularly in young, malnourished males, during dry seasons in Tanzania, Zaire and other parts of East Africa (Howlett et al. 1990; Tylleskar et al. 1991). The disease spectrum varies from hyperreflexia in the legs to severe spastic paraparesis with weakness in the arms. There is good evidence that Konzo results from ingestion of insufficiently processed cassava roots used to make flour. Short-soaking of the cassava roots leads to residual cyanohydrins in the flour and it is likely that this is responsible for the neurological deficit (Tylleskar et al. 1992) Long-standing high cyanide levels result in reactions between cyanide and cysteine residues in albumin yielding aminothiazolidine carboxylic acid which has structural similarities to BOAA (Rosling, 1986). A study from Uppsala carried out extensive electrophysiological testing in two patients with konzo disease that were previously seen in Tanzania (Howlett et al. 1990). In both patients motor and sensory nerve conductions, EMG (including SFEMG), autonomic testing, somatosensory, visual and auditory brainstem-evoked potentials and EEG were all normal. However, repeated efforts to stimulate the motor cortex with the magnetic coil at 100% output, with and without facilitation, failed to elicit any MEPs from either hand or leg muscles. Stimulation of the cervical roots with the coil elicited normal responses.

Based on clinical findings and motor-evoked potential studies evidence points to the motor cortex as the origin of these toxic "myelopathies"; they might be better referred to as toxic disorders of the motor pathways since it seems that it is the corti-comotoneurone that is primarily involved. The exact site of the lesion could be further elucidated by comparing the ability to evoke responses by electrical versus magnetic stimulation. If the lesion is truly one of the corticomotoneurone then it should be possible to elicit a response by electrical (i.e. distal to the cell body) but not magnetic stimulation. On the other hand if the lesion is one of the motor tracts then both magnetic and electrical stimulation of the cortex will fail to elicit a response.

Cervical spondylotic myelopathy (CSM)

This is the most serious manifestation of cervical spondylosis and is the commonest cause of myelopathy over age 60 years (Brain et al. 1952; Brain 1963; laRocca 1988; Lestini and Wiesel 1989). Symptomatic myelopathy does not usually occur unless the spinal cord, visualized by CT myelography, is extensively compressed (Hayashi et al. 1987, 1988). Then the prognosis is poor and the value, if any, of surgical decompression is limited. However, many older subjects with cervical radiculopathy have subtle and difficult to interpret signs, such as easily elicited deep tendon reflexes including finger flexion and slight inversion of the supinator reflex, which are suggestive of a myelopathy.

The treatment of cervical myelopathy is contentious. Even though recent large operative series suggest that surgery is beneficial a significant number of patients undergoing surgery do not improve (Jeffreys 1986; Samii et al. 1989). This, in part, may reflect the considerable neurological deficit usually present before surgery is contemplated. Greater benefit would probably result from judicial intervention at an earlier stage of the disease. The essential requirement is the finding of an object-ive means of detecting early evidence of functional spinal cord compression (Cusick 1988); as the symptomatic deficit is often well advanced before radiographic abnor-malities are apparent by myelography, CT myelography or MRI (Larsson et al. 1989; Lestini and Wiesel 1989).

Somatosensory evoked potentials (SEPs), described in more detail below, evaluate central sensory pathways and, although frequently abnormal in CSM, are usually normal in cervical radiculopathy without myelopathy. This is especially so in the absence of any clinical sensory deficit (Thompson et al. 1987; Green et al. 1988). Very few patients with clinical features suggesting CSM without radiological evi-dence of cord compression have abnormal SEPs. Usually both the cervical and corti-cal SEP responses become abnormal only when a clinical deficit has developed (Aminoff and Eisen 1992). The relatively late development of abnormal SEPs in CSM reflects the late occurrence of sensory impairment clinically. The diagnostic yield of median or ulnar SEPs in CSM is relatively low (25%–50%). Tibial nerve evoked SEPs give a higher yield but have little localizing value (Aminof and Eisen 1992; Green et al. 1988; Yiannikas et al. 1986; Yu and Jones 1985).

Pathological evidence indicates that the corticospinal tracts are affected early in cervical spondylotic myelopathy (CSM) (Brian et al. 1952). This then suggests that transcranial magnetic stimulation is a logical investigative approach. Thus far, expe-rience with magnetic stimulation in cervical spondylosis has mostly described abnormalities associated with clinically overt cervical spondylotic myelopathy (Thompson et al. 1987; Abbruzzese et al. 1988; Masur et al. 1989; Jaskolski et al. 1990; Maertens de Noordhout et al. 1992). In some patients, central conduction time has been shown to improve following surgery (Jaskolski et al. 1990). However, in others surgical decompression did not normalize central motor conduction time indicating permanent damage to the cervical cord.

Comparison with SEPs has shown MEPs to be more sensitive in cervical spondylosis with myelopathy. This is to be expected given that the corticospinal tracts are compressed before and to a greater extent than the dorsal columns from cervical disc disease.

With a view to early diagnosis, Travlos et al. (1992) investigated 18 patients with CT-confirmed cervical radiculopathy but with suggestive clinical myelopathy (brisk deep tendon reflexes in the legs) but without radiological correlates of cord compression. The root level(s) compromised were at C7 ($n = 4$) or more rostral ($n = 14$). MEPs were recorded from hand muscles, which were clinically strong and electromyographically normal (Fig. 11.4). This is important to document in terms of studying the corticospinal pathways in disc degeneration since weakness and wasting of hand muscles can be secondary to cord compression at higher cervical levels (Stark et al. 1981).

Multiple Sclerosis (MS)

The spinal cord is commonly involved in definite multiple sclerosis (MS) and the resultant demyelination of the motor tracts renders magnetic stimulation of considerable interest as a diagnostic tool in suspected MS. In 200 MS suspects with minimal neurological deficit (Kurtzke disability scale < 2.5), magnetic resonance imaging (MRI) was positive in 63% of patients compared to about 50% of cases for SEPs, VEPs and oligoclonal banding and only 27.5% for "double dose" contrast enhanced CT scans (Eisen et al. 1987). Others have confirmed the overall sensitivity of MRI in MS suspects. Of more interest in relation to the potential of magnetic stimulation are findings in 42 patients with progressive myelopathy (spinal MS) with definite neurological deficit (Aminoff and Eisen 1992). In these, the percentage of cases demonstrating abnormal cranial MRI, SEPs, VEPs and oligoclonal banding were 69%, 53%, 47% and 57%, respectively; again indicating the superiority of MRI.

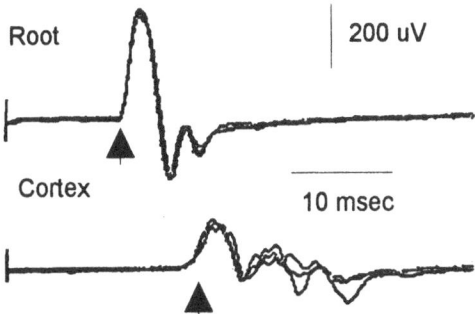

Fig. 11.4. Patient with a right C6 radiculopathy and brisk deep tendon reflexes in both legs. CT scan showed compression of the C6 root but no evidence of cord compression. **Top:** Normal motor evoked potential elicited by stimulation of the lower cervical roots (C8, T1). Latency of the response recorded from the hypothenar muscle complex measured 13.6 ms. **Lower:** Motor evoked potential elicited by stimulation of the left hand area. The potential (also recorded from the hypothenar muscle complex, i.e. below the spinal segment of root compression) is small and delayed in latency (27.4 ms). Central conduction between the motor cortex and lower cervical spine measured 13.8 ms (normal value < 9 ms).

Electrical stimulation of cortex was originally used to study the motor pathways in MS (Cowan et al. 1984; Mills and Murray 1984) but this method has now been largely superseded by transcranial magnetic stimulation (Eisen 1992; Hess et al. 1986; Ingram and Swash 1987). The characteristic abnormality described is slowing of central motor conduction which is frequently marked. Eliciting MEPs from leg muscles is much more uncertain than from hand muscles and most studies in MS have recorded MEPs from hand muscles. Eisen (1992) found that even in a normal population leg MEPs could not be obtained in about 8% of subjects. This makes interpretation in disease difficult. Especially so in suspected MS when abnormal signs may be minimal. Nevertheless, Jones et al. (1991) recorded lower extremity MEPs in 25 patients with definite MS. In seven no response was obtained and in about half of the other limbs studied the MEP was prolonged (they did not consider amplitude measurements). Prolonged latency and central motor conduction time correlated best with the presence of Babinski's sign, leg weakness, and hyperreflexia. The incidence of abnormal tibial SEPs matched that of the MEPs. This contrasts with studies comparing MEPs with median nerve SEPs or with VEPs and BAEPs (Rossini et al. 1989) which showed significantly higher sensitivity of MEPs.

Demyelination induces conduction block, slowed conduction and the inability to sustain rapid trains of impulses. These characteristic physiological disturbances in MS (individually or in combination) account for the delay in central motor conduction, reduced MEP/CMAP ratio and, as has been recently described, increased variability of onset latency of the MEP (Britton et al. 1991). The thenar MEP shown below was recorded from a 23 year woman with MRI confirmed MS. There were no complaints in the arm from which the very slowed MEP was recorded. However, this is the exception; such a gross abnormality is usually associated with significant clinical deficit.

A single cortical stimulus induces repetitive firing of the corticomotoneurone which in turn sets up a series of descending volleys, each separated by about 1.5 ms (Mills 1991). Thus if an anterior horn cell reached threshold with the first volley of the first stimulus but the third volley of the second stimulus the onset latency of the MEP would increase by 3 ms. Assuming a random distribution of the chances of a motor unit reaching threshold due to any of several descending volleys the expected variability in its onset latency (expressed as the mean consecutive discharge) is 0.75 ms (Britton et al. 1991). In MS this value is a significantly prolonged abnormality that was shown to correlate with increased reflexes and impaired fine finger movement.

It is possible to estimate the magnitude of the excitatory postsynaptic potential (EPSP) produced by the descending cortical volley by constructing peristimulus histograms of firing probability of a single motor unit, recorded with a concentric needle electrode, during delivery of magnetic stimuli (Fig. 11.5)

This has been done for both hand and leg muscles (Boniface et al. 1991; Brouwer and Ashby 1991; Brouwer et al. 1991; Mills 1991; Schubert et al. 1991). In normal subjects there are one or more post-stimulus periods, of increased firing probability of the primary and secondary peaks. The peak of increased firing has a mean duration of about 3 ms and may be multimodal with subpeaks of intermodal intervals ranging from 0.6 to 2.4 ms latencies. Subpeaks probably reflect excitatory postsynaptic potentials induced at the anterior horn cell by descending impulses.

In MS the response of single motor units to cortical stimulation is abnormal (Boniface et al. 1991; Mills 1991; Schubert et al. 1991). The primary peak is often absent or delayed in onset and may be increased in duration. Subpeaks may be

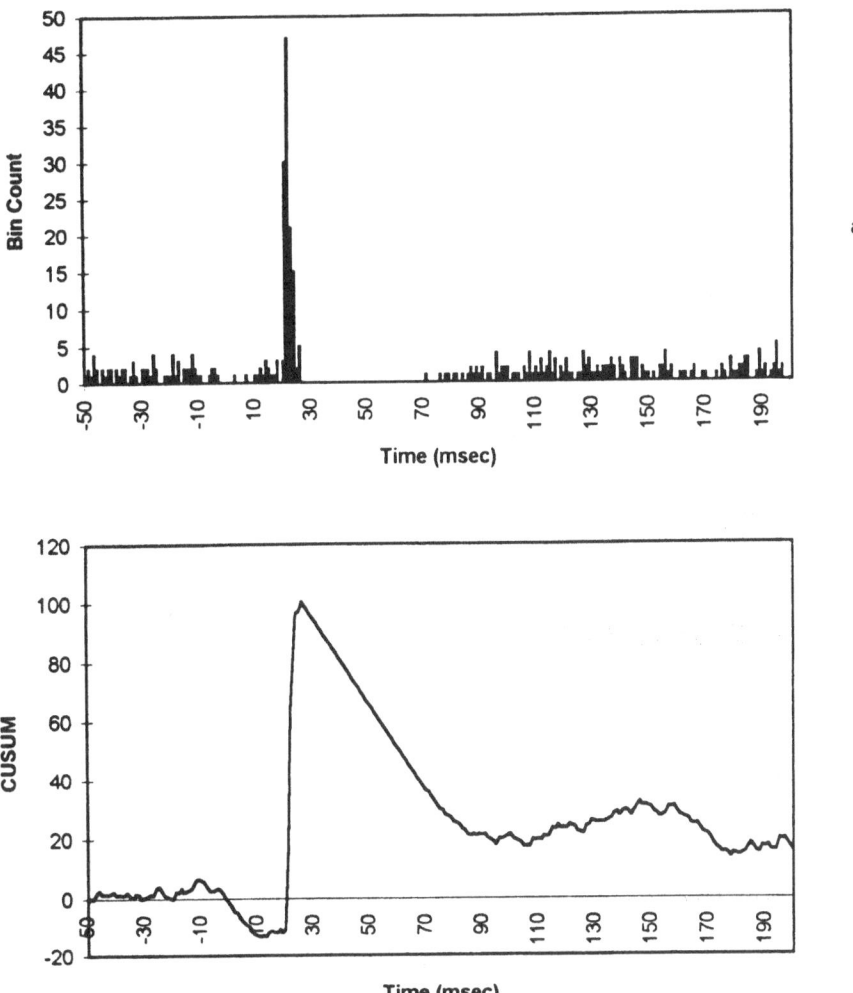

Fig. 11.5. **a** Normal peristimulus time histogram (PSTH). Random cortical stimuli are given at time 0 during the voluntary recruitment of a single motor unit. In the example shown the unit was recorded from the extensor digitorum communis muscle. About 20 ms after the stimulus there is a marked increase in the firing probability of the motor unit followed by a period of complete inhibition. **b** Shows the same changes in firing probability of the motor unit using cumulative sum (CUSUM) analysis. A downward deflection occurs when the firing probability is reduced and an upward deflection when it is increased.

absent; or if present, there is increased intermodal intervals between the subpeaks. These changes are not specific to MS and, for example, have been described following spinal cord injury (Brouwer and Ashby 1991; Brouwer et al. 1991). The possible mechanisms underlying these abnormalities include reduction and dispersion of corticospinal conduction impulse traffic, impaired summation of excitatory post-synaptic potentials at the anterior horn cell and conduction block in corticospinal fibres which may be frequency dependent.

Spinal Motor Neurones

Both alpha and gamma spinal motor neurones are located longitudinally in Rexed lamina IX within the ventral horn. The alpha motoneurones innervating a given muscle (the motor neurone pool) are tightly packed in a cigar-shaped, longitudinal, nuclear columns having a somatotopic arrangement so that motor neurones of functionally related muscles are located near one another. The SMNs are somatopically arranged so that neurones innervating proximal muscles are situated medially whereas those innervating distal muscle are more lateral. Also SMNs to flexor muscles are more dorsal than those to extensor muscles. Alpha motor neurones which innervate the extrafusal muscle fibres are intermingled with the smaller gamma motor neurones which project to the fibres of the muscle spindles.

Voluntary and reflex contraction occur through the orderly firing of motor units according to their size. Small motor neurones (30 μm) are recruited earliest and larger ones (up to 70 μm) are engaged later. The orderly recruitment of motor units allows the CNS to control for any level of muscle force by the production of small twitch and tetanic forces that are fatigue resistant followed by high twitch and tetanic forces that are readily fatigued. The majority of descending and afferent inputs to the SMN are indirect through interneurones. Exceptions include the corticomotoneuronal system described above and the Ia afferent input from muscle spindles.

Diseases of the spinal cord that affect the anterior horn cell are many and estimating the number of functioning SMNs (motor units) innervating a muscle can be very helpful. There are several ways of achieving this. All methods have limitations. For good reviews on motor unit estimating the reader is referred to: Brown et al. 1988; McComas 1991, 1994.

Motor Unit Firing Frequency

This provides an easy but relatively crude estimate of the fall out of motor units. Any loss of motor units, functional or real, due to upper or lower motor neurone lesions, increases the firing rate of remaining motor units. The normal firing rate of a motor unit is about 8–12 Hz depending on the muscle under investigation. Facial muscles including the tongue have the highest rates of firing, followed by distal limb muscles and proximal limb muscles have slower rates of discharge. With training some individuals can learn to drive a motor unit much faster than the "norm". The ratio of the fastest discharge rate of the first recruited motor unit recorded divided by the number of different units recruited at the same time gives a quantitative estimate of motor unit loss. For example, if a motor unit fires at 10 Hz when three other motor units are simultaneously active the ratio would equal 10/3 (3.33). On the other hand if a single motor unit is discharging at a rate of 20 Hz without any other unit being simultaneously recorded the ratio would equal 20/1 (20). Anything above 5 is abnormal. In motor neurone diseases such as amyotrophic lateral sclerosis ratios of ≥ 20 are common.

Incremental Nerve Stimulation

About 25 years ago (McComas et al. 1971) developed the first real physiological method for estimating the number of motor units in vivo in humans. In essence, the stimulus intensity to the motor nerve supplying a muscle was delicately increased in such a way that each increment activated an additional "all or none" response, reflecting an additional motor unit. The average of the differences between the first 15–20 incremental responses gives a value for the average size of the motor unit. And this value, divided into the maximum M-wave (i.e. the maximum compound muscle action potential for the muscle), is a measure of the number of motor units for the muscle (Fig. 11.6).

Although the McComas method was conceptually sound there were several technical problems: such as alternation, which can result in a falsely high count; and the considerable scatter amongst normal values. In the small hand muscles (thenar or hypothenar muscles) values range from 100 to over 40; thus making interpretation of disease states difficult. The variation is not due to technical error but reflects a true biological variation among individuals (McComas 1994). Modifications have been made to the original method in an attempt to address these issues (e.g. Brown 1972; Ballantyne and Hansen 1974; Doherty and Brown 1993). Multiple point stimulation may overcome the problem of alternation. The motor nerve is stimulated at different sites, and only a single, all-or-nothing response is accepted for each of the sites (Kadrie et al. 1976). More recently computerization of McComas' method has been employed to overcome the problem of alternation, simplifying and validating McComas' original observations (Galea et al. 1991; McComas 1991).

The Spike Trigger Averaging Method

The McComas method is less applicable to proximal muscles, but Brown et al. (1988) have developed the spike trigger averaging technique which is equally applicable to motor units counts in proximal and distal muscles. The method involves voluntary

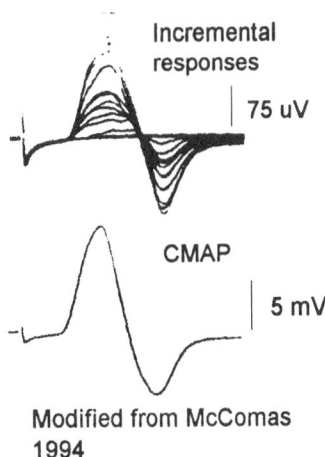

Fig. 11.6. Incremental stimulating method to estimate the number of motor units in a muscle as originally described by McComas. Initial compound motor action potentials evoked by low intensity stimulation of the median nerve. The difference in amplitude between each trace (8 are clearly identifiable) reflects the addition of one motor unit (top traces). The motor unit estimate is derived by dividing the mean difference in the increments into the maximum compound muscle action potential (lower trace). (Modified from McComas 1994.)

activation of a single motor thereby triggering a surface "macro" potential of that unit which is recorded from surface electrodes placed over the muscles endplate. By using a window discriminator (available on most current EMG equipment) it becomes possible to record the macropotential triggered by motor units of a variety of sizes, during moderate voluntary muscle contraction. Several different macropotentials can be measured with the needle in one site. This is not possible using the McComas method. It has the added advantage of being able simultaneously to record the complexity of motor units and the presence fibrillation and positive sharp waves indicating that denervation is present. The motor unit estimate is given by dividing the muscle M-wave by the mean macro amplitude (or area) of 10–20 different macropotentials (Fig. 11.7).

Clinical Applications of Motor Unit Counting

Motor unit estimates have consistently shown a non-linear loss anterior horn cells with ageing. There is a very slow decline up to the 6th–7th decades after which there is a more dramatic loss (30%–50%) of spinal motoneurones (Brown 1972; Campbell et al. 1973; Doherty and Brown 1993; McComas 1994; Brown 1994). In amyotrophic lateral sclerosis (ALS) Dantes and McComas (1991) have shown that once the motoneurone pool is affected, approximately half the neurones cease to function within 6 months with a further halving in the subsequent 6 months. However, relating the number of motor units to their mean amplitude (or twice force) has shown

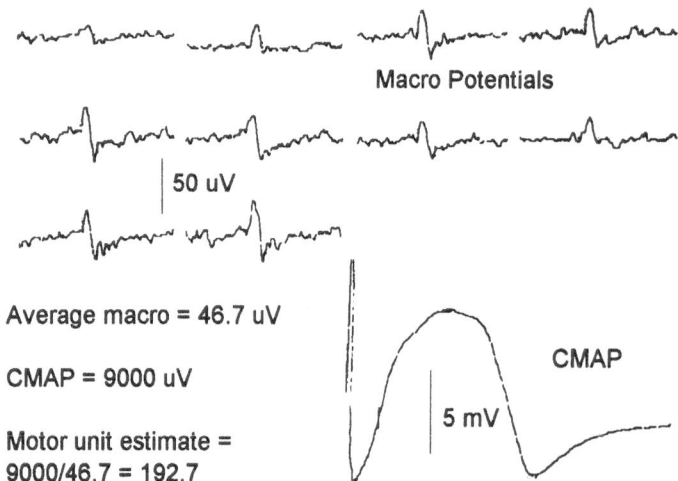

Fig. 11.7. Spike trigger macro-averaging method to estimate the number of motor units in a muscle. A monopolar needle (band pass 1000 hZ to 20 kHz) was used to trigger the spike of a single voluntary contracting motor unit in the extensor indicis proprius muscle. Ten macro potentials are shown recorded with a surface electrode over the muscle endplate. Each is an average of 150–200 sweeps. The average macropotential size as 46.7 µV. When this was divided into the compound muscle action potential (CMAP) (elicited by supramaximal stimulation of the radial nerve) it gave a motor unit estimate measuring 192.7.

that up to 80% of motor units can be lost before there is evidence of clinical weakness indicating that patients with substantial denervation may maintain normal strength and muscle bulk (Dantes and McComas 1991).

It has been recognized for some time that an upper motor neurone lesion, such as that occurring following a motor stroke or high level cord transection can include fibrillation in leg muscles (Brown and Snow 1990). Also the number of functioning motor units in the extensor digitorum brevis (EDB) is reduced after a stroke (McComas et al. 1973). This process takes about 2 months to develop. Over the last decade many neurotrophic growth factors have been identified. It has become apparent that several different factors may be compartmentalized within a "functional system" (Nishi 1994). For example, in the motor unit acidic fibroblast growth factor (FGF) is present in the anterior horn cell, basis FGF in the astrocyte, ciliary nerve trophic factor (CNTF) in the Schwann cell and brain derived neurotrophic factor (BDNF) and FGF-5 in the muscle fibres (Nishi 1994). It is very likely that impairment of such trophic factors is responsible for the loss of functioning motor units and associated muscle denervation.

Detecting a Motor Level by Paraspinal Needle EMG

Evidence for denervation (fibrillation potentials or positive sharp waves) in the paraspinal muscles is proof positive of a lesion that is at least as proximal as the ventral root and the electromyographer must decide if the lesion affects the root or spinal cord. Even in elderly subjects who frequently have asymptomatic degenerative disc disease, paraspinal fibrillation is very uncommon (Travlos et al. 1995). It is unusual for a radiculopathy to involve multiple roots whereas most disorders involving spinal motoneurones do so in a multisegmental, bilateral and often asymmetrical fashion. There may be difficulty distinguishing between a radiculopathy and intrinsic disease involving anterior horn cells in the early stages of some diseases. For example syringomyelia may begin unilaterally with muscle wasting in a C8/T1 distribution. The author has seen several cases of syringomyelia commence in the C5 myotome in the absence of sensory complaints or clinical sensory deficits. In such cases MR imaging is invariably positive.

Ascending Sensory Pathways

The Dorsal Columns

The dorsal columns are made up to two large fibre bundles, the more medial fasciculus gracilis which terminates in the nucleus gracilis and the more lateral fasciculus cuneatus terminating in the nucleus cuneatus. Most of the fibres in the dorsal columns are propriospinal and less than 25% of axons in the fasciculus gracilis extend the full length of the dorsal columns to terminate in the cervical nuclei (Baldissera et al. 1981; Brown 1981). The central projections of primary type II afferents from hair follicles (light touch) and other cutaneous receptors and from the Pacinian corpuscles ascend in the dorsal columns. Group 1a muscle afferents from the upper limbs also travel in the dorsal columns. Those from the lower limbs transfer to the dorsolateral columns. The dorsal column afferents are mediate signals required for complex discriminatory tasks including position sense (for the upper limb), detection of roughness, direction of movement of the skin and for the process of discriminating sensory signals during exploratory movements (Cook and Browder 1965; Wall 1970; Beck 1976). In humans these functions must also be mediated by alternate pathways since lesions restricted to the dorsal columns produce no permanent deficits in the lower limbs and only subtle ones (i.e. impairment of two-point discrimination) in the upper limbs (Cook and Browder 1965). Joint position does not appear to be dependent on dorsal column pathways (Noordenbos and Wall 1976) and surgical lesions of the dorsal columns do not permanently impair vibration perception.

The integrity of the fibre systems traversing the dorsal and dorsolateral columns can be assessed through spinal and short latency somatosensory potentials (SEPs) evoked by mixed or cutaneous nerve stimulation (Aminoff and Eisen 1992). These physiological methods are well tolerated and easily performed. However, they are not disease specific and have poor segmental localizing value. SEPs have also been successfully evoked by a variety of natural stimuli, for example, muscle stretch, thermal stimuli and mechanical tapping (Starr et al. 1981; Kakigi and Shibasaki 1984). Such stimuli relate better to the different functional fibre systems ascending the dorsal columns. Unfortunately the methodology is often tedious to perform and it is doubtful that they will easily lend themselves to routine clinical investigation.

The SEP recorded over the scalp in humans in response to stimulation of a mixed or cutaneous nerve at 2–2.5 times sensory threshold is made up of travelling waves from action potentials in nerve fibres and stationary waves originating at synaptic junctions or where the geometry or density of the volume conductor changes (Aminoff and Eisen 1992). SEPs can be elicited by stimulation of any mixed or cutaneous nerve (e.g. median at the wrist or the posterior tibial nerve at the ankle or the peroneal nerve at the knee). Conventionally the peaks are identified by their polarity and most usual latency. For example, N20 and P40 are the earliest most easily identified negativities and positivities stimulating, respectively, the median nerve at the wrist and the tibial at the ankle. These components reflect arrival of the volley at the primary sensory cortex, and can be used to determine conduction time through the cervical and lumbosacral spinal cords to the sensory cortex. Tibial nerve stimulation evokes potentials which are recordable over the lower spinal cord (Emmerson 1988). The largest (N22), which is most readily recordable over the lower thoracic spine (T11-L1), probably reflects postsynaptic activity in the lumbar grey matter generated in response to inputs from axon collaterals. A global conduction time incorporating the spinal cord can be calculated by the latency difference (cortical P40 - spinal N22). It measures approximately 18 ms (Fig. 11.8). This obviously has limited localizing value since prolongation could reflect a lesion anywhere between the lumbar spine and the cerebral sensory cortex. Nevertheless in the context of a clinically diagnosed cord lesion, without radiological abnormalities, prolongation of (cortical P40 - spinal N22) can be taken to reflect slowing of sensory conduction through the spinal cord. The lumbar spinal potential is often difficult to record without extensive averaging, especially in obese subjects. The SEP can be altered by peripheral nerve disease. For this reason as part of an investigation that includes recording SEPs a peripheral sensory, or mixed nerve, action potential should be simultaneously recorded. There are several conditions which involve both the central and peripheral sensory pathways (diabetes, vitamin B_{12} deficiency and

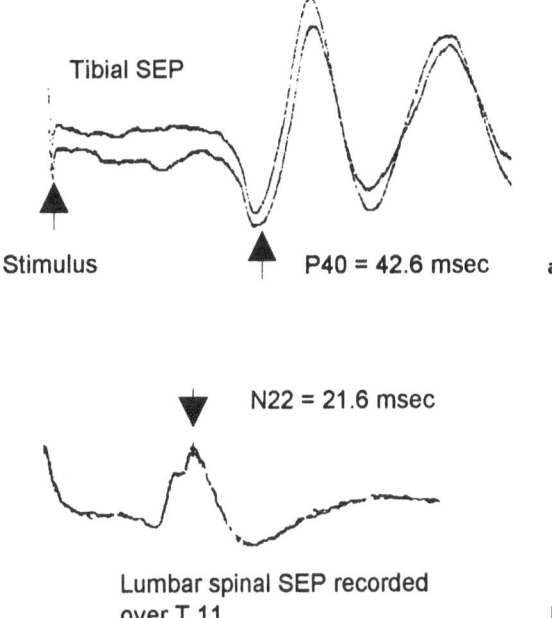

Tibial SEP

Stimulus   P40 = 42.6 msec   a

N22 = 21.6 msec

Lumbar spinal SEP recorded
over T 11   b

Fig. 11.8. **a** Spinal potential evoked by stimulation of the posterior tibial at the ankle. The reference electrode was placed over the iliac crest. **b** Somatosensory evoked potential (SEP) recorded over the scalp at Cz elicited at the same time as the lumbar potential. 500 sweeps were averaged. For clarity different acquisition times were used for recording the lumbar and cortical potentials. The conduction time from the lower spinal cord to the somatosensory cortex is normal at 21 ms.

Friedreich's ataxia) making it important to measure a peripheral sensory nerve action potential with the SEP.

Several smaller "far field potentials" precede the N20 and P40 components of the SEP (Aminoff and Eisen 1992; Emmerson 1988). However, their amplitudes are small and often more than a thousand responses must be averaged for their identification. Furthermore, they may not be present in all normal subjects thus limiting their clinical utility. Identification of far field potentials can be enhanced by restricting the recording bandpass or by digital filtering (Aminoff and Eisen 1992).

With electrodes placed over the cervical spine and a distant reference (earlobe, hand or knee) median nerve stimulation evokes a standing wave N9, generated in the peripheral nerve volley as it reaches the axilla. This probably results from geometrical alteration of the volume conductor at the level of the brachial plexus where there is a marked change in muscle mass (Kimura 1984; Eisen et al. 1986). A travelling wave N11 follows. It increases in latency as it ascends the cervical cord and is thought to reflect the central projections of primary afferents (Aminoff and Eisen 1992). A fixed latency potential (N13/N14) of larger amplitude, that is maximal over C6, arises from synaptic activity in the dorsal horn (Aminoff and Eisen 1992).

In an attempt to attain greater localizing value of short latency SEPs in spinal cord disease Goodridge et al. (1987) developed a method for stimulating the paraspinal muscle afferents. The paraspinal la afferents are stimulated bilaterally and simultaneously at different segmental levels. This method (Fig. 11.9) allows localization over an area of several spinal segments with relative ease. In normal subjects the

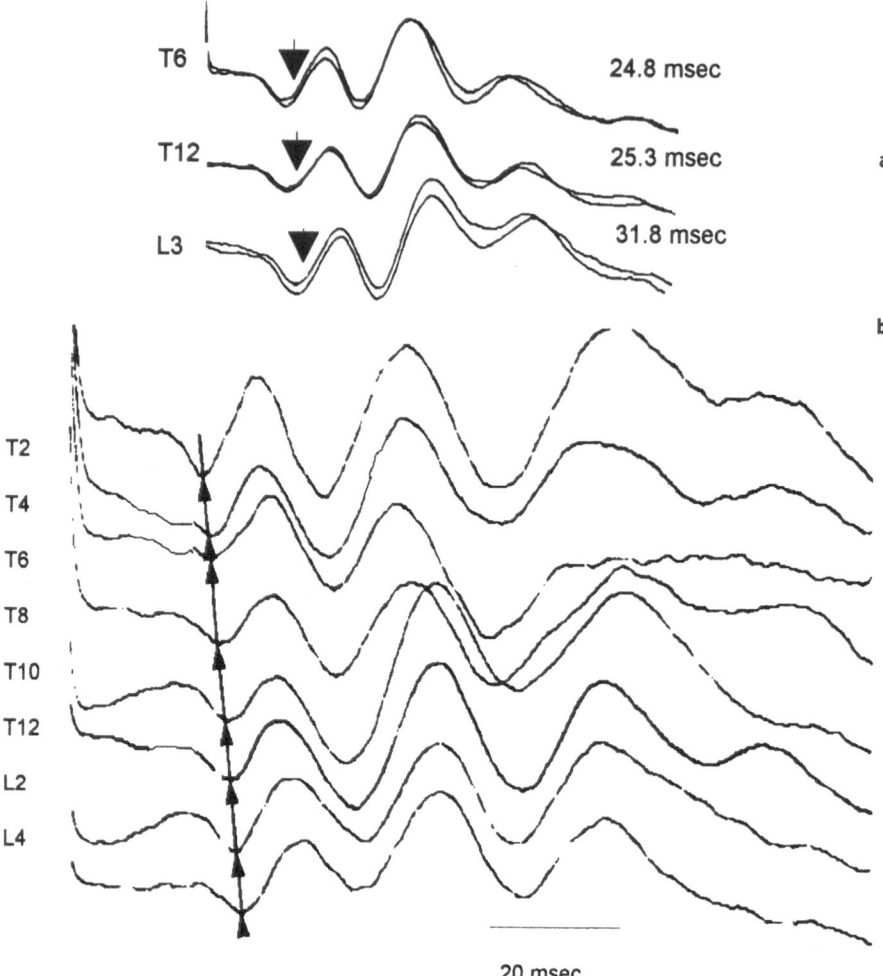

Fig. 11.9. a Paraspinal stimulation to evoke SEPs in a normal subject. Bilateral simultaneous stimulation. Three levels were stimulated and the latencies of the initial positivities are indicated. **b** Same normal subject to show that it is possible to stimulate at many spinal segemental levels. There is a stepwise linear decrease in latency of the first positivity of the SEP from caudal to rostral.

value for spinal cord conduction velocity between T12 and T1 is approximately 64 m/s and the conduction time between these segments is 5.4 ± 1.6 ms (Goodridge et al. 1987). Fig. 11.10 depicts conduction slowing in a patient with an arachnoid cyst at T10 causing spinal cord compression.

Cutaneous Type II Pathways

SEPs can be evoked by stimulating purely cutaneous nerves (for example, the sural, cutaneous branch of the peroneal, saphenous, lateral femoral cutaneus). Stimulating

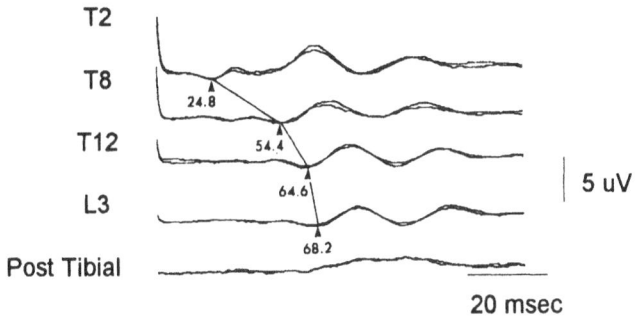

Fig. 11.10. Paraspinal stimulation to evoke SEPs in a patient with a lower thoracic arachnoid cyst. The lowest trace evoked by tibial nerve stimulation shows a very small SEP whose latency could not be determined. At T8, which was proximal to the lesion, there is a marked "jump" in latency (29.6 ms over four spinal segments; this would normally not exceed 5 ms).

a purely cutaneous nerve induces a volley that is less well synchronized than a mixed nerve and because fewer nerve fibres are stimulated the amplitude of the resulting SEP is smaller. Early, "far field components" are seldom recognized. Nevertheless cutaneous SEPs allow one to make inferences about the integrity of the ascending sensory tracts.

SEPs in Spinal Cord Disease

Any lesion resulting in loss or significant diminution of joint position sensation will attenuate or abolish the SEP evoked by mixed nerve stimulation. However, lesions of the spinal cord that selectively interrupt pathways mediating pain and temperature have no effect on the mixed nerve SEP. Following traumatic avulsion of the dorsal root ganglion only the N9 (brachial plexus potential) is preserved. With complete spinal cord transection at C5 or C6, the N11 cervical potential is preserved but all subsequent potentials are lost. The main value of SEPs is in spinal cord disorders that do not have radiological correlates, assessment of spinal cord trauma and intra-operative monitoring of spinal cord function.

Multiple Sclerosis

With the advent of magnetic resonance imaging (MRI) the role of SEPs, and other electrophysiological tests that were previously useful in the diagnosis of MS must be re-evaluated. The sensitivity of MRI and SEPs is similar in definite MS. However, with several years of experience now on record, MRI is more sensitive than any elec-trophysiological test in probable and possible MS and has become the standard against which to measure the efficacy of several drug trials. Nevertheless, a number of patients without clinical evidence of MS have MRI abnormalities of a sort typi-cally seen in MS. Also MRI is still expensive and the relative cost effectiveness SEPs (and VEPs) make them good screening tests before going onto ordering MRI (Fig. 11.11)

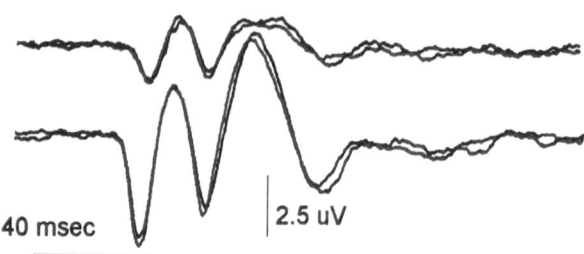

Fig. 11.11. Tibial evoked SEPs in multiple sclerosis. When the asymptomatic leg was stimulated (lower traces) normal SEPs were elicited. The top traces were evoked by stimulation of the symptomatic limb (numbness, loss of position sensation). The SEP is modestly prolonged in latency but markedly reduced in amplitude. Side to side differences should not exceed a difference of 50%. The change probably reflects conduction block in central sensory pathways.

Hereditary Spastic Paraplegia

This group of disorders shares many of the clinical and electrophysiological findings of lathyrism and konzo. They also preferentially affect the legs but unlike konzo and lathyrism the long sensory pathways are involved in addition to the corticospinal tracts. Claus et al. (1990) recorded MEPs from hand muscles in 10 patients with hereditary spastic paraplegia; in eight the responses were normal. Pelosi et al. (1991) recorded leg MEPs in 10 cases and reported abnormalities in all of them (absent responses in six, reduced amplitude in two and delayed central conduction in two). In contrast the arm MEP was normal in all but two patients. Present evidence indicates that in lathyrism, konzo and hereditary spastic paraplegia it is the corticomotoneurone that is primarily affected with a preferential dying forward of the long leg corticospinal fibres.

SEPs are often abnormal, with loss of spinal or cortical components, even when there is no obvious clinical sensory deficit (Aminoff and Eisen 1992). Abnormalities are also seen in spinocerebellar degenerations and Friedreich's ataxia. In this condition it is often not possible to obtain a peripheral sensory nerve action potential (SNAP) despite which it is possible to record a SEP. The potentials are usually small, dispersed and often very prolonged. The ability to record a SEP in the absence of a peripheral response is interesting and is best explained on "central amplification" (Eisen et al. 1982).

Human Immunodeficiency Virus (HIV)

In patients with overt AIDS, spinal cord conduction as measured by SEPs is quite frequently slowed even when there is little evidence of clinical spinal cord disease. It has also been established that SEPs elicited by tibial nerve stimulation may be, or become progressively prolonged over time (2 years) in the absence of clinical AIDS. It remains to be seen if SEPs (or other electrophysiological measures of spinal cord function) will play a meaningful role in the early detection of AIDS (Coats et al. 1990; Smith et al. 1990).

Spinal Cord Trauma

Complete spinal lesions below C7 spare the median but not the ulnar nerve SEP (Perot 1973; Stohr et al. 1982). SEPs can be used to assess the severity of spinal injuries. If potentials can be evoked by stimulation below the level of spinal injury the lesion must be incomplete and the prognosis for functional recovery can be more optimistic (Aminoff and Eisen, 1992). However, an absent SEP does not always signify a complete spinal lesion but recovery is likely to take longer and be incomplete. Perot 1973; Sedgwick et al. 1980)

In recent years transcranial magnetic stimulation has been used to assess spinal injuries (Dimitrijevic et al. 1988). Like SEPs the ability to evoke a motor response at a site distal to the lesion indicates continuity of at least some motor fibres through the lesion. Absence of a recordable MEP may not mean the lesion is complete.

Needle EMG is useful and relevant in the setting of acute and subacute spinal injury. Denervation limited to one or two segments implies a discrete lesion whereas paraspinal and limb muscle denervation (fibrillation and positive sharp waves) over several myotomes, rostral and caudal to the lesion, indicates widespread disruption of motor neurone pools. Loss of sensory nerve action potentials indicates involvement of nerve fibres distal to the dorsal root ganglion cell. Widespread denervation of lower limb musculature in association with a thoracolumbar injury indicates involvement of the cauda equina.

Testing the Integrity of the Phrenic Nerve and Diaphragm

High cervical cord lesions involving C3–C5 are liable to involve the motor neurone pool innervating the diaphragm through the phrenic nerve. With the success of phrenic nerve pacing it is important to demonstrate whether or not the phrenic axons are intact and if the diaphragm has undergone denervation. There are several approaches to stimulating the phrenic nerve. They are percutaneous electrical (Markand et al. 1984) or magnetic stimulation or electrical nerve stimulation through a near nerve needle electrode. The author prefers this last option. Once the technique is mastered it allows selective stimulation of the nerve at a low stimulus intensity and is less uncomfortable than is percutaneous stimulation. The current required for this is often very high inducing spread to the brachial plexus. More importantly the threshold of a regenerating nerve is high and percutaneous stimulation may not be strong enough.

Needle stimulation is achieved by introducing a monopolar needle through an imaginary line drawn from the mid point of the posterior border of the sternocleidomastoid muscle to the cricoid cartilage (MacLean and Mattioni 1981). The needle is advanced in an anteriomedial direction through the fat-pad of the posterior triangle of the neck until it comes to lie nearby the phrenic nerve. The carotid sheath is more anterior and medial. Surface recording electrodes are placed over the xiphoid process (active) and over the intercostal space between the 8th and 9th ribs at the anterior axillary line. The latency to the onset of the compound muscle action potential recorded in this manner is about 8 ms.

The commonly held belief that direct needle EMG of the diaphragm is dangerous because of the risk of puncturing the lung, spleen, liver or colon needs revision. Bolton et al. (1992) have developed methodology that is safe and informative. The recording needle is inserted between the ribs between the anterior axillary and medial clavicular lines and just above the costal margin. Here there is about 1.5 cm distance between the pleural reflection and the lower costal cartilage on which the diaphragm inserts.

Spinal Cord Disorders Involving Positive Neuronal Activity

Stiff Man (person) Syndrome

This has been recognized for over 40 years (Ashby 1987). A prodrome of episodic muscle aching is followed by symmetrical stiffness of trunk, neck and limb musculature. The jaw muscles are spared. There is associated painful muscle spasms easily precipitated by sensory stimuli. Tendon reflexes may be brisk, otherwise the neurological examination is normal and the stiffness is abolished by sleep and much reduced by diazepam and abolished by curare, proximal nerve block, spinal and general anaesthesia indicating the activity is generated proximal to the peripheral nerve (Isaacs 1961; Gordon et al. 1967; Leigh et al. 1980; Sander et al. 1980; Sivak et al. 1993).

Ectopic generation is thought to be due to abnormal function in spinal interneurones, causing depolarization of the anterior horn cells. The potentials resemble those of normal motor units.

Progressive Encephalomyelitis with Rigidity

This is a rare but seriously relentless disorder thought to be viral in origin. It starts with painful muscle spams and stiffness leading to marked rigidity, probably related to interneuronal dysfunction (Ashby 1987). Later myoclonic jerks, tremor, ataxia and occulomotor abnormalities develop indicating the disease is not limited to the spinal cord. In contrast to stiff-man syndrome diazepam has minimal effect. Most neurophysiological studies have been normal but individual experience with the disorder is limited (Whiteley et al. 1976; Howell et al. 1979).

Spinal Myoclonus

Spinal myoclonus most commonly induces involuntary, semirhythmic muscle contractions (Frenken et al. 1974). Contractions affect the same or contiguous segemental myotomes and involve both agonists and antagonists. They persist during sleep and are not abolished by general anaesthesia (Ashby 1987). Animal and human studies have clearly shown that the origin of the activity is in the spinal cord since it persists after complete spinal transection. Nerve conductions are normal and, unlike some myoclonic syndromes of cerebral origin, the SEP is not enhanced. Some cases have, associated with spinal cord tumours or other structural lesions of the spinal cord, show abnormalities on needle electromyography.

Electrophysiological Monitoring During Spinal Cord Surgery

An increasing number of spinal surgeons are seeking intraoperative monitoring of the function of the long ascending and descending tracts. Use of somatosensory evoked potentials (SEPs) is well established. This method is limited by the need for time consuming averaging, making rapid "on line recording" difficult. Also, severe postoperative (motor) disability may occur despite the preservation of good SEPs (Ginsburg et al. 1985).

Early experience with intraoperative motor evoked potential (MEP) monitoring used electrical stimulation (Boyd et al. 1986; Kitagawa et al. 1989; Zentner 1989). It is reasonable to use electrical stimulation of the motor cortex or spinal cord itself with the patient under anaesthesia, when pain is not a relevant issue. Potentials can be recorded either from muscle or over the spinal cord at a site distal to the stimulation site. A major disadvantage of electrical stimulation is that it is painful and not readily accepted in the awake subject making pre- and postoperative comparisons difficult.

Non-painful magnetic stimulation of the cortex is possible in the operative setting (Herdman et al. 1992). However, success in evoking MEPs is very dependent on the anaesthetic used and in particular the number of synapses the volley has to encounter to reach its target (Herdman et al. 1992). With transcranial magnetic stimulation two or three synapses have to be encountered before activating muscle. Ketamine, propofol, fentanyl and etomidate have been found to be accetable agents. The greatest attenuating effect of anaesthetics is at the anterior horn cells. This can be circumvented by recording directly over the spinal cord with epidural electrodes which also precludes the effects of muscle relaxants acting at the neuromuscular junction. Spinal recording is difficult below about T8 and cannot be used to monitor spinal surgery at more caudal levels. One then has to revert to muscle recording.

References

Abbruzzese G, Dall'Agata, D, Morena M et al. (1988) Electrical stimulation of the motor tracts in cervical spondylosis. J Neurol Neurosurg Psychiatry, 51:796–802

Aminoff MJ, Eisen A (1992) Somatosensory evoked potentials. In: Aminoff MJ (ed) Electrodiagnosis in clinical neurology, 3rd edn. Churchill Livingstone, New York, pp 571–603

Ashby P (1987) Clinical neurophysiology of the spinal cord. In: Brown WF, Bolton CF (eds) Clinical electromyography, Butterworths, Boston, pp 453–482

Baldissera F, Hultborn M, Illert M (1981) Integration in spinal neuronal systems. In: Brookhart JM, Mountcastle VB (eds) Handbook of physiology, Section 1. The nervous system, Vol 2. Motor control, part 1. American Physiological Society, Bethesda, MD, pp 509–595

Ballantyne JP, Hansen S (1974) A new method for the estimation of the number of motor units in a muscle. 1. Control subjects and patients with myasthenia gravis. J Neurol Neurosurg Psychiatry 37:907–915

Beck CHM (1976) Dual doral columns: a review. Can J Neurol Sci 3:1–7

Behan WMH, Maia M (1974) Strumpell's familial spastic paraplegia: genetics and neuropathology. J Neurol Neurosurg Psychiatry 37:8–20

Beric A (1993) Transcranial electrical and magnetic stimulation. In: Adv Neurol 63:29–42

Bolton CF, Grand'maison F, Parkes A, Shkrum M (1992) Needle electromyography of the diaphragm. Muscle Nerve 15:678–681

Boniface SJ, Mills KR, Schubert M (1991) Responses of single spinal motoneurons to magnetic stimulation in healthy subjects and patients with multiple sclerosis. Brain 114:643–662

Boyd SG, Rothwell JC, Cowan JMA, Webb PJ et al. (1986) A method for monitoring function in corticospinal pathways during scoliosis surgery with a note on motor conduction velocities. J Neurol Neurosurg Psychiatry 49:252–257

Brian WR, Northfield D, Wilkinson M (1952) The neurological manifestations of cervical spondylosis. Brian 75:187–225

Brain, Lord (1963) Some unsolved problems of cervical spondylosis. Br Med J i:771–777

Britton TC, MeyerB.-U, Benecke R (1991) Variability of cortically evoked motor responses in multiple sclerosis. Electroencephalogr Clin Neurophysiol 81:186–194

Brouwer B, Ashby P (1991) Altered corticospinal projections to lower limb motoneurons in subjects with cerebral palsy. Brain 114:1395–1407

Brouwer B, Bugaresti J, Ashby P (1991) Changes in corticospinal facilitation of lower limb spinal motor neurons after spinal cord lesions. J Neurol Neurosurg Psychiatry 55:20–24

Brown AG (1981) Organization in the spinal cord: The anatomy and physiology of identified neurones. New York, Springer-Verlag

Brown WF (1972) A method for estimating the number of motor units in thenar muscles and changes in motor unit counting with ageing. J Neurol Neurosurg Psychiatry 35:845–852

Brown WF (1994) Neurophysiological changes in aging. 1994 AAEM Plenary Session 1: Aging: Neuromuscular Function and Disease. Johnson Printing Co Inc, pp 17–23

Brown WF, Snow R (1990) Denervation in hemiplegic muscles. Stroke 21:1700–1704

Brown WF, Strong MJ, Snow R (1988) Methods for estimating numbers of motor units in biceps-brachialis muscles and losses of motor units with aging. Muscle Nerve 11:423–432

Calne DB, Eisen A, McGeer E, Spencer P (1986) Alzheimer's disease, Parkinson's disease and motoneurone disease: abiotrophic interaction between aging and environment? Lancet ii:1067–1070

Campbell MJ, McComas AJ, Petito F (1973) Physiological changes in aging muscles. J Neurol Neurosurg Psychiatry 36:174–182

Caramia MD, Cicinelli P, Paradiso C, Marioenzi R et al. (1991) Excitability changes of muscular responses to magnetic brain stimulation in patients with central motor disorders. Electroencephalogr Clin Neurophysiol 81:243–250

Claus D, Waddy HM, Harding AE, Murray NMF, Thomas PK (1990) Hereditary motor and sensory neuropathies and hereditiary spastic paraplegia: a magnetic stimulation study. Ann Neurol 28:43–49

Coats M, Jabbari B, Martin A, Salazar A (1990) Serial evoked potential studies in early human immune deficiency virus infection. Neurology 40:Suppl 1,320

Cook AW, Browder EJ (1965) Function of the posterior columns in man. Arch Neurol 12:72–79

Cowan JMA, Dick JPR, Day BL, Rothwell JC, Thompson PD, Marsden CD (1984) Abnormalities in central motor pathway conduction in multiple sclerosis. Lancet ii:304–307

Cusick JF (1988) Monitoring of cervical spondylotic myelopathy. Spine 13:877–880

Dalakas M, Illa (1991) Post-polio syndrome: concepts in clinical diagnosis, pathogenesis, and etiology. Adv Neurol 56; pp 495–511

Dantes M, McComas AJ (1991) The extent and time-course of motoneuron involvement in amyotrophic lateral sclerosis. Muscle Nerve 14:416–421

Davidoff RA (1984) Handbook of the spinal cord, Vols 1–5, Marcel Dekker, New York

Davidoff RA, Hackman JC (1991) Aspects of spinal cord structure and reflex function. Neurol Clin 9: 533–550

Dimitrijevic MR, Eaton WJ, Sherwood AM, Van Der Linden C (1988) Assessment of corticospinal tract integrity in human chronic spinal cord injury. In: Rossini PM, Marsden CD (eds) Non-invasive stimulation of brain and spinal cord: fundamentals and clinical applications. Alan R Liss New York, pp 243–253

Doherty TJ. Brown WF (1993) The estimated number and relative sizes of thenar motor units as selected by multiple point stimulation in young and older adults. Muscle Nerve 16:355–366

Eisen A, Purves S, Hoirch M (1982) Central nervous system amplification: its potential in the early diagnosis of multiple sclerosis. Neurology 32:359 -

Eisen A, Odusote K, Bozek C, Hoirch M (1986) Far-field potentials from peripheral nerve: generated at sites of muscle mass change. Neurology 36:815–818

Eisen A, Odusote K, Li D, Robertson W et al. (1987) Comparison of resonance imaging with somatosensory testing in MS suspects. Muscle Nerve 10:385–390

Eisen A, Shytbel W, Murphy K, Hoirch M. (1990) Cortical magnetic stimulation in amyotrophic lateral sclerosis Muscle Nerve 13:146–151

Eisen A (1992) Cortical and peripheral nerve magnetic stimulation. Methods Clin Neurophysiol 4:65–84

Eisen A, Kim S, Pant B (1992) Amyotrophic lateral sclerosis (ALS): a phylogenetic disease of the cortico-motoneuron? Muscle Nerve 15:219–228

Eisen A, Pant B, Stewart H (1993) Cortical excitability in amyotrophic lateral sclerosis: a clue to pathogenesis. Can J Neurol Sci 20:1–16

Eisen A (1995) Amyotrophic lateral sclerosis: a multifactorial disease. Muscle Nerve 18:741–752

Emmerson RG (1988) Anatomic and physiologic bases of posterior tibial nerve somatosensory evoked potentials. Neurol Clin 6:735–749

Flament D, Hall EJ, Lemon RN (1992) The development of cortic-motoneuronal projections investigated using magnetic brain stimulation in the infant macaque. J Physiol (Lond) 447:755–768

Frenken CWGM, Notermans SLH, Korten JJ et al. (1974) Myoclonic disorders of spinal origin. Clin Neurol Neurosurg 1:44–53

Galea V, DeBruin H, Cavasin R, McComas AJ (1991) The number and relative sizes of motor units estimated by computer. Muscle Nerve 14:1123–1130

Ginsburg HH, Shetter AG, Raudzens PA (1985) Postoperative paraplegia with preserved intraoperative somatosensory evoked potentials. J Neurosurg 63:296–300

Goodridge A, Eisen A, Hoirch M (1987) Paraspinal stimulation to elicit somatosensory evoked potentials: an approach to physiological localization of spinal lesions. Electroencephalogr Clin Neurophysiol 68:268–276

Gordon EE, Janusko DM, Kaufman L (1967) A critical survey of stiff-man syndrome. Am J Med 42:582–599

Green J, Hamm A, Benfante P, Green S (1988) Clinical effectiveness of dermatomal evoked cerebrally recorded somatosensory responses. Clin Electroencephalogr 19:14–15

Hayashi H, Okada K, Hamada M et al. (1987) Etiologic factors of myelopathy. A radiographic evaluation of the aging changes in the cervical spine. Clin Orthop Related Res 214:200–209

Hayashi H, Okada K, Hashimoto J et al. (1988) Cervical spondylotic myelopathy in the aged patient. A radiographic evaluation of the aging changes in the cervical spine and etiologic factors of myelopathy. Spine 13:618–625

Herdmann J, Lumenta C, Kiprovski K, Krzan M (1992) Magnetic stimulation of the brain in the operating room. In: Lissens MA (ed) Clinical applications of magnetic transcranial stimulation. Peeters Press, Leuven, pp 269–282

Hess CW, Mills KR, Murray NMF (1986) Measurement of central motor conduction times in multiple sclerosis by magnetic stimulation. Lancet ii:355–358

Howell DA, Lees AJ, Toghill PJ (1979) Spinal internuncial neurones in progressive encephalomyelitis with rigidity. J Neurol Neuosurg Psychiatry 42:773–785

Howlett WP, Brubaker GR, Milingi N, Rosling H (1990) Konzo, an epidemic upper motor neuron disease studied in Tanzania. Brain 113:223–235

Hugon J, Lubeau M, Tabarard F, Chazot F, Vallat JM, Dumas M (1987) Centralmotor conduction in motor neuron disease. Ann Neurol 22:544–546

Ingram DA, Swash M (1987) Central motor conduction is abnormal in motor neuron disease. J Neurol Neurosurg Psychiatry 50:159–166

Isaacs H (1961) A syndrome of continuous muscle-fiber activity. J Neurol Neurosurg Psychiatry 24:319–325

Jaskolski DJ, Laing RJ, Jarratt JA, Jukubowski J (1990) Pre- and postoperative motor condution times, measured using magnetic stimulation, in patients with cervical spondylosis. Br J Neurosurg 4:187–192

Jaskolski DJ, Jarratt JA, Jakubowski J (1993) Clinical evaluation of magnetic stimulation cervical spondylosis. Br J Neurosurg III:541–548

Jeffreys RV (1986) The surgical treatment of cervical myelopathy due to spondylosis and disc degeneration. J Neurol neurosurg Psychiatry 49:353–361

Jones SM, Streletz LJ, Raab VE et al. (1991) Lower extremity motor evoked potentials in multiple sclerosis. Arch Neurol 48:944–948

Kadrie HA, Yates SK, Milner-Brown HS, Brown WF (1976) Multiple point electrical stimulation of ulnar and median nerves. J Neurol Neurosurg Psychiatry 39:973–985

Kakigi R, Shibasaki H (1984) Scalp topography of mechanically and electrically evoked somatosensory potentials in man. Electroencephalogr Clin Neurophysiol 59:44–

Kimura J (1984) Field theory: the origin of stationary peaks from a moving source. In: International Symposium on Somatosensory Evoked Potentials. Custom Printing Inc, Rochester, MN, pp 39–50

Kitagawa CJ, Itoh T, Takano T et al. (1989) Motor evoked potential monitoring during upper cervical spine surgery. Spine 14:1078–1083

LaRocca H (1988) Cervical spondylotic myelopathy: natural history. Spine 13:854–855

Larsson EM, Holt S, Cronqvist S, Brandt L (1989) Comparison of myelography, CT myelography and magnetic resonance imaging in cervical spondylosis and disk herniation. Acta Radiol 30:233–239

Leigh PN, Rothwell JC, Traub M et al. (1980) A patient with reflex myoclonus and muscle rigidity: "Jerking stiff man syndrome". J Neuro Neurosurg Psychiatry 43:1125–1131

Lestini WF, Wiesel SW (1989) The pathogensis of cervical spondylosis. Clin Orthop Related Res 239:69–93

Lissens MA (1992) Clinical applications of magnetic transcranial stimulation. University Press, Arendonk, Belgium

MacLean IC, Mattioni TA (1981) Phrenic nerve conduction studies: a new technique and its application in quadraplegic patients. Arch Phys Med Rehabil 62:70–

Maertens de Noordhout A, Remacle JM, Pepin JL, Born JD, Delwaide PJ (1991) Magnetic stimulation of the motor cortex in cervical spondylosis. Neurology 41:75–80

Maertens de Noordhout A, Pepin JL, Gerard P, Delwaide PJ (1992) Facilitation of response to motor cortex stimulation: effects of isometric voluntary contraction. Ann Neurol 32:365–370

Markand ON, Kincaid JC, Pourmand RA et al. (1984) Electrophysiological evaluation of diaphragm by transcutaneous phrenic nerve stimulation. Neurology 34:604–614

Masur H, Elger, CE, Render K et al. (1989) Functional deficits of central sensory and motor pathways in patients with cervical spinal stenosis: a study of SEPs and EMG responses to non-invasive brain stimulation. Electroenceph Clin Neurophysiol 74:450–457

Mayr N, Baumgartner C, Zeitlhofer J, Deeke L (1991) The sensitivity of transcranial cortical magnetic stimulation in detecting pyramidal tract lesions in clinically definite multiple sclerosis. Neurology 41:566–569

McComas AJ (1991) Invited review: motor unit estimation: methods, results, and present status. Muscle Nerve 14:585–597

McComas AJ (1994) Motor unit estimation: anxieties and achievements. Nineteenth Annual Edward H Lambert Lecture of the AAEM. Johnson Printing Co Inc, Rochester, MN, pp 39–48

McComas AJ, Fawcett PRW, Campbell MJ, Sica REP (1971) Electrophysiological estimation of the number of motor units within a human muscle. J Neurol Neurosurg Psychiatry 34:121–131

McComas AJ, Sica REP, Upton ARM, Aguilera N (1973) Functional changes in motoneurones of hemiparetic muscles. J Neurol Neurosurg Psychiatry 36:183–193

Merton PA, Morton HB (1980) Stimulation of cerebral cortex in intact human subject. Nature 285:27–228

Mills KR, Murray NMF (1984) Corticospinal tract conduction times in multiple sclerosis. Ann Neurol 18:601–605

Mills KR (1991) Magnetic brain stimulation: a tool to explore the action of the motor cortex of single human spinal motoneurones. Trends Neurosci 14:401–405

Murray NMF (1993) Motor evoked potentials. In: Aminoff MJ (ed) Electrodiagnosis in clinical neurology, 2nd edn. Churchill Livingstone, New York, pp 605–626

Nishi R (1994) Neurotrophic factors: two are better than one. Science 265:1052–1053

Noordenbos W, Wall PD (1976) Diverse sensory functions with an almost totally divided spinal cord. A case of spinal cord transection with preservation of one anterolateral quadrant. Pain 2:185–195

Pelosi L, Lanzillo B, Perretti A, Santoro L, Blumhardt L, Caruso G. (1991) Motor and somatosensory evoked potentials in hereditary spastic paraplegia. J Neurol Neurosurg Psychiatry 54:1099–1102

Perot PL (1973) The clinical use of somato-sensory evoked potentials in spinal cord injury. Clin Neurosurg 20:367–381

Pezeshkpour GH, Dalakas MC (1988) Long term changes in the spinal cord of patients with old pliomyelitis: signs of continuous disease activity. Arch neurol 45:505–508

Porter R, Lemon R (1993) Corticospinal function and voluntary movement. Monographs of the Physiological Society, Vol 45, Clarendon Press, Oxford

Rosling H (1986) Cassava, cyanide, and epidemic spastic paraparesis. A study in Mozambique on dietary cyanide exposure. Acta Univ Upsal 19:1–52

Rossini PM, Marsden CD (1988) Non-invasive stimulation of the brain and spinal cord: fundamentals and clinical applications. Neurol Neurobiol 41

Rossini PM, Zarola F, Floris R, Bernardi G et al. (1989) Sensory (VEP, BAEP, SEP) and motor evoked potentials, liquoral and magnetic resonance findings in multiple sclerosis. Eur Neurol 29:41–47

Samii M, Vlokening D, Sepehrnia A et al. (1989) Surgical treatment of myeloradiculopathy in cervical spondylosis. A report of 438 operations. Neurosurg Rev 12:285–290

Sander JE, Layzer RB, Golsobel AB (1980) Congenital stiff-man syndrome. Ann Neurol 8:195–197

Schoenen J (1991) Clincial anatomy of the spinal cord. Neurol Clin 9, 503–532

Schriefer TN, Hess CW, Mills KR, Murray NM (1989) Central motor conduction studies in motor neurone disease using magnetic brain stimulation. Electroencephalogr Clin Neurophysiol 74:431–437

Schubert M, Mills KR, Boniface SJ, Konstanzer A, Dengler R (1991) Changes in the responses of motor units to transcranial magnetic stimulation in patients with multiple sclerosis and stroke. EEG EMG Z Elektroenzephalogr Elektromyogr Verwandte Geb 22:28–36

Schwartz MS, Swash M (1992) Neurophysiological investigation of the spinal cord. In Critchley E, Eisen A (eds) Diseases of the spinal cord 1st edn. Springer-Verlag, London, pp 123–140

Sedgwick EM, El-Negamy E, Franel H (1980) Spinal cord potentials in traumatic paraplegia and quadriplegia. J Neurol Neurosurg Psychiatry 43:823–830

Sivak M, Ochoa J, Fernandez JM (1993) Positive manifestations of nerve fiber dysfunction: clinical, electrophysiologic, and pathologic correlates. In: Brown WF, Bolton CF (eds) Clinical electromyography, 2nd edn. Butterworth-Heinemann, Boston pp 117–147

Smith T, Jakobsen J, Trojaborg W (1990) Somatosensory evoked potentials during human immunodeficiency virus (HIV) infection. Electroencephalogr Clin Neurophysiol 75:S142

Spencer PS, Allen CN, Kisby GE, Ludolph AC, Ross SM, Roy DN (1991) Lathyrism and Western Pacific amyotrophic lateral sclerosis: etiology of short and long latency motor system disorders. Adv Neurol 56:287-299

Stark RJ, Kennard C, Swash M (1981) Hand wasting in spondylotic high cord compression: an electromyographic study. Ann Neurol 9:58-62

Starr A, McKeon B, Skuse N, Burke D (1981) Cerebral potentials evoked by muscle stretch in man. Brain 104:149-

Stohr M, Buttner UF, Riffel B et al. (1982) Spinal somatosensory evoked potentials in cervical cord lesions. Electroencephalogr Clin Neurophysiol 54:251-265

Thompson PD, Dick JPR, Asselman P et al. (1987) Examination of motor function in lesions of the spinal cord by stimulation of the motor cortex. Ann Neurol 21:389-396

Travlos A, Pant B, Eisen A (1992) Use of transcranial magnetic stimulation for preclinical detection of cervical spondylotic myelopathy. Arch Phys Med Rehabil 73:442-446

Travlos A, Trueman S, Eisen A (1995) Monopolar needle evaluation of paraspinal musculature in the cervical, thoracic and lumbar regions and the effects of aging. Muscle Nerve 18:196-200

Tylleskar T, Banea M, Bikangi N, Fresco L, Persson LA, Rosling H (1991) Epidemiological evidence from Zaire for a dietary etiology of konzo, an upper motor neuron disease. Bull WHO 69:581-589

Tylleskar T, Banea M, Bikangi N, Cooke RD, Poulter NH, Rosling H (1992) Cassava cyanogens and konzo, an upper motor neuron disease found in Africa. Lancet 339:208-211

Wall PD (1970) The sensory and motor role of impulses travelling in the dorsal columns toward the cerebral cortex. Brain 93:505-524

Whitely AM, Swash M, Urich H (1976) Progressive encephalomyelitis with rigidity. Its relation to "subacute myoclonic spinal neuronitis" and the stiff man syndrome. Brain 99:27-42

Yiannikas C, Shahani BT, Young RR (1986) Short-latency somatosensory-evoked potentials from radial, median, ulnar, and peroneal nerve stimulation in the assessment of cervical spondylosis: comparison with conventional electromyography. Arch Neurol 43:1264-1271

Yu YL, Jones SJ (1985) Somatosensory evoked potentials in cervical spondylosis: correlation of median, ulnar and posterior tibial nerve responses with clinical and radiological findings. Brain 108:273-300

Zentner J (1989) Noninvasive motor evoked potential monitoring during neurosurgical operations on the spinal cord. Neurosurgery 24:709-712

Chapter 12

Radiculopathy due to Diseases other than Disc Disease

A.A. Eisen

By definition a radiculopathy involves the dorsal and/or ventral roots. One or more segmental levels may be affected depending upon the nature of the disease. Some diseases, for example, disc diseases, may involve several roots at the same time or different roots sequentially.

Resulting motor deficit is restricted to those muscles sharing a common innervation through a particular root (a myotome). However, because most muscles derive their innervation through two or more roots, the motor deficit that arises as a result of disease involving a single root is often incomplete and may be extremely mild.

The sensory deficit associated with disease of the dorsal root is restricted to an area of skin innervated through that root (a dermatome). The territory of most dermatomes overlaps so that in a single root lesion the involved area of sensory deficit is usually incomplete. The extent to which different sensory modalities are affected in root lesions depends largely upon the underlying cause. Compressed lesions mainly affect the largest diameter nerve fibres; the Ia and type II cutaneous afferents. This results in loss of the segmental stretch reflex, and altered vibration and touch in the relevant dermatome(s).

The efferent and afferent arcs subserving the monosynaptic stretch reflex leave and enter the spinal cord through the ventral and dorsal roots, respectively. This reflex is usually decreased and may be lost early in a root lesion.

Investigation of radiculopathies should include electromyography, CT scanning and/or MRI. Myelography should only be considered after these non-invasive procedures have failed to confirm the diagnosis. Although there are many causes of radiculopathy (Table 12.1), compressive (entrapment) radiculopathy due to disc degeneration and/or spondylosis is the commonest. This is described elsewhere and in this chapter other causes of radiculopathy and diseases with which they are easily confused will be discussed.

Diabetic Radiculopathies

Radicular-plexopathies (polyradiculopathy) frequently complicate diabetes. Elderly men with type II diabetes are particularly prone to this neuropathy which most fre-

Table 12.1. Some causes of radiculopathy

Diabetes
  Diabetic amyotrophy
  Thoracoabdominal radiculopathy

Sensory neuronopathies (ganglionopathies)
  Subacute
    Lymphoma
    Leukaemia
    Carcinoma
  Acute
    Antibiotics (penicillin)
    Idiopathic

Carcinomatous radiculopathy ("seeding")

Primary tumours of nerve roots
  Schwannoma
  Neurofibromatosis

Infectious/granulomatous radiculopathy
  Lyme disease
  Brucellosis
  Histiocytosis X
  AIDS

Spinal epidural abscess – tuberculosis

Zoster radiculitis

Spinal stenosis

Arachnoiditis

Non-degenerative bony root compression
  Rheumatoid arthritis
  Paget's disease
  Ankylosing spondylitis
  Bony malignancy
  Achondroplasia

Angiomatous malformation of root

Cervical-brachial neuritis

Thoracic outlet syndromes
  Neurogenic thoracic outlet
  Droopy shoulder syndrome

quently involves the myotomes of the anterior thigh (L2, L3, L4) (Wilbourn 1987). Although usually unilateral at onset, many cases go on to involved the contralateral side, not necessarily in a symmetrical fashion. Pain which is typically acute in onset is followed by muscle wasting and weakness, depression or loss of reflexes and sensory loss. Clinical and electrophysiological localization indicate that there may be involvement of root, plexus or nerve or more usually combinations of these. Proximal diabetic radicular-plexopathies often occur on a background of the much commoner diabetic symmetrical polyneuropathy (Asbury 1977; Bastron and Thomas 1981; Brown and Asbury 1984).

Lower lumbar, sacral and cervical roots are affected rarely compared to the upper lumbar myotomes and severe involvement of, for example, the C5, C6 roots should prompt one to seek an alternative cause for the radiculopathy. Diabetic amyotrophy, described originally by Garland (1955), can be reasonably regarded as a specific variant of diabetic polyradiculopathy.

Diabetes can also involve the thoracic roots (thoracic polyradiculopathy, thoraco-abdominal radiculopathy). The usual presenting symptoms are pain and dysaesthesia involving the chest wall or abdomen (Sun and Streib 1981; Streib et al. 1986; Sellman and Mayer 1988; Steward 1989). When pain predominates and is restricted to the abdomen, especially if limited to one quadrant, the disease may be minister-preted as "an acute abdomen". In some cases abdominal swelling due to abdom-inal muscle weakness ensues which may further confound the situation. Electromyography shows active denervation (fibrillation and positive sharp waves) in the paraspinal muscles which are innervated by the diseased roots. Persistent pain, which is often debilitating, frequently responds to anti-inflammatory therapy in combination with phenytoin, carbamazepine or amitriptyline.

Ultimately drugs will be available that will prevent the metabolic derangements causing the complications of diabetes (see below). Meanwhile control of hypergly-caemia, hypertension and obesity is essential. Recognizing the potentially life-endangering threat posed by hypoglycaemia, intensive insulin therapy has been repeatedly shown to be effective in prevention of diabetic complications. Insulin therapy is required for all type I diabetics and may be appropriate therapy for all type II patients who do not become rapidly normoglycaemic with diet and oral sulphonylurea (Flint and Clements 1988).

The chronic complications of diabetes result from the interaction of hypergly-caemia and other metabolic consequences of insulin deficiency as well as poorly understood but independent genetic and environmental factors. Rise in tissue sor-bitol secondary to concentration-dependent activation of polyol pathway activity by glucose and an accompanying fall in tissue myo-inositol and Na-K-ATPase activity have been linked to a self-reinforcing cyclic metabolic defect that accounts for rapidly reversible slowing of conduction in peripheral nerve (Greene 1988; Greene et al. 1988). Treatment aimed at neutralizing this series of events is the obvious approach for the future. Pancreatic transplant has been shown to prevent develop-ment of neuropathy in inbred diabetic rats (Orloff et al. 1988; Sima et al. 1988) and to ameliorate complicating neuropathy in humans (Sutherland et al. 1988; Van der Vliet et al. 1988).

Sensory Neuronopathies (Ganglinopathies)

Sensory neuronopathy is distinguishable from sensory neuropathy by the global, rather than distal, distribution of sensory loss, total areflexia and the absence of recordable sensory nerve action potentials in the face of normal muscle strength and compound motor action potentials, normal motor conduction velocities and needle electromyography (Asbury 1987; Donofrio et al. 1989). These electrophysio-logical features point to the dorsal root ganglion cell as the site of primary pathol-ogy (Fagius et al. 1983). The disease is usually subacute most often being associated with lymphoma, chronic lymphatic leukaemia and carcinoma (in par-ticular oat cell carcinoma); it affects women more frequently than men and may precede the underlying malignancy by several months. Paraesthesia, dysaesthesia, aching in the limbs and ataxia of gait due to impairment of vibration and position sense are the cardinal clinical features. Cutaneous sensation may be relatively preserved.

Rarely an acute form of the disease occurs (Dawson et al. 1988; Knazan et al. 1990). It has most frequently but not invariably been associated with systemic antibiotic therapy especially penicillin. Occasionally, acute sensory neuronopathy has been reported in the absence of associated factors (Knazan et al. 1990). Nosologically it may form part of a broader spectrum of radiculoneuropathies including acute pan-dysautonomia with severe sensory deficit (which involves both dorsal root ganglia and peripheral nerve) and possibly Guillian-Barré syndrome with sensory predominance (Hodson et al. 1984).

Carcinomatous Radiculopathy

A variety of primary tumours may be associated with secondary seeding around the spinal roots. Most common are secondary deposits from primary tumours of the breast, lung, prostate, kidney and lymphomas. When cancer is complicated by seeding of cells within the spinal dural sac pain is predominant occurring in almost every case (Gilbert et al. 1978). The pain is of two types: local and radicular. Most patients complain of local pain which usually is experienced near the site of the lesion as identified myelographically. Radicular pain is localized within one or two vertebral segments of the lesion and is most frequent in the cervical or lumbosacral regions and less common in the thoracic segments. The pain is often bilateral and felt as a girdle radiating from the back to the front of the chest or abdomen. Unlike that associated with herniated intervertebral discs, pain due to carcinomatous seeding is typically made worse by lying down and frequently awakens the patient from sleep.

Carcinomatous radiculopathy of this type is not necessarily associated with signs of spinal cord compression; about 50% of patients presenting with back pain associated with a known cancer have a radiculopathy (Rodichok et al. 1986; Ruff and Lanska 1989).

Primary Tumours of the Spinal Roots

In comparison to secondary tumour invasion of roots, primary spinal root neoplasm is uncommon. The most common benign nerve tumour that affects the spinal roots is a schwannoma (a nerve sheath tumour). They are slowly growing, usually presenting with radicular pain. Although usually solitary they may be multiple in association with neurofibromatosis (von Recklinghausen's disease) where they also may be malignant. Any spinal segment can be involved by schwannomas but they are most frequent in the thoracic segments. If large they can cause secondary cord compression. Neurofibromas are typically associated with von Recklinghausen's disease and can occur on virtually any nerve including the ventral and dorsal spinal roots. Lipomas are other, but rarer, benign tumours recognized as a cause of radiculopathy. Most are within the lumbosacral spinal canal and cause symptoms which vary from discrete intermittent uni- or bilateral sciatica to severe flaccid paraplegia wit sensory and bladder dysfunction (Lassman and James 1967).

Myeloradiculopathies: Infectious and Granulomatous Radiculopathy

There are a variety of inflammatory conditions which result in radiculitis, myelitis and frequently a combination of the two: myeloradiculitis. Many are referred to in Chapter 17. In this section emphasis will be placed on the extent to which these disorders involve the spinal roots.

Lyme Disease

This occurs worldwide as a multisystem disorder caused by recently recognized tick-transmitted spirochaete, *Borrelia burgdorferi*. Transmission is from a bite, usually during summer months, by *Ixodes dammini* or related ixodid ticks (Benhamou et al. 1988; Editorial, Lancet 1989). Typically it induces fever, chills, malaise, headache, a characteristic rash and polyarthritis (stage 1). The acute form is usually benign and responds favourably to therapy with tetracycline. Weeks to months later neurological involvement occurs in about 15% of patients (stage 2). This may happen in the absence of the familiar systemic manifestations or the skin rash typical of stage 1.

The triad of lymphocytic meningitis, cranial nerve involvement and radiculopathy (Bannwarth's syndrome) are the usual neurological features (Pachner and Steere 1985; Midgard and Hofstad 1987; Pachner et al. 1989; Wilder-Smith and Roelke 1989). Facial palsy, often bilateral, thoracic sensory radiculitis, motor radiculitis in the extremities, brachial plexitis, mononeuritis and mononeuritis multiplex are the commonest peripheral nerve manifestations. Rarely, painful and even persistent radiculopathy may be the sole presenting feature.

CSF examination reveals pleocytosis, raised spinal protein levels and oligoclonal bands. The diagnosis is confirmed by demonstrating antibodies to *B. burgdorferi* in the CSF and serum. Neurological manifestations are usually self-limiting resolving in several months but respond to IV penicillin G, 20 million U/day in divided doses over 10 days. In patients allergic to penicillin, tetra-cycline should be tried. Arthritis and acrodermatitis occurring months or years after the initial infection typify stage 3 of the disease. Therapy with third-generation cephalosporins should be considered to treat the late stages of the disease (Czachor and Gleckman 1989). These drugs can, however, cause side effects including bleeding (with use of Moxalactam or Cefoperazone) and a reaction akin to that induced by disulfiram (Antabuse) if taken in association with alcohol. Prolonged therapy is presently expensive.

Brucellosis

The neurological complications of brucellosis are protean and pathogenic mechanisms diverse (Bahemuka et al. 1988; Al Deeb et al. 1989). Neurological manifestations may be the presenting feature and include transient ischaemic attacks and stroke, encephalopathy, motor neurone disease, a cauda equina syndrome and radiculopathy. The disease can be difficult to diagnose and is usually confused with tuberculosis. Serology and culture are superior to radiography and scanning in the diagnosis of brucellosis (Lifeso et al. 1985). There is often a good response to antibiotic therapy but it is important that therapy be continued for a reasonably duration and best monitored with repeated agglutination titres.

Histiocytosis X

This group of diseases encompasses unifocal eosinophilic granuloma, Hand–Schueller–Christian disease (multifocal eosinophilic granuloma) and Letterer–Siwe disease. "X" refers to the frequent but not invariable presence of xanthomata. Common to all three of the histiocytoses is the existence of granulomatous infiltration of histiocytes. There have been several reports of single eosinophilic granulomas causing a compressive radiculopathy (Eil and Adornato 1977; Padovani et al. 1988). Radiotherapy has been found useful in therapy either alone or in addition to surgery.

AIDS

Inflammatory polyradiculopathy infrequently complicates AIDS in the absence of other neurological involvement (Eidelberg et al. 1986; Behar et al. 1987). There is usually progressive, multiple root disease with CSF pleocytosis and elevated protein. The onset is usually insidious and most frequently involves the lumbar and sacral roots leading to a progressive paraparesis and areflexia. A cauda equina syndrome may occur. There may be eventual spread to involve the thoracic and cervical roots. Autopsy studies reveal extensive necrosis, inflammatory infiltrates and focal vasculitis of the involved spinal roots.

Spinal Epidural Abscess

Spinal epidural abscesses are infections in the space between the dura mater and the surrounding vertebral bodies. Purulent liquid or granulomatous tissue, located in the posterior portion of the epidural space of the thoracic or lumbar spine, spans several vertebral levels. The prominent clinical features are fever, spine pain with a radicular distribution and, if untreated, subsequent para-paresis from cord compression. Mild blunt spinal trauma often provides a devitalized site susceptible to transient bacteraemia with subsequent abscess formation. In such cases the infecting organism is frequently S. aureus (Kaufman et al. 1980). Epidural abscess and disc space infection of this type had, until recently, declined markedly in frequency (Verner and Musher 1985; Danner and Hartman 1987). However, with the abundance of drug abuse there has been a resurgence of these conditions especially amongst intravenous drug users and patients with human immunodeficiency virus (HIV) syndrome (Koppel et al. 1988). In many patients so affected, the course is subacute developing over several months with radicular pain commonly occurring. A preceding or associated fever is frequently absent or temperature may be only minimally elevated. The lower thoracic or lumbosacral spines are most commonly involved. Diagnostic evaluation should include spine radiographs, myelography with or without CT, nuclear bone scanning and radioactive gallium scanning. Staphylococcal infection is the commonest infective agent causing abscess amongst drug users.

Spinal tuberculous abscesses usually occur as a single small focus of infection; there is seldom evidence of active TB in another site and chest radiographs may be normal. Compared to bacterial infection, patients are younger (unless the abscess is associated with drug abuse) and back pain is usually much more chronic.

Zoster Radiculitis

Herpes zoster (shingles) represents latent reactivation of the varicella virus which has remained dormant in trigeminal or dorsal root ganglia following childhood chicken-pox. Herpes zoster occurs in about 1% of the population. It is commoner in older subjects and occurs in about 25% of patients with cancer, especially lymphoma, and in immunocompromised patients including those with AIDS (Tenser 1984).

Radicular symptoms (pain, sensory deficit, weakness, depression or loss of appropriate reflexes) usually accompany the presence of vesicles in the relevant dermatome (Burkman et al. 1988). However, they may be absent or scantly and go unnoticed by the patient (zoster sine herpete) (Lewis 1958; Mayo and Booss 1989). Mid thoracic and trigeminal involvement is common, but when lumbosacral roots are involved, especially if there is associated motor deficit, the diagnosis may be easily confused with commoner causes of radiculopathy.

Spinal Stenosis

Mechanical compression of spinal roots from protruding discs or narrowed intervertebral foramina are the commonest causes of radiculopathy. These are largely dealt with elsewhere in this text. Mention here will only be made of spinal stenosis which typically affects elderly men (about 65 years old) more frequently than women. Intermittent *neurogenic* claudication with pain in the hips, thighs or legs brought on by walking are characteristic features (Lipson 1987; Torg and Pavlov 1987; Winter and Jani 1989). However, pain may also be initiated by lying supine and awaken the patient from sleep. Pain or numbness in the feet may also occur and when persistent can mimic and cause confusion with peripheral neuropathy. Most cases of spinal stenosis affect the lumbar spine and roots (L3/4 and L5/S1) at the rostral end of the cauda equina. Often the neurological examination is normal but objective deficit can be precipitated by mild or moderate exertion such as walking a few stairs. Occasionally the cervical cord may be involved. When this happens, transient reversible quadriplegia due to cervical cord neurapaxia occurs. In congenital spinal stenosis the whole spinal canal may be narrowed and cervical cord and cauda equina root compression become evident at a much younger age.

Arachnoiditis

Although this can occur anywhere in the meninges, the lumbosacral region is most commonly affected. The arachnoid becomes thickened and scarred, becoming adherent to the pia and dura. There is secondary obliteration of the meningeal vasculature. Single or multiple spinal roots become entrapped in the adhesions. The underlying mechanism(s) causing arachnoiditis is poorly understood but when experimentally induced in animals it is associated with decreased beta-endorphin in the CSF (Lipman and Haughton 1988).

The causes of arachnoiditis are varied and may follow trauma (including disc herniation) or spinal surgery, intrathecal injections including radiological contrast media or epidural anaesthesia (Sghirlanzoni et al. 1989). The latent period between the original insult and development of symptoms varies from a few months to several years. Spinal meningeal infections, particularly tuberculosis, syphilis and cryptococcosis or rarely cysticercosis, may be also complicated by arachnoiditis as can subarachnoid haemorrhage (Tjandra et al. 1989). Frequently, however, arachnoiditis seems to develop de novo, without apparent cause.

The clinical features of arachnoiditis are those of single or multiple root compression. Later a cauda equina syndrome develops and if the brunt of the disease is rostral to L2/L3 the cord may eventually be compressed. Chronic back pain with radiation down both legs is a prominent feature which early on in the disease may be the only symptom and unaccompanied by objective neurological deficit. Arachnoiditis is usually easily visible on enhanced CT scan. Whereas MRI is superior to CT in visualizing cord enlargement, compression or atrophy, it is not as sensitive as CT for documenting arachnoiditis (Karnaze et al. 1988).

Non-degenerative Bony Compression of Roots

Several conditions other than disc degeneration or degenerative spondylosis may cause radiculopathy from bony encroachment upon the spinal roots. The commonest of these include rheumatoid arthritis, Paget's disease, bony malignancy and achondroplasia. Secondary invasion of bone from primary tumours of the breast, lung, prostate, kidney and bowel are also common. Usually local pain with subsequent radicular pain indicates that there has been vertebral collapse entrapping the root. This may then go on to compression of the cord.

In rheumatoid arthritis and other arthropathies vertebral deformities may result in isolated nerve root compression, subluxation with secondary cord compression and susceptibility to trauma. Lesser trauma than usual can result in fractures of an arthritic spina and extradural haematoma. Ankylosing spondylitis shares similar potential complications. A cauda equina syndrome, commencing as single- or multilevel radiculopathy, at times unilaterally, can occur several years after the onset of the spondylitis. This complication is more common in ankylosing spondylitis than in the other arthropathies (Kramer and Krouth 1978). An unusual cause of mechanical root compression is a synovial cyst associated with the apophyseal joint (Hammer 1988).

Paget's disease is frequently complicated by neurological disturbances (Chen et al. 1979). This chronic progressive disease of bone is characterized by an abnormally rapid rate of bone resorption and unregulated reparative bone formation causing gross deformities of the skeleton. Neurological complications are often serious and given their potential reversibility by therapeutic agents such as calcitonin, mithramycin and etidronate require careful and early recognition. The most common picture associated with spinal root involvement due to Paget's disease is low back pain with radicular spread, leg weakness and sensory changes. In contrast, spinal cord compression is most frequent in the thoracic region where the highest ratio of cord to spinal canal cross-sectional area exists.

Neurological disorders in achondroplasia are produced by structural anomalies of the cranium (resulting in hydrocephalus) and spinal canal (producing spinal and radicular compression). The spinal canal in this disease has a decreased cross-sectional area the intervertebral foramina are narrowed (Blondeau et al. 1984; Lonstein 1988). These changes reduce the area for the dural sac and existing spinal nerves. Cervical-occipital compression is more frequent in childhood and may occur in the first months of life (Hecht et al. 1984). Decompressive surgery is successful in preventing these complications (Shikata et al. 1988). In later years disc degeneration with disc space narrowing and osteophyte formation further complicate an already compromised spinal canal and intervertebral foramina.

Angiomatous Radiculopathy

Angiomatous malformations of the spinal cord usually result in cord compression or ischaemia resulting in long tract signs or sometimes a mixture of upper and lower motor neurone dysfunction (see Chapter 18). Rarely, angiomas may primarily involve the cauda equina or occasionally only a single spinal root (Browne et al. 1976; Gennuso et al. 1989). Extramedullary-intradural haemangioblastomas are often attached to posterior nerve roots and radicular pain, posterior column sensory loss or both are frequent presenting symptoms. Equally unusual is lumbosacral plexopathy or painful radiculopathy secondary to abdominal aneurysm (Lainez et al. 1989).

Brachial Neuritis

Paralytic brachial neuritis (also referred to as neuralgic amyotrophy and the Parsonage-Turner syndrome) can closely mimic cervical radiculopathy and brief commentary is required given the relevance of this disease in the differential diagnosis of cervical root lesions (Parsonage and Turner 1948; Turner and Parsonage 1957).

Characteristically, the syndrome is of acute onset, often with severe pain, accompanied, or more usually followed in several days, by the onset of weakness and subsequent muscle wasting. Mild cases develop pain and weakness but do not go on to develop muscle wasting. The distribution of the pain and weakness is variable, characteristically being poorly localized in terms of peripheral anatomy, involving rather combinations of different peripheral nerves and various components of the brachial plexus. Careful clinical analysis suggests that the lesion in many cases of paralytic brachial neuritis is localized to branching points of the brachial plexus or its major peripheral nerves (England and Summer 1987).

The aetiopathogenesis of this disease is not known, however, about 50% of cases are associated with antecedent events, such as immunization, viral infections, surgery, trauma, pregnancy, drug abuse and collagen vascular diseases. There is a rare familial form (Dunn et al. 1978), some cases of which have proven to have tomaculous neuropathy (Madrid and Bradley 1975) and occasionally the condition is recurrent (Bradley et al. 1975). The majority of patients make a satisfactory, but usually slow, recovery taking one to three years. About 10% of patients do not regain useful function of the involved muscles.

Pathological observations in brachial neuritis are rare (Tsairis et al. 1972). A recent report of two patients with recurrent symptoms who, because of developing a tender supraclavicular mass underwent surgery, showed macroscopic fusiform segmental swelling of the trunks of the brachial plexus. Microscopically the lesions were characterized by oedema, onion bulb formation and marked focal chronic inflammatory infiltrates with lymphoid follicle formation, limited to the endoneurial compartment (Cusimano et al. 1988).

Thoracic Outlet Syndromes

The concept of thoracic outlet has evolved over the past century. Controversy surrounds virtually every aspect of it (Cuetter and Bartoszek 1989). However, in the context of the present chapter the critical issue lies in the differential diagnosis of root lesions, especially involvement of C8, T1 cervical roots. Pragmatically it can be argued that most, if not all, thoracic outlet syndromes are of two types. The very rare *true neurogenic thoracic outlet syndrome* and the very common *droopy shoulder syndrome*.

Neurogenic thoracic outlet syndrome has been well delineated (Gilliatt 1976; Gilliat et al. 1978). It is rare and the author has seen fewer than 20 cases in 25 years of neurological and electromyographic practice. Typically it affects young women and presents with painless, partial, thenar wasting. But in contradistinction to carpal tunnel syndrome, sensory complaints, when they occur, involve the medial aspect of the forearm and ulnar side of the hand. The symptoms are directly due to pressure or stretching of the lower trunk or C8, T1 roots from a fibrous band attached to a supernumerary rib or elongated C7 transverse process. When extra ribs are present, they often occur bilaterally, but usually it is the less prominent rib (with the longer fibrous band) that is the one responsible for symptoms. X-ray or CT scan does not invariably reveal an extra rib or elongated C7 transverse process and therefore normal radiological studies do not rule out neurogenic thoracic outlet syndrome.

Electrophysiological studies are helpful in the diagnosis and localization of the lesion (Wilbourn 1982, 1988). A constellation of characteristic abnormalities have evolved. They are:

1. A much reduced median motor compound action potential in the face of a normal median sensory compound action potential.
2. A reduced or absent ulnar sensory compound action potential in the face of a normal or only modestly reduced ulnar motor compound action potential.
3. A prolonged or absent ulnar F wave.
4. A prolonged and/or small ulnar somatosensory evoked potential.
5. Needle EMG evidence for chronic partial denervation in the C8 and T1 supplied muscles.

In contrast to the above, the droopy shoulder syndrome, a term coined by Swift and Nichols (1984), is common and accounts for many if not most other cases of thoracic outlet syndrome. This syndrome is virtually limited to women. The following are the criteria for droopy shoulder syndrome:

1. Pain or paraesthesia occurring in the shoulder, arm, forearm or hand.
2. Long, graceful and swan-like neck; low set shoulders, and horizontal or downsloping clavicles.

3. Exacerbation of symptoms on palpation of brachial plexus or passive downward traction of the arms.
4. Immediate relief of symptoms by passive shoulder elevation.
5. Absence of vascular phenomena, muscle atrophy, sensory loss or reflex changes.
6. Normal electrophysiological studies.
7. The second thoracic or lower vertebrae are visible above the shoulders on lateral cervical spine X-rays.

Electrophysiological Investigation of Radiculopathies

CT scanning and MRI give excellent visualization of the nerve root and spinal cord and it is relevant to ask what, if any, is the role of electrophysiology in an era of these advanced radiological techniques. The presence of a radiological and clinical defect do not always go hand in hand. In older subjects silent radiological defects commonly occur in the absence of clinically obvious disease. In contrast, many of the inflammatory radiculopathies are not accompanied by radiological abnormalities. Radiological abnormalities give little or no information regarding severity and potential for prognosis and when several segmental levels are involved it is often not possible to determine on radiological grounds which or how many levels have clinical relevance.

Several different electrophysiological techniques are available for the assessment of root lesions (Tonzola et al. 1981; Eisen 1987; Wilbourn and Aminoff 1988). Each will be discussed briefly.

Motor and Sensory Conductions

Usually, these are normal in roots lesions, If axonal destruction or loss has been marked there may be moderate slowing of motor conduction velocity in relevant nerves. More importantly, axonal loss is accompanied by reduced amplitude of the compound muscle action potential and side-to-side comparison of homologous muscles is useful in unilateral lesions. A reduction of greater than 50% indicates that there has been a considerable loss of axons and consequently, if spontaneous recovery is to be anticipated, it is likely to be delayed and incomplete. In the majority of root lesions, those due to mechanical causes, the dorsal root ganglion lies distal to the site of compression or entrapment. As a result the sensory nerve action potential remains normal. A reduced, or absent sensory nerve action potential indicates that either the lesion is distal to be the dorsal root or that one is dealing with a true ganglionopathy in which there has been ganglion cell loss.

Needle Electromyography

This is by far the most useful of the various electrophysiological tests available for assessing root lesions. It is rare for other tests to be abnormal in the face of a normal needle EMG. The presence of fibrillation or positive sharp waves is proof positive that there is ongoing, or previous, axonal damage with resulting muscle denervation. This then becomes an important issue in prognosis (not available through imaging). Unfortunately fibrillation takes time to develop. It develops first in the paraspinal muscles which are innervated directly from the spinal root through the medial branch of its posterior primary ramus. In these muscles it can take up to a week to 10 days before fibrillation becomes evident. In distal limb muscles development of fibrillization can take as long as 6 weeks. Paraspinal needle EMG is not only a useful prognostic feature but is also valuable in localization. In the lumbosacral region there is reasonable specificity as to segmental level especially in the deeper muscle layers (multifidi). In the cervical region there is considerably more overlap and segmental specificity is limited. For this reason it is common for quite severe cervical root lesions to occur without the developing fibrillation.

Proximal Conduction Studies

Various methods have been employed specifically to evaluate conduction slowing and/or block through the root. In single root lesions conduction block is reflected clinically by depression or loss of the relevant deep tendon reflex but because of shared innervation muscle weakness, if present, is modest and incomplete. Two methods in particular have prove of limited value in the assessment of radiculopathies. They are the *F response* and *somatosensory evoked potentials*. It is beyond the scope of this chapter to detail these techniques and controversies surrounding their use for which the reader is referred to more comprehensive texts. Essentially the F response is an antidromically induced excitation of the anterior horn cell resulting from supramaximal stimulation of a peripheral motor nerve. In root lesions its latency is sometimes prolonged or it may become unrecordable. The somatosensory evoked potential (SEP), is the measurable cortical response to a sensory, predominantly Ia afferent, stimulus. Because its impulse traffic traverses the root it can be used to assess conduction through the dorsal root fibres. Both techniques suffer from the fact that they attempt to measure slowed conduction or block through a very short segment of nerve, the root, diluted in a long length of normally conducing distal stretch of nerve. One other technique, the H reflex, shares the same limitation and additionally can only be easily applied to lesions of the S1 or the L5 roots.

Electrophysiological Confirmation of Root Avulsion

Root avulsion is important to diagnose since it precludes any attempt at neurosurgical reconstruction. Radiological confirmation using myelography usually delineates the extent of root injury. However, pseudomeningoceles with intact roots and root avulsion without characteristic radiological changes both occur. Electrophysiologically, root avulsion is associated with paraspinal and limb muscle denervation in the relevant myotome(s). A normal sensory nerve action potential in the presence of an anaesthetic and paretic limb reflects that the dorsal root has been separated from its central connections. For the same reason the histamine response (skin flare induced by intradermal histamine) remains intact. Absence of a SEP and inability to record a muscle action potential using cortical (magnetic) stimulation are further proof that the dorsal and ventral roots have been severed.

References

Al Deeb SM, Yaqub BA, Sharif HS, et al. (1989) Neurobrucellosis: clinical characteristics, diagnosis, and outcome. Neurology 39:498–501

Asbury AK (1977) Proximal diabetic neuropathy. An Neurol 2:179–180

Asbury AK (1987) Sensory neuropathy. Semi Neurol 7:58–66

Bahemuka M, Shemena AR, Panayiotopoulos CP, et al. (1988) Neurological syndromes of brucellosis. J. Neurol Neurosurg Psychiatry 51:1017–1021

Bastron JA, Thomas JE (1981) Diabetic polyradiculopathy. Mayo Clin Proc 56:725–732

Behar R, Wiley C, McCutchan JA (1987) Cytomegalovirus polyadiculoneuropathy in acquired immune deficiency syndrome. Neurology 37:557–561

Benhamou CI, Grauvain JB, Calamy G, Lemaire JF (1988) Lyme disease: clinical, biological and developmental aspects. 29 cases in the Orleans region. Rev Rhum Mal Osteoartic 55:647–653

Blondeau M, Brunet D, Blanche JM, et al. (1984) Compression of he cervical spinal cord in achondroplasia. Sem Hop Paris 60:771–775

Bradley WG, Madrid R, Thrush DC (1975) Recurrent brachial plexus neuropathy. Brain 98:381–398

Brown MJ, Asbury AK (1984) Diabetic neuropathy. Ann Neurol 15:2–12

Browne TR, Adams RD, Roberson GH (1976) Hemangioblastoma of the spinal cord. Review and report of five cases. Arch Neurol 33:435–441

Burkman KA, Gaines Jr RW, Kshani SR, Smith RD (1988) Herpes zoster: a consideration in the differential diagnosis of radiculopathy. Arch Phys Med Rehabil 69:132–134

Chen J, Rhee RSC, Wallach S, et al. (1979) Neurologic disturbance in Paget disease of bone: response to calcitonin. Neurology 29:448–457

Cuetter AC, Bartoszek DM (1989) The thoracic outlet syndrome: controversies, overdiagnosis, overtreatment and recommendations for management. Muscle Nerve 12:410–419

Cusimano MD, Bilbao JM, Cohen SM (1988) Hypertrophic brachial plexus neuritis: a pathological study of two cases. Ann Neurol 24:615–622

Czachor JS, Gleckman RA (1989) Third-generation cephalosporins. A plea to save them for specific infections. Postgrad Med 85:169–172, 175–176

Danner RL, Hartman BJ (1987) Update of spinal epidural abscess: thirty-five cases and review of the literature. Rev Infect Dis 9:265–274

Dawson DM, Samuels MA, Morris J (1988) Sensory form of acute polyneuritis. Neurology 38:1728–1731

Donofrio PD, Alessi AG, Albers JW, Knapp RH, Blaivas M (1989) Electrodiagnostic evolution of carcinomatous sensory neuronopathy. Muscle Nerve 12:508–513

Dunn HG, Daube JR, Gomez MR (1978) Heredofamilial brachial plexus neuropathy (hereditary neuralgic amyotrophy with brachial predilection) in childhood. Dev Med Child Neurol 20:28–46

Editorial (1989) Lancet 2:198–199

Edidelberg D, Sotrel A, Vogel H, Walker P, Kleefield J, Crumpacker CS (1986) Progressive polyradiculopathy in acquired immune deficiency syndrome. Neurology 36:912–916

Eil C, Adornator BT (1977) Radicular compression in multifocal eosinophilic granuloma. Successful treatment with radiotherapy. Arch Neurol 34:786–787

Eisen A (1987) Radiculopathies and plexopathies. In: Brown WF, Bolton CF (eds) Clinical electromyography. Butterworths, Boston, Toronto, pp 51–73

England JD, Sumner AJ (1987) Neuralgic amyotrophy: an increasingly diverse entity. Muscle Nerve 10:60–68

Fagius J, Westerberg CE, Olsson Y (1983) Acute pandysautonomia and severe sensory deficit with poor recovery. A clinical, neurophysiological and pathological case study. J Neurol Neurosurg Psychiatry 46:725–733

Flint MA, Clements RS (1988) Prevention of the complications of diabetes. Prim Care 15:277–284

Garland H (1955) Diabetic amyotrophy. Br Med J 2:1287–1290

Gennuso R, Zappulla RA, Strenger SW (1989) A localized lumbar spinal root arteriovenous malformation presenting with radicular signs and symtoms. Spine 14:543–546

Gilbert RW, Kim JH, Posner JB (1978) Epidural spinal cord compression from metastatic tumor: diagnosis and treatment. Ann Neurol 3:40–51

Gilliatt RW (1976) Thoracic outlet compression syndrome. Br Med J 1:1274–1275

Gilliatt RW, Willison RG, Dietz V, Williams IR (1978) Peripheral nerve conduction in patients with cervical rib and band. Ann Neurol 4:124–129

Greene D (1988) The pathogenesis and prevention of diabetic neuropathy and nephropathy. Metabolism 37:25–29

Greene DA, Lattimer SA, Sima AA (1988) Pathogenesis and prevention of diabetic neuropathy. Diabetes Metab Rev 4:201–221

Hammer AJ (1988) Synovial cyst: an unusual cause of nerve root compression. A case report. S Afr Med J 73:44–45

Hecht JT, Butler IJ, Scott CT (1984) Long-term neurological sequelae in achondroplasia. Eur J Pediatr 143:58–60

Hodson AK, Hurwitz BJ, Albrecht R (1984) Dysautonomia in Guillain-Barrle syndrome with dorsal root ganglioneuropathy, Wallerian degeneration, and fatal myocarditis. Ann Neurol 15:88–95

Karnaze MG, Gado MH, Sartor KJ, Hodges FJ (1988) Comparison of MR and CT myelography in imaging the cervical and thoracic spine. Am J Roentgenol 150:397–403

Kaufman DM, Kaplan JG, Litman N (1980) Infections agents in spinal epidural abscesses. Neurology 30:844–850

Knazam M, Bohlega S, Berry K, Eisen A (1990) Acute sensory neuronopathy with preserved SEPs and long-latency reflexes. Muscle Nerve 13:381–384

Koppel BS, tuchman AJ, Mangiardi JR, Daras M, Weitzner I (1988) Epidural spinal infection in intravenous drug Abusers. Arch Neurol 45:1331–1337

Kramer LD, Krouth GJ (1978) Computerized tomography. An adjunct to early diagnosis in the cauda equina syndrome of ankylosing spondylitis. Arch Neurol 35:116–118

Lainez JM, Yaya R, Lluch V, et al. (1989) Lumbosacral plexopathy caused by aneurysms of the abdominal aorta. Med clin (Barc) 92:462–464

Lassman LP, James CCM (1967) Lumbosacral lipomas: critical survey of 26 cases submitted to laminectomy. J Neurol Neurosurg Psychiatry 30:174–181

Lewis GW (1958) Zoster sine herpete. Br Med J 2:418–421

Lifeso RM, Harder E, McCorkell SJ (1985) Spinal brucellosis. J Bone Joint Surg (Br) 67:345–351

Lipman Bt, Haughton VM (1988) Diminished cerebrospinal and fluid beta-endorphin concentration in monkeys with arachnoiditis. Invest Radiol 23:190–192

Lipson SJ (1987) Spinal stenosis. Rheum Dis Clin North Am 14:613–618

Lonstein JE (1988) Treatment of kyphosis and lumbar stenosis in achondroplasia. Basic Life Sci 48:283–292

Madrid R, Bradley WG (1975) The pathology of tomaculous neuropathy: studies on the formation of the abnormal myelin sheath. J Neurol Sci 25:415–448

Mayo DR, Booss J (1989) Varicella zoster-associated neurological disease without skin lesions. Arch Neurol 46:313–315

Midgard A, Hofstad H (1987) Unusual manifestations of nervous system Borrelia burgdorferi infection. Arch Neurol 44:781–783

Orloff MJ, Macedo A, Greenleaf GE (1988) Effect of pancreas transplantation on diabetic somatic neuropathy. Surgery 104:437–444

Pachner AR, Steere AC (1985) The triad of neurological manifestations of Lyme disease: meningitis, cranial neuritis and radiculoneuritis. Neurology 35:47–53

Pachner AR, Duray P, Steere AC (1989) Central nervous system manifestations of Lyme disease. Arch Neurol 46:790–795

Padovani R, Cavallo M, Tonelli MP, et al. (1988) Histiocytosis-X: a rare cause of radiculopathy. Neurosurgery 22:1077–1079

Parsonage MJ, Turner JWA (1948) Neurologic amyotrophy: the shoulder-girdle syndrome. Lancet 1:973–978

Rodichok LD, Ruckdeschel JC, Harper GR, et al. (1986) Early detection and treatment of spinal epidural metastases: the role of myelography. Ann Neurol 20:696–702

Ruff RL, Lanska DJ (1989) Epidural metastases in prospectively evaluated veterans with cancer and back pain. Cancer 63:2234–2241

Sellman MS, Mayer RF (1988) thoracoabdominal radiculopathy. South Med J 81:199–201

Sghirlanzoni A, Marazzi R, Pareyson D, et al. (1989) Epidural anaesthesia and spinal arachnoiditis. Anaesthesia 44:317–321

Shikata J, Yamamuro T, Iida H, et al. (1988) Surgical treatment of achondroplastic dwarfs with paraplegia. Surg Neurol 29:125–130

Sima AA, Zhang WX, Tze WJ, et al. (1988) Diabetic neuropathy in STZ-induced diabetic rat and effect of allogenic islet cell transplantation. Morphometric analysis. Diabetes 37:1129–1136

Stewart JD (1989) Diabetic truncal neuropathy: topography of the sensory deficit. Ann Neurol 25:233–238

Streib EW, Sun SF, Paustian FF, Gallagher TF, Shipp JC, Ecklund RE (1986) Diabetic thoracic radiculopathy: electrodiagnostic study. Muscle Nerve 9:548–553

Sun SF, Streib EW (1981) Diabetic thoracoabdominal neuropathy: clinical and eletromyographic features. Ann Neurol 9:75–79

Sutherland DE, Kendall DM, Moudry KC, et al. (1988) Pancreas transplantation in nonuremic, type I diabetic recipients. Surgery 104:453–464

Swift TR, Nichols FT (1984) The droopy shoulder syndrome. Neurology 34:212–215

Tenser RB (1984) Herpes simplex and herpes zoster: nervous system involvement. Neurol Clin 2:215–240

Tjandra JJ, Varma TR, Weeks RD (1989) Spinal arachnoiditis following subarachnoid haemorrhage. Aust NZ J Surg 59:84–87

Tonzola RJ, Ackel AA, Shahani BT, Young RR (1981) Usefulness of electrophysiological studies in the diagnosis of lumbosacral root disease. Ann Neurol 9:305–308

Torg JS, Pavlov H (1987) Cervical spinal stenosis with cord neurapraxia and transient quadriplegia. Clin Sports Med 6:115–133

Tsairis P, Dyck P, Mulder DW (1972) Natural history of brachial plexus neuropathy. Arch Neurol 27:109–117

Turner JWA, Parsonage MJ (1957) Neurologic amyotrophy (paralytic brachial neuritis). Lancet 2:209–212

Van der Vilet JA, Navarro X, Kennedy WR, et al. (1988)a The effect of pancreas transplantation on diabetic polyneuropathy. Transplantation 45:368–370

Verner EF, Musher DM (1985) Spinal epidural abscess. Med Clin North Am 69:375–384

Wilbourn AJ (1982) True neurogenic thoracic outlet syndrome. American association of electromyography and electrodiagnosis, Rochester MN

Wilbourn AJ (1987) The diabetic neuropathies. In: Brown WF, Bolton CF (eds) Clinical electromyography. Butterworths, Boston, Toronto, pp 329–364

Wilbourn AJ (1988) Thoracic outlet syndrome surgery causing severe brachial plexopathy. Muscle Nerve 11:66–74

Wilbourn AJ, Aminoff MJ (1988) The electrophysiologic examination in patients with radiculopathies. AAEE minimonograph 32. Muscle Nerve 11:1099–1114

Wilder-Smith E, Roelke U (1989) Meningopolyradiculitis (Bannwarth syndrome) as a primary manifestation of a centrocytic-centroblastic lymphoma. J Neurol 236:168–169

Winter M, Jani L (1989) The narrowed spinal canal. Dtsch Med Wochenschr 114:756–758

Chapter 13

Autonomic Dysfunction in Spinal Cord Disease

R.D. Fealey

Anatomical Considerations

Cortical, hypothalamic and brainstem projections directly or indirectly influence autonomic centres in the intermediolateral cell columns of the T1 to L2 or L3 cord segments with both inhibitory and facilitatory inputs to the sympathetic centres and the S2 to S4 sacral parasympathetic centres. Vagal afferent and efferent projections from the nuclei of the tractus solitarius and ambiguus in the medulla are not directly involved by spinal cord disease whereas sympathoexcitatory neurones of the rostral ventrolateral medulla are partially or completely prevented from reaching their target neurones in the intermediolateral cell columns. This relative absence of sympathetic activation may lead to a relative overactivity of vagal activity especially if the functional disconnection is relatively acute and complete; an example is the occurrence of profound bradycardia and cardiac arrest with tracheal suction in the recently injured quadraplegic.

The level of last functioning cord segment is important in cardiovascular autonomic disturbances: lesions above the splanchnic sympathetic outflow (T5 to T9) regularly cause orthostatic hypotension and, in the chronic stage of cord injury are associated with paroxysmal hypertensive episodes (autonomic dysreflexia). Lesions below T9 cause little or no disturbance of blood pressure regulation. (Fealey et al. 1984; Mathias and Frankel 1992).

Disconnection from hypothalamic centres in the preoptic and anterior hypothalamic area markedly affects thermoregulatory (sweating, vasodilation and shivering) responses (Pollock et al 1951; Fealey 1993; Kihara et al. 1995) and loss of connectivity with the pontine micturition centre profoundly affects synergistic parasympathetic, sympathetic and striated urethral sphincter function leading to urinary bladder storage and emptying abnormalities.

Gastrointestinal activity appears to be less profoundly affected by supraspinal disconnection because of the intrinsic intramural plexuses of the gut, although there can be profound effects initially (ileus, gastrointestinal haemorrhage). Lesions of the midthoracic cord affecting the splanchnic sympathetic outflow are sometimes associated with loss of the "sympathetic inhibitory brake" producing diarrhoea and excessive, uncoordinated, segmental intestinal contractility (Fealey et al. 1984).

Autonomic Disturbances in Upper Spinal Cord Injury or Disease

Traumatic cervical spinal cord injury (SCI) is the most common form of myelopathy producing profound disturbances of autonomic function. Acute transverse myelopathy can also be due to inflammatory, ischaemic or rapidly expanding compressive lesions.

Common autonomic disturbances in these conditions are next discussed.

Spinal Shock

Analogous to the absent deep tendon and superficial reflexes and skeletal muscle hypotonia, spinal autonomic reflexes are also absent after acute cervical myelopathy. The large bowel and urinary bladder are atonic and faecal and urinary retention, distention and overflow incontinence occur; cutaneous vasodilation occurs and there is systemic and postural hypotension and a propensity to poikilothermia as shivering and sweating in response to low and high environmental temperatures cannot occur. The upper gastrointestinal tract may also be atonic (paralytic ileus) and oesophageal, gastric and duodenal ulceration can occur. Gastric distention can limit diaphragmatic excursion and increase the risk of aspiration and cause hypoxia and retained secretions. There is often profound bradycardia in response to tracheal suction and hypoxia. There is an increased incidence of neurogenic pulmonary oedema with excessive extravascular lung water and vascular permeability requiring meticulous management of volume status (Hickey et al. 1995). This state typically lasts from several days to several weeks. Treatment measures are straightforward but very important (Table 13.1).

Syndromes of Chronic Cervical Cord Transection

Orthostatic Hypotension

In the chronic stages of upper (above T4) spinal cord disconnection from supraspinal centres autonomic cardiovascular disturbances still persist. Severe orthostatic hypotension occurs although ameliorated by the gradual development of compensatory changes in the renin–angiotensin–aldosterone axis with repeated exposure to the headup position. The patient may suddenly lose consciousness with rapid tilt up or if left upright beyond sitting tolerance. Eating, drinking, medication dosing and bacteraemia are other occasions when symptomatic orthostatic hypotension may occur. Treatment measures for this complication consist of: (a) tilt back down with legs elevated for immediate control; (b) use of thigh length Ace wraps or elastic garment and/or lumbosacral corset with sheepskin lining (one specifically designed for spinal cord injury) as preventative measures; (c) checking fluid and electrolyte status, blood count and urine culture etc. for adverse change; (d) gradually acclimating the patient to sitting by small increments in the "up" time and (e) in some cases using small doses of the mineralocorticoid florinef 0.1 mg each morning (Chan 1993).

Table 13.1.   Treatment of the autonomic dysfunction of spinal shock

Respiratory measures

1. Monitor PaO_2; endotracheal intubation for hypoventilation, to manage secretions, to prevent atelectasis, to allow hyperoxygenation prior to suction; i.v. atropine is given to reduce secretions and inhibit reflex bradycardia
2. Use NG tube to eliminate gastric distension and restriction on diaphragm movement
3. Be diligent for neurogenic pulmonary oedema

Cardiovascular measures

1. Monitor pulmonary artery pressure for hypotensive volume replacement
2. Avoid head up position in bed; elevate legs for postural hypotensive syncope
3. i.v. atropine use to counteract reflex bradycardia during turning and trachael suction, rarely a demand pacemaker may be necessary
4. Parenteral (i.e. dopamine drip) or p.o. (i.e. 15 mg ephedrine) pressor Rx, can be used if volume expansion and supine posture do not restore blood pressure

Thermoregulatory measures

1. Monitor central (oral) temperature; environmental temperature should be adjusted to maintain normal body temperature
2. Protect vasodilated dry skin from pressure-induced injury with sheepskin

Gastrointestinal measures

1. Monitor for abdominal distension (ileus); NG decompression tube can reduce gastric respiratory compromise if present and monitor for GI haemorrhage;
2. Begin bowel care programme to reduce incidence of rectal impaction and distension; monitor for return of anal reflex and end of spinal shock
3. Use H2 blocker RX prophylaxis; monitor for metabolic alkalosis due to NG suction

Genitourinary measures

1. Initiate indwelling urinary catheter to decompress bladder, check for infection and monitor urine output volumes
2. Begin bladder rehabilitation measures of intermittent catheterization, a fluid schedule with and in between meals; monitor for infection, Rx. with appropriate antibiotics if severe; chronic prophylaxis with trimethoprim-sulfaoxazole is sometimes required

Autonomic Dysreflexia (Hyperreflexia)

A frequently seen complication of paroxysmal hypertension occurs in most patients with complete upper spinal cord trans-section. When triggered by stimuli below the level of the lesion this phenomenon is termed "autonomic dysreflexia" or "autonomic hyperreflexia". The development of severe hypertension and headache mimics a phaeochromocytoma but catecholamine levels are not elevated (Mathias and Frankel 1992). Hypertension does not develop when the upper level of the cord lesion is below the fifth thoracic segment, when the lesion is multifocal with a long longitudinal extent or at times when the lesion is incomplete. These observations suggest that lack of supraspinal regulation of the intact but isolated splanchnic sympathetic outflow from the 5th to 9th thoracic segment permits the development of autonomic dysreflexia. Recent evidence (Lee et al. 1995) suggests additional mechanisms such as increased numbers of spinal and microvascular alpha adrenoreceptors, the accumulation of substance P and reduction of gamma amino benzoic acid, noradrenaline and 5-hydroxytryptamine below the lesion may be operating. Causes of and treatment measures for this unique spinal cord syndrome are given in the Table 13.2 and 13.3. Hawkins et al. (1994) have reported

Table 13.2.   Causes of autonomic dysreflexia

Site/structure	Condition
Ureter	calculus
Urinary bladder	distension, dyssynergic bladder contraction
uterus	labour, menstruation
rectum/anus	impaction, fissure, haemorrhoid, enema
stomach	gastritis, ulcer distension
gallbladder	cholecystitis
cutaneous	pressure sores, burns, ingrown toenail
other	fractures, orgasm, extensor spasms

Table 13.3.   Treatment measures for autonomic dysrefiexia

Acute autonomic dysreflexia (AAD)

1 Immediate intervention
  a. Elevate head of bed; monitor BP and pulse q-5 min.
  b. Remove all tight clothing, braces, drainage bags etc.
  c. Check for distended bladder or rectal impaction (under topical anaesthesia)
  d. Replace catheter; dissimpact if BP < 200/130

2 Drug intervention
  a. None if BP < 140/100
  b. For BP >140/100 but < 180/120; nifedipine (if no excess sensitivity) 10 mg capsule chewed; effect expected in 20–30 min; Mecamylamine 2.5 mg to 5 mg p.o. and then t.i.d. is alternative
  c. For BP >180/120: start i.v. D5W infusion; Transfer for ICU; stat bloods; first can try nifedipine as above; if life threatening situation use nitroprusside or diazoxide i.v., 3 μg/kg/min, 1–3 mg/kg respectively.

Recurrent autonomic dysreflexia (AD)

1 Attend to the primary problem known to cause AD
  a. reduce fluid intake, catheterize more frequently if AD is due to distension
  b. treat symptomatic bladder infection; suppress bladder spasms the latter with ditropan 5 mg t.i.d.
  c. use cystoscopy to search for stones, laceration, cystitis if AD continues
  d. alter diet and use stool softeners

2 Pharmocologic Rx.
  a. Nifedipine 10 mg p.o. or sublinqual 30 min. prior to procedures causing AD
  b. Phenoxybenzamine (Dibenzyline) 10–40 mg/day in divided doses
  c. Mecamylamine (Inversine) 2.5–5 mg p.o. t.i.d.; contraindicated in uraemia.
  d. Terazocin (Hytrin) an α-1 blocker 1–5 mg/day has been advocated recently.
  e. Clonidine a centrally acting α-2 agonist has been used as a prophylactic drug to prevent AD especially during bladder stimulation
  f. Prazocin another α-1 blocker, 3 mg. b.i.d. has also been more effective than placebo in reducing blood pressure rise and symptoms of AD

a patient who was cured of his recurrent dysreflexia and after surgical repair of prolapsed haemorrhoids. Thyberg et al. (1994) have recently demonstrated the effectiveness of nifedipine in the specific case of cystometry-induced hypertension.

Neurogenic Bladder

In spinal cord diseases the level of the neurological deficit is predictive of the altered physiology and associated treatment strategies. With acute myelopathy there is urinary retention and detrusor areflexia as previously mentioned. Prevention of bladder overdistention via intermittent catheterization and maintainence of a fluid schedule are simple measures that are instituted early on. In the chronic stages, bladder dysfunction is characterized by detrusor hyperreflexia and detrusor sphincter dyssynergia in lesions above the lumbosacral cord and cauda equina. The bladder has uninhibited contractions and uncoordinated sphincter activity resulting in a small "spastic" bladder with both incontinence and incomplete voluntary voiding. Bladder distension will often trigger autonomic dysreflexia in cord lesions above T5. Treatment measures therefore focus on keeping the bladder decompressed, inhibiting spasms and trying to reduce sphincter resistance. Table 13.4 gives details of the pharmacological methods to do this.

When the neurological disorder affects the conus medularis and cauda equina the bladder is hypotonic and areflexic. The striated urethral sphincter is often lax. Treatment measures are aimed at keeping the bladder from getting overstretched, getting as complete emptying as possible and pharmacologically trying to keep the internal smooth sphincter competent. Such measures are given in Table 13.5.

Table 13.4. Treatment of "spastic" neurogenic bladder

Oxybutinin hydrochloride (Ditropan)	Start 2.5 mg. b.i.d.; increase as tolerated to 5.0 mg t.i.d.; give p.o. on an empty stomach.; 5.0 mg. can also be dissolved in saline and instilled into the bladder directly by catheter.
Imipramine hydrochloride	10–25 mg po q.i.d.
Propantheline bromide (Pro-Banthine)	7.5 mg three times a day
Alpha adrenergic blockers	Phenoxybenzamine 5–10 mg po b.i.d. or Prazocin 1–2 mg po t.i.d. increasing slowing if necessary; used only with documented sphincter dyssynergia

Table 13.5. Treatment of hypotonic neurogenic bladder

Crede manoeuvre	Used when low outflow resistance co-exists; done while sitting; works best in those with thin abdominal walls
Clean intermittent self-catheterization	14-Fr clear polyvinyl or red rubber catheters used upon each am and h. and q-4h in between; catheters, hands, urethral meatus cleansed with soap and water beforehand; used with a fluid intake schedule of 1800 ml/24 h: 400 ml at 8 am 12 noon and 6 pm, 200 ml. q-2-h in between
Bethanechol	25–100 mg po q.i.d. with voiding
Urecholine	15–20 min later q.i.d.
Alpha adrenergic blockers	Phenoxyoenzamine 5–10 mg po b.i.d. Prazocin 1–2 mg po t.i.d. increasing slowing if necessary; used only in combination with above methods

Gastrointestinal Dysfunction

Disorders of the spinal cord more commonly produce colonic and anorectal dysfunction with decrease in colon compliance, loss of the gastrocolic reflex activity. Reflex rectal stimulation is often required for stool evacuation in those with intact conus and cauda equina. Loss of voluntary control of the external sphincter is especially problematic when diarrhoea occurs due to dietary or infectious causes. The common elements of management therefore involve bulk elements in the diet and scheduled enemas or stimulant suppositories. Table 13.6 gives details of some of the commonly used regimens.

Less commonly, diarrhoea and increased intestinal motility and luminal transit speed occurs with thoracic cord lesion. The osmotic load of tube feedings and laxatives and effects of bacterial overgrowth can cause diarrhoea in the spinal cord compromised patient. In that case the treatment measures detailed in Table 13.7 can be used.

Thermoregulatory Disorders

With cervical spinal cord interruption a major portion of muscle mass cannot be activated, making thermogenesis due to shivering insufficient to prevent hypothermia in cold environments. The appreciation of cold by skin afferents is reduced

Table 13.6. Treatment of neurogenic constipation

Bulk laxative and stool softener	Psyllium hydrophilic mucilloid (Metamucil), 1 tsp to 1 tbl t.i.d.; colase 100 mg po qd
Osmotic laxative	Milk of magnesia 2 tabs 2–4× daily Lactulose 10–20 ml up to 4× daily
Bisacodyl (Dulcolax)	First rule out fecal impaction; 2 tabs p.o. hs for an am evacuation; one suppository 15–60 min before evacuation
Metoclopramide (Reglan)	5–10 mg po t.i.d. given 30 min before meals
Cisapride (Propulcid)	20 mg p.o. qid, given 30 min before meals and hs.

Table 13.7. Treatment of neurogenic diarrhoea

Dietary	Rarely malabsorbtion exists and Viokase (pancreatic enzyme concentrate) is given with meals
Antibiotics	Used when intestinal bacterial overgrowth is diagnosed or suspected; 250 mg of tetracycline once or twice at onset of diarrhoea or metronidazole 250 mg po t.i.d. for 7 days often help
Codeine phosphate	30 mg po q-4h prn
Loperamide (Immodium)	One cap contains 2 mg; dose is 2 caps stat then one cap following each unformed stool but not exceeding 8 caps a day
Diphenoxylate (Lomotil)	One tablet contains 2.5 mg; dose is 2 tabs po q.i.d. pm
Clonidine (catapress)	0.1 mg po b.i.d. to start; increase prn to 0.3 mg po t.i.d.
Octreotide (Sandostatin)	25 µg sub q b.i.d. initially; up to 100–200 µg t.i.d. may be required

adding to the difficulty in recognizing temperature extremes and initiating appropriate counter manoeuvres. The ability to constrict cutaneous vessels is impaired (more so in acute lesions) enhancing body heat loss and hypothermia. Low-reading thermometers (i.e. rectal thermometers) are essential to recognize and manage hypothermia. Treatment consists of external (heating blankets etc.) and internal (warm drinks, infusion of warmed saline) heating and avoidance of vasodilator drugs and cold environments. Nifedipine, commonly used for treatment of dysreflexia, has been reported to induce hypothermia (Menard and Hahn 1991). Hyperthermia typically occurs in cervical and high thoracic cord complete lesions during infections or in high environmental temperatures. Thermoregulatory sweating with evaporative heat loss is dependent on high central (core, blood) and integrated mean skin temperature activation of hypothalamic-bulbospinal pathways to the intermediolateral cell columns in the thoracolumbar cord. Interruption of these connections leads to large areas of impaired sweating. Coupled with impaired active and passive vasodilatation in these same lesions it is not surprising that hyperthermia is common when environmental temperatures are high. Treatment therefore consists of proper environmental temperature maintainence and for symptomatic hyperthermia tepid sponge baths while blowing air over the body surface. Severe (105.8°F(41°C) or greater) hyperpyrexia may require ice-bath immersion, cooled fluid irrigation of bladder and i.v. infusion and aspirin. Chlorpromazine, diazepam and rarely dantrium may be needed. Table 13.8 gives a management plan for mild and severe hyperthermia (Ingall 1993).

Paroxysmal sweating in body areas below the last innervated segment often occurs in high cord complete lesions. Generally this is part of autonomic dysreflexia often caused by a distended bladder or rectum. Rarely this may occur in high environmental temperatures as either a direct effect of heat on the skin or via a somatosympathetic reflex through the isolated cord segments. In patients with thoracic cord lesions perilesional hyperhidrosis can occur sometimes requiring local application of topical anticholinergic agents (e.g. a 20% Drysol solution) to control the sweat output.

Table 13.8.   Prevention and treatment of hyperthermia

Heat intolerance treatment	Heat stroke treatment
1. Avoid hot/humid environments	1. Establish Dx. criteria: (a) core temp. >41 °C or 105.8°F; (b) impaired CNS state; (c) dry, hot ashen or pink skin
2. Be outdoors early am or late pm	2. Immediately remove from hot environment
3. Avoid strenuous activity in heat	3. Surface cool to core temp. of 39.0°C
4. Set house thermostat lower	4. Correct hypovolemia with isotonic saline
5. Wear head covering but loose, light breathable clothing	5. Treat possible complications: DIC, shock rhabdomyolysis, renal failure, seizures
6. Keep well hydrated (2–3 l/day)	6. Use diazepam to control shivering and seizures
7. Avoid alcohol, diuretic, neuroleptic and anticholinergic drugs if possible	

Other Disorders

Multiple Sclerosis

Patients with chronic multiple sclerosis affecting the spinal cord commonly have involvement of descending inhibitory tracts to the sacral parasympathetic outflow resulting in urinary frequency and urge incontinence. Constipation and sexual dysfunction often occur. Detrusor hyperreflexia and detrusor-sphincter dyssynergia is revealed by cystometry. Thermoregulatory sweating abnormalities occur in almost half the patients carefully studied and the extent of anhidrosis correlates positively with the Kurtzke disability score and pyramidal tract involvement (Noronha et al. 1968). Spinal reflex sweating with bladder distention (and clinically important autonomic dysreflexia) does not occur, most likely due to the longitudinal distribution of cervical and thoracic cord lexions as well as the less than complete interruption of descending inhibitory pathways.

Syringomyelia

A cervical or upper thoracic syrinx can occasionally produce symptomatic autonomic dysfunction. Direct compression of the descending bulbospinal pathways by the syrinx or associated Chiari malformation may produce unilateral or bilateral Horner's syndrome, segmental hyperhidrosis followed by anhidrosis of the trunk and upper limbs often accompanied by vasomotor and trophic changes and sensory loss in the hands. When more extensive cavities are present orthostatic hypotension and neurogenic bowel and bladder dysfunction can occur. Autonomic dysreflexia generally does not occur. Cardiovagal function is intact unless extensive syringobulbia is present. Baroreceptor failure with wide swings in blood pressure can occur if the nucleus and tractus solitarius are involved. Glasauer and Czyrny (1994) have described hyperhidrosis as a presenting symptom of post-traumatic syringomyelia.

Primary Autonomic Failure

Involvement of the intermediolateral cell columns and sacral parasympathetic nuclei of Onuf in the spinal cord with marked depletion of autonomic cytons characterizes the syndromes of pure autonomic failure and Shy-Drager syndrome. Segmental to global anhidrosis, marked orthostatic hypotension with inadequate cardioacceleration, supine hypertension without autonomic dysreflexia, urinary incontinence and impotence regularly occur upon autonomic testing (Fealey et al. 1989; Sandroni et al 1991). Occasionally the patient may be bothered by compensatory hyperhidrosis in an area of preserved sweating. Autonomic testing utilizing a combination of thermoregulatory and a peripheral sweat test such as the QSART (quantitative sudomotor axon reflex test) can often be used to delineate involvement of the intermediolateral cells of the spinal cord as the former will show anhidrosis in areas where the latter is normal.

References

Chan CW (1993) Spinal cord injury. In: Sinaki M (ed) Basic clinical rehabilitation medicine. Mosby, St Louis, pp 183–194

Fealey RD (1993) The thermoregulatory sweat test. In: Low P (ed) Clinical autonomic disorders (evaluation and management), Little, Brown, Boston, pp 217–229

Fealey RD, Szurszewski JH, Merritt JL, DiMagno EP (1984) Effect of traumatic spinal cord transection on human upper gastrointestinal motility and gastric emptying. Gastroenterology 87:69–75

Fealey RD, Low PA, Thomas JE (1989) Thermoregulatory sweating abnormalities in diabetes mellitus. Mayo Clin Proc 64:617–628

Glasauer FE, Czyrny JJ (1994) Hyperhidrosis as the presenting symptom in post-traumatic syringomyelia. Paraplegia 32:423–429

Hawkins RL, Jr, Bailey HR, Donnovan WH (1994) Autonomic dysreflexia resulting from prolapsed hemorrhoids. Report of a case. Dis Colon Rectum 37:492–493

Hickey R, Sloan TB, Albin MS (1995) Acute spinal cord trauma. In: Shoremaker, Ayres, Grenvik, Holbrook (eds) Text book of critical care, 3rd edn. WB Saunders, Philadelphia, pp 1457–1465

Ingall TJ (1993) Hyperthermia and hypothermia. In: Low P (ed) Clinical autonomic disorders (evaluation and management). Little Brown, Boston, pp 713–729

Kihara M, Fealey R, Takahashi A, Schmelzer J (1995) Sudomotor dysfunction and its investigation. In Korczyn A (ed) Handbook of autonomic nervous system dysfunction. Marcel Dekker, New York, pp 523–533

Lee BY, Karmakar MG, Herz BL, Sturgill RA (1995) Autonomic dysreflexia revisited. (Review) J Spinal Cord Med 18:75–87

Mathias CJ, Frankel HL (1992) Autonomic disturbances in spinal cord lesions. In: Bannister R, Mathias CJ (eds) Autonomic failure: a textbook of clinical disorders of the autonomic nervous system, 3rd edn. Oxford Medical Publications, Oxford, pp 839–881

Menard MR, Hahn G (1991) Acute and chronic hypothermia in a man with spinal cord injury: environmental and pharmacologic causes Arch Phys Med Rehabi 72:421–424

Noronha MJ, Vas CJ, Aziz H (1968) Autonomic dysfunction (sweating responses) in multiple sclerosis. J Neurol Neurosurg Psychiatry 31:19–22

Pollock L, Boshes B, Chor J, Finkelman I, Arieff A, Brown M (1951) Defects in regulatory mechanisms of autonomic function in injuries to spinal cord. J Neurophysiol 14:85–93

Sandroni P, Ahlskog JE, Fealey RD, Low PA (1991) Autonomic involvement in extra-pyramidal and cerebellar disorders. Clin Autonomic Res 1:147–155

Thyberg M, Ertzgaard P, Gylling M, Granerus G (1994) Effect of nifedipine on cystometry-induced elevation of blood pressure in patients with a reflex urinary bladder after high spinal cord injury. Paraplegia 32:308–313

Chapter 14

Trauma to the Cervical Spine

J.R. Johnson

Trauma to the cervical spine can be divided up into soft tissue injuries, such as whiplash injuries and other ligamentous damage and fractures, and/or dislocations. Because injuries in the upper cervical region, i.e. C1/2 have many characteristics relating to the aetiology and treatment that set them apart from the rest of the cervical spine, they are normally considered separately from injuries from C3 downwards. In the lower cervical spine, whatever the force is, the resultant deformity is often transitional which implies ligament failure. Damage to the ligament complex is therefore an important component of cervical injuries and an accurate assessment of this damage is essential in diagnosis.

Initial diagnosis is made on the basis of history, examination and plain lateral radiographs of the cervical spine. Once the initial assessment has been made, more sophisticated imaging techniques such as CT scanning and MRI may be necessary to make a final decision on the management. The incidence of cervical spine trauma based on work by Dvorak in Switzerland is probably in the order of one per thousand population for the year. Of these only 13% will have a cervical spine fracture with or without a spinal cord lesion.

Soft Tissue Injuries of the Cervical Spine

Acute Neck Sprain

In 1989 Porter coined the term acute neck sprain which has now been generally adopted in the English literature to get away from the rather more emotive term of "whiplash injury". This is because the majority of injuries are associated with some form of road traffic accident and therefore have a compensation and/or litigation aspect.

The incidence of soft tissue neck injuries is difficult to assess. In the United States the incidence of hyperextension neck injuries in all road traffic accidents is around 3%. Galasko et al. (1993) found a progressive increase in soft tissue injuries to the spine between 1982 and 1991. They found an incidence of neck injuries in all road traffic accidents of 7.7% before the introduction of the compulsory seat belts. This rose to 20% in the 12 months after the introduction of seat belts. However, the incidences continued to rise and there has been a steady rise to about 45% up to end of 1991. Around 50% of injuries occurred in rear end collision. Mackay (1970) found that direct rear end impacts probably only represent about 8% of major road traffic accidents and he felt that the term "whiplash" should probably only been used for these pure, hyperflexion injuries. Galasko et al. found that not only was the incidence of neck injuries increasing, but that neck injuries were accounting for an increasing proportion of all injuries occurring in road traffic accidents. Clearly although there was an increase in neck injuries after the introduction of seat belts, this increase has continued and therefore cannot be put down entirely to this factor alone.

The underlying pathophysiology of acute neck sprain is not clearly understood despite numerous animal and in vitro studies (MacNab, 1971; La Rocca, 1977; White 1990).

Saternus and Thrun (1987) in an analysis of the cervical spines of patients dying as a result of severe injuries, found a high percentage of damage to soft tissues, mainly ligamentous ruptures.

Most acute neck sprains occur as result of road traffic accidents. Dvorak and Valach (1989) found 55% of these patients were injured in a car accident and 45% by other means, usually sports injuries and falls or diving. The most common cause of acute sprain in the road traffic accident group were head-on and rear-end collisions.

The natural history of neck pain following acute cervical injury is that 50% of patients will have significant pain at 8 months and 18% at 3 years. In the past it has been assumed that the majority of soft tissue injuries would be fully healed by 2 years and the work by Parmar and Raymakers (1993) suggests that 3 years may be a better time to assess patients, certainly from the point of view of medicolegal assessment. They also found that after 3 years the proportion of patients in each grade of pain remains constant, suggesting that there was unlikely to be any improvement in the more severely graded patients.

There were some prognostic factors which were that patients over the age of 45 years tended to have pain that lasted for longer. Drivers tended to outnumber front seat passengers in terms of developing acute neck strains but the front seat passengers tended to have pain for longer.

It is quite common for patients not to get immediate pain following these accidents and in Dvorak and Valach 's series only 50% of the injured patients consulted their physicians in the first 12 hours followed by another 40% within the first 3 days. Parmar and Raymakers (1993) found there was a clear statistical difference indicating a quicker recovery and better end result for those patients whose pain was only noticed after 12 hours. Patients with either a clinical history or X-ray changes of spondylosis tended to suffer pain for longer but it did not affect the final severity or level of pain at the end of the review period.

Medicolegal Aspects

Parmar and Raymakers (1993) found that over age 45 years, a history of neck pain and signs of radiological spondylosis were all associated with the worst prognosis. Similar findings have been reported by Hohl (1974) and Norris and Watt (1983). They did not find any relationship with the influence of compensation claims. The majority of patients were free of significant pain before settlement of their claims and only four improved after receiving compensation. The generally held belief that compensation neurosis developed after this type of neck sprain is not borne out in their study. The concluded that 3 years from injury was a reasonable time to make a full medicolegal assessment. This was also confirmed by Robinson and Cassar-Pullicino (1993) who found no correlation between patient satisfaction in Court and resolution of symptoms. Again, they found the patients with the worst prognosis were those who had pre-existing degenerative changes in their cervical spine.

Clinical Assessment

The most frequent complaints of patients are those of neck pain and pain on rotation of the spine. Pain radiating into the shoulders is quite common as is dizziness. Paraesthesia, neurological symptoms and signs in the upper limb are uncommon. On examination pain on rotation of the head and neck stiffness are the most common signs.

Assessment of patients following the initial clinical assessment, anteroposterior and lateral radiographs of the entire cervical spine should always be performed.

Treatment

This normally consists of a soft collar for the first few days together with painkillers or analgesia or anti-inflammatory tablets. Early physiotherapy, i.e. around 4–6 weeks, has been found helpful in various studies. If symptoms are no better after a period of 6-weeks in a collar with anti-inflammatories, then flexion/extension views may be helpful together with electromyographic studies if there is radicular pain. After this 6 week period it is safe to undergo physiotherapy and generally early physiotherapy has been recommended. If symptoms persist beyond 6 months, it may be reasonable to investigate further with magnetic resonance imaging (MRI) or CT scanning.

There is no doubt that the organized approach to the management will get patients back to work earlier. In the industrial setting, although neck injuries are only about 20% as common as low back injuries, the amount of time lost from work is significantly higher with neck injuries compared to the back.

In general all patients should be able to return to work by 6 weeks after injury and should be encouraged to do so even if mild symptoms persist.

Fractures and Fracture Dislocations

Incidence

Ryan and Henderson (1992) reviewed all the cervical fractures and fracture dislocations admitted to a regional centre and found 717 cases representing about 1 per 100 000 population per year. The levels most frequently injured were C2, C5 and C6 in that order respectively. Combined C1/C2 fractures were common, an association first described by Jefferson (1920) who found that 77% of C1 fractures were associated with C2 fractures (53% with odontoid fractures and 24% with hangman's fractures).

Odontoid fractures are the commonest cervical injury in the over 70 age population. Multilevel injuries are not uncommon and Ryan and Henderson (1992) recommended that if a fracture of the upper cervical spine is seen on X-ray, further fractures in the lower cervical spine should be excluded.

A report in the United States in 1981 estimated that 6000 deaths occur annually from fatal cervical spine injuries in road traffic accidents. About 500–600 patients become quadriplegic from road traffic accidents and the highest incidence of this injury occurs amongst 16–25 year olds. In the United States probably half of the spinal cord injuries that occur are as a result of road traffic accidents which is in line with the Swiss figure.

Classification

In the cervical spine there is a clear relationship between the mechanism of injury and the resultant damage to the spine. Holdsworth (1963) described a two column concept where the anterior column equals the anterior elements, i.e. the anterior longitudinal ligament, the vertebral body, the intervertebral disc and the posterior longitudinal ligament and a second column, the posterior elements comprising everything behind the posterior longitudinal ligament. Louis (1983) described a different concept of three columns or pillars. The anterior pillar was the vertebral body and there were two pillars of the facet joints posteriorly, connected by the lamina and the spinous process. Denis (1983) redefined the spinal columns to include the middle column. This consisted of the posterior wall of the vertebral body, the posterior longitudinal ligament and the posterior part of the annulus fibrosus. The basic principles are that in flexion, the anterior column is compressed and the posterior column is distracted. Conversely hyperextension force causes simultaneous distraction of the anterior column and compression of the posterior column.

Many classification have been proposed for cervical spine injuries. Most have been based on the mechanism of injury. In the cervical spine this is probably a reasonable concept as biomechanical and cadaver studies have shown the mechanisms of injury to be of major importance. Harris et al. (1986) suggested a classification based on injuries, or groups of injuries (Table 14.1).

Flexion Injuries

1. Anterior subluxation (Fig. 14.1): this is usually a soft tissue injury to the posterior ligamentous complex. It is often associated with late instability due to the failure of the posterior ligaments to heal. This mechanism is involved in unilateral facet dislocations (see below).
2. Bilateral facet dislocation (Fig 14.2): most of these involve complete disruption of the posterior complex. This allows a 50% slip of the vertebral body and is not a stable injury.
3. Simple wedge fracture (Fig. 14.3): this is caused by hyperflexion compacting one vertebra into the vertebra below.

Table 14.1. Cervical spine injuries: mechanism of injury

I. Flexion
    A. Anterior subluxation (hyperflexion sprain)
    B. Bilateral interfacetal dislocation
    C. Simple wedge (compression) fracture
    D. Clay-shoveler (coal-shoveler) fracture
    E. Flexion teardrop fracture

II. Flexion-rotation
    A. Unilateral and interfacetal dislocation

III. Extension-rotation
    A. Pillar fracture

IV. Vertical compression
    A. Jefferson bursting fracture of atlas
    B. Burst (bursting, dispersion, axial loading) fracture

V. Hyperextension
    A. Hyperextension dislocation
    B. Avulsion fracture of anterior arch of atlas
    C. Extension teardrop fracture of axis
    D. Fracture of posterior arch of atlas
    E. Laminar fracture
    F. Traumatic spondylolisthesis (hangman's fracture)
    G. Hypextension fracture-dislocation

VI. Lateral Flexion
    A. Uncinate process fracture

VII. Diverse or imprecisely understood mechanisms
    A. Atlanto-occipital dissociation
    B. Odontoid fractures

From Harris et al. (1986).

4. Clay shoveler's fracture (Fig. 14.4): this is the avulsion of either C7, C6 or T1. These levels are given in the order of common occurrence.
5. Flexion tear drop fracture (Fig. 14.5): in these injuries there is complete disruption of all the ligaments and the disc at the level of injury and therefore the injury is often associated with an anterior cervical cord syndrome with complete paraplegia but some sensory preservation.

Flexion and Rotation Injuries

1. Unilateral facet dislocation (Fig. 14.6) – caused by a combination of flexion and rotation which gives the so called "locked" facet. This is a stable injury but it may be associated with a facet fracture. In these cases the forward displacement is usually only about 25% of the vertebral body.

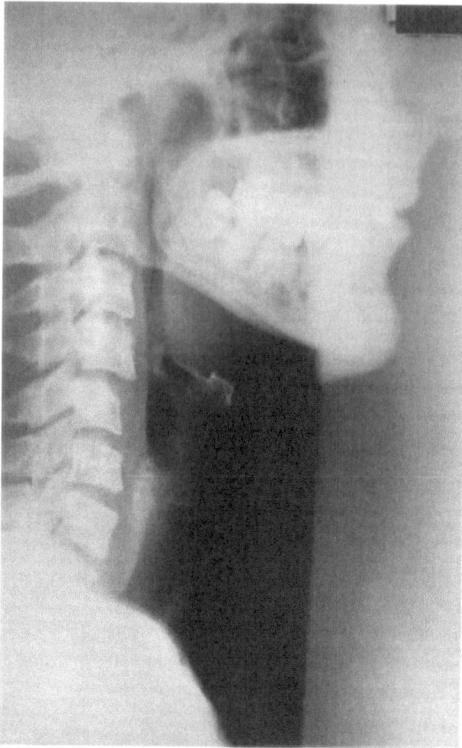

Fig. 14.1. Anterior subluxation of C4 on C5.

Hyperextension of Rotation Injuries

1. The pillar fracture – a vertical fracture of the lateral articular mass.
2. The vertical compression fracture: this is a burst fracture that occurs similarly in the thoracolumbar and other parts of the spine and particular fractures, e.g. the Jefferson fracture at C1 (see below).

Extension Injuries

1. Hyperextension dislocation (more distraction than extension injury) (Fig. 14.7): this injury is commoner in the older age group and often occurs with a force onto the face. The injury causes disruption of the anterior longitudinal ligament and of the disc. There is sometimes separation of the posterior longitudinal ligament from the lower of the injured vertebrae. Because of this the cord can be pinched anteriorly and also posteriorly by buckling of the ligamentum flavum and inversion of the lamina.
2. Extension tear drop fracture of the axis: an injury that occurs in elderly patients with cervical spondylosis or osteoporosis.

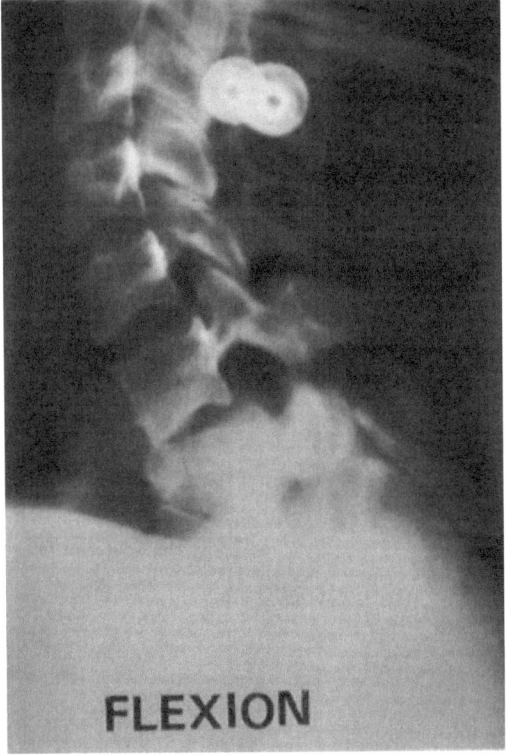

Fig. 14.2. Bilateral facet dislocation of C7 on T1.

3. A lamina fracture (compression/extension type): an uncommon fracture usually occurring in the elderly.
4. Hangman's fracture (see below).
5. Hyperextension fracture (compression/extension): despite the fact this is a hyperextension injury, it may look like a flexion injury on the lateral X-ray as there is some transitional forces.

Lateral Flexion

This rarely occurs on its own and is often associated with other injuries, for example C1 or C2 fractures. The only isolated injury of this type is the rare uncinate process fracture.

Imprecisely Defined Mechanisms

1. Atlanto-occipital dissociation
2. Odontoid fractures

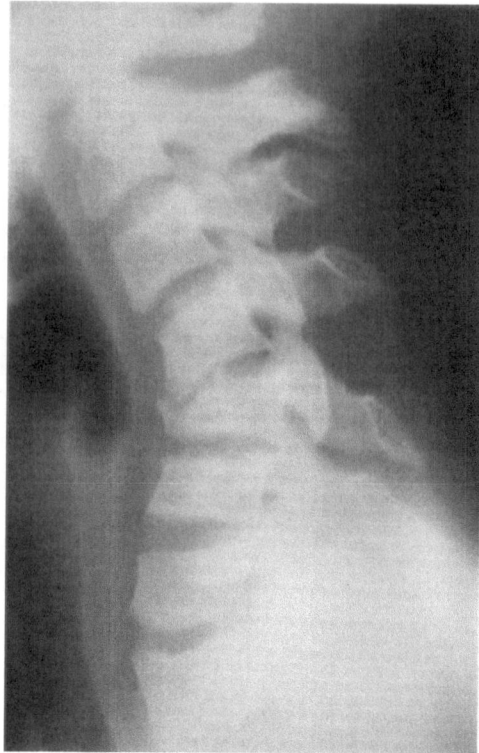

Fig. 14.3. Flexion wedge compression fracture C5.

Both these are discussed below.

Upper Cervical Spine Injuries (C1/2)

As has already been stated, injuries to the upper cervical spine have different characteristics from those at lower levels. This is probably because the force of injury is
applied directly to the base of the skull and there is therefore a shorter lever arm.
Many of these injuries are associated with head injuries and if they are not immediately fatal, the overall prognosis is usually good. There is a low incidence of permanent neurological deficit. The bony injuries stabilize quickly and surgical
intervention is not often required.

Obviously posterior fusions compromise movement of the upper cervical spine to
a greater degree than the rest of the spine because the occiput/C1 motion segment
provides 50% of cervical flexion/extension. Similarly the motion of segment C1/C2
provides 50% of rotation.

Primary ligamentous injuries may require stabilization at a later stage and careful
assessment is essential because of the associated head injuries and multiple injuries

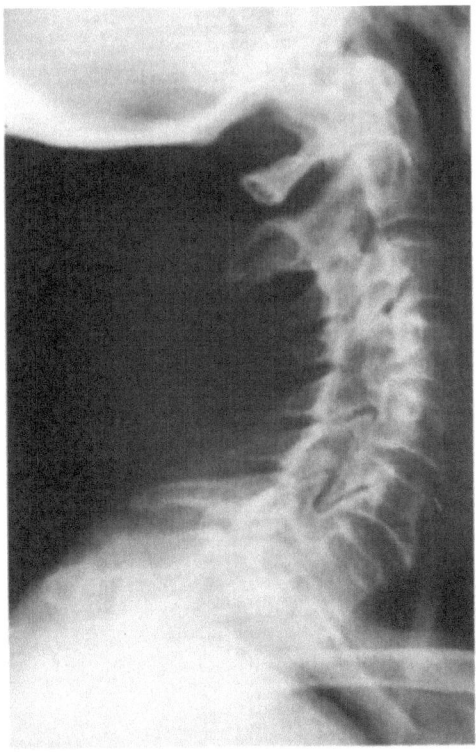

Fig. 14.4.   Clay shoveler's fracture of D1.

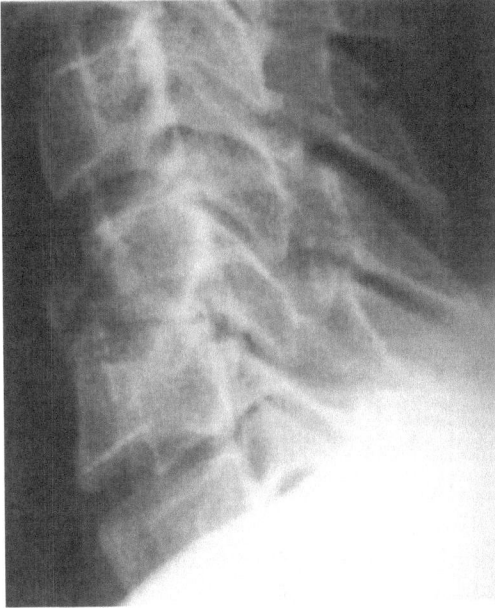

Fig. 14.5.   Flexion tear drop fracture of C5.

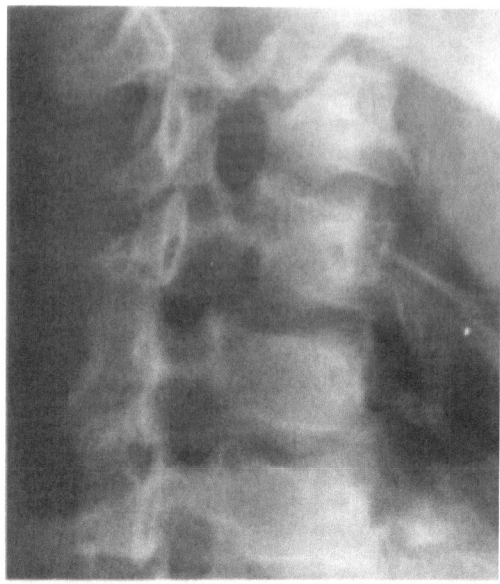

Fig. 14.6.   Unilateral facet dislocation C4/5.

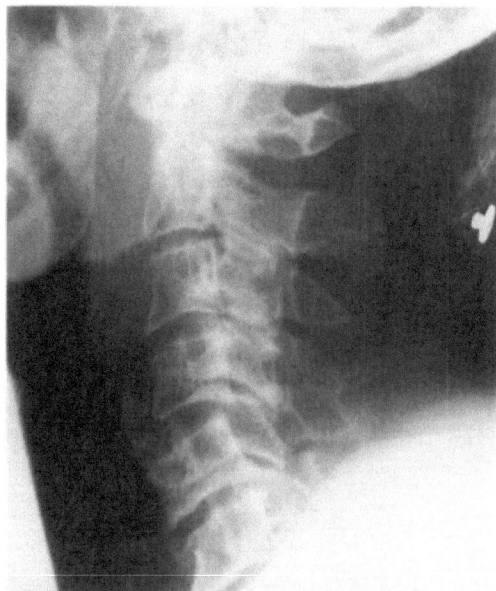

Fig. 14.7.   Hyperextension dislocation C4/5.

to other organs. General principles applied to spinal cord injuries (see Chapter X) apply to these injuries.

Although the majority of injuries occur to a normal cervical spine, there is a small group of patients who have a pathological upper cervical spine for other reasons, e.g.

rheumatoid arthritis. There are also other inflammatory arthropathies associated with ligamentous laxity and also anomalies in this part of the neck associated with Down's syndrome and the mucopolysaccharide group of diseases. In this group of patients with abnormal necks, a relatively minor accident may cause neurological damage.

Initial Management and Assessment

Podolsky et al. (1983) suggested that between 3% and 25% of spinal cord injuries occurred after the initial injury, either during transit or early in the course of treatment. However, since then there have been great strides in emergency medical care with the arrival of highly skilled paramedics at the scene of the accident and general adoption of the Advanced Trauma Life Support training which has come from the United States. All patients are considered as having possible cervical spine injuries, particularly if they are unconscious and hard neck collars are used to stabilize the patient together with sand bags. Following initial assessment and resuscitation, lateral cervical spine X-rays are normally performed and are a good basic screening test for a cervical injury. Films that do not include all seven cervical vertebrae should be regarded as inadequate. In cases of doubtful fractures, particularly in the upper cervical region, CT scanning may be valuable in the further assessment of these injuries.

There is some controversy about the place of steroids in patients with neurological impairment. However, there is general agreement on early stabilization with light traction.

Condylar Fractures

These usually occur in association with fractures of the base of the skull. The alar ligaments are usually intact and therefore these fractures are stable. They are often difficult to diagnose, particularly in the unconscious patient and CT scanning may be helpful.

Occipito-Atlantal Dislocation

This is an uncommon injury and when it does occur it is invariably fatal. In one series between 1977 and 1984, only one patient survived a complete occiput C1 dislocation (Levine and Edwards 1985). There have been several case reports of patients surviving this particular injury. If the patient does survive, the recommended course of treatment is to reduce the dislocation by gentle traction following which skin callipers are applied. Patients are then mobilized in the halo vest. Normally patients will require a later occipitocervical fusion but this should be postponed until it is clear that there are no underlying respiratory or cardiovascular problems.

Fractures of the Atlas

These are often associated with other cervical spine fractures, particularly of the axis. They are sometimes difficult to diagnose on plain radiographs and CT scanning can be very helpful in delineating the type of ring fracture. Three major fractures have been described; the first is a posterior arch fracture. This usually occurs at the junction of the posterior arch with the lateral mass. The second is a less common type of fracture which just involves the lateral mass on one side only although occasionally there is a posterior arch fracture on the same or opposite side. The third type is the burst injury or Jefferson fracture (Fig. 14.8). This usually has four fractures, two in the posterior arch and two in the anterior arch.

Acute fractures are often associated with a retropharyngeal soft tissue shadow and this in itself can be a useful diagnostic sign.

Treatment depends on the type of fracture. An isolated posterior arch fracture is quite stable and may be treated with a simple collar. However, as so many fractures are associated with other cervical injuries, especially fracture of C2, treatment may well depend on the type of dens fracture at C2.

The mechanism of injury of the Jefferson fracture is vertical compression and therefore reduction is best achieved by traction. This should be applied for 6–8 weeks before application of a halo vest for a further 4–6 weeks.

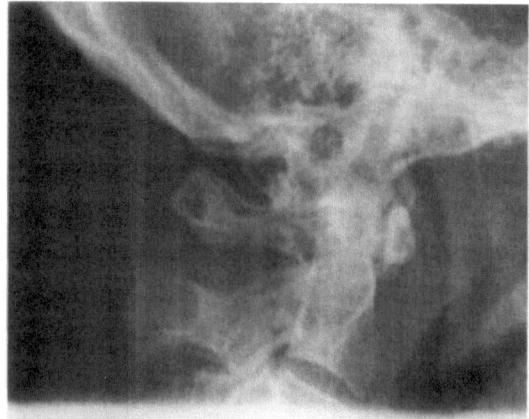

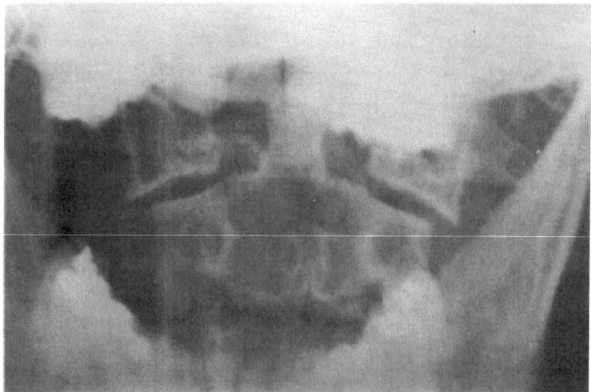

Fig. 14.8. Jefferson fracture, anteroposterior and lateral views.

Rupture of the Transverse Ligament

This injury is rare and allows forward subluxation of the atlas. It tends to occur in older patients and often results from a fall with a blow to the occiput.

The ligament may rupture in the middle or at the side. The latter type is often associated with a flake fracture from the lateral mass which may be visible on transoral radiograph views. Diagnosis is normally by flexion/extension views on lateral radiograph. This injury cannot be treated conservatively and surgical stabilization is always necessary. There is general agreement that a period of traction to allow any swelling to go down is advisable before surgery. Stabilization is usually achieved by a C1/C2 Gallie type fusion, i.e. wiring from the C1 arch to the spinous process of C2.

Rotatory Subluxation and Dislocation of C1–C2 (Fig. 14.9)

These dislocations rarely occur in adults and when they do are different from those in children. In children they are often associated with a viral illness and resolve with conservative treatment. In adults the injury normally occurs after road traffic accidents and is often missed. The diagnosis is based on the open mouth view and is characterized by the so called "wink" sign on the open mouth view. This is an overriding of the C1/2 joint on one side with a normal configuration on the other. Acute cases may be manipulated with traction using a halo ring but in later cases open reduction followed by a C1/C2 fusion may be necessary.

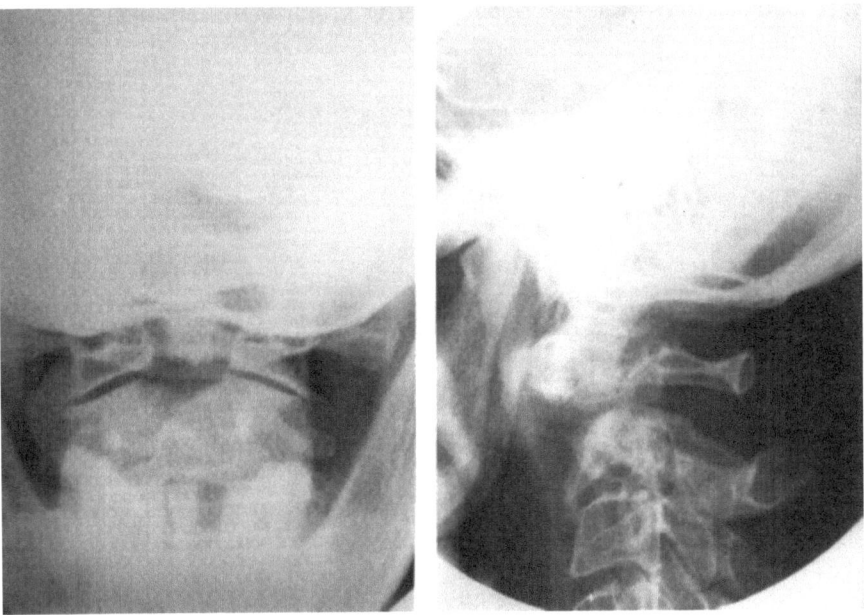

Fig. 14.9. Fracture of the odontoid with secondary dislocation of the atlanto-axial joint, anteroposterior and lateral views.

Fractures of the Odontoid (Dens) (Fig. 14.10)

The treatment of odontoid fractures is based on the level of injury to the dens. This has been classified by Anderson and D'Alonzo (1974) into three types.

Type 1:   An avulsion fracture of the tip of the dens. This is a benign injury and does not need surgical treatment.

Type 2:   Fractures which occur above the junction of the body of the axis, to the base of the odontoid and it is these fractures that are prone to non-union, probably due to the lack of blood supply.

Type 3:   Fractures which extend downwards into the cancellous body of the axis. These are usually treated conservatively as they rarely fail to unite.

The main controversy associated with these fractures is the incidence of non-union. The incidence of non-union seems to depend partly on the degree of initial displacement but also on the adequacy of reduction, the age of the patient and the type of immobilization. If the initial displacement is more than 5 mm, non-union is more likely. Non-union rates have been described from 5% to 64% in fractures treated conservatively. Non-union rates have fallen since the change from a Minerva type of plaster cast to a halo vest immobilization.

In most cases initial treatment consists of immobilizing on skull traction until adequate radiographs have been obtained. Type 1 fractures can be treated in a collar, as can basal Type 3 fractures. For undisplaced fractures a well-fitting Somi type brace is all that is necessary. If there is a displaced fracture, immobilization is best in a halo jacket.

Type 2 fractures, because of their association with non-unions, are usually treated surgically. Posterior atlanto-axial fusion is usually entirely satisfactory although other methods have been described. Anterior stabilization can be achieved by a

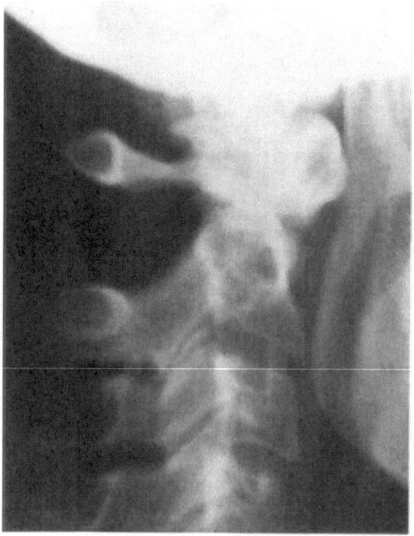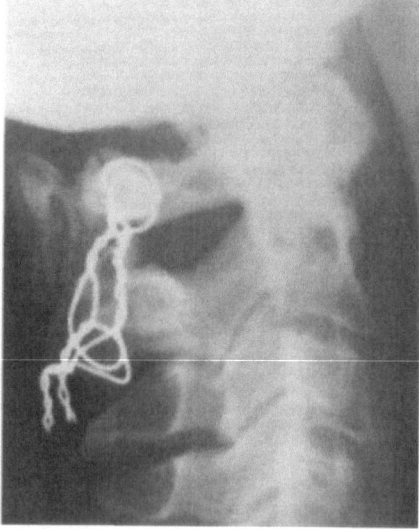

Fig. 14.10.   Fracture of the odontoid before and after posteror fusion.

screw from the base of C2 up through and into the odontoid using X-ray control. However, this method carries a significant morbidity and should only be carried out by surgeons familiar with this approach.

Atlanto-Axial Instability

The first description of atlanto-axial instability is attributed to Sir Charles Bell in 1830. Pilcher (1910) described an unsuccessful attempt to reduce subluxation by surgery. Anterior subluxation is more common than posterior. Pain in the occipital region with an abnormal posture may be the only presenting symptoms. Other neurological signs have been reported in addition to various vascular complications. The diagnosis may be difficult in patients with rheumatoid arthritis or other congenital deformities like the Klippel–Feil syndrome. Treatment depends on the patient's age, the amount of pain and the degree of neurological deficit. Treatment is normally surgical as the instability cannot be controlled any other way.

Atlanto-Axial Injuries

These cases present with awry neck or torticollis type of deformity and may not be recognized straightaway; if not the damage to ligaments causes fibrosis. Fielding and Hawkins (1977) described four types of fixed rotation.

Type 1: The transverse ligament is intact so that anterior subluxation of the atlas does not occur. The dens acts as a pivot permitting rotation. Reduction is achieved with traction.

Type 2: This is associated with anterior atlanto-axial instability because of a deficiency of the transverse ligament. This requires surgical stabilization.

Type 3: This is rare and is characterized by deficiency of both the transverse and capsular ligaments.

Type 4: There is rotatory fixation with posterior displacement which is extremely rare as there is a deficient odontoid process. Diagnosis is based on a history of injury. In addition there may be a difficulty in swallowing and an inability to open the jaw fully. The torticollis may only be noticed later. The most useful radiograph is the open mouth view although it is not always possible to carry this out in the acute phase because of the difficulty in opening the jaw fully. Manual traction using a halter may be successful in early cases although it may be necessary to apply skull traction to reduce the late cases. If this fails a posterior atlanto-axial fusion is sometimes necessary.

Traumatic Spondylolisthesis of the Axis (Hangman's Fracture) (Fig. 14.11)

This fracture was originally described for neck injuries relating to judicial hanging although nowadays it is much more likely to be associated with road traffic or diving accidents caused by hyperextension and axial compression. In judicial hanging a submental or near submental knot is used and the lesion is produced by a violent

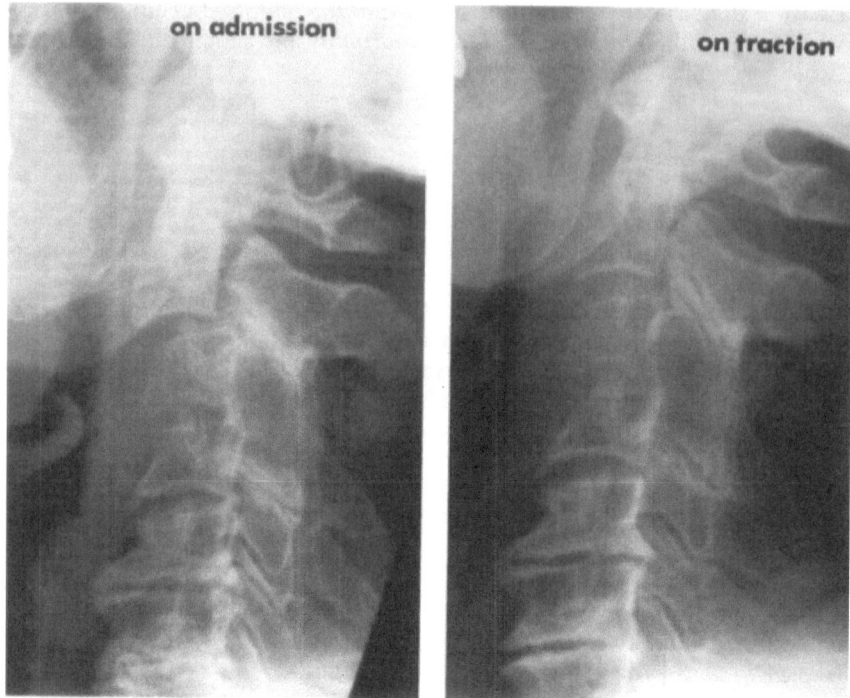

Fig. 14.11. Hangman's fracture on admission and reduced picture on traction.

jerk which throws the head backwards and snaps the pedicles off the axis. Death is instantaneous because of the extreme distraction of the spinal cord.

Using lateral radiographs, these fractures can be classified into four types depending on the degree of displacement and the angular deformity.

Type 1:   These are all undisplaced fractures and those with no angulation. There is a low incidence of neurological deficit. This fracture is normally stable and can be treated conservatively in a soft collar.

Type 2:   This consists of a fracture involving both pedicles with more than 3 mm of translation slip and some angulation. This fracture should be treated with traction in slight extension. A halo vest may not maintain the reduction and it is recommended that traction is continued for 4–6 weeks until the fracture is sticky and that this is then followed by the halo vest for the final 4–5 weeks.

Type 2a: This is a similar fracture with angulation rather than translation. In this case the injury is an extension injury and reduction can best be achieved by gentle axial compression under X-ray control followed by the application of a halo jacket.

Type 3:   This has severe angulation and translation and is often associated with a greater or lesser neurological deficit. These fractures may require surgical stabilization which is best achieved by the anterior approach with an anterior interbody fusion to prevent any loss of rotation.

Combined Injuries

As has already been stated, it is not uncommon to have multiple C1 and C2 injuries. The general principles of treatment here are to regard each injury separately in relationship to stability and possible treatment and it may be necessary to allow a C1 fracture to heal before stabilizing C1/2.

Injuries to the Mid and Lower Cervical Spine (C3–C7)

The basic principle with these fractures first is to obtain a healed fracture in good alignment but secondly to prevent future injury or encroachment on the spinal cord or nerve roots. One of the problems is with posterior ligamentous ruptures which are often not diagnosed on routine lateral radiographs. It is not uncommon to find late instability and progressive subluxation in patients who have had ligamentous ruptures missed on the initial radiographs. White (1990) suggested a stretch test in which 30–40 pounds of traction on a cervical halter is carried out under direct supervision in the X-ray department using lateral radiographs. Ligamentous disruption does not heal well, even if held in a reduced position for a prolonged period of time.

Mechanism of Injury

Unlike in the upper cervical spine, the fractures and dislocations that occur lower down are a result of indirect forces rather than direct forces on the head. These days the majority of injuries are either caused by being thrown forwards, head first in a road traffic accident or from diving injuries. The resulting injury is either a burst fracture from an axial load in compression or a dislocation with rupture of the ligaments which occurs with more complex mechanisms. Using AP and lateral radiographs, the injury can be assessed by looking at the three columns. CT scanning may be useful as an additional deciding factor as to which columns are involved and therefore whether the fracture is unstable or not.

Stability

Isolated body fractures tend to be stable. However, if the posterior ligaments are injured in addition an unstable injury can result. Careful assessment is necessary to exclude ligament damage.

Fracture Classification

1. Wedge compression fractures (Fig. 14.3) this includes burst fractures of the vertebral bodies which are stable once the fracture is consolidated. Initially they

may be potentially unstable and may cause pressure on the spinal cord. This may require surgical decompression at an early stage.

2. Hyperextension/dislocation (Fig. 14.7).

3. Hyperflexion injuries often associated with road traffic accident and occasionally diving. These are often associated with spinal cord damage.

4. Ligament injuries: posterior ligamentous tears may allow unilateral or bilateral facet dislocation to occur. The traditional unilateral facet (Fig. 14.6) dislocation or locked facet is often very difficult to reduce with traction. If there is a fracture of the facet, then a closed reduction can occur more easily. If there is no evidence of nerve root impingement, the unilateral locked facet can be left and will heal without instability, even in the dislocated position. However, patients may complain of limitation of rotation and chronic pain and the normal treatment is an attempted closed reduction or open reduction if the closed treatment is not successful. Open reduction is relatively easy within 2 weeks of injury but may be much more difficult after this time. It may be necessary to leave the locked facet, even in cases with some nerve root irritation and perform a secondary foraminotomy. There is a tendency for these to lead to chronic instability and a successful reduction should be followed-up with an interspinous wiring.

5. Bilateral facet dislocation (Fig. 14.2) usually implies damage to the posterior annulus and disc as well as to the posterior longitudinal ligaments. Although they normally respond to closed traction methods, they are very unstable once reduced and require an early posterior fusion.

6. Pedicle fractures produce a posterior facet dislocation of a different type. These are unstable fractures often associated with neurological damage. Re-alignment is normally achieved with skull traction but for mobilisation purposes it may be justified to use an anterior grafting and plating.

Surgery

Posterior fusion is normally achieved by trans-spinous wiring with good effect.

Anterior fusion is achieved using a Smith–Robinson type unicortical crest graft together with an AO type anterior cervical locking plate (Fig. 14.12). Even in the quadriplegic patient this allows early mobilization and rehabilitation of these patients.

Posterior Fusion

This technique is used for facet fractures, dislocations and chronic subluxation. The patient is usually stabilized on traction on the table, the face resting on a suitable head rest. Under image intensifier control any reductions are performed and the posterior cervical spine exposed. The obstructing tip of the dislocated superior facet may need to be removed and then wires are passed through the base of the spinous process. Bone graft is then taken from the iliac crest and applied over the decorticated lamina and facets.

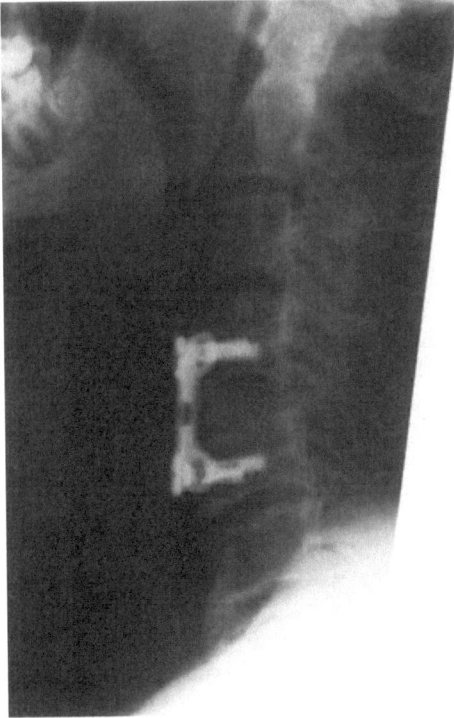

Fig. 14.12. Smith–Robinson anterior fusion with AO locking plate, C4/5.

Anterior Fusion

This is indicated for comminuted anterior body fractures and for patients on whom decompression is going to be necessary. In the lower cervical spine, the left-sided approach offers better exposure and is less likely to damage the recurrent laryngeal nerve. The usual approach is along the medial border of sternomastoid and down through the space between the carotid sheath and the oesophagus. Cloward type retractors are used to expose the anterior spine. A needle is placed in the disc to identify the level and checked with lateral radiographs. A tricortical Smith–Robinson type graft is used following removal of the disc and a locking type plate may be used to stabilize the relevant levels (Fig. 14.12).

Cervical Trauma in Children

Cervical injuries in children are rare but when they do occur usually involve the upper cervical spine, probably due to the relatively large skull on the smaller neck.

Birth Injuries

Rarely the spinal column can be stretched on delivery. True incidences are unknown as most of the infants who sustain a serious spinal cord injury, die shortly after birth or are even stillborn. If the child survives, a variety of neurological syndromes may occur which have to be differentiated from amyotonia congenita and infantile spinal muscular atrophy.

Fractures

Neck fractures in the child are rare. However, when they do occur even with some neurological damage, they carry a good prognosis. Treatment with a moulded plaster collar is all that is normally necessary.

Fracture of C2 in children under 7 years occasionally occurs after road traffic accidents and may be missed on X-ray (Fig. 14.13). Most will unite satisfactorily with a period of bed rest followed by a soft collar.

Ligamentous Injuries

It is not uncommon to see an anterior displacement of the 2nd on 3rd cervical vertebra following a minor injury. Bailey (1952) described this as pseudosubluxation and showed it was of no significance. Another not uncommon abnormality is that the arch of the atlas may override on the dens in as many as 20% of normal children.

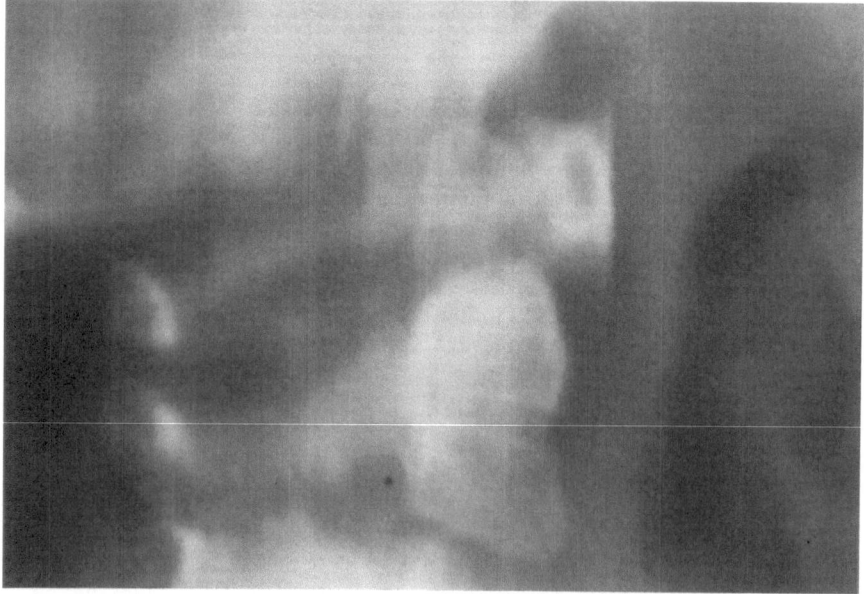

Fig. 14.13. Tomogram of fractured odontoid in a 3-year-old child.

True traumatic subluxation is rare and really only occurs as a result of a severe injury, either in a road traffic accident or in sport.

Pseudosubluxation may be diagnosed after a minor neck injury. If there was any doubt about the diagnosis, a period of halter traction should be applied for a few days and then further radiographs taken in flexion and extension. Ligamentous laxity may also occur due to hyperaemic softening of the ligaments secondary to infection in the aura-pharynx. This may lead to a torticollis (Grisel 1930).

Down's Syndrome

Down's syndrome is associated with a generalized ligamentous laxity and there is often a symptomless atlanto-axial instability, the incidence being about 12%–15%. The true incidence of neurological impairment is not known. However, many Down's syndrome patients complain of neck discomfort, transient weakness of a limb or of grip. The Department of Health and Social Security (Acheson 1986) suggested that although patients with Down's syndrome were at risk from deceleration injuries in day to day activities, they should not be deprived unnecessarily of any reasonable activity that they enjoyed. Davidson (1988) pointed out that most of these patients develop warning clinical signs that would alert the physician. The current view is that parents of children with Down's syndrome should be warned about the possible dangers of competitive sports. Operative intervention is not advised on prophylactic grounds, particularly as the operative risks are significant.

Os-Odontoidium

This is a rare abnormality and there is a lot of discussion in the literature as to whether this is traumatic or a true skeletal anomaly. There have been two reports of a normally developing odontoid process demonstrated radiologically at the age of 2 years subsequently disappearing (Freiberger et al. 1965; Fielding, 1965). This anomaly may be associated with varying degrees of instability of the atlanto-axial joint. Spierings and Braakman (1982) suggested that the important measurement is the sagittal diameter of the spinal canal between the posterior border of the axis and the posterior atlantal arch in flexion. If there is a sagittal diameter of 14 mm or less, cord compression behind the odontoid may occur. Often patients present with quite mild neck pain or shoulder pain. Even if patients present with paresis of the upper limbs which they may do, they normally respond to conservative treatment with skull traction.

References

Acheson ED (1986) Atlanto-axial instability in people with Down's syndrome. Department of Health and Social Security. Circular letter CMO (86):9; London
Anderson LD, D'Alonzo RT (1974) Fractures of the odontoid process of the axis. J Bone Joint Surg 56A:1663–1674
Bailey DK (1952) The normal cervical spine in infants and children. Radiology 59:712–719

Bell C (1830) The nervous system of the human body. Longman, Rees, Orme, Brown & Green, London

Davidson RG (1988) Atlanto-axial instability in individuals with Down's syndrome: a fresh look at the evidence. Paediatrics 81:857–865

Denis F (1983) The three column spine and its significance in the classification of acute thoracolumbar spinal injuries. Spine 8:817–831

Dvorak J, Valach H (1989) Cervical spine injuries in Switzerland. J Manual Med 4:7–16

Fielding JW (1965) Disappearance of the central portion of the odontoid process: a case report. J Bone Joint Surg 47A:1228–1230

Freiberger RH, Wilson PD, Nicholas JA (1965) Acquired absence of the odontoid process: a case report. J Bone Joint Surg 47A:1231–1236

Galasko CSB, Murray PM, Pitcher M et al. (1993) Neck sprains after road traffic accidents; a modern epidemic. Injury 24:155–157

Grisel P (1930) Enucleation de l'atlas et torticollis naso pharyngien. Presse Med 38:50–53

Harris JH Jr, Edeiken-Monroe B, Kopaniky DR (1986) A practical classification of acute cervical spine injuries. Orthop Clin North Am 17:15–30

Hohl M (1974) Soft tissue injuries of the neck in automobile accidents. J Bone Joint Surg 56A:1675

Holdsworth F (1963) Fractures, dislocations and fracture dislocations of the spine. J Bone Joint Surg 45:6–20

Jefferson G (1920) Fractures of the atlas vertebra; report of four cases, and a review of those previously recorded. Br J Surg 7:407

La Rocca H (1977) Acceleration injuries of the neck. Clin Neurosurg 25:209

Levine AM, Edwards CC (1985) The management of traumatic spondylolisthesis of the axis. J Bone Joint Surg 67A:217–226

Louis R (1983) Surgery of the spine: surgical anatomy and operative approaches. Springer-Verlag, Berlin

Mackay GM (1970) The nature of collisions. Technical Aspects Road Safety 43:1

MacNab I (1971) The "whiplash syndrome". Orthop Clin North Am 2:389

Norris SH, Watt I (1983) The prognosis of neck injuries resulting from rear-end vehicle collisions. J Bone Joint Surg 65B:608

Parmar HV, Raymakers R (1993) Neck injuries from rear impact road traffic accidents: prognosis in persons seeking compensation. Injury 24:75–78

Pilcher LS (1910) Atlanto-axoid fracture dislocation. Ann Surg 51:208–211

Podolsky S, Baraff LJ, Simon RR (1983) Efficacy of cervical spine immobilization methods. J Trauma 23:461–465

Robinson DD, Cassar-Pullicino VN (1993) Acute neck sprain after road traffic accident: a long-term clinical and radiological review. Injury 24:79–82

Ryan MD, Henderson JJ (1992) The epidemiology of fractures and fracture dislocations of the cervical spine. Injury 23:38–40

Saternus KS, Thrun C (1987) Traumatology of the alar ligaments. Aktuel Traumatol 36:214–218

Spierings EL, Braakman R (1982) The management of os odontoideum: analysis of 37 cases. J Bont Joint Surg 64B:422–428

White A (1990) Clinical biomechanics of spine, 2nd edn. Lippincott, Philadelphia

White AA, Southwick WO, Panjabi MM (1976) Clinical instability in the lower cervical spine: a review of past and current concepts. Spine 1:15–27

Chapter 15

Disc and Degenerative Disease: Stenosis, Spondylosis and Subluxation

C.H.G. Davis

More than a century ago, Godlee removed the first brain tumour (Davis and Bradford 1986); yet it was over 50 years later before the first extruded lumbar inter-vertebral disc was excised (Mixter and Barr 1934). Since the Second World War degenerative and disc disease affecting the contents of the spinal column, i.e. the spinal cord and cauda equina, has received increasing recognition and appears to be ever more common. As late as the 1930s, sciatica was thought to originate within the sciatic nerve and was treated with bizarre methods such as high pressure oxygen insufflation.

A static anatomical view of the vertebral column is relevant only to the narrow and relatively immobile thoracic canal. Degenerative disease occurs particularly in the lumbar region and within the more capacious and mobile cervical spine where the cervical nerve roots are able to move up to 3 cm within their dural sheaths during everyday life (Adams and Logue 1971). Although lacking the remarkable mobility of the upper cervical spine, the lumbar canal is also relatively mobile and capacious. Occasionally, narrowing of the cervical or lumbar canals may arise as a result of congenital or acquired disease, or from a combination of pathologies. In the cervical spine, degenerative changes may compress both the spinal cord and/or the exiting nerve roots. In the lumbar region, the spinal cord terminates at L2, (unless there is spinal dysraphism), and the single nerve roots, which run a long angulated course, are more at risk from degenerative disease than the main bulk of the cauda equina.

There is often considerable confusion over the nomenclature of degenerative disease. Spondylosis, disc disease and degenerative or osteoarthritic changes are interchangeable terms and are applied to radiological rather than to symptomatic features. "Radiculopathy" is commonly used to indicate neural compression of the cervical nerve roots and "sciatica" to indicate compression of the lower lumbar or first sacral nerve roots; yet it is highly probable that most pain in the upper and lower limbs associated with spinal degenerative disease does not arise from neural compression but from facet joints, the discs or soft tissues. "Stenosis" in its radio-logical sense is used to describe a narrowing of the axial plane of the spinal column by bone or soft tissue, or by subluxation.

Pathophysiology

The pathophysiology of spinal degenerative disease is reasonably understood and may indeed be considered to be part of the natural process of ageing. Clinical and radiological investigators tend to concentrate their attention on a particular problem as it arises and thus gain a static image which may not relate clearly to a patient's symptoms and signs. The function and efficiency of the spinal column depends on the mobility and integrated movements of the various soft tissues, joints and bones which also serve to protect the spinal cord and its emerging nerve roots. These tissues, particularly where the spine is most mobile, are also involved in the degenerative changes along with the intervertebral discs.

An intervertebral disc consists of three parts.

1. The annulus fibrosus with its tough fibrous tissue acts as a restraint between the vertebral bodies and contains the nucleus pulposus of the disc. The annulus can be penetrated by ruptured degenerative nuclear material posteriorly giving rise to central and lateral protrusions and extrusions.

2. The nucleus pulposus likewise contains a tough fibrous material and is compressible within the annulus fibrosus.

3. The hyaline cartilage end plates of the adjacent vertebral bodies are attached to the annulus peripherally.

When the nucleus of an intervertebral disc degenerates it assumes the quality of "crabmeat" tending to collapse on itself and so loses its ability to act as an hydrostatic shock absorber. As a disc space collapses and disc protrusions and extrusions occur, the annulus fibrosus has to take the additional strain which is transmitted to the hyaline cartilage end plates, and stimulates the formation of osteophytes (Findlay 1987). A vicious cycle is set up resulting in further collapse of the disc space. Facet joints at the same level are thrown out of alignment, and additional tension is placed on the adjacent joints, disc spaces, ligaments and muscles. Pain may arise from distortion of soft tissues, facet joints and disc spaces (discogenic pain) and may be referred to distant sites, particularly if nerve roots are also compressed.

Cervical Spondylosis and Disc Disease

Although the cervical spine does not carry the weight of the lumbar spine it should not be forgotten that the cranium and its contents weigh something in the region of 6.5 kg and that the cervical spine is constantly moving through a greater range of movement than other parts of the vertebral column. The upper cervical spine (C1–C3) is chiefly responsible for rotatory movements. At this level the spinal canal is at its widest, spondylotic disease is rare, and impingement on the spinal cord is unusual.

Anterior osteophyte formation rarely causes any problem except for the occasional case of dysphagia. However, lateral osteophyte and degenerative changes in the associated joints may predispose to neurological symptomatology where there is concomitant vascular disease as, for example, through compression of athero-sclerotic or ectatic vertebral arteries.

Posterior disc protrusion with osteophyte formation will impinge either on the spinal cord causing a myelopathy or in the region of the exit root canal causing a radiculopathy; a combination of both is often demonstrable radiologically but not usually clinically (Brain et al. 1952; Adams and Logue 1971; Nurick 1972; Ogino et al. 1983; Yu et al. 1986a, b, 1987). Degenerative changes can result in fusion of vertebrae as a disc space collapses, and this in turn may place additional strain on the cervical spine. Subluxation is not uncommon, and may be either fixed or mobile.

It is well known that C4/5 and C5/6 levels are most commonly affected in degener-ative disease and that C6/7 is less often involved. In the elderly, and particularly the very old, it has become increasingly recognized that the C3/4 level is frequently affected, possibly due to degeneration of the cervical spine resulting in spontaneous fusions at lower levels thereby leaving C3/4 as the only flexion-extension joint. Lateral disc protrusion is usually the only recognized change at C7/T1. Above C3 spondylitic changes may give rise to occipital neuralgia but surgery on the canal itself is rarely required.

Some people are born with a congenitally narrow cervical spine but symptoms rarely develop until the ligaments flavum becomes thickened with advancing age. At this stage cervical canal stenosis may be diagnosed radiologically, and radicu-lopathy and myelopathy present clinically. It is not uncommon for canal stenosis to exist in both the cervical and lumbar regions, i.e. tandem stenosis.

Radiological features of the degenerative cervical spine disease are present in more than 50% of the middle aged and elderly and indeed by the age of 80 there are very few members of the population who do not exhibit such radiological changes.

Predisposing Factors

It is generally accepted that wear and tear, and trauma, are common factors in the development of degenerative arthritis in associated with joints. As far as the cervical spine is concerned, there is no question that severe trauma can result in degenera-tive changes occurring very rapidly, often in a period of months. Similarly, an ante-rior bone graft will produce vertebral fusion within 6–8 weeks. However, the majority of patients with symptomatic spondylosis have not suffered severe trauma, but careful questioning may reveal moderate trauma or repeated minor trauma. Manual workers such as miners often develop radiological signs of degenerative disease particularly as age advances. It is known that repeated moderate trauma may result in the speedy development of radiological spondylotic changes. The best example of this is to be found among National Hunt jockeys who suffer flexion injuries on several occasions through every riding season. Although none of these injuries on its own may require hospital admission, the cumulative effect of this trauma may become symptomatic within 5–10 years.

The time lag between trauma and the development of symptomatic disease may be several years. In the author's personal series of 300 patients requiring anterior cervical decompression, 78 were members of the Armed Services undertaking parachute jumps in the Second World War. None of these patients remembers suf-fering severe neck pain at any time. This extraordinarily high proportion of para-chutists in an otherwise normal population would suggest that repeated moderate trauma may lead to degenerative changes 30–40 years later. This is also evidence that patients who experience what is generally thought to be minor trauma such as whiplash injuries may continue with symptomatic spondylotic symptoms after litigation has been settled. Patients with continual trauma such as those suffering from spasmodic torticollis and dystonia rapidly develop radiculopathy and myelopathy. It would thus seem that trauma is certainly the most common factor in the development of the degenerative process although the time interval may be extremely variable and it is impossible to predict which patients will be affected.

There are other predisposing factors. Patients with a congenitally narrow spinal canal such as achondroplastics (Spillane 1952) have a high incidence of cervical myelopathy. Patients with neurological disability affecting the lower limbs, e.g. following spinal cord injury or multiple sclerosis, tend to throw excessive strain on the cervical spine. Patients with congenital fusions (Klippel–Feil syndrome) and those who have had cervical spine surgery in childhood also tend to develop degenerative disease.

Cervical Radiculopathy

Natural History and Symptoms

It is important to recognize the natural history of cervical radiculopathy before embarking on unnecessary treatment and investigations. The majority of patients who suffer an acute neck pain do not have an acute disc protrusion. There are three types of presentation of cervical radiculopathy.

First, there is the acute cervical disc protrusion with radiculopathy (Findlay 1987). An acute disc protrusion may be extremely painful and is often associated with trauma. Although a history of trauma is usually obtained, the symptoms may not develop for hours or even days after the event. The patient complains of severe pain at the back of the neck immobilizing his neck and limbs and preventing sleep. Any movement is painful and the pain is made worse by coughing, sneezing and straining. There may also be a complaint of root pain in the appropriate derma-tone radiating down the ipsilateral upper limb. Often there are paraesthesiae distally and weakness and sensory loss appropriate to the degree of nerve root compression.

Second – and much more common – is the subacute and relapsing or chronic variety of radiculopathy. As in the first category this may occur at any age. The symptoms are not as acute or severe as the acute lateral disc protrusion of the younger patient and are associated with a chronic relapsing course. The episodes tend to last days, and on occasions weeks, and then clear completely. There may be intervals of months or years between episodes and after several attacks the patient may complain of a constant neck pain which is relieved by rest.

Third – and more rare – is the silent radiculopathy occurring predominantly in the elderly. These patients may present with a sudden neurological deficit in an arm associated with little pain in the neck. Usually a history of previous neck problems is obtained, though these systems may not have caused medical consultation.

Signs

The patient with an acute cervical disc protrusion is usually in extreme pain, is unable to move his cervical spine, and holds his or her shoulder elevated on the ipsilateral side. Neck movements, coughing or straining results in radicular pain in the dermatomal distribution with spinothalamic sensory loss. The reflexes are absent or may be exaggerated at the affected level, depending on the exact anatomical site of the lateral disc protrusion in relation to the nerve root. A full neurological examination is mandatory and particular attention must be paid to the lower limbs to exclude a concomitant myelopathy.

The patient with a chronic relapsing radiculopathy is usually not in severe pain. The examination findings are similar to those for a patient with an acute cervical disc except that the neck movements are less severely affected. It is very common to find tender "fibrotic nodules" around the medial side of the scapula in the distribution of the appropriate dermatome. The older patient with a silent radiculopathy may have an obvious root neuropraxia accompanied by weakness, wasting or sensory loss.

Management, Differential Diagnosis and Investigation

Cervical radiculopathy is usually a benign disease. Hospitalization and surgery are rarely required. Symptoms often remit when treated with simple analgesics and rest, with or without a cervical collar. Investigation and management will depend on available facilities but must be complementary. There is no point in ordering an MR scan for a patient who has a mild neck problem.

Neurophysiological investigations are rarely necessary unless there is doubt as to the diagnosis – as may occur with a brachial plexus lesion or if multiple sclerosis, motor neurone disease, or other diffuse neurological conditions are suspected. Proximal nerve lesions at the nerve root may summate and be combined with more distal lesions, e.g. ulnar nerve compression at the medial epicondyle. Traumatic lesions to the neck may be combined with a brachial plexus lesion, and at other times it may be necessary to exclude the presence of a spinal tumour or infection involving the meninges.

In the presence of clinical evidence of radiculopathy or coexisting myelopthy, it is essential to perform detailed radiological investigations (Fig. 15.1). Plain radiographs (anteroposterior, lateral and oblique views) may confirm the level of involvement but do not alter management. Myelography, with or without CT scanning, or MRI is essential where there is weakness, wasting or objective sensory loss. Reflex changes on their own do not necessitate further investigation provided the patient is watched carefully.

A relative indication for further investigation is pain. The pain may be severe or less severe but episodic. If the patient's lifestyle is adversely affected and the symptoms are not improving or are worsening, either myelography or MR scanning is indicated.

Myelography still remains the best investigation for displaying nerve root compression in the cervical spine. With myelography it is possible to obtain flexion and extension views thus reproducing to a certain extent the physiological parameters for that patient. CT scanning (Yu et al. 1986a, b) without myelography is time consuming as it may be difficult to pinpoint which level to image and interpretation

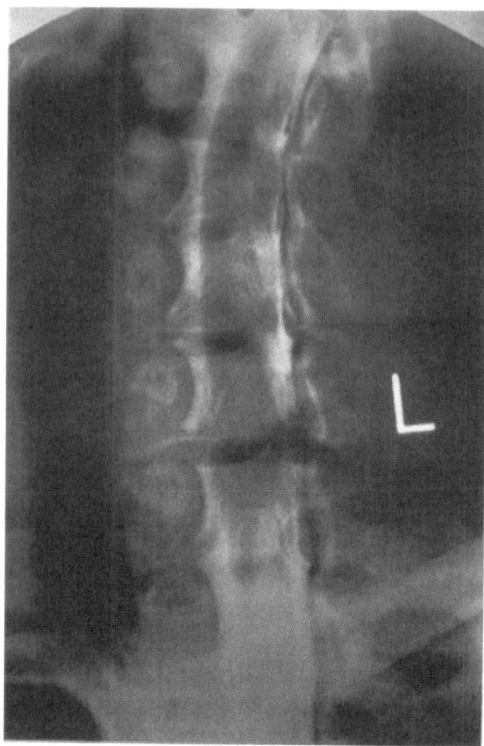

Fig. 15.1.   Cervical radiculopathy. Myelogram oblique view; left lateral C6/7 disc protrusion.

may be open to question. MR scanning (Modic et al. 1983), though ideal for imaging the spinal cord, requires axial views to image the nerve roots, and at present is not as accurate as myelography. It is essential when the possibility of surgery arises that lateral plain radiographs in flexion and extension are obtained to show the degree of stability of the cervical spine.

Most patients respond to periods of analgesia and rest using a collar. Patients vary in their acceptance of collars. A substantial number will discard them after a few weeks; others become "addicts". There is some evidence that wearing a collar for very long periods results in a weakening of the cervical musculature. Isometric neck exercises are particularly useful in the management of painful radiculopathies as they encourage strengthening of the musculature without movement. Vigorous exercising and manipulation are to be avoided if a root lesion is suspected (Davis 1985). The length of time for which the patient should be observed prior to surgical referral will vary tremendously.

Surgery

The indications for surgery for cervical radiculopathy are progressive neurological signs and/or pain which has failed conservative treatment and when radiologically demonstrable nerve compression fits neurological symptoms and signs.

Where there is instability or subluxation, anterior discectomy by the anterior approach, using the natural plane between the carotid sheath and contents laterally, and pharynx and larynx medially, combined in most instances with fusion using autologous bone grafts (the Cloward procedure with the microscope), has found considerable favour (Cloward 1958; Lunsford et al. 1980; Grisoli et al. 1989). Some surgeons favour microdiscectomy without fusion. If there is instability without displacement, either the anterior approach or posterior approach (Henderson et al. 1983), i.e. foraminotomy with hemilaminectomy, will give similar results. Using the posterior approach, it is often not possible to remove disc material but an adequate nerve root decompression appears to achieve the same relief of symptoms.

Surgery for radiculopathy provides good relief in perhaps 75% of cases. The reason for lack of success in approximately a quarter of those operated upon may be that the nerve root has been irreparably damaged prior to operation. A more likely explanation arises from our lack of understanding of the mechanism of neck and upper limb pain. Where more than one intervertebral disc space is involved it may be necessary to perform a surgical procedure at several levels though care must be taken not to destabilize the spine. Fusion will throw additional strain over the coming years on the joints above and below perhaps resulting in later complications. Patients must be informed of the risks and the chances of success with any surgical procedure. In the older patient who has suffered a complete nerve root lesion of the silent variety, the outlook is ominous and it is debatable where decompression has any place.

Cervical Spondylotic Myelopathy

Pathophysiology, Natural History and Symptoms

Cervical myelopathy tends to affect middle-aged and older patients, though younger patients can be affected by soft disc protrusions often traumatic in origin. As with cervical radiculopathy, patients with a congenitally narrow canal with hypertrophy of the ligamentum flavum (stenosis), neurological disease affecting the central nervous system, or spinal cord injury, are prone to develop myelopathy (Brain et al. 1952; Nurick 1972; Kojima et al. 1989).

Cervical myelopathy due to disc protrusion and osteophyte formation, is not only the direct result of compression of the spinal cord but can also arise from vascular insufficiency, possibly due to compression of the anterior spinal artery. The presence of vascular changes may explain the occurrence of physical signs at a higher level than that demonstrated radiologically. Demyelination may also occur from compression, particularly in the older age group.

There are three clinical patterns of cervical spondylotic myelopathy. In the elderly especially, an acute episode may have a vascular basis. The patient awakes to find that he/she is unsteady in the lower limbs and has weakness with sensory loss in the hands. The patient may then remain on a plateau, perhaps with further acute episodes over months or years. The second form of myelopathy is an insidious progression over several months. The third and most common form is a mixture of episodic and progressive deterioration. However, some patients may appear to go into remission. All too often a careful history and examination will reveal that this is only an apparent remission. Where symptoms and signs continue for months or years, the results of decompressive laminectomy are disappointing. Thus, in the 1950s, neurologists were loath to send these patients for operation (Brain et al. 1952).

The symptoms of a cervical myelopathy are unsteadiness of gait usually affecting both lower limbs, difficulty with fine finger movement (e.g. doing up buttons, dropping objects), sensory loss in the hands, and uncomfortable peripheral dysaesthesiae. As the condition worsens there is a spastic quadriparesis with further sensory loss. Patients may occasionally present with a Brown–Sequard syndrome simulating a vascular accident. The initial complaints often appear to exceed recognizable neurological signs. Neck pain is not necessarily a feature of cervical myelopathy and is an unreliable prognostic indicator.

Signs

Neck movements are often normal. Neurological examination of the upper limbs will reveal weakness in the fingers with a lack of fine finger movement. When dressing, patients may fail to do up buttons whilst looking straight ahead. Wasting of the small muscles of the hand, if present, is more often due to disuse than to specific root involvement. Sensory loss to pinprick is often patchy and may suggest a peripheral neuropathy. Joint position sense is preserved except when the myelopathy affects the C3/4 level: the anatomy of this particular lesion is ill understood. Reflexes are increased below the highest level of cord compression but may be absent at the actual cervical level. In the lower limbs there is nearly always spasticity, with or without clonus, and the patient is unsteady. The unsteadiness in not just due to a spastic gait but appears to be out of proportion to any weakness or sensory loss that may be found. Careful neurological examination will give earlier diagnosis and consequently better results from treatment.

The differential diagnosis includes extradural and extramedullary spinal tumours, which are usually more dramatically painful; hereditary spastic paraparesis and spinocerebellar degeneration; subacute combined degeneration due to vitamin B_{12} deficiency; late onset demyelinating disease; and amyotrophic lateral sclerosis (motor neurone disease) with spasticity in the lower limbs and wasting of the upper limbs.

Investigation and Management

Surgery is the treatment of choice for cervical myelopathy. The results of surgery and the risks accompanying such procedures outweigh the dangers of leaving cervical myelopathy to progress. There is little place for conservative treatment unless the patient's general condition precludes anaesthesia. Myelography (Fig. 15.2a and b) with or without CT or MR scanning is mandatory (Modic et al. 1983; Yu et al. 1986a, b). Except where there is generalized cervical canal stenosis, compression usually arises at a single intravertebral space.

Surgery

If a single level of anterior compression can be identified, anterior decompression is required. A posterior decompression could result in spinal cord infarction if there is

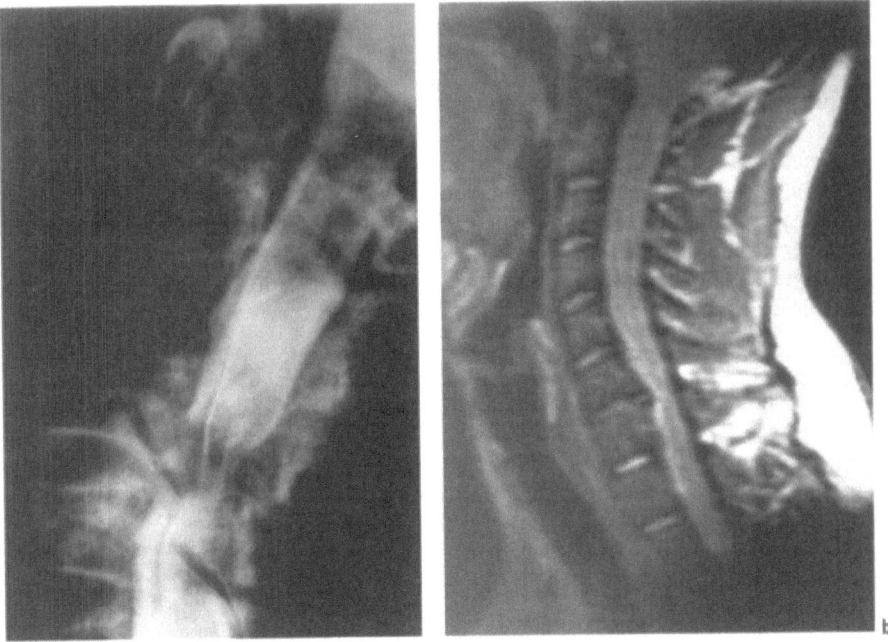

Fig. 15.2. Cervical myelopathy. **a** Myelogram lateral view; C3/4 disc protrusion. **b** MRI scan sagittal view; C6/7 protrusion.

considerable cord compression anteriorly from discs and bony excretions. If more than one level is involved or there is subluxation or instability, the anterior approach should also be used using microdiscectomy or the Cloward (1958) procedure. If there is cervical canal stenosis with ligamentous hypertrophy then the posterior approach – usually with cervical decompression from C3 to C7 inclusive – is required. A wide and lengthy decompressive laminectomy should be avoided in the younger age group as this can lead to deformity later in life. Where there is a combination of anterior and posterior compression then choices have to be made according to the exact anatomical problems relating to each individual patient (Symon and Lavender 1967; Jeffreys 1986). It is wise to remind the patient that not only does surgery near the spinal cord carry a morbidity and mortality but also late complication can occur from fusion.

Anterior spinal cord decompression for myelopathy should result in at least 80% of patients being stabilized as far as their neurological condition is concerned, though it must be admitted that surgeons tend to be overenthusiastic about their results. Not all the 80% will exhibit a marked neurological improvement. Cervical decompressive laminectomy for stenosis also given reasonably favourable results. However, both the anterior and posterior approach carry a small risk of further neurological deterioration in 5% of cases and it is essential that only surgeons with experience operate in this field. The practice of a posterior approach with dural opening and division of the dentate ligaments has largely fallen into disuse as it has not been shown to carry superior results.

Thoracic Spine

The thoracic spine does not move and is rarely affected by degenerative disease causing compression of neural structures. Despite the high incidence of osteoporosis with vertebral body collapse, which can be considered an element in the degenerative process in women, an association with spinal cord compression is virtually unknown. The thoracic canal may be narrowed in achondroplasia (Spillane 1952), and ossification of the ligamentum flavum occurs in association with parathyroid disease (Kojima et al. 1989). These are rarities, but thoracic disc protrusion can occur and the condition is extremely difficult to diagnose without radiological confirmation.

Thoracic Disc Protrusion

This usually involves the lower thoracic spine and may present at any age. More often than not there is no preceding history of trauma or pain, thus the diagnosis is often extremely difficult. The patient usually presents with an insidious paraparesis of upper motor neurone type with pyramidal features. As compression progresses, sensory signs occur.

Disc calcification is seen with plain radiographs in at least 50% of cases. MR imaging is the investigation of choice where available; otherwise myelography should be combined with CT scanning (Figs. 15.3 and 15.4). It is important that axial

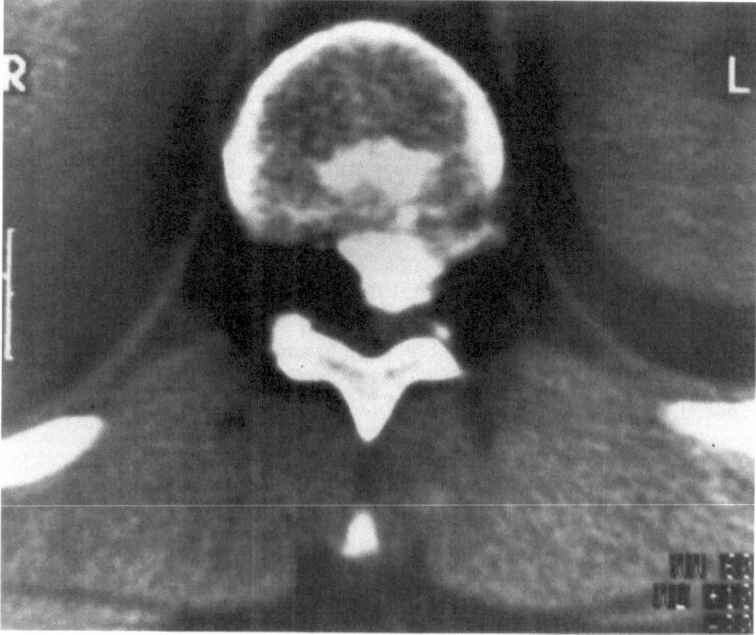

Fig. 15.3.   Thoracic myelopathy. CT scan axial view; calcified disc protrusion.

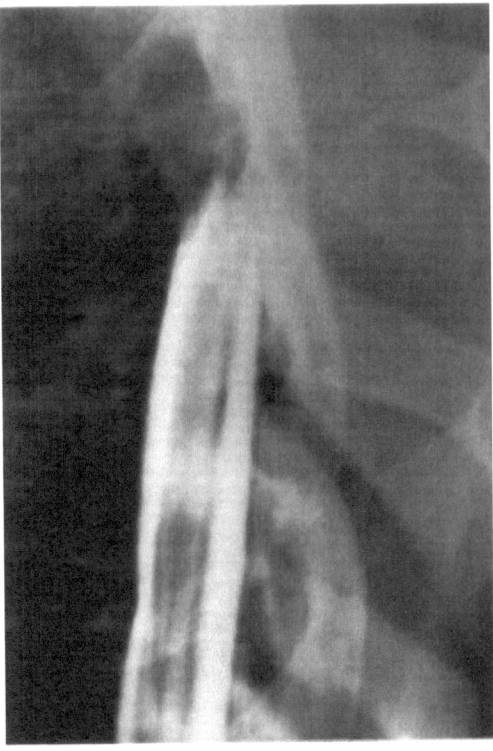

Fig. 15.4.   Thoracic myelopathy. Myelogram lateral view; thoracic disc protrusion.

views are taken to show in which direction the disc is protruded, i.e. laterally or centrolaterally. The thoracic disc protrusions usually consists of a firm extruded fragment which may penetrate the dura and indeed the spinal cord itself.

Surgery is required for thoracic disc protrusion (Findlay 1987). Conservative treatment will not prevent the development of a progressive irreversible disability once signs of cord compression have appeared. There is considerable controversy over the approach to thoracic disc protrusions and no surgeon can claim excellent results. It has always been considered surprising that such a small lesion can cause such disability. It is believed that part of the disability is due to direct compression of the anterior spinal artery. Other anterolaterally placed masses such as intradural tumours, e.g. meningiomas, usually reach a much larger size before causing an equivalent neurological deficit.

Laminectomy alone is liable to worsen the patient's condition. For centrolaterally placed discs a variety of approaches may be used: anterior thoracic, anterolateral (costotransversectomy), posterolateral with pediculectomy, or hemilaminectomy and intradural lateral excision. If the disc protrusion is central and known to be within the spinal cord substance then either the anterior transthoracic or anterolateral approach may be used. It may be impossible to remove disc material from within the spinal cord itself.

Lumbar Spondylosis and Disc Disease

Pathophysiology and Natural History

The pathophysiology of lumbar degenerative disease is similar to that of the cervical spine. Although the L4/5 and L5/S1 levels are the most mobile and are most frequently affected, the upper lumbar spine may be also involved, particularly in lumbar canal stenosis (Verbiest 1954). The lumbar spine has to bear the weight of the upper parts of the body and in consequence the bones, joints, ligaments and soft tissues are larger and stronger. The degenerative process probably starts in many cases at an early age, e.g. during adolescence, with degeneration of the nucleus pulposus of the intervertebral disc followed by disc protrusion and/or extrusion. From the clinical point of view the most important direction of protrusion is posteriorly in a central or lateral direction, initially stretching the annulus fibrosus and eventually tearing it (Maurice-Williams 1981; Findlay 1987). Anterior disc protrusion is of no consequence but extra posterolateral disc protrusion is now recognized as an uncommon cause of nerve root compression outside the spinal canal. As the process progresses, osteophyte formation begins in much the same manner as in the cervical spine. The facet joints become malaligned and overgrown, and there is thickening of the ligamentum flavum. In patients with a congenitally narrow canal (Critchley 1982; Ganz 1990), this process may occur throughout the lumbar spine and the canal loses its rounded appearance and assumes a "trefoil" axial shape. To a degree this is part of the natural process of ageing. Fortunately the lumbar spinal canal below L2 contains only the nerve roots of the cauda equina. Neural compression is thus mainly limited to the intervertebral exit root foraminae. Disc protrusion can affect either sex and may be related to obvious trauma. Lumbar canal stenosis is predominantly a disease affecting male manual workers around the age of retirement.

There are various predisposing factors to the development of lumbar degenerative disease. Patients with a congenitally narrow spinal canal, congenital spondylolisthesis or spinal dysraphism are at risk of developing lumbar canal stenosis. Pre-existing neurological conditions such as multiple sclerosis, shortening of one of the lower limbs, or kyphoscoliosis, are also more likely to result in lumbar degenerative disease (spondylosis) due to the assymmetrical forces exerted on the lower lumbar spine.

Low back pain and pain in one or both of the lower limbs is normally attributed to lumbar disc disease. However, it must be emphasized that the lumbar disc is only one element of the lumbar spine liable to damage or disruption. The facet joints, ligaments and muscles may also show degenerative changes, with or without lumbar disc disease. Neural compression occurs in a minority of patients. Positive neurological signs are found only in a small percentage of those affected.

The differential diagnosis of lumbar disc disease must include infection (e.g. septic arthritis of the hip), tumours of the sacrum and pelvis, spinal intradural tumours (e.g. neuromas), sacroiliac disease, and extradural metastases of the lumbosacral bony spine.

Classification of Lumbar Degenerative Disease

For the purposes of classification, lumbar degenerative disease has been divided into seven varieties, although these may overlap.

1. Acute lumbar disc protrusion
2. Chronic lumbar disc protrusion and foraminal exit canal stenosis
3. Acute lumbar disc protrusion with neurological compression
4. Focal lumbar stenosis, lumbar spondylolisis, and spondylolisthesis
5. The failed back and pain syndromes
6. Lumbar canal stenosis
7. Extralateral (outside the spinal canal) lumbar disc protrusion

Acute Lumbar Disc Protrusion

The history of an acute lumbar disc protrusion is often of greater help in determining the diagnosis and management than the clinical examination (Maurice-Williams 1981). The onset begins with severe lumbar pain across the lower part of the lumbar spine. This is typically the case with a central disc protrusion at L4/5 level, but a more lateral protrusion is classically accompanied by sciatic pain radiating down one or both legs. If symptoms arise acutely, triggered by bending, twisting or lifting, the onset of pain is abrupt and the patient may be stuck in a particular position unable to straighten up.

Characteristically the pain of a lumbar disc protrusion is made worse by movement of the lumbar spine, by coughing and by sneezing. It is relieved by resting. Most patients get greatest relief when lying flat on their back, but others – particularly if an upper lumbar nerve root is involved – find it easier to lie in a lateral posture or prone with their hip flexed. The low back pain of an acute lumbar disc is mainly in the midline. Pain localized slightly to one side of the midline may suggest facet joint involvement or other pathology such as a tumour. At rest the pain is felt as a deep ache, but when the erector spinae muscles are thrown into spasm a sharp pain may radiate up the spine to the neck and the back may become acutely tender to touch. With time the patient may enter a chronic stage with a functional scoliosis and will limp when attempting to walk.

The "acute" lumbar disc is a disease of young and middle-aged adults. In the majority of cases of acute lumbar disc protrusion, a previous history of back strain is common. Indeed, the history may go back to injuries in the teens or during pregnancy. In the older age group the presentation is less likely to be acute but rather a combination of degenerative changes and chronic disc problems. The "sciatica" is a sharp pain, usually in the L5 or S1 distribution, radiating across the buttock passing down the outer border of the lower limb to the external malleolus and foot, often the gaps in the appropriate neurotome and associated with paraesthesiae distally. The pain is made worse by movement of the lumbar spine and by flexion of the hip and dorsiflexion at the ankle, i.e. the straight leg raising test. The sciatic pain does not usually come on for some hours or sometimes days after the disc has prolapsed. In some cases, sciatica may be a more prominent feature than low back pain. The sudden disappearance of sciatica accompanied by a complain of numbness or weakness, e.g. a footdrop, is frequently a sinister sign requiring urgent attention. A history of previous trauma, as opposed to backstrain, is present in 50% of patients and almost invariably associated with the patient's occupation. Nurses and others required to do heavy lifting should be specifically taught how to do so and should be encouraged to use any lifting aids available.

Signs, Investigations and Management

The patient with an acute lumbar disc protrusion may require opiate analgesia. Examination is often limited by the severity of the pain and hospital admission may be required for assessment. The test procedure used are in part mechanical looking for tension signs, and in part neurological.

Postural examination will reveal the presence of thoracolumbar scoliosis and spasm of the erector spinae muscles. Spinal movements may be assessed by marking the palpable spines and measuring the interspinous distances on flexion. Patients may compensate by moving or elevating a hip at the same time holding the lumbar spine immobile. In severe cases the patient may be bedridden. Straight leg raising is nearly always reduced on the appropriate side with lateral disc protrusions but may be normal with a central disc protrusion or extrusion. Dorsiflexion of the ankle, thereby stretching the sciatic nerve, will worsen sciatic pain; and high disc protrusions at L3/4 can be recognized by the femoral stretch test. With experience it is possible to differentiate between a reduction in straight leg raising and spasm of the hamstrings (common with chronic disc protrusions) and arrive at a recordable clinical examination which can be compared with subsequent observations (Maurice-Williams 1981).

Neurological examination of the lower limbs is mandatory. A brief examination of the cranial nerves and upper limbs is required to exclude other neurological conditions. Localized muscle weakness and sensory loss in the appropriate dermatomes should be recorded. The reflexes in the lower limbs should be elicited and compared, if necessary asking the patient to kneel on a hard chair to obtain the ankle jerks. The lower sacral nerve root must be examined with the patient turned on to his/her side. A rectal examination is also advisable to exclude the possibility of a tumour. Changes in neurological signs may indicate increased damage to the nerve root despite lessening of pain as the illness evolves.

The diagnosis of an acute lumbar disc protrusion where symptoms are severe and the signs demonstrable is usually not in doubt. However, it must be remembered that tumours within and without the spinal canal or of the pelvis and sacrum can present in a similar manner, though usually the history is more chronic.

In the United Kingdom it is generally accepted that a conservative course should be followed in the management of acute lumbar disc disease unless there is an indication to investigate early, e.g. the diagnosis is in doubt or there are hard neurological signs. However, this policy is questionable when considerations such as loss of employment and earnings are evaluated, and may do no more than mask delays in hospital referral. Early surgery may be helpful for sedentary workers but risk the livelihood of manual workers. In the majority of cases bed rest at home, analgesia and sometimes sedation, is usually enough to overcome an acute attack. If the pain is uncontrollable, hospital admission may be required. If there are positive neurological signs or the pain cannot be relieved, further investigation as a prelude to invasive treatment is required. Plain radiographs alone will not suffice. Myelography (Begg et al. 1946) with or without CT scanning or MRI may be performed according to the availability of these investigations and the certainty of diagnosis (Fig. 15.5).

If a small disc protrusion is found or the investigations prove to be negative, inpatient care with analgesia, epidural anaesthesia and facet joint anaesthetic blocks will be required. Manipulation may help occasionally. Referral to a pain clinic or a second opinion may be needed at this stage and the patient should be reassured that a positive approach to his complaint is being adopted and that he will not be forced into unnecessary treatment. Wrong decisions made at an early stage may prove difficult or impossible to rectify.

Invasive Treatment of Acute Lumbar Disc Protrusion

Before embarking on invasive treatment it is essential to take into account any psychological factors or pending litigation. The surgeon must get to know his patient well and explain thoroughly the positive and negative aspects of lumbar spine surgery and/or chemolysis. On occasion it may be useful to obtain a second opinion

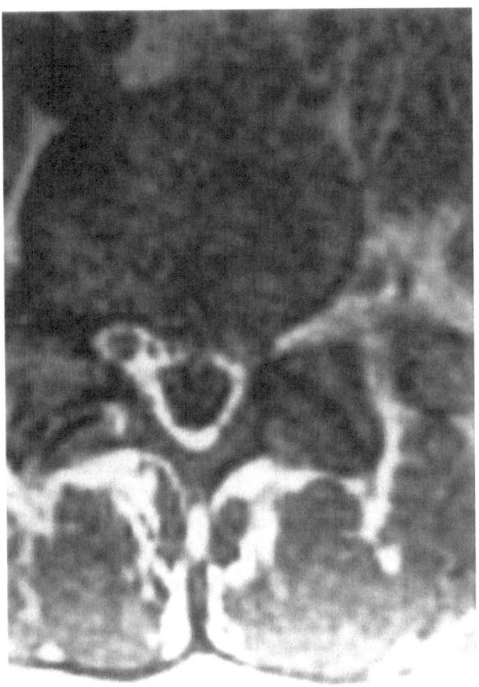

Fig. 15.5.   Lumbar disc protrusion. MRI scan axial view; right lateral disc protrusion.

but this may often serve to cloud the patient's mind. A joint decision needs to be reached between patient and surgeon.

Chemonucleolysis is the least invasive procedure for soft protruded lumbar discs (McCulloch 1977). The procedure offers a 50% success rate for patients with low back pain, sciatica and a proven protrusion (but not for an extrusion as shown by CT scanning). However, it is not a completely safe procedure, neither is it painless. Under image intensification, chymopapain is injected into the ipsilateral side of the disc protrusion with the patient mildly sedated. The L5/S1 space is more difficult to inject than L4/5. Post-treatment analgesia is usually required for a few days before the patient is mobilized in a brace. Manual work must not be undertaken for 6 weeks post-treatment.

An alternative therapy is percutaneous lumbar discectomy using a rotating sucking side-cutting needle or laser either under X-ray control or endoscopic visualization to evacuate the contents of a disc protrusion. Patients with a large disc protrusion or an extruded fragment are not suitable for such treatment. Percutaneous discectomy has gained some popularity in North America, whereas the United Kingdom more conservative management is preferred. Open surgery aimed at early mobilization by means of microdiscectomy or fenestration procedures can be used for lateral disc protrusions. Patients should have a least 6–8 weeks off work and 12 weeks if heavy manual work is contemplated. It must be remembered that disc protrusions requiring surgery not only result in a focal lesion but also result in some derangement of the lumbar spine.

The results of surgery for large protrusions or extruded fragments are excellent with regard to pain relief, although the abolition of all low back pain cannot be guaranteed (O'Connell 1951). With a small disc protrusion, surgical results are less favourable. The risks of surgery, e.g. neuropraxia, infection, and nerve root scarring, should always be considered. Patients should be carefully selected for surgery and appropriate facilities for physiotherapy should be available. With centrolateral or central protrusions, bilaterial microdiscectomies, bilaterial fenestration operations, or a partial laminectomy of the L4/5 level may be indicated.

Chronic Lumbar Disc Protrusions and Foraminal Exit Canal Stenosis

Most patients with low back problems have more chronic symptoms punctuated by occasional relapses. There is often a background of low back pain, and each attack lasts days or weeks. Neurological signs may be absent and tension signs less obvious than expected from the patient's complaints. There is often a functional thoracolumbar scoliosis and unilateral facet joint pain causing the patient to limp. Pain from a facet joint may radiate into the ipsilateral leg as a dull ache but rarely extends below the knee. The pain is relieved by rest and lacks the characteristics of true sciatica. If the patient limps, a pelvic tilt will develop thereby throwing increased strain on to the contralateral leg which may also become painful. Hamstring spasm is common and may be mistaken for a true reduction in straight leg raising. A thorough neurological examination should be undertaken with each relapse to exclude the possibility of a slow-growing tumour in the spinal canal such as an ependymoma (Davis and Barnard 1985). As the patient's disease becomes more chronic the pain threshold drops and symptoms may summate warranting further radiological investigation. Many of the patients have a degree of exit root canal stenosis (Epstein et al. 1972; Crock 1981) due to bony overgrowth of the facet joints and osteophyte formation without soft disc protrusions.

It is essential that a psychological profile of the patient is understood. The role of a clinical psychologist is revealing sexual, marital, financial and other problems is not to be underestimated. The radiological investigations are the same as for an acute disc but the results of surgery are far less satisfactory.

Acute Disc Protrusion with Neurological Compression

A rare, but serious, manifestation of lumbar or lumbosacral disc protrusion is neurological compression. A central disc protrusion – most commonly at L4/5 – may cause acute compression of the cauda equina. Usually an extruded fragment affects all the roots of the cauda equina below the appropriate level giving rise to a lower motor neurone type of paraparesis with sphincter involvement. Symptoms may develop rapidly, and sometimes silently. A lateral disc protrusion causing compression of the L5 or S1 nerve root may produce an acute, and often painless, footdrop. If the clinical diagnosis is uncertain, neuropraxia may be differentiated from a lateral popliteal nerve palsy by nerve conduction studies.

Both acute cauda equina compression and acute footdrop need urgent admission and removal of the disc as an emergency measure (Jennett 1956) (Fig. 15.6). Unfortunately the results of surgery are not good if neurological signs have been

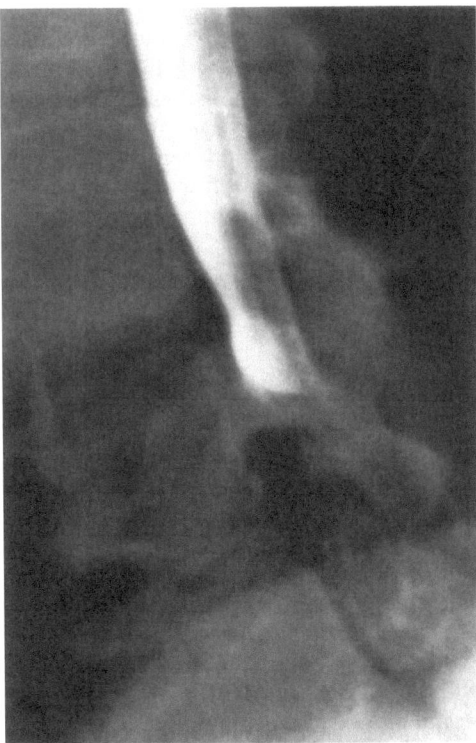

Fig. 15.6.   Acute cauda equina compression. Lumbar myelogram lateral view; L4/5 disc protrusion migrating behind body of L4.

present for more than 48 hours. Neural regeneration is poor with complete lesions, and in older patients there may be little point in offering surgery.

Focal Lumbar Stenosis, Lumbar Spondylolisis and Spondylolisthesis

Two types of vertebral subluxation are particularly associated with the lower end of the lumbar spine.

With the congenital variety there is an absence of the pars interarticularis, i.e. incomplete formation of part of the pedicle. Patients may present at a young age with bilateral sciatica or acute neurological compression. The absence of bone may not appear obvious on lateral radiographs, but at operation one is often surprised by the presence of large bilateral defects, which unless replaced by a fibrous union may allow the lamina to hang loose.

In the acquired mature onset focal spondylolisis with focal stenosis the spine is usually stable. There is often a long history of low back pain with bilateral sciatica and neurogenic claudication. Symptoms develop in middle age with women more often affected than men. An element of stenosis usually exists at the affected level, which is commonly L4/5. The aetiology is probably of disc space narrowing at L5/S1 earlier in life followed by fusion; thus setting up a process of strain with excessive mobility of the proximal joint.

With both varieties intervertebral body subluxation can be seen radiographically and the degree of instability of the spine assessed by flexion/extension views (Fig. 15.7). Further investigation by myelography or MRI is mandatory prior to surgery which is the treatment of choice. A fusion operation is required for the younger patient with congenital spondylolisthesis, either by anterior interbody fusion or preferably by a posterior approach with instrumentation as well as an autologous bone graft. If more than half the anteroposterior surface of the vertebral body has slipped, the patient should be dealt with as an emergency. In the mature spondylolisis with focal stenosis, local decompression with undercutting facetectomy may be undertaken provided stability is assessed pre- and postoperatively. Both conditions respond well to surgical treatment (Stauffer and Coventry 1972; Epstein et al. 1983; Markwalder and Reulen 1989).

The Failed Back and Pain Syndromes

With any longstanding chronic pain syndrome there are a minority of patients who fail to respond to treatment. This is particularly so with respect to the lumbar spine. Often the doctor is tempted to blame the patient's psyche and, indeed, there is no question that psychological evaluation can be most useful in assessing the patient's symptoms. Recurrent or continuing symptoms of low back pain and sciatica may be attributed to nerve root damage, reverberating circuits and changes in receptor sites within the spinal cord and brain; or to exaggeration of symptoms due to impending litigation, work avoidance, marital or sexual problems, etc. It is incumbent upon specialists who deal with lumbar degenerative disease to offer a service not only to their potentially successful patients, but also their failures.

The degree to which one investigates patients with pain syndromes and those with poor surgical results will depend on personal preference. However, with the increasing availability of non-invasive investigations, e.g. MR scanning, it is not unreason-

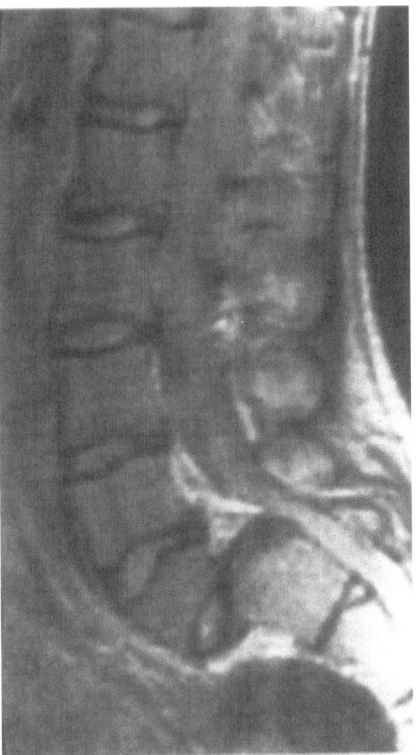

Fig. 15.7. Spondylolisthesis. MRI sagittal view; congenital L4/5 spondylolisthesis.

able to ascertain that the patient has not suffered a recurrent disc protrusion at the previous surgical site, or even at another level. Once radiological investigation has excluded an obvious surgical target then evaluation by a clinical psychologist and pain specialist in a multidisciplinary approach may be most useful. Further conservative treatment such as epidural anaesthesia, acupuncture or antidepressants may be useful in the first instance and dorsal column stimulation and even deep brain stimulation helpful in a minority of carefully selected patients. Cordotomy and rhizotomy have no place in the treatment of benign pain as a recurrence of symptoms is inevitable within two years.

Lumbar Canal Stenosis

Lumbar canal stenosis is an underdiagnosed condition affecting the middle aged and elderly (Verbiest 1954; Blau and Logue 1961; Jones and Thompson 1968; Kavanagh et al. 1968; Critchley 1982). Such patients are considered to have a congenitally narrow lumbar canal. Achondroplastics are similarly affected (Spillane 1952). As the patient ages multiple disc protrusions with osteophytosis occur in conjunction with overgrown facet joints, and the ligamentum flavum becomes hypertrophied (Jones and Thompson 1968; Sortland et al. 1977). The lumbar spine canal assumes a typical trefoil shape with a narrow anteroposterior diameter (Fig. 15.8).

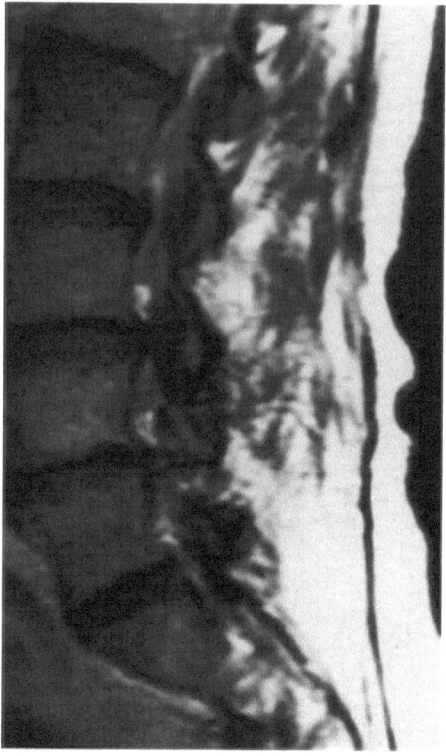

Fig. 15.8.   Lumbar canal stenosis. MRI sagittal view; L3/4 and L4/5 canal stenosis.

The patient has two complaints. First, sciatic pain related to exercise (Verbiest 1954). Such pain is often bilateral and due to exit root canal stenosis. Second, typical neurogenic claudication where one or both the lower limbs become weak and floppy after walking a set distance (Blau and Logue 1961). These symptoms are relieved by sitting down and resting for 5–10 minutes and the patient is then able to walk a similar distance (Kavanagh et al. 1968). The vascular supply to the cauda equina is presumed to be affected and claudication may be eased by flexion opening up the exit root canals thereby relieving the compression caused by overgrowth of the ligamentum flavum (Ganz 1990). The patient tends to walk with the back flexed. Occasionally as the disease progresses, the nerve roots become entrapped causing concomitant neurological signs. The natural history of lumbar canal stenosis is of the patient adapting to his disability. Walking distance becomes less and less and the patient walks slower and slower. Often this deterioration is in a stepwise manner, i.e. he/she may find that the walking distance is 200 yards then deteriorates to 150 yards after a period of some months. Back pain is usually not a major feature of this disease. Eventually the patient's lifestyle changes to one of immobility and may become housebound, but rarely totally immobile or paralysed. However, in general, the main feature of lumbar canal stenosis with claudication of the cauda equina is the absence of physical signs at rest, although an exercise test may reveal absent ankle reflexes. Straight leg raising is nearly always normal. Lumbar canal stenosis usually affects the L4/5 and L3/4 levels but later extends throughout the whole lumbar spine as the disease progresses.

Lumbar canal stenosis is treated by surgical decompression, usually with laminectomy at the affected level and undercutting facetectomy (Verbiest 1977; Critchley 1982; Ganz 1990). The results of surgery are good with 80% of patients being relieved of their symptoms. However, if there is severe sciatica at rest with objective neurological signs, the results of decompression are not nearly as favourable. In patients with tandem stenosis, lumbar decompression may unmask upper motor neurone signs due to a disguised cervical myelopathy.

In elder patients or those with the medical condition precluding surgery, calcitonin may ameliorate symptomatology (Eskola et al. 1992).

Extralateral Lumbar Disc Protrusion

It has become appreciated that extralateral lumbar disc protrusions may actually involve the nerve root one level above that expected (Frankhauser and de Tribolet 1987; Abdullah et al. 1988; Jane et al. 1990). Extralateral disc protrusions (sometimes called far lateral or extreme lateral) probably account for at least 10% of lumbar disc protrusions requiring surgery. Unfortunately the majority of physicians, surgeons and indeed radiologists are completely unaware that this can be a symptomatic condition. The age group of both males and females affected by this condition tends to be slightly older than the average, i.e. middle aged and older. A disc protrusion presses on the affected nerve root either pushing it laterally or against the front of the facet joint. There may be a lateral disc protrusion at the same level and therefore two roots may be affected. The commonest affected levels are L4/5 and L3/4 affecting the L4 and L3 nerve roots. Next in frequency is L2/3; L5/S1 is rarely affected because of its different anatomy. The patient, therefore, may present with anterior thigh pain, normal straight leg raising, absent knee reflex and appropriate sensory loss (Porchet et al. 1994). Such symptoms may be ignored as the symptomatology associated with sciatica is absent. The patient finds relief from his pain by lying on his side or sitting slightly flexed. Extension of the spine may be painful and lying in the supine position tends to exaggerate the pain. There are similarities in the symptomatology between an extralateral lumbar disc protrusion and facet joint pain. Indeed injections around the facet joint may relieve the pain temporarily. When the symptomatology of a lumbar disc protrusion has not been confirmed by a myelogram or axial CT scanning of the L4/5 and L5/S1 interspaces then further CT scanning or an MR scan should be performed to look for an extralateral protrusion. Surgical treatment may be confined to a lateral approach completely outside the lumbar canal (Jane et al. 1990). On theoretical grounds both percutaneous discectomy could be an ideal treatment and even be used when an extralateral disc protrusion is completely extruded; however, the author believes that complete facetectomy is required as well as disc excision. Surgery inside the spinal canal for a lateral disc protrusion will inevitably worsen an extralateral disc protrusion as the disc space collapses causing more extralateral disc protrusion at the same level and may be a cause of some failed surgical procedures. Myelography is of no help in the diagnosis of this condition which is best seen on an axial CT scan (Fig. 15.9). When the diagnosis of an acute lumbar disc protrusion is expected but routine investigations are negative, axial CT scanning of adjacent intervertebral levels should be undertaken, if necessary at several levels. Surgical treatment may

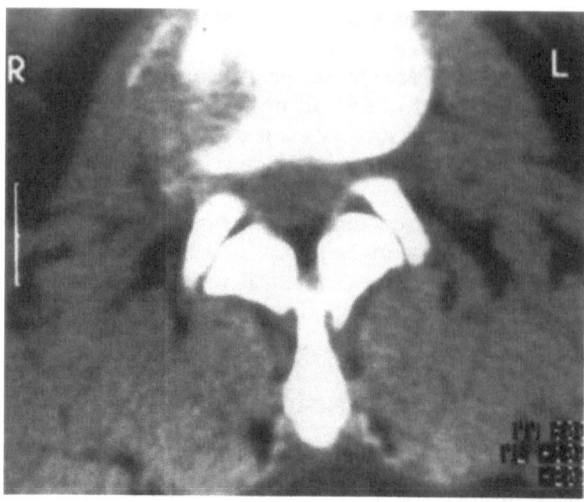

Fig. 15.9. Extralateral disc protrusion. CT scan axial view; right extralateral disc protrusion.

be confined to a lateral approach completely outside the lumbar canal (Jane et al. 1990).

Acknowledgements
I would like to thank Dr C. Coutinho of the Neuro-Radiology Department, Royal Preston Hospital and Professor J. Edwards of the University of Liverpool for supplying the illustrative radiographs.

References

Abdullah AF, Wolber PGH, Warfield JR, Gunani IK (1988) Surgical management of extreme lateral lumbar disc herniations; review of 138 cases. Neurosurgery 22:648–653

Adams CBT, Logue V (1971) Studies in cervical spondylotic myelopathy. II The movement and contour of the spine in relation to the neural complications of cervical spondylosis. Brain 94:569–586

Begg AC, Falconer MA, McGeorge M (1946) Myelography in lumbar intervertebral disk lesions. A correlation with operative findings. Br J Surg 34:141–157

Blau JN, Logue V (1961) Intermittent claudications of the cauda equina. An unusual syndrome resulting from central protrusion of a lumbar intervertebral disc. Lancet i:1081–1086

Brain WR, Northfield D, Wilkinson M (1952) The neurological manifestations of cervical spondylosis. Brain 75: 187–225

Cloward RB (1958) The anterior approach for removal of ruptured cervical disks. J Neurosurg 15:602–614

Critchley EMR (1982) Lumbar spinal stenosis. Br Med J 284:1588–1589

Crock HV (1981) Normal and pathological anatomy of the lumbar spinal nerve root canals. J Bone Joint Surg (Br) 63B:487–490

Davis C (1985) Osteopathic manipulation resulting in damage to spinal cord. Br Med J 291:1540–1541

Davis C, Barnard RO (1985) Malignant behaviour of myxopapillary ependymoma. J Neurosurg 62:925–929

Davis C, Bradford R (1986) A surgical history of Maida Vale Hospital. In: Walker MD, Thomas DGT (eds) Biology of brain tumour. Martinus Nijhoff, Netherlands, pp 245–249

Epstein JA, Epstein BS, Rosenthal Ad, Carras R, Lavine LS (1972) Sciatica caused by nerve root entrapment in the lateral recess: the superior facet syndrome. J Neurosurg 36:584–589

Epstein NE, Epstein JA, Carras R, Lavine LS (1983) Degenerative spondylolisthesis with an intact neural arch: a review of 60 cases with an analysis of clinical findings and the development of surgical management. Neurosurgery 13:555–561

Eskola A, Pohjolainen T, Alaranta H, Soini J, Tallorth K, Slatis P (1992) Calcitonin treatment in lumbar spinal stenosis: a randomized, placebo-controlled, double-blind, cross-over study with one year follow-up. Calcif Tissue Int 50:400–403

Findlay FG (1987) Spinal degenerative disease. In: Miller JD (ed) Northfield's surgery of the central nervous system. Blackwell Scientific, Oxford, pp 760–794

Frankhauser H, de Tribolet N (1987) Extreme lateral lumbar disc herniation. Br J Neurosurg 1:111–129

Ganz JC (1990) Lumbar spinal stenosis: postoperative results in terms of preoperative posture-related pain. J Neurosurg 72:71–74

Grisoli F, Graziani N, Fabrizi AP, Peragut JC, Vincentelli F, Diaz-Vasquez P (1989) Anterior discectomy without fusion for treatment of cervical lateral soft disc extrusion: a follow-up of 120 cases. Neurosurgery 24:853–859

Henderson CM, Hennessy RG, Shuey HM, Shackelford EG (1983) Posterior-lateral foraminectomy as an exclusive operative technique for cervical radiculopathy: a review of 846 consecutively operated cases. Neurosurgery 13:504–512

Jane JA, Haworth CS, Broaddus WC, Lee JH, Malik J (1990) A neurosurgical approach to far-lateral disc herniation. J Neurosurg 72:143–144

Jeffreys RV (1986) The surgical treatment of cervical myelopathy due to spondylosis and disc degeneration. J Neurol Neurosurg Psychiatry 49:353–361

Jennett WB (1956) A study of 25 cases of compression of the cauda equina by prolapsed intervertebral discs. J Neurol Neurosurg Psychiatry 19:109–116

Jones RAC, Thompson JLG (1968) The narrow spinal canal. A clinical and radiological review. J Bone Joint Surg (Br) 50B:595–605

Kavanagh GJ, Svien HJ, Holman CB et al. (1968) "Pseudoclaudication" syndrome produced by compression of the cauda equina. JAMA 206:2477–2481

Kojima T, Waga S, Kubo Y, Kanamaru K, Shimosaka S, Shimizu T (1989) Anterior cervical vertebrectomy and interbody fusion for multi-level spondylosis and ossification of the posterior longitudinal ligament. Neurosurgery 24:864–872

Lunsford LD, Bissonette DJ, Jannetta PJ, Sheptak PE, Zorub DS (1980) Anterior surgery for cervical disc disease. Part I: treatment of lateral cervical disc herniation in 253 cases. J Neurosurg 53:1–11

Markwalder TM, Reulen HJ (1989) Translaminar screw fixation in lumbar spine pathology: technical note. Acta Neurochir 99:58–60

Maurice-Williams RS (1981) Spinal degenerative disease. Wright, Bristol.

McCulloch JA (1977) Chemonucleolysis. J Bone Joint Surg (Br) 59B:45–52

Mixter WJ, Barr JS (1934) Rupture of the intervertebral disc with involvement of the spinal canal. N Engl J Med 211:210–215

Modic MT, Weinstein MA, Pavlicek W, Boumphrey F, Starnes D, Duchesneau PM (1983) Magnetic resonance imaging of the cervical spine: technical and clinical observations. AJR 141:1129–1136

Nurick S (1972) The pathogenesis of the spinal cord disorder associated with cervical spondylosis. Brain 95:87–100

O'Connell JEA (1951) Protrusions of the lumbar intervertebral discs: a clinical review based on five hundred cases treated by excision of the protrusion. J Bone Joint Surg (Br) 33B:8–30

Ogino H, Tada K, Okada K et al. (1983) Canal diameter, anteroposterior compression ratio, and spondylotic myelopathy of the cervical spine. Spine 8:1–15

Porchet F, Frankhauser H, De-Tribolet N (1994) Extreme lateral lumbar disc herniation: clinical presentation in 1978 patients. Acta Neurochir 127:203–209

Sortland O, Magnaes B, Hauge T (1977) Functional myelography with metrizamide in the diagnosis of lumbar spinal stenosis. Acta Radiol (suppl) 355:42–54

Spillane JD (1952) Three cases of achondroplasia with neurological complications. J Neurol Neurosurg Psychiatry 15:246–252

Stauffer RN, Coventry MB (1972) Posterolateral lumbar-spine fusion: analysis of Mayo Clinic series. J Bone Joint Surg (Am) 54A:1195–1204

Symon L, Lavender P (1967) The surgical treatment of cervical spondylotic myelopathy. Neurology 17:117–127

Verbiest H (1954) A radicular syndrome for developmental narrowing of the lumbar vertebral canal. J bone Joint Surg (Br) 36B:230–237

Verbiest H (1977) Results of surgical treatment of idiopathic developmental stenosis of the lumbar vertebral canal. A review of twenty-seven years' experience. J Bone Joint Surg (Br) 59B:181–188

Yu YL, du Boulay GH, Stevens JM, Kendall BE (1986a) Computer-assisted myelography in cervical spondylotic myelopathy and radiculopathy: clinical correlations and pathogenetic mechanisms. Brain 109:259–278

Yu YL, du Boulay GH, Stevens JM, Kendall BE (1986b) Computed tomography in cervical spondylotic myelopathy and radiculopathy: visualization of structure, myelographic comparison, cord measurements and clinical utility. Neuroradiology 28:221–236

Yu YL, Woo E, Huang CY (1987) Cervical spondylotic myelopathy and radiculopathy. Acta Neurol Scand 75:367–373

Chapter 16

Craniocervical Anomalies and Non-traumatic Syringomyelia

R.A. Metcalfe and R.A. Johnston

The majority of cases of syringomyelia are associated with abnormalities in the region of the foramen magnum but the reverse is not so and the true prevalence of structural anomalies in this region is unknown. It is difficult and somewhat artificial to analyse these disorders separately for many are found together in the same patient. There is also little genuine consensus of opinion about the cause of the anomalies or of related syringomyelia. In this review we have attempted to shed a little light by considering first the anomalies themselves and then proceeding to a more detailed discussion of syringomyelia and its surgical management.

Chiari Malformations

Chiari (1891, 1896) described a number of cases of childhood hydrocephalus with particular reference to changes which he observed in the cerebellum and lower brain stem. He divided his cases into four groups, only the first two being of contemporary relevance. Arnold (1894) presented a single case of Chiari's Type II deformity and his name has been frequently associated with the condition without evident justification. The chauvinistic reader might prefer the term Cleland-Chiari syndrome since the original description was by the Englishman John Cleland (1883). In the interests of simplicity only Chiari's name will be used in this article. Other authors have avoided eponyms in favour of descriptive titles – e.g. *primary cerebellar ectopia* (Spillane et al. 1957) and *hindbrain herniation* (Williams 1986). The problem with these terms is that they both imply that the primary defect relates to the hindbrain not the surrounding structures. This has not actually been established beyond doubt.

Baker (1963) showed that the conditions was easily missed if myelography in the supine position was not performed and after this both recognition of the disorder and frequency of publications increased. This chapter will concentrate on recent publications but the reader interested in the older literature is referred to the papers by Gardner (1965), Conway (1967), Appleby et al. (1968) and Banerji and Millar (1974).

There are two components to the malformation:

1. A tongue of cerebellum posterior to the medulla and spinal cord extending through the foramen magnum.
2. Downward displacement of the medulla and sometimes the caudal portion of the fourth ventricle relative to the foramen magnum.

The mildest, Chiari Type I, refers to patients who have cerebellar tonsillar descent through the foramen magnum but no evidence of spina bifida or other dysraphism. In Type II, the herniation is more severe and is associated with spina bifida and pronounced medullary descent. The distinction is artificial but the more subtle Type I form is of interest in that it presents commonly in adult life (Mohr et al. 1977; Paul et al. 1983), is often unaccompanied by other disorders and indeed is sometimes encountered as an incidental finding at myelography and MRI. The prevalence of tonsillar herniation is unknown. The largest published series from the Cleveland Clinic (Levy et al. 1983) reports an average annual incidence of 3.5 new cases each year in a large neurosurgical department. This figure is likely to be an underestimate and increased availability of MRI will probably result in a higher proportion of cases, both symptomatic and incidental, being discovered.

Aetiology

There is considerable divergence of opinion about the aetiology. One theory proposes a primary distortion of neuronal tissue secondary to a failure of embryonic development of the hindbrain structures including cerebellum, medulla, fourth ventricle and also the occipital bone and cervical spine. This is the most widely held view (Salam and Adams 1978). Other suggestions include downward pressure from hydrocephalus and tethering of the spinal cord by a myelomeningocele. This latter suggestion elaborated by Roth (1986) requires that the normal craniocaudal skeletal development is prevented by tethering of the spinal cord at the level of the meningomyelocele and a compensatory reversal of growth direction results in the posterior fossa contents being assimilated into the spinal canal. It is an attractive concept which does not explain those Chiari malformations which are not associated with cord tethering. A careful neuropathological analysis of 25 children with severe Chiari II malformation including myelomeningocele and hyhrocephalus demonstrated a wide range of associated malformations, including hypoplastic cranial nerve nuclei, cerebellar dysplasia, fusion of the thalami and agenesis of the corpus callosum (Gilbert et al. 1986). The authors reasonably suggest that the Chiari malformation is part of a spectrum of malformations caused by an unknown influence on the development of the central nervous system.

Recently a case has been advanced for a distortion of the bones forming the posterior fossa (occipital dysplasia) as the primary event with subsequent crowding of the posterior fossa structures leading to secondary neuronal distortion. Thus Marin-Padilla and Marin-Padilla (1981) treated pregnant hamsters with high dose Vitamin A on the eighth day of gestation and produced an underdeveloped basichondrocranium and cerebellar descent. Schady et al. (1987) made careful measurements of lateral skull radiographs of patients with the Chiari I malformation and found a high incidence of bony abnormalities in the posterior fossa. This positive result does not of course exclude the possibility that the bone changes are secondary to neural maldevelopment but a low incidence would have argued against the Marin-Padillas' assertion. Battersby and Williams (1982) advance the notion that distortion of the occipital bone during a traumatic birth may contribute to hindbrain herniation secondary to basilar impression.

Familial syringomyelia usually occurs on the basis of a craniocervical disorder (Schliep 1978). Coria et al. (1983) described three generations of a family affected by occipital dysplasia and Chiari I malformation, postulating an autosomal dominant disorder with variable phenotypic expression, the bony abnormality being primary. It seems unlikely that a genetic factor is present in all cases but the hypothesis can now be tested with the advent of MRI.

Clinical Features

The more severe Type II Chiari malformations present as a rule in infancy with major deformities, spina bifida and hydrocephalus. Syringomyelia may present later in life and sometimes in patients who have forgotten or never been told about surgery on the spine early in life. Although Williams (1986) has emphasized the artificiality of the distinction between the two varieties, the clinical description given here refers primarily to the milder Type I herniation which presents in adult life.

Symptoms

Headache and neck pain are the commonest complaints followed by sensory disturbance in the arms, gait disorder and lower cranial nerve dysfunction (Paul et al. 1983; Levy et al. 1983). Nightingale and Williams (1987) draw attention to the clinical characteristics of "hindbrain hernia headache" – severe occipital headache provoked by measures which increase the pressure differential between head and neck. Rarely, syncope may also be the presenting feature of hindbrain herniation, perhaps related to impaction at the foramen magnum (Hampton et al. 1982). One case of central sleep apnoea in association with a Chiari malformation has been reported with clinical improvement after occipital decompression (Balk et al. 1985). Bullock et al. (1988) report two cases of central respiratory failure in the context of syringomyelia and a Chiari malformation.

Signs

The most common features on examination are: lower limb hyperreflexia, weakness and wasting in the arm and hand, nystagmus, dissociated sensory loss, lower cranial nerve palsy and a gait disorder due to varying combinations of cerebellar, posterior column and pyramidal tract disturbance.

Clinical Syndromes

All the recent papers on the adult Chiari malformation use slightly different classifications of the clinical manifestations but there are five main components which may present separately or in combination:

1. Syringomyelia – most probably related to obstruction of CSF flow from the fourth ventricle with subsequent development of fluid-filled cavities in the substance of the spinal cord.
2. Paraparesis – related to direct pressure on the spinal cord.
3. Cerebellar syndrome – usually a truncal ataxia due to disturbance of midline cerebellar function and spinocerebellar pathways.

4. Raised intracranial pressure – headache often exacerbated by exertion and presumed to relate to plugging of the foramen magnum with intermittent intracranial hypertension.
5. Cranial nerve disorder – this could relate to either syringobulbia or cranial nerve distortion due to the cephalad course of the lower cranial nerves frequently seen in the Chiari malformation.

Oculomotor Features

The classical disorder, downbeating nystagmus, was described by Cogan (1968) but a wide range of other features have been documented including side-beat, periodic alternating, divergent, gaze-evoked and rebound nystagmus, impaired saccadic, pursuit and vergence eye movements and internuclear ophthalmoplegia (Leigh and Zee 1983). One case of see-saw nystagmus has also been reported (Zimmerman et al. 1986). In practice the presence of genunine downbeating nystagmus should lead to a thorough search for a foramen magnum lesion. Oscillopsia is a frequent complaint and both this and the abnormal eye signs tend slowly to improve after surgical decompression.

Misdiagnosis

Foramen magnum disorders presenting with vague headache and odd sensory complaints without clear physical signs are quite likely to be misdiagnosed. Neurosis, multiple sclerosis and motor neurone disease are common errors (Levy et al. 1983).

Investigation

Plain Radiology

Plain radiology has no real place in the investigation of the patient suspected of having a foramen magnum syndrome but the results are interesting and of some relevance to the aetiology.

The frequency of detection of bony abnormalities related to Chiari malformations depends on how hard one looks. Platybasia, basilar impression, concavity of the clivus and enlargement of the foramen magnum have all been reported, the largest series describing skull abnormalities in 36% of cases (Levy et al. 1983). Careful measurement of lateral skull radiographs increases this proportion to two-thirds (Schady et al. 1987). Cervical spine views may show assimilation of the atlas, a widened canal, altered cervical curvature (increased, decreased or reversed) or spina bifida. These changes are seen in 35% of cases (Levy et al. 1983).

Imaging

The hazardous and invasive investigations of oily contrast medium myelography, pneumoencephalography and vertebral angiography were superceded by water-

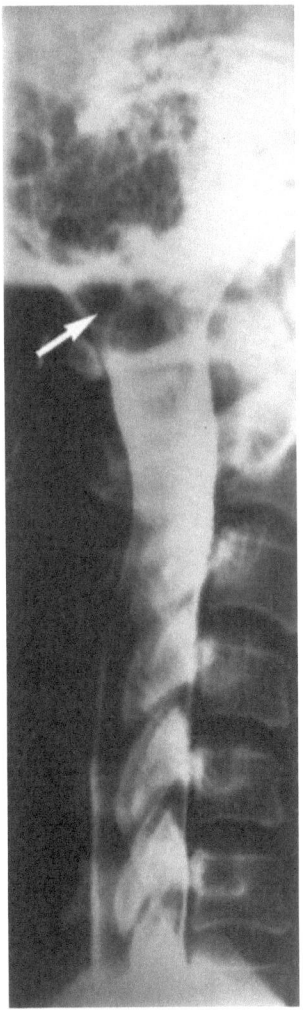

Fig. 16.1. Lateral view of myelogram demonstrating cerebellar tonsillar herniation below foramen magnum (arrow). (Radiograph by courtesy of Professor I. Isherwood.)

soluble supine myelography with or without CT and this in turn by magnetic resonance imaging (Bosley et al. 1985). There is already an extensive literature on MRI in this region all of which confirms that MRI is now the investigation of choice (McManus and Bartlett 1986), although imaging abnormalities do not necessarily correlate with clinical features (Wolpert et al. 1988). A study of the position of cerebellar tonsils in the normal population compared with the Chiari malformation (Aboulezz et al. 1985) suggests that extension of the tonsils up to 3 mm below the foramen magnum is normal but clearly pathological beyond 5 mm. Barkovitch et al. (1986) produced similar findings. MRI's superiority is likely to be enhanced with further technical developments and the use of gadolinium as a contrast agent. Fig. 16.1 shows a water-soluble contrast supine myelogram and Fig. 16.2 the results of MRI in a similar patient.

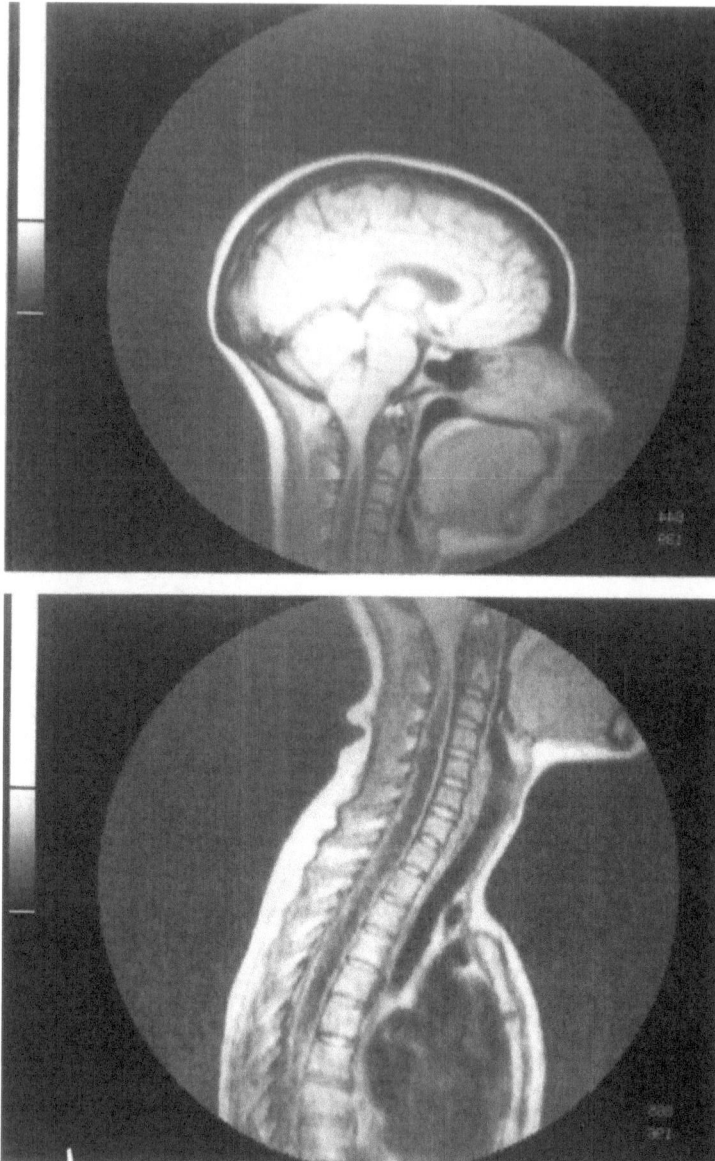

Fig. 16.2. Upper figure: MRI demonstrating Chiari I malformation with associated syringomyelia. Lower figure: MRI of the same patient demonstrating the extensive syrinx formation. (Radiograph by courtesy of Professor I. Isherwood.)

Management

There are no controlled data available on this topic and even the natural history is difficult to establish in an area where there is such a wide range of severity and type

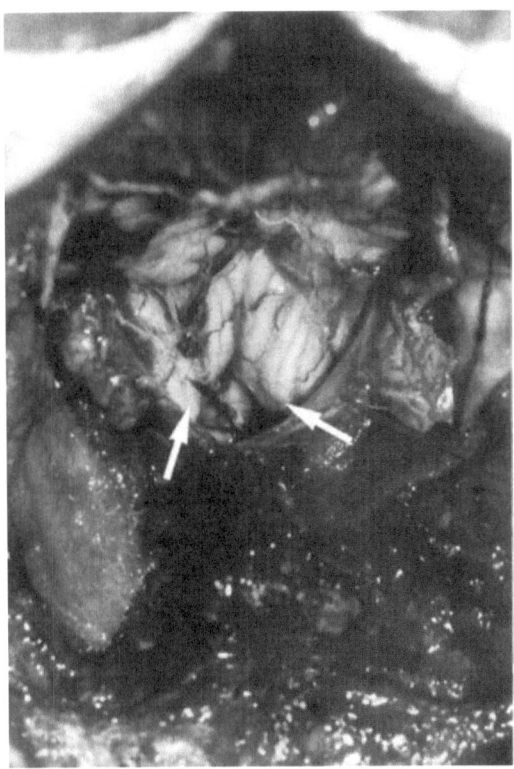

Fig. 16.3.   Operative view of a Chiari I malformation. The dura has been opened and the tips of the cerebellar tonsils are arrowed. (Illustration by courtesy of Mr. R A. Johnston.)

of presentation. The management of *symptomatic* adult Chiari malformations without syrinx tends to be similar to that of syringomyelia – i.e. surgical in the presumption that the condition is likely to worsen with the passage of time and that operation stands a reasonable chance of stabilizing the condition and in some case results in sustained improvement. Fig. 16.3 shows a view of a Chiari I malformation at operation.

Paul et al. (1983) reported the results of suboccipital decompression and C1–C3 laminectomy in 71 patients presenting in adult life; 65% had a central cord syndrome, 22% evidence of foramen magnum compression and 11% a pure cerebellar syndrome. At operation 41% had evidence of arachnoiditis in addition to tonsillar herniation, 30% had a constricting dural band at the foramen magnum or C1 and a variety of bony abnormalities were described, not all of which were evident on radiology. Respiratory depression was the most frequent operative complication (14%) and one patient died from this. About three-quarters of the whole group showed initial improvement but 20% subsequently relapsed, usually within 2–3 years of operation. Patients with a purely cerebellar presentation did not relapse.

Levy et al. (1983) reported a series of 127 patients who had had a similar procedure with or without an attempt to plug the central canal of the spinal cord with muscle. Of these patients, 21 had no evidence of tonsillar descent at operation and in this group arachnoiditis was a universal finding often associated with a kinked brain stem or occlusion of the foramen of Magendie. In general the results were similar to those described by Paul with about half showing long-term benefit, a quarter unchanged and the remainder deteriorating. The attempt to block the central canal produced neither obvious benefit nor complication. The results of Saez et al. (1976) are in broad agreement with both these publications.

Dandy-Walker Syndrome

Although not strictly a craniocervical anomaly, it seems appropriate to mention this unusual disorder here since it may form part of the spectrum of hindbrain developmental disorders which include the Chiari malformation. Brown (1977) defines six major features: hydrocephalus; defective development of the cerebellar vermis: cyst-like enlargement of the fourth ventricle; enlargement of the posterior fossa: elevated location of the transverse sinuses and the tentorium; and usually lack of patency of the foraminae of Luschka and Magendie.

The syndrome was properly delineated in separate publications by Dandy and Blackfan (1914) and Taggert and Walker (1942). Gardner postulated a relationship between the Chiari malformations and the Dandy-Walker syndrome, suggesting that they both represented "failure of the outlets of the fourth ventricle to develop normally in the rhombic roof of the embryo" (Gardner et al. 1972; Gardner 1973). In his view if CSF, unable to exit from the fourth ventricle was retrained in the lateral ventricles, then a small posterior fossa resulted with herniation through the foramen magnum. Retention in and hence expansion of the fourth ventricle would cause an enlarged posterior fossa with the Dandy-Walker cyst. This may explain some cases where there is evident hydrocephalus but cannot easily explain the small or distorted posterior fossa seen in the Chiari malformations without hydrocephalus. Barkovich et al. (1989) have studied 31 patients with posterior fossa CSF collections using MRI and conclude that the Dandy-Walker syndrome is part of a spectrum of posterior fossa development anomalies which include mega-cisterna magna.

Clinically the syndrome usually presents at birth or in infancy with dydrocephalus (about 60%), in childhood or adolescence with raised intracranial pressure (35%) and the remainder in adult life. There seems to be a female excess in most series (Brown 1977). A variety of associated anomalies have been reported but syringomyelia occurs rarely. Management is by shunting to control intracranial pressure.

Bony Abnormalities at the Craniocervical Junction

A variety of different measurements have been applied to lateral skull radio-graphs in order to define disorders of the skull base (McRae 1953; Schmidt et al. 1978; Schady et al. 1987). Fig. 16.4 is taken from the paper by Schady et al. and demonstrates most of them. The reader is referred to the exhaustive account of Schmidt et al. (1978) for more details. *Platybasia* means flattening of the skull base with an

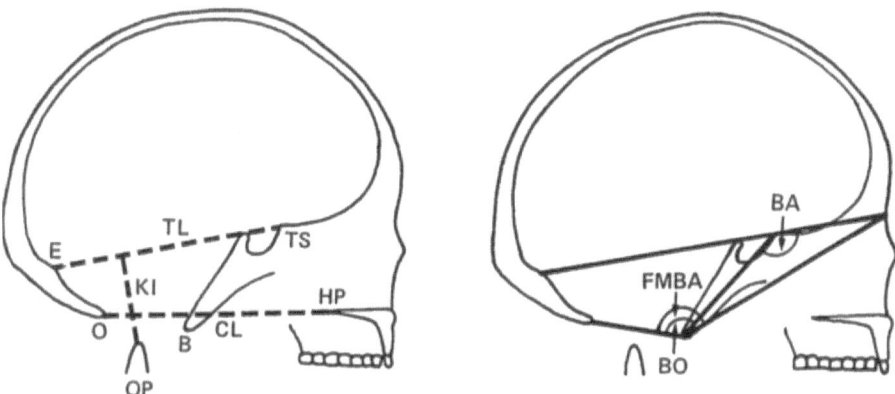

Fig. 16.4. Diagram to illustrate some of the relevant measurements indicating platybasia and basilar impression (the position of the odontoid peg has been shifted posteriorly to aid clarity). Key to abbreviations: B, Basion; E, Endinion; O, Opisthion; OP, Odontoid Peg; TL, Twining's line; TS, Tuberculum Sella; KI, Klaus Index; CL, Chamberlain's Line; HP, Hard Palate; BA, Basal Angle; BO, Boogaard's Angle; FMBA, Foramen Magnum Basilar Angle. (Reproduced by courtesy of Dr. W. Schady.)

increase in the basal angle (BA in the diagram), the angle between the planes of clivus and the floor of the anterior fossa. *Basilar invagination* or *impression* implies an upward bulging of the margins of the foramen magnum. In practice, the anterior margin of the foramen magnum is often displaced upwards to a greater degree than the posterior margin, thus increasing Boogaard's angle (BO), the angle between the plane of the clivus and the plane of the foramen magnum. The position of the odontoid peg relative to Chamberlain's line (CL) and Twining's line (TL) may also be used to indicate basilar impression. Hypoplasia of the occipital condyles is perhaps the mildest example of occipital dysplasia and marked asymmetries of development of the occipital bone are also recognized to occur (Schmidt et al. 1978).

The majority of cases of platybasia and basilar impression are congenital or possibly acquired during birth but a number of primary bone disorders can produce a secondary invagination during adult life. These include: Paget's disease, rickets, osteomalacia, hypothyroidism, osteogenesis imperfecta, fibrous dysplasia, gargoylism, achondroplasia and cleidocranial dysostosis. The proportion of cases of secondary basilar impression is probably between 4% and 8% of the total (Schmidt et al. 1978).

Occipitalization of the Atlas

Some degree of bony union between skull and atlas was recognized in 28 cases out of 66 discussed by McRae (1953). This was *not* commonly associated with platybasia and basilar impression but neurological symptoms and signs similar to those seen in the Chiari malformation were present in two-thirds. McRae reports the presence of the Chiari malformation and dural bands which may well contribute to symptomatology. A high, long or posteriorly angulated odontoid process was usually associated with symptoms.

Clinical Features

The proportion of cases of basilar impression presenting as a clinical problem varies in series depending largely on the derivation of patients. Series from departments attached to neuroscience units will naturally produce a higher frequency of patients with clinical problems. In the English literature, Moreton's (1943) figure of 20% symptomatic is representative of a general radiological series compared with McRae's (1953) suggestion of 62% in patients derived from a neurological institute. Peak onset appears to be in the fifth decade.

A number of authors have commented on the general appearance of many patients with basilar impression. These features are by no means invariable but the presence of a short neck should alert the clinician to the possible association. Neurological symptoms and signs cannot in general be distinguished from those outlined in the discussion of the Chiari malformation for the very good reason that the pathophysiology is essentially the same. However De Barros et al. (1968) felt that a pure pyramidal syndrome was more common in isolated basilar impression.

Association with Chiari Malformation and Syringomyelia

De Barros et al. (1968) reported a series of 66 patients with neurologically symptomatic basilar impression; 33 were subjected to surgical decompression and the Chiari malformation was found in 76% of these. Syringomyelia is also found in association with basilar impression but much less frequently; a figure of 15%–20% seems reasonable but clearly very much dependent upon the derivation of cases (Schmidt et al. 1978).

Management

There are no recent series on the management of bony craniocervical anomalies. The asymptomatic patient clearly presents no problem but a progressing and disabling neurological disorder usually requires surgical decompression. The outlook is clearly less good than for the Chiari malformation and will depend upon the degree of deformation of bone and neural tissue. The coexistence of the Chiari malformation may be protective by acting as a cushion between bone and medulla (De Barros et al. 1968) and in the same way the presence of a wide spinal canal may be helpful in reducing the likelihood of impaction in the Chiari malformation.

Birth Injury

The effects of perinatal trauma have been studied in basilar impression (Battersby and Williams 1982) and in syringomyelia (Williams 1977; Newman et al. 1981). The Chiari malformation has not been studied specifically but as the reader will be aware, there is a great deal of overlap and many of the cases cited in these three studies also had tonsillar herniation. Battersby and Williams derived a birth score based on such factors as prolonged labour, high birth weight, use of forceps and breech delivery and found a history of birth frauma to be four times more likely in patients with basilar impression than in control subjects. This study followed on from the earlier publication of Williams (1977) in syringomyelia. Overriding of the lateral and squamous portions of the occipital bones (occipital osteodiastasis) during birth is proposed as one of the mechanisms leading to foramen magnum distortion and syringomyelia.

Newman et al. (1981) from data in their similar study suggest that traumatic birth is common in cases of syringomyelia and *either* Chiari malformation *or* basal arachnoiditis but no association was found with the Chiari malformation presenting in other ways. this finding requires confirmation but, if correct, suggests that birth trauma is a factor precipitating syringomyelia in individuals prone to this condition by virtue of the Chiari malformation.

Klippel-Feil Syndrome

This disorder, first described in 1912 by Klippel and Feil, consists of the clinical features of limited neck movements, a low hairline and a very short neck and radiology demonstrating fusion of vertebrae. considerable variation in the degree of severity exists, a familial tendency has been recognized and the defect is generally thought to represent a defect of mesodermal segmentation, probably occurring before the eighth week of gestation. Many associated abnormalities have been described including hydrocephalus, syringomyelia and syringobulbia. Deafness is fairly common and a curious form of synkinesis or mirror movements of the arms has also been recognized (Wilkinson 1978).

Syringomyelia

The majority of cases of cord syrinx formation are related to obstruction to the outflow of CSF from the fourth ventricle and as such are associated with either craniocervical anomalies or arachnoiditis. As with the anomalies themselves the terminology is confused and confusing. Hydromyelia is used interchangeably with syringomyelia by some authors but by others to describe dilatation of the central canal without the formation of fluid-filled cavities outside the canal in the substance of the cord. Some prefer the combined term syringohydromyelia but the simple terms syringomyelia and syrinx will be used here to describe all fluid-filled cavities within the cord. The majority of syrinx, presenting usually with a central cord syndrome, are secondary to obstruction of the foramen magnum ("communicating syringomyelia" in the terminology of Barnett et al. 1973). A small proportion are post-traumatic, relate to local arachnoiditis around the cord or are cystic central cord tumours ("non-communicating syringomyelia" according to Barnett et al. 1973). A variety of other disorders have been described in which syrinx formation has occurred. These include intradural extramedullary tumours, vertebral body fractures and disc protrusions. these relatively rare causes of syrinx formation are outside the scope of this article and will not be considered further here.

Aetiology

Like many neurological conditions whose origins are obscure, syringomyelia was first regarded as a degenerative disorder. This term prevented proper thought and active enquiry into its origins for many years. Gardner (1965, 1967) provided the first rational concept when he proposed his *hydrodynamic theory*. This asserted that the condition arose from an obstruction to the outflow of CSF from the fourth ventricle with a patent central canal (which normally closes early in embryonic life) providing an ingress for CSF at raised pressure into the substance of the cord. Arterial pulsations transmitted to the CSF were thought to be the source of the pressure differential. Foster and Hudgson (1973) reasonably nominate cord cavitation, ventricular outflow obstruction and a communication between cavity and fourth ventricle as *Gardner's triad*. They point out that whilst it may not be possible to demonstrate a communication between syrinx and ventricle at operation or post mortem, this does not mean that such a channel was never present.

In a development of this concept, Williams (1969, 1970, 1972) suggested that the major hydrodynamic event was a transfer of CSF from the spinal into the cranial subarachnoid space past the occluding cerebellar tonsils during Valsalva manouevres. The tonsils then re-impact in the foramen magnum leaving a pressure differential between cranial and spinal compartments. The presence of a patent canal leading from the fourth ventricle then encourages tracking of this CSF at raised pressure into the spinal cord. As Foster and Hudgson (1973) point out, this does not really explain every case of communicating syringomyelia especially those with adhesive arachnoiditis around the foramen magnum but the two concepts are not mutually exclusive and both mechanisms may operate.

There is a lack of pathological evidence of a connection between syrinx cavity and either a patent canal or the fourth ventricle itself. Protagonists of the hydrodynamic theory protest that a connection may have been present at some stage which was subsequently sealed off but this awkward fact remains a problem. Ball and Dayan (1972) avoided this difficulty by suggesting that fluid in the spinal subarachnoid space under increased pressure as a result of foramen magnum block ,tracked into the substance of the spinal cord along the Virchow-Robin spaces and thus formed syrinx cavities independent of the central canal.

A number of authors have considered ischaemia of the cord to be important in the aetiology (see Foster and Hudgson (1973) for a discussion). Logue and Rice Edwards (1981) regard syringomyelia and the Chiari malformation as associated conditions without a causal link and point out that most of the improvement seen after operation is attributable to decompression of cerebellum and spinal cord rather than an improvement in syringomyelia. MRI of the syrinx before and after operation has however demonstrated reduction in syrinx size, at least initially (Grant et al. 1987a). Prevention of progression of syringomyelia would seen to be the important point here and a definite benefit is difficult to establish given the impossibility of performing a controlled study.

Clinical Features

The two large series of Barnett et al. (1973) and Logue and Rice Edwards (1981) are remarkably similar in the clinical features which they describe. Both describe patients from the era when investigations were not free of hazard and thus the clinical suspicion of syringomyelia had to be strong, i.e. usually a presentation conforming to the classical description. Mean duration of disease before diagnosis was 7.8 years in Logue's series. One must suspect that ready availability of MRI will alter our concepts of the clinical presentation and many more asymptomatic syrinx will be revealed.

Symptoms

Both series point out the extreme variability of both presentation and progression. Onset or deterioration of symptoms in relation to minor trauma, coughing or sneezing is commonplace. Stiffness of the legs, numb hands, pain in the neck and arms and headache are the common principal complaints. Others presented with symptoms of brain stem or lower cranial nerve involvement.

Signs

General appearance A substantial minority of Barnett's patients had one or more of the following: large head, short neck, scoliosis, Morvan's acrodystrophy of the hands, a *main succulente* or a Charcot joint.

Neurological signs About 75% of cases had classical syringomyelia with features of a central cord syndrome. The dissociated anaesthesia can be unilateral or bilateral, usually in a "cape", "*cuirasse*" or "suspended" distribution affecting the cervical and dorsal segments. Sensory loss which does not respect the conventional dermatomes may lead the unwary to conclude that a functional component is present. Spinothalamic sensory loss only affecting the leg caused by involvement of sensory long tracts rather than crossing fibres may be seen. Loss of all modalities of sensation in an arm due to root entry zone disease are also recognized to occur. Dissociated sensory loss involving the head and tending to spare the snout regions are a later feature. Somewhat surprisingly, in both series, joint position sense was found to be commonly impaired in both arms and legs. Barnett attributes this to cervical cord compression or upward extension of the syrinx whilst Logue found that proprioceptive loss in the hips is commoner than distal joint loss. This interesting observation is deserving of further study.

As for the sensory changes, lower motor neurone features in the upper limbs are a rule which is frequently broken with either preserved reflexes or frank upper motor neurone changes in the arms. Nine of Logue's 75 patients had complete preservation of upper limb reflexes. Normally the first dorsal segment of the spinal cord is involved early in the disease process producing intrinsic hand muscle wasting and a claw hand. Unless a lumbar syrinx is present, only upper motor neurone signs are found in the legs with a substantial number having no lower limb abnormality. Rarely, a patient may present with lower motor neurone features in the leg. Bladder, bowel and sexual dysfunction occur relatively late in most cases.

Roughly 25% of patients in these two series had symptoms attributable to brain stem involvement. What proportion of these features are truly due to syringobulbia rather than brain stem and lower cranial nerve distortion secondary to the Chiari malformation is another issue which should be resolvable in the future by MRI.

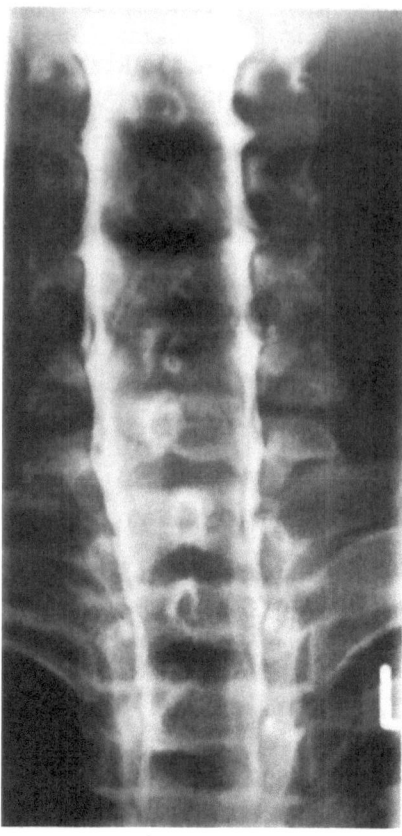

Fig. 16.5. Myelogram demonstrating enlarged cervical spinal cord containing a syrinx. (Radiograph by courtesy of Professor I. Isherwood.)

In general the oculomotor disorders seen in syringomyelia are due to a coexistent Chiari malformation and have already been described. the series of both Logue and Barnett mention nystagmus, commonly rotary or vertical in their patients. Clearly true syringopontis might produce a wide range of disorders of gaze but clear correlation of pathology with clinical signs is difficult to obtain. A unilateral Horner's syndrome is not uncommon and usually occurs in association with T1 lower motor neurone signs.

Differential Diagnosis

The patient presenting with a classical central cord syndrome, with or without features of the Chiari malformation, does not usually present much problem to the clinician. The real difficulty here lies with the radiologist who has to differentiate a communicating syrinx from intramedullary tumour, syrinx related to local arachnoiditis or that seen after spinal cord trauma.

Just as the Chiari malformation may present in subtle and insidious ways, so the diagnosis of syringomyelia can be difficult in the early stages. Pain is an early symptom and if unaccompanied by other complaints or definite signs, may be dismissed. Lower motor neurone signs in the arms with atypical sensory signs and a spastic paraparesis may be mistaken for cervical spondylosis in the elderly and multiple sclerosis in the young. Amyotrophy with complete absence of sensory changes can lead to the diagnosis of motor neuron disease being entertained.

Imaging

A full review of imaging of syringomyelia is beyond the scope of this article. The field is rapidly changing and the plethora of papers appearing in the radiological journals is testimony to this. Water-soluble contrast myelography in the supine position will usually demonstrate a Chiari malformation (Fig. 16.1) and sometimes a spinal cord of increased diameter (Fig. 16.5). CT of the spinal cord after myelography will often demonstrate the accumulation of contrast in the syrinx cavity, though there is debate about how it gets there. This is often best seen with delayed CT. There is however no doubt that MRI is the investigation of choice on grounds of image quality and the non-invasive nature of the procedure (Fig. 16.2). Patients suspected of syringomyelia should be referred to an appropriately equipped centre. Unfortunately a few patients are quite unable to tolerate the procedure because of the claustrophobia which is induced by the confined space within the scanner. The presence of aneurysm clips or cardiac pacemakers are also contraindications. MRI produces sagittal images which demonstrate the longitudinal extent of syrinx cavities and the degree of hindbrain or cerebellar herniation. A correlation of syrinx size with clinical features has not been demonstrated (Grant et al. 1987b). The presence of severe degrees of scoliosis may make it difficult to obtain these images. T1-weighted or proton density images provide the best anatomical demonstration of disordered anatomy (Sherman et al. 1986). The advent of gadolinium-DTPA as an intravenous contrast agent may contribute to the recognition of arachnoiditis and help in the differentiation of communicating syringomyelia from cavities related to intramedullary tumours.

Surgical Management of Syringomyelia

A variety of surgical procedures to treat syringomyelia have evolved over many years (Matsumoto, 1989). These developed in response to neuroanatomical abnormalities such as hindbrain hernia, to unproven hypotheses such as the persistence of an embryonic connection between the fourth ventricle through the obex to a preserved central spinal canal, or simply as a means of draining the fluid-filled cavity in the spinal cord. The origin and progression of syringomyelia has proved extremely difficult to investigate, but more recently the use of differential CSF pressure monitoring (Williams 1981) and in particular the use of phase-contrast magnetic resonance (MR) imaging with intraoperative ultrasound (Oldfield et al. 1994) have produced a relatively simple and acceptable pathogenetic mechanism to explain syringomyelia.

The commonest neuroanatomical abnormality associated with syringmyelia is herniation of the cerebellar tonsils below the foramen magnum. With the increasing use of MR scanning this has been revealed as a much more common abnormality than was first thought to be the case. However, there are degrees of herniation and it is probable that only the more severe instances of tonsillar displacement, perhaps together with the actual diameter of the foramen magnum result in formation of a syrinx. Oldfield et al. used phase-contrast and phase-contrast cine MR imaging with intraoperative ultrasound to examine the flow of cerebrospinal fluid within the intracranial compartment, at the foramen magnum and within the spinal cord of patients with syringomyelia. They discovered a pulsatile CSF flow mechanism such that during cardiac systole when the brain became filled with blood, a pressure wave was transmitted to the intracranial CSF. This wave failed to egress through the foramen magnum which was blocked by the herniated tonsils which instead acted as a piston transmitting the pressure wave to the spinal cord. During cardiac systole they noted caudad movement of spinal CSF and also fluid within the syrinx. During cardiac diastole they noted craniad movement of spinal CSF and syrinx fluid. Thus there is a frequent compressive force transmitted to the upper part of the spinal cord causing upward and downward flow of fluid inside and outwith the spinal cord. To some extent this complements Williams' hypothesis concerning "suck and slosh" in that gravity and posture probably also have a significant influence in the upward and downward enlargement and elongation of a syrinx. This feature was recognized many years ago when the diagnosis of syringomyelia was made using myelography with the patient in alternate head-up and head-down positions.

It is known that the perivascular spaces of a spinal cord with syringomyelia are enlarged and there is good evidence using markers and isotope labelled proteins that this is the mechanism for the movement of fluid from the spinal CSF compartment to the interior of the spinal cord (Lee Olszewski 1960; Ikata et al. 1988). There is little evidence from MR studies that an anatomical communication persists between the floor of the fourth ventricle and the syrinx, although this is seen occasionally. The hypothesis which led to surgical plugging of the obex is no longer tenable and there is no clinical evidence that it is a useful exercise.

The development of syringomyelia following spinal cord injury or in relation to arachnoiditis, however caused, is less clear but the same hypothesis of turbulent or pulsatile CSF movement outside the spinal cord can be applied providing to some extent a unified hypothesis for the pathogenesis and progression of a syrinx.

Surgical treatment can be classified into definitive procedures to neutralize the abnormality which is generating the syrinx or into secondary procedures which largely comprise various forms of syrinx drainage. Relatively few patients with cerebellar herniation, which is by far the commonest associated neuroanatomical abnormality, also have ventricular enlargement. This hydrocephalus may in itself be the source of neurological dysfunction as well as being a secondary effect of the foramen magnum compression and constriction. If hydrocephalus is present most authorities recommend the use of a ventriculoperitoneal CSF diversion system as the initial form of surgical treatment. In some cases this may bring about a resolution or diminution of the syringomyelia which is easily evaluated in the postoperative period using MR imaging. The original approach by Gardner to decompress the foramen magnum posteriorly remains the mainstay of surgical treatment and is highly successful in producing reduction in size of the syrinx. The purpose of the foramen magnum decompression can now be considered as relief of the pulsatile pressure mechanism on the upper spinal cord and spinal CSF.

A foramen magnum decompression is carried out with the patient in the prone position and the cervical spine in neutral alignment or very slight flexion. A midline incision is made between the inion and the C3 or C4 spinal process. Dissection is carried out through the midline to expose the suboccipital bone and the posterior arches of C1 and C2. Occasionally the tonsillar herniation will extend below C2 and the dissection is extended accordingly. Muscle dissection is carried out using standard techniques including fine-point needle diathermy in the occipital region, almost as far as the foramen magnum. The muscles are then dissected off the C2 neural arch leaving the muscle tissue over the C1 arch and foramen magnum for final dissection. Vertebral abnormalities are sometimes encountered in this region such as an assimilated or partially assimilated atlas vertebra or a spina bifida of the C1 arch. Such abnormalities should be anticipated and appropriate care taken with dissection. Location of the posterior spinous process of C1 can be achieved using a blunt probe and the muscle dissection carried out bilaterally from this starting point. Care should be taken not to rupture the posterior atlanto-occipital membrane through unguarded use of cutting diathermy. In this context it is often helpful and wise to leave a small layer of muscle or fascial tissue between the membrane and the dissecting instrument in the lateral recesses of the dissection, which should be carried out laterally as far as the posterior aspect of the lateral mass of C1. At this point usually some venous bleeding from the plexus around the vertebral artery is encountered. This is difficult to stop using conventional or bipolar diathermy, but is easily controlled using a small haemostatic pack with gentle pressure for a few minutes.

A posterior suboccipital craniectomy is carried out. The conventional method using a craniotome is to create two suboccipital burrholes which are joined and extended using bone-removing punches or a high-speed drill. The craniectomy is extended laterally and downwards to the posterior rim of the foramen magnum which is much thicker than the squamous suboccipital bone. Careful extradural dissection is needed at this stage and the posterior rim is removed to the lateral surface of the dura on each side. The posterior arch of C1 and if necessary C2 is also removed bilaterally.

The purpose of the operation is to alter CSF flow and for this reason the dura must be opened. The dura at the level of the foramen magnum is often considerably thicker than normal and to some extent may act itself as a constrictive agent. It is at this level that the twin layers of the cranial dura blend into the single layer of the spinal dura. The dura can be opened in a "Y" shape with the vertical extension taken at least 1 cm below the lowest point of the cerebellar tonsils. The arachnoid layer does not require to be opened. At this stage the dura can be sutured back to surrounding tissues and left open, with the muscles closed in multiple layers above this. An alternative is to create a duroplasty by suturing in a suitably tailored gusset of fascia lata or synthetic dural material.

In the postoperative period the complication rate is relatively low. Some patients will suffer from low pressure headaches as a result of the newly altered CSF flow characteristics. These are self-resolving, usually within the first seven days after surgery. Of course it is not always possible to carry out the duroplasty or dural opening without a tear in the arachnoid layer. This may lead to leakage of CSF into the muscle layers which will form a pseudomeningocele. On one occasion when this procedure was carried out a tension pseudomeningocele formed causing a temporary quadriparesis six days after the operation. Re-exploration was carried out as an emergency. The dural substitute was still in place but did not form a watertight seal and was removed. The wound was closed and the quadriparesis resolved completely. If the arachnoid integrity can be maintained this is probably the optimal situation. Should a leak occur, however, the possibility of a one-way flow of CSF forming a significant pseudomeningocele exists and it may be that a large opening in the arachnoid is a safer proposition than a small leak.

The follow-up for a patient having this surgery is by MR imaging usually several weeks or a small number of months later and this investigation is often rewarded by substantial reduction in size of the syrinx, usually but not invariably, associated with cessation in the progress of neurological symptoms or even an improvement.

The incidence of post-traumatic syringmyelia is usually quoted in the region of 3% of patients with spinal cord injury. With the increases in MR scanning it is likely that this incidence will also increase, although only a fraction of cases of post-traumatic syringomyelia are clinically significant. Until relatively recently the most common surgical option has been to employ a direct drainage procedure from the syrinx into the subarachnoid space, the pleural cavity or the peritoneal cavity. However, applying the hypothesis quoted earlier concerning turbulent flow of CSF at the site of trauma due to the development of arachnoid adhesions, the definitive surgical solution might well be to carry out a laminectomy and an arachnoid dissection to eliminate the turbulent CSF flow. Sgouros and Williams (1995) have produced data which confirm the advantage of laminectomy alone over drainage procedures. The same argument should apply to cases of arachnoiditis due to a variety of other causes such as infection, haemorrhage or tumour.

In practice there is a small number of cases where there is no definitive neuroanatomical abnormality nor any evidence of arachnoiditis and also some cases in whom adequate decompression of the foramen magnum fails to achieve decompression of the syrinx. It is to this group of patients that the second-line procedure of direct syrinx drainage should be first applied. The main options are syringopleural or syringosubarachnoid shunting. Sgouros and Williams (1995) have shown relatively little difference between the effectiveness or either type of CSF diversion. The problem with all shunting devices and systems is that the tubing may become dislodged, obstructed or non-functional due to initial collapse of the syrinx. It may even excite an extramedullary arachnoid reaction and in effect be counterproductive. For both types of shunt, approximately 50% of devices continue to function after 10 years with the greatest number of failures occurring within the first 12 months.

Spinal cord transection, myelotomy, terminal ventriculostomy and the insertion of "wicks" into the syrinx have all been tried in the past and are associated with poor results (Sgouros and William 1995).

Conclusion

This brief chapter has attempted to identify a number of different clinical strands in a rather complex web of disorders. The central feature is a malformation at the foramen magnum producing a fascinating variety of effects which remain ill-understood and partly because of that lack of understanding, are difficult to manage. Fig. 16.6 is an attempt to illustrate some of the factors which may be important in the development of the clinical syndromes described. The relative importance of genetic, developmental and acquired factors is likely to remain unclear for some time and the challenge for treatment probably lies in the detection of people at risk for syrinx development and a better understanding of the pathophysiology involved, the hope being that early and appropriate intervention will help prevent the awful decline that was previously the lot of the patient with syringomyelia.

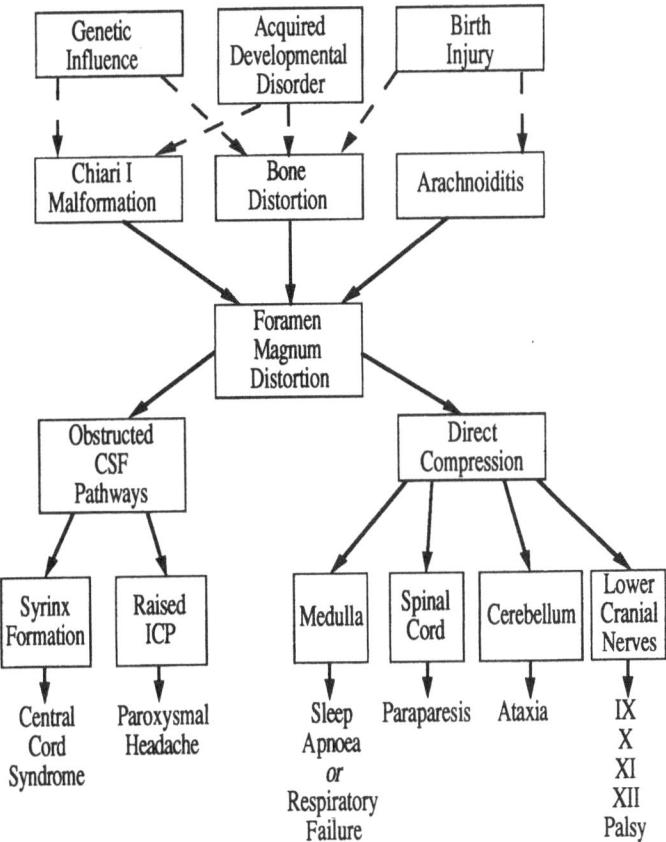

Fig. 16.6. A diagrammatic representation of some of the potential interreacting factors in the production of foramen syndromes.

Acknowledgements We are grateful to Professor Ian Isherwood of the Department of Diagnostic Radiology at Manchester University for the radiological illustrations. Drs. Ian Bone and Donald Hadley reviewed the manuscript and provided much helpful comment. Any errors are our own.

References

Aboulezz AO, Sartor K, Geyer CA, Gado MH (1985) Position of cerebellar tonsils in the normal population and in patients with the Chiari malformation: a quantitative approach with MR imaging. J Comput Assist Tomogr 9(6):1033–1036

Appleby A, Foster JB, Hankinson J, Hudgson P (1968) The diagnosis and management of the Chiari anomalies in adult life. Brain 91:131–140

Arnold J (1894) Myelocyste, Transposition von Gewebskeimen und Sympodie. Beitr Path Anat 16:1

Baker HL (1963) Myelographic examination of the posterior fossa with a positive contrast medium. Radiology 81:791

Balk RA, Hiller FC, Lucas EA, Scrima L, Wilson FJ, Wooten V (1985) Sleep apnoea and the Arnold-Chiari malformation. Am Rev Respir Dis 132(4):929–930

Ball MJ, Dayan AD (1972) Pathogenesis of syringomyelia. Lancet 2:799

Banerji NK, Millar JHD (1974) Chiari malformation presenting in adult life – its relationship to syringomyelia. Brain 97:157–168

Barkovich AJ, Wippold FJ, Sherman JL, Citrin CM (1986) Significance of cerebellar tonsillar position on MR. AJNR 7:795–799

Barkovich AJ, Bent OK, Norman D, Edwards MS (1989) Revised classification of posterior fossa cysts and cystlike malformations based on the results of multiplanar MR imaging. AJNR 10:977–988

Barnett HJM, Foster JB, Hudgson P (1973) Syringomyelia. Saunders, London

Battersby RDE, Williams B (1982) Birth injury: a possible contributory factor in the aetiology of primary basilar impression. J Neurol Neurosurg Psychiatry 45:879–883

Bosley TM, Cohen DA, Schatz NJ, et al. (1985) Comparison of metrizamide computed tomography and magnetic resonance imaging in the evaluation of lesions at the cervicomedullary junction. Neurology 35:485–492

Brown JR (1977) The Dandy-Walker syndrome. In: Vinken PJ, Bruyn GW (eds) Handbook of clinical neurology vol 30. Elsevier/North-Holland, Amsterdam, pp 623–646

Bullock R, Todd NV, Easton J, Hadley D (1988) Isolated central respiratory failure due to syringomyelia and Arnold-Chiari malformation. Br Med J 297:1448–1449

Chiari H (1891) Über Veränderungen des Kleinhirns infolge Hydrocephalie des Grosshirns. Dtsch Med Wschr 17:1172–1175

Chiari H (1896) Über Veränderungen des Kleinhirns, des Pons und Medulla oblongata infolge von kongenitaler Hydrocephalie des Grosshirns. Denkschr Akad Wiss Wien 63:71

Cleland J (1883) Contribution to the study of spina bifida, encephalocoele and anencephalus. J Anat Physiol 17:257

Cogan DG (1968) Downbeating nystagmus. Arch Ophthalmol 80:757

Conway LW (1967) Hydrodynamic studies in syringomyelia. J Neurosurg 27:501–514

Coria F, Quintana F, Rebollo M, Combarros O, Berciano J (1983) Occipital dysplasia and Chiari type I deformity in a family. Clinical and radiological study of three generations. J Neurol Sci 62: 147–158

Dandy WE, Blackfan KD (1914) Internal hydrocephalus: an experimental, clinical and pathological study. Amer J Dis Child 8:406–482

De Barros MC, Farias W, Ataide L, Lins S (1968) Basilar impression and Arnold Chiari malformation. J Neurol Neurosurg Psychiatry 31:596–605

Foster JB, Hudgson P (1973) The pathogenesis of communicating syringomyelia. In: Barnett HJM, Foster JB, Hudgson P (eds) Syringomyelia. Saunders, London, pp 104–123

Gardner WJ (1965) Hydrodynamic mechanisms of syringomyelia: its relationship to myelocele. J Neurol Neurosurg Psychiatry 28:247–256

Gardner WJ (1967) Myelocele: rupture of the neural tube? Clin Neurosurg 15:57

Gardner WJ (1973) The Dandy Walker malformation. The dysraphic states from syringomyelia to anencephaly. Excerpta Medica, Amsterdam, pp 127–143

Gardner WJ, Smith JL, Padget DH (1972) The relationship of Arnold-Chiari and Dandy-Walker malformations. J Neurosurg 36:481–486

Gilbert JN, Jones KL, Rorke LB, Chernoff GF, James HE (1986) Central nervous system anomalies associated with meningomyelocoele, hydrocephalus and the Arnold-Chiari malformation: reappraisal of theories regarding the pathogenesis of posterior neural tube closure defects. Neurosurgery 18(5):559–564

Grant R, Hadley DM, Lang D, et al. (1987a) MRI measurement of syrinx size before and after operation. J Neurol Neurosurg Psychiatry 50:1685–1687

Grant R, Hadley DM, Macpherson P, et al. (1987b) Syringomyelia: cyst measurement by magnetic resonance imaging and comparison with symptoms, signs and disability. J Neurol Neurosurg Psychiatry 50:1008–1014

Hampton F, Williams B, Loizou LA (1982) Syncope as a presenting feature of hindbrain herniation with syringomyelia. J Neurol Neurosurg Psychiatry 45:919–922

Ikata T, Masaki A, Kashiwaguchi S (1988) Clinical and experimental studies on permeability of tracers in normal spinal cord and syringomyelia. Spine 13:737–741

Lee JC, Olszewski J (1960) Penetration of radioactive bovine albumen from cerebrospinal fluid into brain tissue. Neurology 10:814–822

Leigh JR, Zee DS (1983) Diagnosis of central disorders of ocular motility. The neurology of eye movement. Davis, Philadelphia, pp 216–217

Marin-Padilla M, Marin-Padilla TM (1981) Morphogenesis of experimentally induced Arnold-Chiari malformation. J Neurol Sci 50:29–55

Matsumoto T, Symon L (1989) Surgical management of syringomyelia – current results. Surg Neurol 32:258–265

McManus D, Bartlett P (1986) The role of nuclear magnetic resonance imaging in the diagnosis of the Arnold Chiari malformation. Radiography 52:275–80

McRae DL (1953) Bony abnormalities in the region of the foramen magnum: correlation of the anatomic and neurological findings. Acta Radiol [Stockh] 40:335–354

Mohr PD, Strang FA, Sambrook M, Boddie HG (1977) The clinical and surgical features of 40 patients with primary cerebellar ectopia (adult Chiari malformation). Quart J Med 181:85–96

Moreton RD (1943) Basilar invagination: so-called platybasia. Proc Mayo Clin 18:353

Newman PK, Terenty TR, Foster JB (1981) Some observations on the pathogenesis of syringomyelia. J Neurol Neurosurg Psychiatry 44:964–969

Nightingale S, Williams B (1987) Hindbrain hernia headache. Lancet 1:731–734

Oldfield EH, Muraszko K, Shawker TH, Patronas NJ (1994) Pathophysiology of syringomyelia associated with Chiari I malformation of the cerebellar tonsils. J Neurosurg 80:3–15

Paul KS, Lye RH, Strang FA, Dutton J (1983) Arnold Chiari malformation – review of 71 cases. J Neurosurg 58:183–187

Roth M (1986) Cranio-cervical growth collision: another explanation of the Arnold-Chiari malformation and of basilar impression. Neuroradiology 28:187–194

Saez RJ, Onofrio BM, Yangihara T (1976) Experience with Arnold-Chiari malformation 1960–1970. J Neurosurg 45:416–422

Salam MZ, Adams RD (1978) The Arnold-Chiari malformation. In: Vinken PJ, Bruyn GW (eds) Handbook of clinical neurology vol 32. Elsevier/North-Holland, Amsterdam, pp 99–110

Schady W, Metcalfe RA, Butler P (1987) The incidence of craniocervical bony anomalies in the adult Chiari malformation. J Neurol Sci 82:193–203

Schliep G (1978) Syringomyelia and syringobulbia. In: Vinken PJ, Bruyn GW (eds) Handbook of clinical neurology vol 32. Elsevier/North-Holland, Amsterdam, pp 255–327

Schmidt H, Sartor K, Heckl RW (1978) Bone malformations of the craniocervical region. In: Vinken PJ, Bruyn GW (eds) Handbook of clinical neurology vol 32. Elsevier/North-Holland, Amsterdam, pp 1–98

Sgouros S, Williams B (1995) A critical appraisal of drainage in syringomyelia. J Neurosurg 82:1–10

Sherman JL, Barkovich AJ, Citrin CM (1986) The MR appearances of syringomyelia: new observations. AJNR 7:985–995

Spillane JD, Pallis C, Jones AM (1957) Developmental abnormalities in the region of the foramen magnum. Brain 80:11

Taggert JK, Walker AE (1942) Congenital atresia of the foramens of Luschka and Magendie. Arch Neurol Psychiatry (Chic) 48:583–612

Van Calenbergh F, van Denburgh R (1993) Syringo-peritoneal shunting: results and problems in a consecutive series. Acta Neurochir 123:203–205

Wilkinson M (1978) The Klippel-Feil syndrome. In: Vinken PJ, Bruyn GW (eds) Handbook of clinical neurology vol 32. Elsevier/North-Holland, Amsterdam, pp 111–122

Williams B (1969) Hypothesis: the distending force in the production of "communicating syringomyelia". Lancet 2:189

Williams B (1970) Current concepts of syringomyelia. Br J Hosp Med 4:331

Williams B (1972) Combined cisternal and lumbar pressure recordings in the sitting position using differential manometry. J Neurol Neurosurg Psychiatry 35:142

Willams B (1977) Difficult labour as a cause of communicating syringomyelia. Lancet 2:51–53

Williams B (1981) Simultaneous cerebral and spinal fluid pressure recordings. 2. Cerebrospinal dissociation with lesions at the foramen magnum post-op. Acta Neurochir 59:123–142

Wolpert SM, Scott RM, Platenberg C, Runge VM (1988) The clinical significance of hindbrain herniation and deformity as shown on MR images of patients with Chiari II malformation. AJNR 9(6):1075–1080

Zimmerman CF, Roach ES, Troost BT (1986) See-saw nystagmus associated with the Chiari malformation. Arch Neurol 43(3):299–300

Chapter 17

Rheumatoid Arthritis of the Cervical Spine

M. Dvorak and R.W. McGraw

Introduction

Rheumatoid arthritis (RA) is an inflammatory arthritis that causes destruction of the joint capsules, ligaments, and supporting bones. It is primarily due to a synovitis that affects all the synovial joints, including the more than 30 separate joints in the cervical spine.

There has not been consistent agreement about the screening of rheumatoid patients with cervical involvement, their prognosis given non-operative treatment, or the indications and outcome of surgical treatment. With a clear understanding of the clinical anatomy, pathology, and the results of various forms of treatment, clinicians can make informed decisions about the management of these often complex patients.

Pathoanatomy and Neuroanatomy

The pathology of RA in the cervical spine involves an inflammatory synovitis with lymphocyte infiltration in the acute phase. Ligaments and joints are damaged and slowly destroyed by a proliferative synovitis that degrades hyaline cartilage; erodes and necroses subchondral bone; and weakens, infiltrates, and disrupts supporting ligaments.

The inflammatory rheumatoid process may lead to destruction of the transverse atlantal ligament and other supporting ligaments at C1-2, eventually causing atlantoaxial subluxation (AAS). If the rheumatoid process begins to destroy the supporting subchondral bone of the C1 lateral masses, it may cause rotatory subluxation, lateral subluxation and eventually vertical migration of the odontoid (VMO), depending on the pattern of erosion and its symmetry. In the subaxial spine, i.e. from C3 to C7, destruction of the facet joint capsules, facet articular cartilage and subchondral bone, uncovertebral joints of Luschka and supporting ligaments may lead to subaxial subluxation (SAS). These three forms of subluxation lead to different clinical presentations, each with its own natural history.

The neuroanatomy and clinical neuropathology has been reviewed by Zeidman and Ducker (1994). The amount of space required by neural structures in the cervical spine is estimated to be greater than 14 mm at C1–2 and at least 12–13 mm in the subaxial spine. The transverse diameter of the cervical spinal cord is normally 17 mm, but the transverse dimension of the spinal canal is rarely affected by this disease process. Decrease in the required space may be due to bony encroachment secondary to subluxation and altered anatomy or to compression by soft tissue pannus.

Neurological symptoms may occur when any of the following structures are compressed.

C2 Posterior Primary Ramus

The dorsal ramus of C2, also known as the greater occipital nerve, exits under the C1 posterior arch. Compression or irritation of this nerve may result in numbness or pain in the occipital region.

V Cranial Nerve

The spinal ganglion of the trigeminal nerve, which extends within the spinal cord to the level of the body of C2, is also at risk with C1–C2 subluxation (Thompson and Meyer 1985). Irritation of the spinal ganglion most commonly results in numbness in the sensory distribution of the first division of the trigeminal nerve and an absent corneal reflex.

Corticospinal Tracts

Severe cord compression at C1–2 may result in a cruciate type of paralysis as described by Bell (1970). This may affect the decussation of the pyramidal tracts leading to profound proximal upper extremity weakness. Dysfunction of the lower cranial nerves leading to difficulty swallowing, absent gag reflex and weakness in the tongue and sternocleidomastoid and trapezius muscles are concomitant effects in Bell's paralysis.

Cord compression at C1–2 may eventually progress to a profound central cord syndrome of incomplete quadriplegia and finally to complete respirator dependent pentaplegia. The sacral fibres of the corticospinal tract may also be affected which may lead to a neurogenic bowel and bladder, initially atonic, and later spastic.

Dorsal Columns and Spinothalamic Tracts

The primary afferent sensory pathways include the dorsal columns and anterior and lateral spinothalmic tracts. Initially, irritation or compression of these tracts may result in subtle symptoms including local neck pain, impaired vibration sense in the feet, and numb and clumsy hands, a syndrome described by Chang et al. (1992). Who postulated that this clumsy hand syndrome was due to lesions identified in the cuneate funiculus.

Pathological Changes in the Compressed Spinal Cord

Chronic mechanical compression of the spinal cord in the rheumatoid cervical spine has been shown, in a postmortem analysis (Delamarter and Bohlman 1994), to produce flattening of the spinal cord, thickening of the dural sac, scarring and gliosis. In the severely compressed spinal cord, axonal degeneration, atrophy, and necrosis can be seen. Vascular compromise, characterized by ischaemic changes in the central part of the spinal cord, can be seen in patients with less severe mechanical compression. Delamarter and Bohlman (1994) noted that, in two patients with severe myelopathy, no histopathological abnormality could be identified. They postulated a concussion of the spinal cord as the probable aetiology of the severe neurological deficit.

Compression of the upper cervical spinal cord as a result of rheumatoid VMO has been reported to cause syringomyelia (Tumiati and Casoli 1991).

Clinical Presentation

Up to 88% of patients with rheumatoid arthritis complain of some neck pain. The pain is most commonly occipital but may have a pattern of local referred pain. Patients may complain of numbness in the back of the head (related to greater occipital nerve compression) or numbness in the face (related to trigeminal nerve compression). Previous injury to the nerves from halo pins and surgical exposures may also be responsible for paraesthesia in the distribution of the greater occipital nerve. Patients may report subjective sensations of instability or "clunking". The most subtle neurological symptom, and often an early symptom, is a sensation of subjective weakness or clumsiness in the hands with paraesthesia in the hands and/or feet.

In patients with RA, symptoms of pain or neurological dysfunction are often overlooked in the presence of what is frequently severe peripheral disease. Gait disturbances and weakness in the hands as well as urinary dysfunction may be attributed by the clinician to the effects of peripheral arthritis or other medical problems. Numbness and tingling may often be confused with peripheral neuropathy and peripheral nerve entrapment syndromes (i.e. carpal tunnel syndrome) which are also common in rheumatoid arthritis.

Some factors known to correlate with rheumatoid cervical involvement include: peripheral erosive disease (especially progressive peripheral periarticular erosions), corticosteroid therapy, seropositive disease, subcutaneous nodules, and the presence of mutilating peripheral articular disease (Agarwal et al. 1993). Progression of disease in the metaearpal-phalangeal joints and carpal bones has also been correlated with disease activity in the cervical spine.

Clinical Symptoms and Signs

In patients with RA, range of motion of the cervical spine may be limited by pain. The clinician must be alert for presence of Lhermittes sign at the extremes of flexion.

The cranial nerves must be examined with specific care and attention to involvement in the distribution of the 5th cranial nerve as well as the lower cranial nerves (IX to XII).

Since motor testing is difficult and unreliable, a careful and precise sensory examination is mandatory. Pain and temperature sensation (lateral spinothalamic tracts), as well as joint position sense and vibration (posterior or dorsal columns) are all at risk of being affected. Peripheral nerve entrapment syndromes and peripheral neuropathy are not unusual in rheumatoid patients. Electrodiagnostic evaluation is often necessary to differentiate between these diagnoses and spinal cord involvement. Great diligence is also required for the examination of the perineum where symptoms of perineal numbness or loss of voluntary or resting tone of the anal sphincter may suggest neurological involvement.

Evaluation of reflexes is rarely hampered by severe peripheral disease. The presence of increased tone, combined with brisk reflexes in the presence of a normal jaw jerk reflex is highly suggestive of upper motor neurone involvement at the C1–C2 level. Absence of superficial reflexes such as the cremasteric and abdominal reflexes may also suggest corticospinal long-tract involvement. Evaluation of the plantar response and Hoffman reflex may help to identify dysfunction of the descending corticospinal tract.

Finally, gait must be evaluated for ataxia, and the Rhomberg sign tested, in the knowledge that it is often difficult to differentiate gait disturbances caused by the effects of peripheral arthritis from those caused by neurological involvement.

Ranawat's neurological function classification (Ranawat et al. 1979) has been found to be useful in clinical evaluation as well as in determining treatment and predicting neurological outcome (Boden et al. 1993). This classification uses three major categories:

Class 1 – normal
Class 2 – subjective weakness, hyper-reflexia, paraesthesia
Class 3 – objective weakness with long tract signs
      (a) Ambulatory
      (b) Non-ambulatory

Diagnostic Modalities

Conventional Radiographs

The radiographic views that are most useful in this group are an open mouth view, used to visualize the odontoid and lateral masses; and lateral neutral, flexion and extension views. Oblique views are rarely useful. Radiographic evidence of instability in the cervical spine has been reported in up to 86% of all rheumatoid arthritis patients (Pellicci et al. 1981). Subluxation may occur at C1–C2 (AAS) or in the subaxial spine (C3–7) (SAS), or erosion of the C1 lateral masses in association with AAS may eventually lead to vertical migration of the odontoid.

Atlanto Axial Subluxation

The most common radiographic measure of AAS if the atlantodental interval (ADI) which is normally less than 3 mm in adults. An ADI greater than 3.5 mm is likely abnormal and subluxation greater than 10–12 mm is indicative of destruction of not only the transverse ligament but the alar and apical ligaments (Fielding et al. 1974). A more recently developed measure (Boden et al. 1993) is the posterior atlantodental interval (PADI) which is measured from the posterior wall of the dens to the anterior aspect of the C1 lamina. The sensitivity (97%) and negative predictive value (94%) for PADI in predicting development of paralysis make it an ideal measurement for screening purposes (Fig. 17.1).

Subaxial Subluxation

Plain radiographs (particularly flexion/extension lateral views) may help predict myelopathy in the presence of SAS. Any degree of measurable forward subluxation of one vertebra on its more caudal neighbour is significant and can lead to progressive subluxation and myelopathy.

Vertical Migration of the Odontoid

VMO is often difficult to diagnose from plain radiographs. This difficulty is highlighted by the plethora of radiographic measurements proposed to diagnose VMO. Difficulty in visualizing key landmarks, such as the margins of the foramen

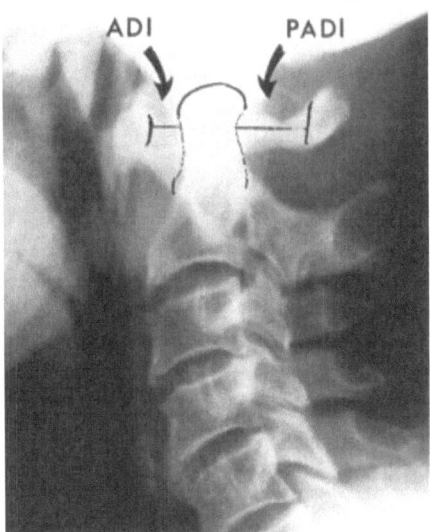

Fig. 17.1. Lateral radiograph showing atlantodental interval (ADI) and posterior atlantodental interval (PADI).

magnum, the hard palate, the pedicle of C2, and particularly the tip of the odontoid, makes many of these measurement techniques impractical. Furthermore, depending on which method is used, the same patient may or may not meet the diagnostic criteria. We have found it most useful to compare the same measurement on serial plain radiographs.

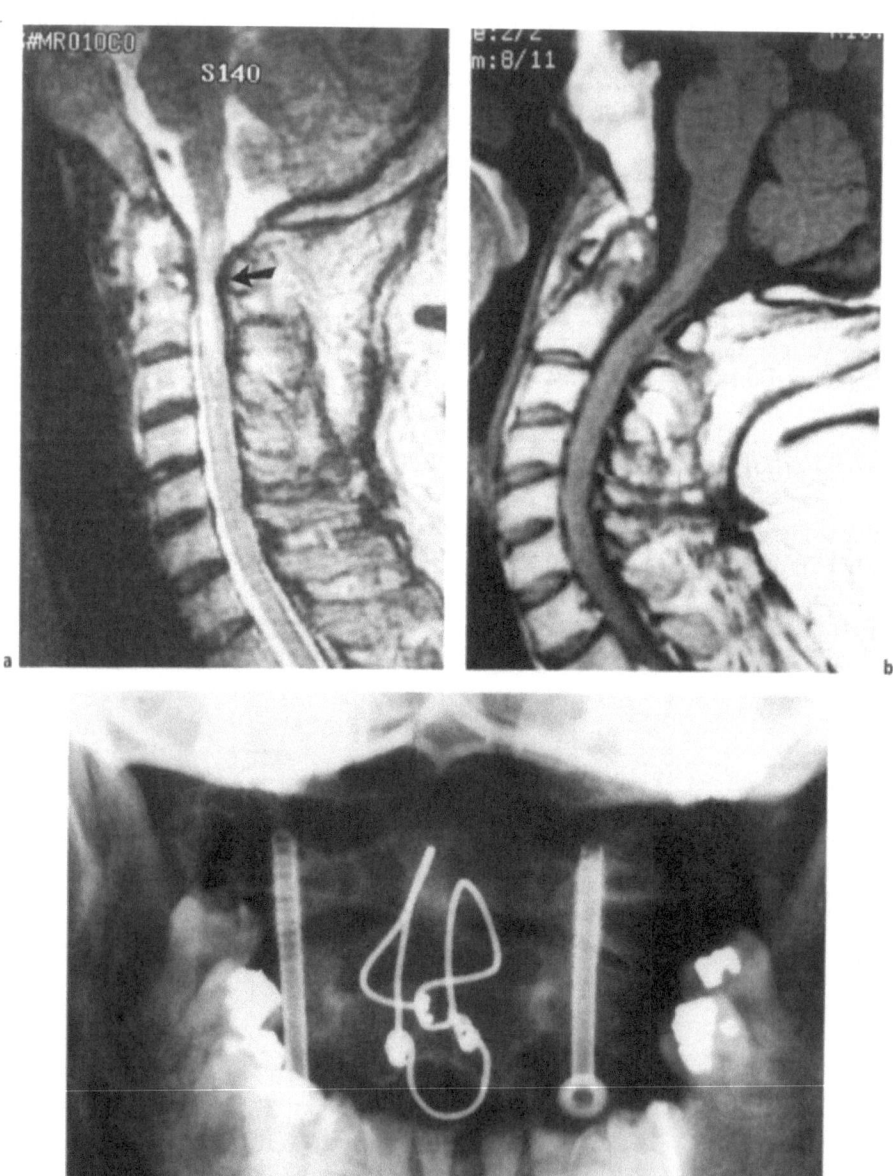

Fig. 17.2. A 35-year-old patient with chronic central cord syndrome and quadriparesis. Flexion MRI (**a**) clearly identifies neural compression (*arrow*) and extension MRI (**b**) reveals adequate decompression. Postoperative open mouth view (**c**) and lateral (**d**) plain radiographs show transarticular screw fixation of C1–C2.

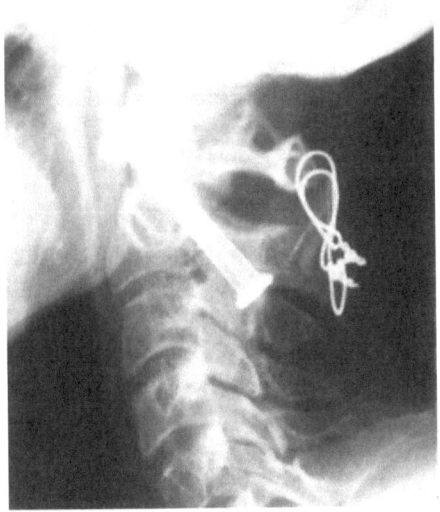

Fig. 17.2. *(Continued)*

A particularly ominous finding is a decrease in ADI in the neutral position on serial measurement. This change, which might be interpreted as "improvement", actually indicates that the C1 arch is settling into a more caudal position relative to C2, an early sign of VMO (Rana 1989).

CT Scan, Tomography and Magnetic Resonance Imaging (MRI)

Braunstein et al. (1984) suggest that CT scanning is particularly affective in identifying cord compression when clinical myelopathy is being investigated. Intrathecally enhanced CT scanning has essentially been replaced by MRI. Lateral tomography may provide enhanced bone detail, but it is the author's impression that modern CT scanning with sagittal or coronal reformatting, provides as good bone detail as tomography, which we rarely perform today (see Fig. 17.3b).

MRI has vastly improved our ability to image both the spinal cord and adjacent structures that may be compressing it. Compression and physical distortion of the spinal cord as seen on MRI have been shown to be associated with clinical myelopathy (Breedveld et al. 1987). MRI scans performed in flexion have been reported to provide more information than similar scans performed with the patient's cervical spine in neutral alignment (Roca et al. 1993): cord compression, angulation and distortion are evident on flexion MRI scans although they may not be apparent in neutral studies.

In one study of flexion MRI scanning and motor-evoked potential monitoring, spinal cord diameter was measured directly and in all patients with myelopathy the spinal cord diameter was less than 6 mm (Dvorak et al. 1989).

The full range of C1–2 instability may not be reproduced on MRI in flexion and extension due to the confines of the magnet. The interpretation of flexion MRI must include evaluation of maximal forward flexion plain films. Despite this limitation, the authors agree that flexion and extension MRI scanning is critical in the presurgical evaluation of many patients (Fig. 17.2).

A cervical medullary angle of less than 135° (normally 135–175°) on MRI imaging is associated with clinical evidence of myelopathy (Bundschuh and Modic 1987). Bundschuh and Modic (1987) also noted that signal change within the spinal cord on serial MRI is correlated with clinical evidence of myelopathy.

Electrodiagnostic testing

Dvorak et al. (1989) showed that even in the absence of clinical evidence of myelopathy there may still be neurophysiological evidence of conduction abnormalities as evidenced by a delay in the central motor latency on motor evoked potential monitoring. As previously mentioned, electrodiagnostic testing including motor evoked potentials, electromyography (EMG) and somatosensory evoked potentials may assist in clarifying a difficult diagnosis.

Treatment Considerations

Natural History

To identify those patients who require surgical treatment and minimize the investigations and screening studies performed on others, a comprehensive knowledge of the natural history is essential. Most studies that claim to describe natural history, in fact, report on non-operative management, as the majority of these patients are prescribed medical treatment for their rheumatoid disease with or without external support for the cervical spine.

Risk of Developing Cervical Subluxation

The prevalence of rheumatoid cervical subluxation in a community-based rheumatoid arthritis population has been reported as: AAS > 4 mm in 33%, VMO in 14% and SAS in 21%. Other authors have identified some form of cervical instability in up to 71% of radiographic surveys (Pellicci et al. 1981). The timing of onset of cervical instability is variable, from about 2 years up to 25 years after diagnosis.

Once present, subluxation progresses in 35%–80% of patients. Mathews (1974) noted that, at 5 year follow-up, 17% of patients with AAS and 33% of patients with VMO had deteriorated radiographically.

About 6%–10% of patients with AAS progress to VMO (Smith et al. 1972; Mathews 1974; Pellicci et al. 1981; Rana 1989).

Risk of Progression of Myelopathy

Pellicci et al. (1981) noted that, at 5-year follow-up, 36% of his patients had deteriorated at least one Ranawat grade (1981) (90% treated conservatively, and 10% surgically).

Weissman et al. (1982) identified risk factors for progression of neurological findings in rheumatoid patients: AAS of greater than 9 mm is highly suggestive of cord compression and neurological compromise; and males and patients with VMO and lateral C1-2 subluxation are more likely to exhibit neurological features. Factors not correlated with cervical cord compression include seropositivity, rheumatoid nodules, age of onset of RA, age of detection of subluxation or disease severity.

Mathews (1974) noted patients with VMO were more likely to develop clinical myelopathy, with up to 50% deteriorating neurologically, compared to the overall rate of 15%.

More recently, Boden et al. (1993) analysed 73 patients with rheumatoid cervical spine involvement with an average follow-up of 7 years. In their patients 57% developed clinical myelopathy. The most sensitive (97%) indicator of paralysis at 7-year follow-up, with a high negative predictive value (94%), was a posterior atlantodental interval (PADI) of less than 14 mm.

Risk of Mortality

In Rana's (1989) review 5% of the patients died and had their death directly attributed to their cervical rheumatoid disease.

Marks and Sharp (1981) reviewed the clinical presentation and outcome of 31 patients with rheumatoid cervical myelopathy. Within 6 months of presentation 15 of these 31 patients were dead. Four other patients died later. All patients who were untreated died; 50% of those patients treated with a cervical collar only died. The only treatment which provided an opportunity for survival was surgical fusion.

Other autopsy studies (Meijers et al. 1974; Delamarter and Bohlman 1994) reveal a rate of up to 10% of fatal medullary brainstem compression in patients with RA who die. Delamarter and Bohlman also noted that spinal cord compression was found to be the cause of death in 10 of 11 patients with myelopathy and RA.

Bracing

Kauppi and Anttila (1995) found a stiff cervical collar restricted the amount of AAS by 30% but was only effective in half of their patients. Patients with an increased atlantoaxial interval in neutral position did not benefit from application of a stiff collar. There is no evidence that external bracing in any way modifies the natural history of atlantoaxial or other cervical instabilities in rheumatoid patients although cervical orthoses are often prescribed (Pellicci et al. 1981).

Summary

Once a patient develops myelopathy, the prognosis is 50% mortality in 6 months if left untreated. Once myelopathy develops it is very likely to progress. Mortality is higher in patients with severe comorbid conditions especially severe extra-articular rheumatoid arthritis and interstitial lung disease.

Therefore, as soon as neurological dysfunction is recognized, surgery should be recommended. Patients who have been identified as being at high risk for developing neurological dysfunction (i.e. those with AAS > 9 mm, PADI < 14 mm, spinal cord sagittal diameter on MRI of less than 6 mm, AP spinal canal < 13 mm in the subaxial spine, cervical medullary angle < 135° or signal change in the cervical cord on serial MRI images) may also be candidates for surgical stabilization. Some of these patients who clinically do not appear to have myelopathy may have subtle findings on neurophysiological testing.

Surgical Treatment Recommendations

General Considerations

Surgical decisions must be made with tremendous care in this patient group. Patients with rheumatoid cervical spine involvement often have other general medical problems related to their systemic rheumatoid disease and its medical treatment. Pulmonary fibrosis as well as medical complications of long-term steroid use are common. These patients often have had extensive previous hospitalizations and multiple surgical procedures, and further surgery is best avoided unless strongly indicated.

Local complications related to treatment of the cervical spine are related to generalized osteoporosis and poor bone quality. This affects the surgical fixation techniques available for stabilization. These patients have friable skin which poorly tolerates pressure. They are less likely to tolerate a standard halo thoracic brace, due both to skin friability and deformities such as increased thoracic kyphosis. Some of the newer designs in light weight halo thoracic vests are better tolerated. Surgical techniques which minimize reliance on postoperative external bracing and immobilization are therefore preferred.

Atlanto Axial Subluxation (AAS)

Indications for surgery in AAS have varied tremendously. Some authors have considered an atlantoaxial interval greater than 6 mm (Papadopoulos 1991) as a strong indication for surgery, while other authors have stated that surgery should be deferred until the AAS reaches 9 or 10 mm (Weissman 1982; Rana 1989; Clark 1992, 1994). This traditional indication has not been critically validated and the poor reliability of utilizing the ADI in either predicting paralysis or as in indication for surgery has been clearly shown (Boden et al. 1993; Boden 1994).

The only absolute surgical indication is progressive neurological compromise secondary to AAS with demonstrated cord compression due to pannus or bony instability (Thompson and Meyer 1985, Rana 1989, Santavirta et al. 1991; Boden et al. 1993; Boden 1994; Clark 1994).

Relative surgical indications include intractable mechanical pain or "impending" myelopathy, including radiographic evidence of cord compression with minimal or possibly subclinical evidence of myelopathy. Since we know that patients can have conduction abnormalities on neurophysiological testing without objective neurological abnormalities and that AAS may progress in a significant proportion of patients, it is reasonable to stabilize and decompress patients on whom imaging reveals evidence of cord compression at the site of AAS (i.e. a cervical medullary angle

< 135°, space available for the spinal cord < 13 mm, deformity of the cervical spinal cord, cord < 6 mm sagittal diameter, or signal change within the spinal cord).

Mobile vs. Fixed Deformity

Patients considered for surgery can be divided into two groups. The first group consists of those patients with a mobile subluxation which can be easily reduced. The reduction may either be spontaneous on extension of the spine as noted in preoperative flexion/extension lateral cervical spine views, or it may require several days of preoperative traction. Traction may be provided through either a halo ring or with tongs (Gardner Wells or Cone Barton). Often placement of a rolled towel or bolster under the neck may facilitate the extension required to reduce a patient in traction. Careful clinical neurological monitoring as well as radiographic monitoring is required while attempting a closed reduction in traction. More than 10 or 15 kg (20 or 30 lbs) is rarely necessary to effect an appropriate reduction at the C1–C2 level.

For the patient whose subluxation reduces anatomically and whose neurological status improves following reduction, a simple in situ posterior fusion of C1–C2 is indicated (Fig. 17.2). Patients whose subluxations do not completely reduce in traction, require careful evaluation of the degree and quality of neurological compression. They may require a direct decompressive procedure as well as a fusion. If, after 3 or 4 days of halo or tong traction, a deformity is not completely reduced, repeat neurological imaging (MRI) is recommended. This possibility should be anticipated and thus MR compatible tongs and halo rings should be used.

If the neurological compression is due to soft tissue pannus and not bony compression and the neurological function is stable, a successful posterior in situ fusion will result in resolution, resorption, and decrease in size of the granulomatous pannus (Milbrink and Nyman 1990). Thus, given primarily soft tissue pannus compression, direct anterior decompression is not necessary and an effective stabilizing procedure will result in indirect decompression of the cervical spinal cord. There is, however, the risk of intraoperative manipulation of the spine with further extrusion of the pannus and worsening of the neurological deficit.

In the case of bony compression of the cervical cord in the presence of a fixed irreducible AAS, surgical options include anterior resection of the odontoid with an associated C1–C2 fusion, or a posterior decompressive laminectomy and fusion. Stanley et al. (1994) treated 25 patients with AAS with a posterior decompression and fusion. Clinical improvement was noted in 75% and mortality was 8%. No neurological deterioration was noted. This procedure is made more effective with the addition of C1–2 transarticular screw fixation (Magerl and Seemann 1987). Transarticular C1–C2 screw fixation does not rely on an intact posterior arch of C1 and can easily be performed following a posterior laminectomy of C1.

Because of the complication rate associated with the Halifax interlaminar clamp, this procedure is not recommended (Statham et al. 1993)). In addition, the Sonntag fusion appears to have a very high rate of non-union, as does a Gallie type fusion without postoperative halo immobilization.

At the authors' institution we prefer the Magerl technique of transarticular C1–2 screw fixation, augmented by a posterior "Gallie-type" arthrodesis (Fig. 17.2c, d). In 11 patients with RA, we have a 100% successful arthrodesis rate with no neurological deterioration. The transarticular screw technique has the benefits of providing excellent fixation without entering the spinal canal (as is the case with wires and clamps). This technique does not rely on an intact posterior arch of C1 or C2, nor does it rely on an intact odontoid, and the majority of our patients are treated not with a halo but with a removable cervical orthosis (SOMI). It is this lack of required Halo immobilization in the presence of a high fusion rate that is particularly attractive in the rheumatoid patient who often poorly tolerates the halo ring and vest.

In most papers, neurological improvement following surgery is good. The results outlined by Peppelman et al. (1993) suggest that almost 95% of patients can improve at least one Ranawat class. Neurological symptoms and recovery appeared to be related to the severity of the neurological deficit prior to surgery and are also related to the type of instability.

A survey of the results of surgery is given in Table 17.1.

Vertical Migration of the Odontoid

VMO comprises up to 22% of cervical subluxations (Weissman et al. 1982; Boden 1994). VMO is clearly associated with a higher morbidity than simple AAS. The risk of developing a neurological deficit with VMO is greater and once that deficit develops it is less likely to resolve with treatment (Weissman et al. 1982). Mortality is also higher with VMO, as is the radiographic risk of progression (Sherk 1978; Weissman et al. 1982; Slätis et al. 1989). An absolute indication for surgery in VMO is compression of the spinal cord or brainstem with progressive neurological deficit. Relative indications include progressive VMO or impending spinal cord compression.

Because of the poor prognosis for neurological recovery and the probability of progression in patients with VMO, the authors contend that if a patient develops progressive VMO with an increase of more that 5 mm on serial radiographs, even in the absence of neurological compression prophylactic stabilization should be considered. In many of these patients, if caught early, VMO may be successfully stabilized with an atlantoaxial arthrodesis and extension of the fusion to the occiput may

Table 17.1. Results of surgery

Reference	Procedure	n	Result	Pseudoarthrosis rate	Mortality
Ranawat et al. (1979)	Posterior fusion	20%	35%		
Thompson and Meyer (1985)	Occiput–C1 fusion	10	84% satisfactory	1 of 10	1 of 10
McGraw and Rusch (1973)	Modified Gallie	7	Excellent	0%	0%
Stirrat and Fyfe (1993)	Posterior C1–2 fusion	17	12%		
Santavirta et al. (1991)	Gallie fusion	24	50%		
Peppelman et al. (1993)	Gallie fusion	55	95% neurologically improved	14%	
Clark (1994)	C1–2 fusion	20	12%		
Statham et al. (1993)	Halifax interlaminar clamp	45	30% complication		
Papadopoulos (1991)	Sonntag fusion	17	24%		
Vanden Berge et al. (1991)	Occiput–C2 fusion	22	88% improved	35%	9%
Dvorak (preliminary results)	Magerl screw xation	11	0% neurological deterioration	0%	0%

be avoided. If successful, the C1–2 arthrodesis is protective against further VMO, and carries with it less surgical morbidity, and is less disabling for the patient.

In the case of VMO with neurological symptoms, if the deformity is reducible, and in our experience the majority of these deformities can be reduced with halo traction, then an occiput to C2 fusion is indicated. Irreducible deformities are not common, and we would agree with Stirrat and Fyfe (1993) that odontoid resection is rarely necessary.

Newer techniques of plate and screw fixation, which maintain reduction with rigid internal fixation, have a high fusion rate and minimize reliance upon external orthoses. At the authors institution, a "gamma" shaped plate is fixed to the midline of the occiput with screws and extended caudally to incorporate two transarticular C1–2 screws (Fig. 17.3). This has been performed in seven patients to date, not all rheumatoid, with no pseudarthroses, no neurological deterioration, and excellent

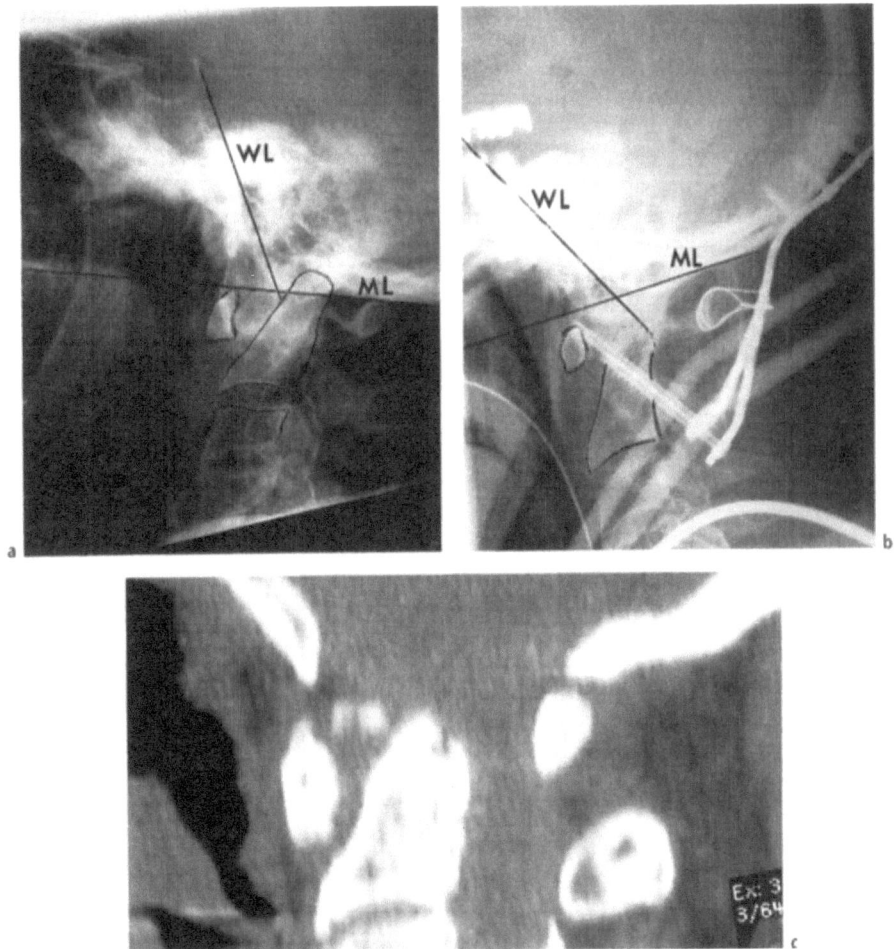

Fig. 17.3. Vertical migration of the odontoid in a patient with RA followed for a number of years with asymptomatic AAS. McGregor's line (McGregor 1948) and Wachenheim's line (Clark 1992) (labelled ML and WL respectively) are seen on preoperative (**a**) and postoperative (**b**) lateral films. Sagittal reformatted CT scans (**c**) are useful.

maintenance of reduction. We would strongly recommend this technique as being superior to other fixation techniques.

Subaxial Subluxation

Subaxial subluxation (SAS) has been reported in 15%–20% of rheumatoid patients with cervical subluxation (Grantham and Lipson 1989). Typically, it develops as an anterior multiple level subluxation, most commonly occurring at C3–4 and developing into a "staircase", or "stepladder" type deformity. Other forms of SAS include subluxations below previous fusions (Fig. 17.4), anterior spondylodiscitis with cord compression, and subaxial hyperlordosis.

Stirrat and Fyfe (1993) have clearly identified the difficulties in treating SAS. One third of their patients required more than one operative procedure, the mortality was 17%, and half the patients were non-ambulatory postoperatively. In Peppelman et al.'s (1993) review, 13 of the 15 patients with worsening or recurrent neurological findings were found to have SAS. Santavirta et al. (1990) reviewed 16 patients treated surgically for SAS and recommended posterior decompression and fusion for the treatment of SAS with progressive neurological compromise. Their results were good with recurrent deformity at adjacent levels in three patients (19%).

The natural history of SAS has not been clearly defined. Oda et al. (1995) found that patients with concomitant VMO tended to have more severe SAS. Progression of SAS was strongly correlated with disease severity, disc space narrowing, erosion of the endplates, erosion and fracture of the spinous processes, and adjacent fusions.

Progressive neurological deficit in association with SAS is an indication for surgical treatment. Posterior decompression and fusion is the most commonly recommended procedure. This can often be complicated by the poor quality of the eroded

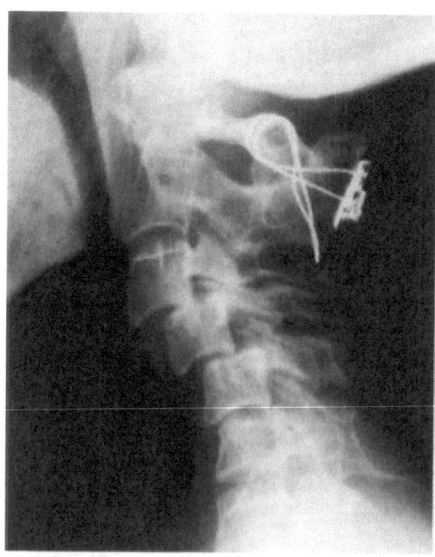

Fig. 17.4. Development of SAS in a patient 8 years after a successful C1–2 arthrodesis utilizing the McGraw–Rusch (1973) (modified Gallie) fusion technique.

and subluxed lateral masses and the position of the fusion in tension, as opposed to compression. This has prompted the authors to combine anterior and posterior fusions with posterior laminectomy and decompression in an attempt to obtain a circumferential fusion with the highest possible chance of solid stable fusion (Fig. 17.5). Other authors have recommended a more aggressive approach to the treatment of SAS particularly in the presence of adjacent cervical fusions (Kraus et al. 1991). Once a substantial deformity has developed, the opportunity for performing a simple, single stage stabilizing procedure has been lost. There may therefore be a rationale for a more aggressive approach to surgical treatment of SAS, especially in

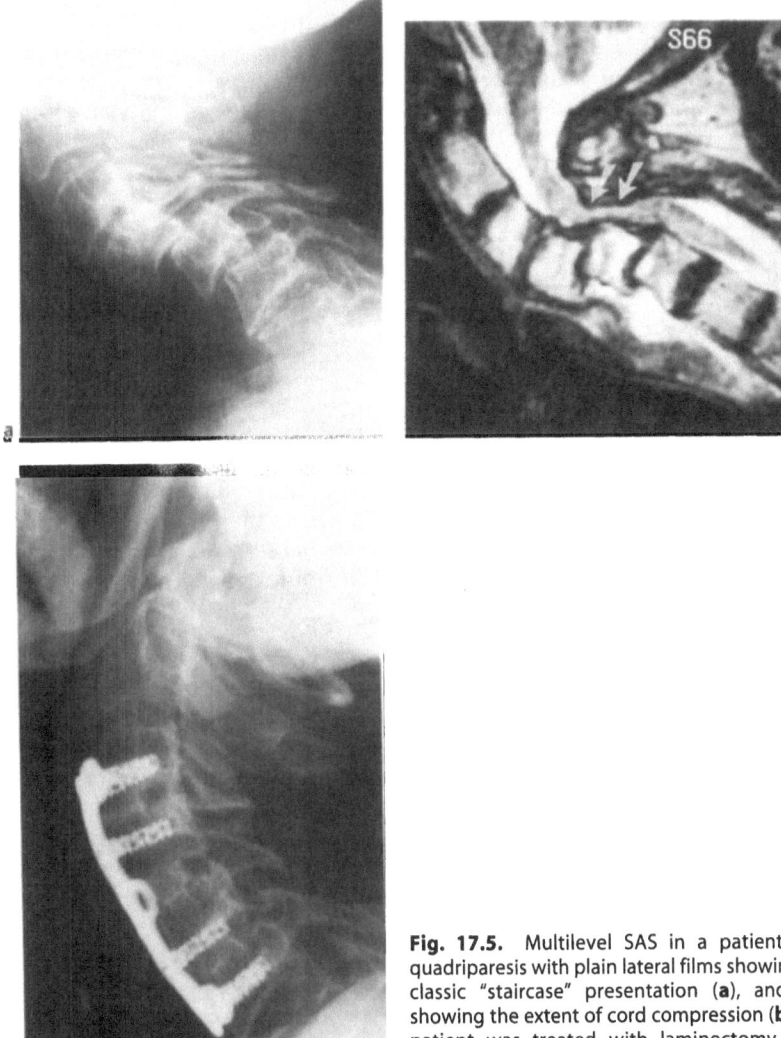

Fig. 17.5. Multilevel SAS in a patient with quadriparesis with plain lateral films showing the classic "staircase" presentation (**a**), and MRI showing the extent of cord compression (**b**). The patient was treated with laminectomy, then reduction in traction, and anterior fusion and plating (**c**).

the patient who has a pre-existing occiput to C2 fusion or in the patient who may not be compliant with regular follow-up advice.

Recurrence of Deformity Following Previous Fusion

Kraus et al. (1991) and Agarwal et al. (1992) reported that recurrence of cervical instability following a successful previous fusion occurred in 5.5% patients. Interestingly, Agarwal et al. found that no patient with a successful C1–2 fusion progressed to develop VMO. It was felt that successful C1–2 arthrodesis protected the patient from further progression and development of VMO. This finding suggests that a posterior C1–2 fusion is indicated for AAS and that extension of the fusion to the occiput is unnecessary. Those patients with a successful C1–2 fusion who developed SAS required surgery an average of 9 years after the first fusion. In patients with a successful occipitocervical fusion, however, the risk of developing SAS was 36% and SAS developed more rapidly (average of 2.6 years after fusion).

Screening in the Rheumatoid Cervical Spine

Predicting Paralysis

Boden et al. (1993) developed a reliable screening tool for predicting paralysis and for identifying patients who require further investigation. The posterior atlantodental interval (PADI) has a sensitivity of 97% and a negative predictive value of 94% (Boden et al. 1993; Boden 1994). Thus, if the PADI is greater than 14 mm, paraplegia is very unlikely to ensue. This makes the PADI a reliable screening measurement. This measurement, easily made on plain lateral flexion/extension views, should replace reliance on the atlantodental interval.

Preoperative Screening of Rheumatoid Arthritis Patients

Campbell et al. (1995) questioned the usefulness of routine preoperative cervical spine radiographs in rheumatoid patients undergoing elective orthopaedic procedures. He noted an incidence of 5.5% of unsuspected subluxation and reported that in no case did this change anaesthetic management. The patient population studied had relatively mild rheumatoid disease, and the overall 15% incidence of radiographic abnormalities is well below other reported prevalence rates. Abandoning preoperative cervical screening in rheumatoid patients is not justified by this report. Collins et al. (1991) found a 61% incidence of subluxation in preoperative screening and half of these patients were asymptomatic. Preoperative flexion/extension lateral radiographs are recommended in all rheumatoid patients undergoing surgical procedures.

Summary

The three major deformities in the cervical rheumatoid spine are atlantoaxial subluxation (AAS), vertical migration of the odontoid (VMO), and subaxial subluxation (SAS). These instability patterns, although they often occur together, have different natural histories and require individualized treatment approaches.

AAS is often benign and only requires treatment when neurological structures are compromised, when neurological compromise is impending or highly predictable, or when pain is severe and refractory to other treatment modalities.

VMO has a more sinister prognosis and the treatment is more difficult, with less predictable outcome. VMO appears to result from severe progression of AAS and early recognition and more aggressive surgical treatment may be justified.

SAS may also be a cause of cervical myelopathy. It is often seen in patients with coexistent instability in the upper cervical spine (treated or untreated). Once it progresses to neurological compromise, it is often difficult to treat surgically and the neurological outcome is less predictable. Careful follow-up in high risk groups (i.e. patients with occiput–C2 fusions, and radiographic risk factors) may be justified, and early surgical intervention may be appropriate.

References

Agarwal AK, Peppelman WC, Kraus DR et al. (1992) Recurrence of cervical spine instability in rheumatoid arthritis following previous fusion: Can disease progression be prevented by early surgery? J Rheumatol 19:1364–1370

Agarwal AK, Peppelman WC, Kraus DR, Eisenbeis CH (1993) The cervical spine in rheumatoid arthritis. Br Med J 306:79–80

Bell HS (1970) Paralysis of both arms from injury of the upper portion of the pyramidal decussation: "cruciate paralysis". J Neurosurg 33:376–380.

Boden SD (1994) Rheumatoid arthritis of the cervical spine. Surgical decision making based on predictors of paralysis and recovery. Spine 19:2275–2280

Boden SD, Dodge LD, Bohlman HH, Rechtine GR (1993) Rheumatoid arthritis of the cervical spine. A long-term analysis with predictors of paralysis and recovery. J Bone Joint Surg 75A:1282–1297

Braunstein EM, Weissman BN, Seltzer SE, Sosman JL, Wong A, Zamani A (1984) Computed tomography and conventional radiographs of the craniocervical region in rheumatoid arthritis. Arthritis Rheum 27:26–31

Breedveld FC, Algra PR, Vielvoye CJ, Cats A (1987) Magnetic resonance imaging in the evaluation of patients with rheumatoid arthritis and subluxations of the cervical spine. Arthritis Rheum 30:624–629

Bundschuh CV, Modic MT (1987) Rheumatoid arthritis of the cervical spine. Orthop Trans 11:7

Campbell RSD, Wou P, Watt I (1995) A continuing role for pre-operative cervical spine radiography in rheumatoid arthritis? Clin Radiol 50:157–159

Chang MH, Liao KK, Cheung SC, Kong KW, Chang SP (1992) "Numb, clumsy hands" and tactile agnosia secondary to high cervical spondylotic myelopathy: a clinical and electrophysiological correlation. Acta Neurol Scand 86:622–625

Clark CR (1992) Rheumatoid arthritis: surgical considerations. In: Rothman RH, Simeone FA (eds) The spine. WB Saunders, Toronto, pp 1429–1444

Clark CR (1994) Rheumatoid involvement of the cervical spine. An overview. Spine 19:2257–2258

Collins DN, Barnes CL, FitzRandolph RL (1991) Cervical spine instability in rheumatoid patients having total hip or knee arthroplasty. Clin Orthop 272:127–135

Delamarter RB, Bohlman HH (1994) Postmortem osseus and neuropathologic analysis of the rheumatoid cervical spine. Spine 19:2267-2274

Dvorak J, Grob D, Baumgartner H, Gschwend N, Grauer W, Larsson S (1989) Functional evaluation of the spinal cord by magnetic resonance imaging in patients with rheumatoid arthritis and instability of upper cervical spine. Spine 14:1057-1064

Fielding JW, Cochran GVB, Lawsing JF, Hohl M (1974) Tears of the transverse ligament of the atlas - a clinical and biomechanical study. J Bone Joint Surg 56A:1683-1691

Grantham SA, Lipson SJ (1989) Rheumatoid arthritis and other noninfectious inflammatory diseases. In: Sherk HH et al. (eds) The cervical spine. JP Lippincott, Philadelphia

Kauppi M, Anttila P (1995) A stiff collar can restrict atlantoaxial instability in rheumatoid cervical spine in selected cases. Ann Rheum Dis 54:305-307

Kraus DR, Peppelman WC, Agarwal AK, DeLeeuw HW, Donaldson WF (1991) Incidence of subaxial subluxation in patients with generalized rheumatoid arthritis who have had previous occiput cervical fusions. Spine 16(Suppl):S486-S489

Magerl F Seemann PS (1987) Stable posterior fusion of the atlas and axis by transarticular screw fixation. In: Kehr P, Weidner A (eds) Cervical spine 1. Springer-Verlag Wien, New York, pp 322-327

Marks JS, Sharp J (1981) Rheumatoid cervical myelopathy. Q J Med 199:307-319

Mathews JA (1974) Atlanto-axial subluxation in rheumatoid arthritis. A five year follow-up study. Ann Rheum Dis 33:526-531

McGraw RW, Rusch RM (1973) Atlantoaxial arthrodesis. J Bone Joint Surg 55B:482-489

McGregor M (1948) The significance of certain measurements of the skull in the diagnosis of basilar impression. Br J. Radiol 21:171-178

Meijers KA, vanBeusekam GT, Luyendijk W, Duijfjes F (1974) Dislocation of the cervical spine with cord compression in rheumatoid arthritis. J Bone Joint Surg 56B:668-680

Milbrink J, Nyman (1990) Posterior stabilization of the cervical spine in rheumatoid arthritis: clinical results and magnetic resonance imaging correlation. J Spinal Disord 3:308-315

Oda T, Fujiwara K, Yonenobu K, Azuma B, Ochi T (1995) Natural course of cervical spine lesions in rheumatoid arthritis. Spine 20:1128-1135

Papdopoulus SM, Dickman CA, Sonntag VKH (1991) Atlantoaxial stabilization in rheumatoid arthritis. J Neurosurg 74:1-7

Pellicci PM, Ranawat CS, Tsairis P, Bryan WJ (1981) A prospective study of the progression of rheumatoid arthritis of the cervical spine. J Bone Joint Surg 63A:342-350

Peppelman WC, Kraus DR, Donaldson WF, Agarwal A (1993) Cervical spine surgery in rheumatoid arthritis: improvement of neurologic deficit after cervical spine fusion. Spine 18:2375-2379

Rana NA (1989) Natural history of atlanto-axial subluxation in rheumatoid arthritis. Spine 14:1054-1056

Ranawat CS, O'Leary P, Pellicci P, Tsairis P, Marchisello P, Dorr L (1979) Cervical fusion in rheumatoid arthritis. J Bone Joint Surg 61A:1003-1010

Roca A, Bernreuter WK, Alarcon GS (1993) Functional magenetic resonance imaging should be included in the evaluation of the cervical spine in patients with rheumatoid arthritis. J Rheumatol 20:1485-1488

Santavirta S, Konttinen YT, Sandelin J, Slätis P (1990) Operations for the unstable cervical spine in rheumatoid arthritis. Acta Orthop Scand 61:106-110

Santavirta S, Konttinen YT, Laasonen E, Honkanen V, Antti-Poika I, Kauppi M (1991) Ten-year results of operations for rheumatoid cervical spine disorders. J Bone Joint Surg 73B:116-120

Sherk HH (1978) Atlanto-axial instability and acquired basilar invagination in rheumatoid arthritis. Orthop Clin North Am 9:1053-1063

Slätis P, Santavirta S, Sandelin J, Konttinen YT (1989) Cranial subluxation of the odontoid process in rheumatoid arthritis J Bone Joint Surg 71A:189-195

Smith PH, Benn RT, Sharp J (1972) Natural history of rheumatoid cervical luxations. Ann Rheum Dis 31:431-439

Statham P, O'Sullivan M, Russell T (1993) The Halifax interlaminar clamp for posterior cervical fusion: initial experience in the United Kingdom. Neurosurgery 32:396-399

Stanley D, Laing RJ, Forster DM, Getty CJ (1994) Posterior decompression and fusion in rheumatoid disease of the cervical spine. J Spinal Disord 7:439-443

Stirrat AN, Fyfe IS (1993) Surgery of the rheumatoid cervical spine. Correlation of the pathoogy and prognosis. Clin Orthop 293:135-143

Thompson RCJr, Meyer TJ (1985) Posterior surgical stabilization for atlantoaxial subluxation in rheumatoid arthritis. Spine 10:597-601

Tumiati B, Casoli P (1991) Syringomyelia in a patients with rheumatoid subluxation of the cervical spine. J Rheumatol 18:1403-1405

Vanden Berghe A, Ackerman C, Veys E, Verjans P, Uyttendaele D, Claessens H (1991) Acta Orthop Belg 57(Suppl 1):94–98

Weissman BNW, Aliabadi P, Weinfeld MS, Thomas WH, Sosman JL (1982) Prognostic features of atlantoaxial subluxation in rheumatoid arthritis. Radiology 144:745–751

Zeidman SM, Ducker TB (1994) Rheumatoid arthritis. Neuroanatomy, compression and grading of deficits. Spine 19:2259–2266

Chapter 18

Meningitic Disorders and Myelopathies

E.M.R. Critchley

The spinal cord is that part of the central nervous system lying within the vertebral canal. It extends as an oval tube from the medulla oblongata at the foramen magnum to the L1-2 interspace or the upper part of the L2 vertebra. Its enveloping membranes are confluent with those covering the surface of the brain. The pia mater is intimately adherent to the cord with fine septa penetrating into the parenchyma. The arachnoid mater covers the cord more loosely, extending laterally over the dorsal ganglia and emergent roots, and downwards over the nerves of the cauda equina where it is attached to the sacrum at S2. CSF, secreted in the main by the choroid plexuses within the ventricular system of the brain, is contained within the transparent arachnoid membrane. Externally, the dura mater forms a tougher, opaque membrane over the surface of the brain and spinal cord. At spinal level it is tethered laterally by the dentate ligaments and ensheathes the arachnoid, pia, spinal cord and upper part of the cauda equina before ending at S2-3.

Any inflammatory, irritative or infiltrative disorder of the leptomeninges (pia mater and arachnoid) will cause a meningitic reaction – meningitis – with thickening of the meninges and exudation of cells and protein into the CSF of the subarachnoid space. Almost invariably, the meningeal reaction also involves the dura and spreads into the substance of the brain and spinal cord producing local inflammatory, infiltrative or arteritic changes. Viral diseases, predominantly but not invariably, invade the brain producing an encephalitis. Some secondary changes occur elsewhere but the pyogenic reaction is minimal. Where a bacterial infection clearly involves the substance of the brain, terms such as encephalomyelitis or myeloencephalitis are used; but even where there has been little encephalitic reaction, a bacterial meningitic infection will result in systemic changes such as pyrexia and leucocytosis; cerebral irritation with headache, epilepsy, cranial nerve palsies or photophobia; as well as cerebrospinal and spinal manifestations. There are two valid reasons that explain the undue emphasis usually given to the spinal component of meningitis: the clinical recognition of its presence by means of tests which depend essentially upon the presence of muscle spasm over the irritated meninges, and the use of a lumbar puncture needle, penetrating the lower subarachnoid space, in diagnosis, and sometimes therapeutically, in the management of meningitis.

Most spinal infections result from haematogenous spread. The meninges may be invaded directly as happens with disseminated military tuberculosis, via the choroid plexus with bacteria entering the CSF directly, or as a result of septic emboli lodging in the smaller arteries causing mycotic aneurysms to develop and rupture.

Ascending vascular spread via the venous plexuses of blood vessels around the cord is a rare but well-documented cause of infection. Next most common after blood-borne infection is direct spread from local sites of infection such as bone, the sinuses and middle ear. In the case of certain viral infections neural spread from the nasopharynx and other infected tissues may also occur. Lastly, direct penetration of the meninges can occur aided by dysraphism, fractures or the introduction of conta-minants – bacteria, chemicals, or the development of dermoids – via a lumbar punc-ture needle. Repeated episodes of meningitis raise questions of additional factors such as dural tears with CSF leakage, dermal sinuses, unhealed fractures, midline deformities and immunodeficient states.

An acute epidural abscess is likely to be the result of a blood-borne infection but at least 50% of chronic abscesses and granulomas develop from contiguous infection from neighboring bones. Most epidural abscesses are caused by staphylococci but brucella, typhoid and Gram-negative infections due to *E. coli*, pseudomonas or proteus may also present with the formation of an epidural abscess. Such abscesses are mostly seen over several segments of the thoracic spine. Partial compression of the cord may result, accompanied by excessive secretion of protein into the CSF to give Froin's syndrome with a thick, yellow, gelatinous and proteinaceous spinal fluid; but such classical signs suggest delayed diagnosis.

Subdural infection usually arises via the paranasal sinuses where the adherent dura becomes infected and the infection spreads on to its inner more vascular layer. Once the dura has been penetrated, the leptomeninges offer little resistance and fungal infections in particular spread locally to produce a combination of chronic meningitis, thrombophlebitis, microabscesses and granulomata.

The CSF offers an excellent culture medium for many organisms but the innate vascularity of the meninges enables a rapid blood-borne cellular response to develop. Where the infection is bacterial, the resultant pyogenic exudation shows a predominantly polymorphonuclear pleocytosis; if the infection is viral a lympho-cytic pleocytosis is more usual. These cellular changes are accompanied by a seepage of protein into the CSF rendering it more sticky and eventually impeding flow. If the meningitis becomes chronic, as may happen with subacute or partially treated infections, fibroblasts proliferate and adhesions develop blocking the basal cisterns, sealing off the foramina of Lushka and Magendie, or matting together the roots of the cauda equina. Later complications include the development of hydrocephalus, arachnoid cysts at various levels, and a progressive spinal arachnoiditis. Spinal arachnoiditis occurs particularly as a response to the injection of toxic chemicals. Radio-opaque contrast media have been especially inculpated in the past but the combination of aetiological factors required is far from clear with the suggestion that there should be some evidence of infection as well as irritation. Thus certain non-infective causes of chronic meningitis such as neoplasia, sarcoidosis, Behçet's and chronic benign lymphocytic meningitis (Mollaret's meningitis), are associated with a low incidence of arachnoiditis whereas chronic infections with tuberculosis, brucellosis and fungi frequently cause widespread arachnoid reactions.

Meningitis may be overlooked and obscured by other disease manifestations in the very young and very old. At the extremes of life the differential diagnosis of unexplained pyrexia, failure to thrive or inanition require an examination of the CSF. Chronic infections may present insidiously in all age groups, but especially in the immunocompromised individual. Nonetheless, most forms of meningitis present with a tetrad of headache, fever, increasing drowsiness and meningeal irrita-tion. Headache is almost invariable and usually severe, continuous and increasing in intensity, especially at the back of the head and neck. Its presence may be indicated in young children and in those too ill to complain by other accompanying features such as photophobia, vomiting and papilloedema. Even taking these characteristics into account it is a lesser diagnostic feature than meningeal irritability.

The neck is the most mobile part of the spinal column and any muscular spasm in response to irritation due to meningitis, raised intracranial pressure or blood in the CSF is best seen as nuchal rigidity developing within a few hours. In its extreme form, nuchal rigidity encompasses the whole length of the spine with opisthotonus due to extreme hyperextension of the back. However, nuchal rigidity can be missed in the early stages, with overwhelming infection, or in the presence of disc pathology. Neck rigidity essentially occurs in the sagittal plane and can be elicited by placing a hand behind the head and trying to flex the neck passively. The presence of rigidity primarily in the sagittal plane is helpful in separating meningeal irritation from limited movements due to cervical spondylosis or to meningism occurring as a result of swollen neck glands or throat infections in children. A useful test in a child or young person is to see whether they can flex their head to touch their knees, or to "kiss the knees".

There are more formal tests. Kernig's test is useful in children and young adults. Extension of the knee with the hip flexed produces spasm and pain in the hamstrings. In the elderly, Brudzinski's set of signs of meningeal irritation is obtained more readily. Firstly, there may be spontaneous flexion of the knees and hips with attempted flexion of the neck, and secondly, extension of the knee with the hip flexed results in flexion of the other knee, or occasionally in extension.

Investigation of Acute Meningitis

Whenever possible a CT or ultrasound scan should be performed before a lumbar puncture. If the patient is drowsy, has had fits, or there is any suspicion of raised intracranial pressure a CT scan is mandatory. Even so, unless the meningitis is part of a septicaemia and the diagnosis can be obtained by blood culture, or in the course of an endemic a pathognomonic rash of meningococcal meningitis has been observed, examination of the CSF is required in order to make an accurate diagnosis and enable the clinician to contend with an unusual organism, an unusual strain, antibiotic resistance or antibiotic hypersensitivity necessitating a change in treatment as the meningitis progresses (Addy 1987). A CT scan should alert the clinician to the presence of a cerebral abscess, which may have ruptured to produce meningitis, to raised intracranial pressure from cerebral oedema complicating purulent bacterial infections or in the later stages to hydrocephalus, arachnoid cysts or secondary abscess formation. Drowsiness and coma, altered conscious levels due to fits, shock and disseminated intravascular coagulation may all develop and require urgent action.

It is accepted practice to start therapy with broad spectrum antibiotics whilst awaiting the outcome of CSF examination and to modify the treatment once the organism is known. The problem is how to minimize the risks of obtaining CSF in the presence of the complications mentioned. If there is any suspicion of raised intracranial pressure, the clinician may either elect to give a bolus of mannitol 2g/kg intravenously before the CSF is examined or to obtain CSF from the cerebral ventricles. In the event of hydrocephalus a needle or catheter can be introduced into the ventricles via an open or bulging fontanelle or, in older children and adults, via burr holes. The catheter can then be used to withdraw CSF for examination, to relieve the increase in intracranial pressure and to continue to monitor intracranial pressure. If there is raised intracranial pressure but slit-like ventricles the clinician will have to decide between treating empirically with antibiotics or inserting a subarachnoid screw to monitor intracranial pressure before beginning treatment (Brown and Steer 1986; Newton 1987).

Neonatal meningitis, resulting from intrapartum infection with *E. coli*, group B streptococci or *Listeria*, carries a mortality of 20%–50%. Later infections up to three months after delivery are usually from exogenous contaminants such as *Staphylococcus aureus*, pseudomonas and *Klebsiella* with a lesser mortality of 10%–20%. In childhood the prevalent organisms are *Neisseria meningitis* and *Haemophilus influenzae* and in the elderly, *Streptococcus pneumoniae* and *E. coli*. A detailed discussion of the management of meningitis is outside the scope of this book and can be found in Critchley (1988) or Wood and Anderson (1988).

Tuberculous Infections

Tuberculous (TB) infection of the CNS may take on many protean forms but it is essential to recognize that the onset of TB meningitis may be as acute as any other type of bacterial or viral infection. The difference often lies in the subsequent progress. Instead of reaching a plateau or showing regression, the infection may fulminate and the patient becomes increasingly stuporose. Meningeal involvement is always secondary to TB infection elsewhere and may develop on a background of myalgia, anorexia, generalized malaise, low grade fever and intermittent headache. The onset of meningeal signs can be accompanied by headache, nerve palsies and drowsiness. If unsuccessfully treated a third phase follows with progressive neurological defects, coma and decerebration. Infants can present with full fontanelles and vomiting, children with abdominal pain and fits, and adults with focal features – an apparent stroke, a painful or paralysed eye, acute hydrocephalus or acute cerebral oedema (Tandon and Pathak 1973). Acute TB meningitis used to be the scourge of children under six years of age in developing countries. Even after the introduction of effective antibiotics, there was a 35% mortality with much attendant morbidity. Despite a perceptible shift from younger children to older children and young adults as the major risk group the mortality still remains unacceptably high.

Inflammation, exudation, giant cell proliferation and caseation are features of a fully developed TB meningitis; but many patients begin with a serous meningitis related to the haematogenous dissemination of miliary tuberculosis secondary to the breakdown of a silent Ghon focus in the lungs or gastrointestinal tract. In about 75% of these patients the chest X-ray will show miliary tubercles with enlarged mediastinal lymph nodes. Very occasionally tubercles may be seen with the ophthalmoscope in the choroidal layer of the eye appearing as rounded, white patches about half the size of the optic disc. Miliary tubercles are secreted via the choroid plexus and become scattered over the leptomeninges. At first the CSF is clear and in all respects normal, but changes rapidly within one or two days into an opalescent fluid capable of forming a fine, fibrinous clot on standing. The white cell count rises to 100–200/mm³, initially with a slight preponderance of polymorphs over lymphocytes but the ratio is soon reversed. The protein content may exceed 15 g/l and the sugar fall below 40% of the blood sugar level. The cornerstone of successful management is early diagnosis: any delay in the onset of treatment weighs on the prognosis. Rather than await the identification of acid-fast bacilli or the outcome of cultures and guinea-pig inoculation tests, therapy should be started on clinical suspicion and backed up by a thorough search for organisms in the lumbar CSF and even ventricular fluid.

Meningitis may be associated with any form of underlying systemic tuberculosis (Rich 1952) and its various forms described with reference to the main pathological characteristics e.g. focal plaques with caseation, acute inflammatory caseous meningitis or proliferative meningitis. TB as a disease is highly dependent upon the state of resistance of the host, the presence of infection elsewhere, the state of nutrition, and the immune responses. The onset of meningitis may be protracted over several months. The patient may have no discernible fever but complain of malaise, apathy, listlessness, anorexia, weight loss, occasional vomiting and focal symptoms. The complications of a chronic, slowly progressive meningitis include the development of arachnoiditis, subdural empyemata, and perivascular arteritic inflammatory changes involving infarction and granuloma formation within the spinal cord.

Caseous changes may remain focal at any site within the nervous system with the production of tuberculomata. A further breakdown in resistance may present with meningitis after a long latent period. Similarly, tuberculous spinal osteomyelitis secondary to haematogenous spread may involve one or more vertebral bodies and discs with minimal symptoms until an acute paraplegia develops secondary to vertebral collapse or direct extension leads to epidural granuloma or abscess formation, or even to meningitis. The differential diagnosis of a progressive paraplegia in the presence of TB includes: (1) vertebral collapse, (2) cord compression secondary to an epidural abscess or granuloma, (3) cord ischaemia and infarction secondary to arteritis or thrombophlebitis in the neighborhood of a tuberculous infection, (4) an expanding subdural empyema, or (5) arachnoiditis or a high CSF protein resulting in a spinal block.

Neurobrucellosis

The intraspinal manifestations of brucellosis mimic closely those of TB and fungal infections. Systemic brucellosis primarily involves the whole of the reticuloendothelial system with secondary involvement of bone. Organisms enter and proliferate within the cytoplasm of macrophages, thus the acute stage may be followed by a protracted, subclinical or relapsing illness. Non-specific symptoms such as headache, back pain and low grade fever can persist for months or years. In the acute stages meningism can arise from tender, enlarged cervical lymph nodes and occasionally there may be an acute serious meningitis which responds readily to tetracycline.

Four main intraspinal manifestations of brucellosis can occur with chronic infection, often presenting in combination.

Spinal Brucellosis or Spondylitis

Infection of a disc is most liable to occur in the lumbosacral or lower thoracic spine with spread to the adjacent vertebral bodies. Local tenderness and pain are common and the spine may become deformed with sciatica and radicular pains resulting from root compression. Vertebral erosion may lead to collapse with compression of the cord or cauda equina and the development of paraplegia. Alternatively, local spread can affect the meninges with epidural abscess formation also producing compression.

Chronic Lymphocytic Meningitis

The lymphocytic meningitis closely resembles that of TB with normal or reduced sugar levels and a greatly raised protein. Chronic meningitis may also affect the brain – meningoencephalitis, or the cord – meningomyelitis. Cerebral oedema or basal adhesions may result in a raised intracranial pressure with papilloedema and headache. Similarly, the high protein and arachnoid adhesions may result in a spinal block with paraplegia.

Radiculopathy

A Guillain–Barré like syndrome is described with radiculopathy, peripheral neuropathy and autonomic manifestations.

Myelopathy

The cord itself may be involved with demyelination, e.g. progressive ataxic quadriparesis (Al Deeb et al. 1989), acute transverse myelopathy, infarction or other vascular manifestations. In AIDS or other immune-deficient states, brucellosis may appear as an opportunistic infection.

The presence of chronic infection may be confirmed by a raised ESR and standard brucella agglutination tests. Identification of the organism can be difficult but may be achieved from blood or marrow culture or CSF. The accepted treatment of neuro-brucellosis is one or more six-week course of oral tetracycline 2–3 g daily or co-trimoxazole b.d. with intramuscular streptomycin 1 g daily, gentamicin 6 mg/kg or rifampicin, but eradication cannot be guaranteed.

Sarcoidosis

About 5% of patients with sarcoidosis develop symptomatic nervous system disease, sometimes in isolation and sometimes in a setting of extraneural sarcoidosis. The percentage is higher if ocular manifestations – uveitis, conjunctivitis, scleral scarring and choroidoretinitis – are also included. The majority of neurological manifestations, amounting to 75% of the total, are peripheral, typically involving the facial nerve, singly, bilaterally or in Heerfordt's triad of uveoparotid fever. Other cranial nerves may be affected singly or as a cranial polyneuritis. Peripheral manifestations may develop unevenly with the evolution of mononeuritis multiplex or produce a combination of neuropathy and radiculopathy as in the Guillain–Barré syndrome.

Twenty-five per cent of neurosarcoidosis involves the CNS. Disease manifestations are seen relatively early in the course of the systemic illness, notably with the development of diabetes insipidus or other neuroendocrine dysfunction. The predominant lesion is a basal granulomatous meningitis blocking the basal cisterns and invading the parenchyma, infiltrating and compressing structures at the base of the brain. Leptomeningeal granulomata may be patchy rather than continuous. Their presence may account for the development or cranial nerve palsies and for symptomatic spinal cord sarcoidosis. Thus brainstem and spinal neurosarcoidosis can frequently masquerade as multiple sclerosis or transient ischaemic attacks in vertebrobasilar territory. A low grade or subclinical lymphocytic meningitis possibly occurs more frequently than a granulomatous meningitis; thus at least 75% of patients with neurosarcoidosis, perhaps presenting with a hypothalamic granuloma, will be shown to have a raised spinal fluid protein and a lymphocytic pleocytosis.

The pathology of the spinal lesions is little different from that of the more overt lesions at the base of the brain, but if they arise in isolation they can present much diagnostic difficulty. Isolated intra- or extramedullary granulomas in the cervical cord, or less commonly in the thoracic and lumbar cord, can present similarly to ependymomas or gliomas at the same site. Compression of the cord can develop from within, from without or from multiple parenchymatous granulomata associated with adhesive arachnoiditis. Granulomatous vasculitis and local infiltration can produce primary segmental demyelination, axonal degeneration, multiple small infarcts and, ultimately, necrosis of the cord. A common clinical presentation is of progressive paraplegia, especially at the thoracic level. the myelographic appearance is that of cord compression, but unless the diagnosis appears certain from the presence of other systemic manifestations it is advisable to confirm the sarcoid lesion by biopsy before treating with high-dose steroids. An improvement may be confirmed radiographically but a careful follow-up is required to exclude yeast, tubercle or fungal infection which may mimic neurosarcoidosis or be alighted as opportunistic infections by prolonged treatment with corticosteroids.

Neurosyphilis

Early Presentations

Spirochaetal invasion of the meninges can occur in the primary and secondary stages and at any time before the onset of the tertiary stage. The result is usually a clinically silent lymphocytic meningeal reaction in which a positive diagnosis from the CSF is only possible in 10%–15% of cases. Subsequently the lymphocytosis disappears and the fluid returns to normal. Later however, a brisk symptomatic meningeal reaction can occur, occasionally associated with optic neuritis, or cranial and spinal nerve lesions. The CSF is abnormal with positive treponemal reactions, a raised protein and a prolific cytosis with up to 1000/μl lymphocytes, polymorphs and plasma cells. A reduction of the CSF sugar content can make the differential diagnosis from TB meningitis dependent on the treponemal tests. If untreated at this stage the meningitis may continue to develop with granulomatous involvement of the meninges, adhesions and endarteritis.

Congenital Syphilis

Before two years of age, neurological signs are rare. However, hydrocephalus can develop secondarily to an acute or subacute meningitis. Later onset congenital syphilis has the same spectrum as the adult variety of the disease. A high proportion of meningeal and vascular forms are noted, cervical pachymeningitis is described but congenital tabes is extremely rare.

Meningovascular Syphilis

Meningovascular syphilis assaults the brain or spinal cord or both together. The essential lesion is an arteritis, sometimes with intermittent symptoms as in so-called cerebral congestive attacks. Fits and hemiplegia may be more permanent or there can be a relentless progression of symptoms. Arteritis of the meninges causes widespread, diffuse thickening of the pia arachnoid. Pachymeningitis cervicalis hypertrophica differs from cervical spondylosis in that the brunt of the thickening involves the pia arachnoid rather than dura and ligamentum flavum. A painful radiculopathy of the upper limbs may develop from root compression with a less marked spastic weakness of the legs. In addition, meningovascular syphilis involving the cervical region may produce tabetic amyotrophy or amyotrophic meningomyelitis resembling motor neurone disease (ALS). The features in common are an asymmetric wasting of the shoulder girdles and upper limbs with spasticity of the lower limbs, but distinct differences exist in that an appreciable proportion of patients have Argyll Robertson pupils, impaired vibration sense in the lower limbs and loss of sphincter control.

In meningovascular syphilis the cellular and protein changes in the CSF are less marked than in the earlier acute symptomatic meningitis but there is infiltration of the Virchow–Robin spaces by lymphocytes and plasma cells, an obliterative endarteritis and spinal arachnoiditis. The end result of a diffuse syphilitic spinal arachnoiditis can be: root symptoms with small gummata along the nerve roots, arachnoid cysts, vascular occlusion, and a slow strangulation of the cord under a swollen pia arachnoid with obliteration of small penetrating arteries thereby producing a concentric peripheral rim of demyelination and infarction – a syphilitic halo (Hughes 1978).

At the beginning of the century, spinal meningovascular syphilis was a major cause of transverse myelitis. The syndromes tended to be subacute or chronically progressive and invariably involved a combination of leptomeningeal exudation with granulomata, and a pan- or endarteritis. Erb's syphilitic paraplegia is a progressive form of meningomyelitis of the thoracic region with radicular pains, intense spasticity, some loss of vibration and position sense and severe sphincter impairment. Other manifestations may be thrombosis of major arteries such as the anterior spinal artery, infarction of a lateral branch of the anterior spinal artery causing a hemitransection akin to the Brown–Séquard syndrome, or multiple scattered lesions that bear a macroscopic resemblance to multiple sclerosis – so-called syphilitic sclerosis.

Tabes Dorsalis

Two to five per cent of patients with syphilis ultimately develop tabes or taboparesis 10, 15, 20 or more years after the primary infection. Tabes dorsalis is regarded as a parenchymatous affliction of the cord but this is not strictly true. There is a meningeal cellular reaction and vascular changes are rarely absent. Concentric lesions occur round the dorsal roots which appear pinkish and gelatinous. As a result, retrograde degeneration affects Lissauer's tracts and the posterior columns of the spinal cord. The cord shrinks and appears flattened in its antero–posterior diameter.

Most clinical manifestations which develop slowly in the fullness of time depend on this insidious sensory degeneration. Irritative sensory changes account for: (1) lightening pains or "screws" in the legs and trunk occurring as clusters of lancinating agony which can respond to carbamazepine 100 mg t.d.s., (2) laryngeal, gastric, rectal or bladder crises with pain concentrated upon a viscus, (3) areas of skin hyperaesthesia which gradually become hypoanaesthetic. These involve the nose and upper lip (Duchenne's tabetic mask), the breast plate area of the trunk, ulnar borders of the forearms and the fronts of the shins. Sensory loss mainly affects the lower limbs with (1) Romberg's sign of ataxia dependent on eye closure, (2) hyporeflexia, areflexia, and sluggish or absent plantar responses, (3) muscle hypotonia, (4) a sensation of walking on cotton wool, (5) impaired and delayed responses to Achilles tendon pressure, (6) neuropathic arthropathies producing Charcot's joints, and (7) trophic skin ulceration over pressure points.

Visceral sensory impairment can result in constipation, impotence, paralytic ileus or bladder retention, cysts and overflow. Clumsiness and pseudoathetosis may be present in the upper limbs. Involvement of sympathetic afferents may account for bilateral ptosis with compensatory puckering of the brows and synechial degeneration of the iris with adhesions causing the irregularity of the Argyll Robertson pupil. Ependymitis and gliosis, affecting the oculomotor fibres in the pretectal region dorsal to the Edinger Westphal nucleus, prevent the response to light but spare the ventral fibres which subserve accommodation (Harriman 1976). Treatment of tabes dorsalis is essentially symptomatic and does not affect the progression of the disease.

Neoplastic Meningomyelitis

The comparative frequency of neoplastic meningitis contrasts with the occasional finding of solitary leukaemic or lymphomatous deposits lodged within the meninges and with the exceedingly rare event of haematogenous metastases thriving within the spinal cord. Diffuse or multifocal infiltration of the leptomeninges by tumour cells can envelop the whole spinal cord, nerve roots and basal cisterns of the brain, with or without associated intraparenchymal lesions (Olsen et al. 1974). Apart from primary neuroectodermal tumours and haematopoietic malignancies, the other tumours that commonly lead to meningeal spread include primary lesions in the lung, breast, gastrointestinal tract and malignant melanoma (Moseley et al. 1989). In a series of 216 patients with malignant melanoma, leptomeningeal infiltration was seen in 24% of cases, thus occurring in 44% of patients with CNS metastatic disease (Patel et al. 1978). In a separate clinicopathological study, leptomeningeal metastases were seen at necropsy in 70% of those with CNS disease (Amer et al. 1978). Although the proportion of patients developing neoplastic meningitis from primary lesions elsewhere is much smaller than with malignant melanoma, the generalization can be made that neoplastic meningitis develops insidiously and some patients remain asymptomatic. Others develop root pains, sensory loss or paraparesis, and the progression can be potentially lethal, compressing, strangling or necrosing the cord.

Neoplastic meningitis may be apparent from myelography, CT scanning or MRI, and the CSF findings may mimic those of TB meningitis. Examination for mitotic cells in the CSF can be most helpful in the diagnosis and management of malignant disease even in the absence of a definite neoplastic meningitis. Unfortunately, conventional CSF cytological methods are frequently unsatisfactory with a reported rate of detection as low as 20% in some series (Bigner and Johston 1981). A frequent fault is to report malignant cells as lymphocytes. However, with the addition of monoclonal antibody immunocytology to conventional techniques, cytological accuracy is enhanced and the type of malignant cell can also be determined (Moseley et al. 1989).

Cord lesions secondary to neoplasia are uncommon. Intraparenchymal infiltration by leukaemic cells leading to a myelopathy and radiculopathy is recorded (Norris 1979) but of greater interest is the possibility of changes due to the remote effects of carcinoma. Acute or subacute necrotizing myelopathies with progressive glial involvement, a reactive astrocytosis and eventual necrosis may cause death from respiratory insufficiency. The other condition believed to be a remote effect of carcinoma is amyotrophic myelopathy. The neurological effects of this syndrome are usually indistinguishable from motor neurone disease (ALS) but in some patients fewer anterior horn cells are destroyed and there appears to be a cellular reaction verging on frank infiltration of the spared ventral horns and CNS ganglia (suggesting a definite similarity to poliomyelitis). The course is relatively benign (Norris 1979). Historically, the first association between malignancy and ALS involved gastric neoplasms but of the recorded cases over 80% arise from bronchial endothelium and reticuloendothelial tissue. Some improvement in the amyotrophy can follow successful removal of the neoplasm.

Acute Transverse Myelopathy

Myelopathy refers to pathology of the substance of the cord. The term, acute transverse myelopathy, is a useful anatomical formulation for disease syndromes involving the cord bilaterally, at or up to a horizontal segmental level which may lie in the sacral, lumbar, thoracic or cervical portion of the cord. The term also implies a monophasic illness with the onset of symptoms and signs developing over a period of 2 hours to 14 days and resulting in a diagnostic triad of: complete sensory loss below the level of involvement, an initially flaccid paraparesis or quadriparesis, and severe impairment of sphincter function.

Myelopathies may occur as part of a more widespread disease process. Where this is so, spinal cord involvement may accompany or be overshadowed by other manifestations such as encephalitis, peripheral neuropathy or polyradiculopathy. However, rapidly developing transverse lesions of the spinal cord, occurring as the sole manifestation of a disease process, often present a difficult diagnostic and therapeutic problem.

The probable diagnosis of acute transverse myelopathy is made more likely if there is a preceding history of an exanthema, vaccination or an upper respiratory tract infection. The alternative diagnosis of MS may be suggested if the patient has had previous neurological symptoms. With recurrent episodes, recurring at exactly the same level each time, a third diagnosis, namely a spinal arteriovenous malformation, is also possible. However, the immediate differential diagnosis is the exclusion of cord compression either from an intrinsic tumour or from an extradural tumour or abscess. Unless these conditions can be excluded beyond reasonable doubt, the definitive test is lumbar myelography. Unfortunately, examination of the spinal fluid without myelography provides little useful information.

Initially the cord lesion is limited longitudinally to a few segments and the full thickness of the cord is not usually involved. The lesion is not necessarily stable but may progress rostrally spreading as an ascending myelitis. Radiographic support for the diagnosis of acute transverse myelitis comes from the finding of a spinal cord of normal calibre; but this is not invariably so. With the rapid development of transverse myelopathy, oedematous swelling of the cord may trap and compress radicular veins within the cord causing further congestion so that the clinical level in effect marks the upper boundary of this drainage. Where swelling has occurred an attempt may be made to establish the nature of the lesions by MR imaging. But if this is not possible or the findings remain uncertain, surgical decompression and biopsy may be the only way to exclude other intrinsic lesions. Decompression rarely has an adverse effect on the course of the disease and has been used in the past to establish whether the disease has progressed to necrosis or if recovery is still possible.

Acute transverse myelopathy as an isolated event remains a relatively rare but probably underdiagnosed condition. Berman et al. (1981) found 62 patients who fulfilled the necessary diagnostic criteria in Israel over a 20-year period from 1955–1975; thus giving an incidence of 1.34 per million. Transverse myelitis (or myelopathy) is often classified as a demyelinative condition developing as a result of secondary non-specific hypersensitivity phenomena similar pathologically to the lesions of acute disseminated encephalomyopathy. In this form it may be indistinguishable from spinal multiple sclerosis; thus Lipton and Teasdall in 1973 reported a follow-up study of 34 patients: 7 of whom were diagnosed 5 to 42 years later as having multiple sclerosis. Nowadays the proportion developing multiple sclerosis can be further reduced by means of visual, auditory and upper limb somatosensory evoked potentials, by MR imaging or CT scanning of the brain or by MR imaging of the spinal cord.

Viral Aetiology

In recognizing that acute transverse myelography is essentially an anatomical formulation we recognize that there may be many disparate causes and that the natural history of one form may not coincide with another. Between 20% and 40%

of cases have a probable viral origin (Tyler et al. 1986) and represent the most typical picture of transverse myelitis. The diagnosis of a viral infection is never straightforward. In a classical paper (Wells 1971) investigated 19 patients from the Cardiff area of South Wales who had developed an acute neurological disorder with predominant spinal and radicular symptoms following an upper respiratory infection during the winter of 1969–1970. Serological tests showed that the infection was probably due to influenza A virus in eight cases and to other viruses (including adenovirus and herpes zoster) in six, while in five cases the studies were negative. It was not possible to isolate a virus or to culture it from the blood in any case. The interval between the onset of the febrile illness and the development of neurological complications varied from 1 to 112 days, and it was indeed so variable that it was difficult to draw any valid conclusions whether the neurological state resulted from direct viral invasion or from an autoimmune or hypersensitivity process, though the latter seemed more probable. It is also possible that some symbiosis between viruses can occur; thus Boiardi et al. (1986) reported the recurrence of herpes zoster myelitis in combination with a Coxsackie infection; and cases of transverse myelitis have been reported in the past during epidemics of poliomyelitis (Foley and Beresford 1974).

Transverse myelitis can develop over hours or days. The sequence of events is usually similar. Both sexes are equally affected and there is little variation with age. The most common site of affliction is the upper or mid-thoracic cord. There may be an acute pyrexia and radiculopathy or back pain localized over a few spinal segments, soon followed by symptoms of spinal cord transection. A low grade temperature may persist for several days. Bilateral paraesthesiae start in the feet and ascend with numbness and sensory impairment until a discrete sensory level is reached. Sphincter dysfunction occurs with urinary retention and loss of bowel control. There follows a progressive flaccid weakness of the lower limbs and abdominal muscles. With high dorsal lesions assisted ventilation is required. The paresis may remain flaccid if the spinal cord starts to necrose. More often the initial flaccid weakness gives way to an increasingly spastic paraplegia.

The CSF can be normal, or mildly abnormal with a pleocytosis and a slightly raised protein. Occasionally it is frankly xanthochromic with high level of protein often exceeding 10 g/l and up to 200 lymphocytes. Such abnormal findings usually occur when the onset is apoplectic. A clinical state of spinal shock develops, as seen after traumatic transection, and the cord becomes oedematous. The presence of an acute spinal block may be confirmed by myelography, with or without CT, but the differential diagnosis is more clearly revealed by MRI which may give an abnormal signal over the full extent of the lesion.

With milder degrees of myelopathy, not affecting the full thickness of the cord, various patterns of sensory loss may be seen. Thus vibration and joint position sensation may be spared suggesting that there has been segmental occlusion of the anterior spinal artery. Occlusion of the anterior spinal artery mainly involves anterior horn cells and corticospinal tracts; spinothalamic sensation is lost at the beginning but tends to recover and dorsal column sensation is spared. It may also be difficult to differentiate transverse myelopathy from an acute ascending polyradiculopathy unless an ascending sensory level is present on the trunk thereby indicating that the spinal cord is affected. As with acute disseminated encephalomyelitis, the pathology of the cord can vary from patchy perivenous demyelination to a severe necrotizing, haemorrhagic form. The cord may appear oedematous and hyperaemic with perivascular cuffing, arteritis and yet more extensive vascular involvement, and there may be an inflammatory cellular exudation involving the leptomeninges.

There is a tendency to compare the natural history of acute transverse myelopathy with that of an isolated spinal plaque of MS with recovery within approximately six weeks. Such a supposition can be very misleading. Full recovery is not invariable: Lipton and Teasdall (1973) reported a mortality of 14.5%, a reasonable recovery may occur in just over 33% often spread over three or more months, with residual deficits in about 25% (Berman et al. 1981; Lancet 1986); 23% progress to the Foix-Alajouanine syndrome (Foix and Alajouanine 1926) of subacute necrosis of the spinal cord (Berman et al. 1981).

After the initial stage the majority of patients pass to a stable plateau phase lasting days or weeks before proceeding imperceptibly into a phase of recovery. Improvement may take place over several months, often with a mild residual disability which fails to clear. Those who fail to make a good recovery may develop osteomalacia with necrotic softening and cavitation of the whole extent of the cord below the lesion. Once this occurs further recovery is unlikely. A small number of patients make a delayed but complete functional recovery apart from the persistence of hyperreflexia and extensor plantar responses.

Three mechanisms have been postulated to explain the viral pathogenesis of acute transverse myelopathy:

1. Viral invasion of the spinal cord – the mechanism which most probably explains myelopathy in AIDS
2. A toxic myelopathy – extremely hard to prove or disprove
3. A delayed hypersensitivity reaction – this is the most probable explanation of myelopathy following vaccination (Bitzen 1987)

Of the neurotropic viruses, the DNA viruses are more prone to cause myelopathy than the RNA viruses. Table 18.1 shows those included in causing myelitis in humans.

Table 18.1. Viruses which cause myelitis in humans

DNA viruses	
Enveloped:	Herpes viruses (simplex, simiae, varicella-zoster), Epstein-Barr and cytomegalovirus
	Pox viruses: vaccinia and variola
Non-enveloped:	Hepatitis B
RNA viruses	
Non-enveloped:	Picornaviruses: Coxsackie, ECHO, polio
	Other enteroviruses: hepatitis A, encephalomyocarditis virus
Enveloped:	Togaviruses: arborviruses, tick-borne encephalitis, rubella
	Retroviruses: HTLV-1, HTLV-111 (HIV)
	Orthomyxoviruses: influenza
	Paramyxoviruses: measles, mumps
	Bunyaviruses: Californian encephalitis
	Arenaviruses: lymphocytic choriomeningitis
	Rhabdoviruses: rabies

(After Tyler et al. 1986.)

Herpes Viruses

These are most commonly incriminated in sporadic cases. Broadbent (1866) described muscle wasting with zoster infections. As the intercostal muscles are most frequently involved, wasting may be difficult to quantify clinically. Zoster myelopathy can lead to dysfunction of the bladder and anus (Jellinek and Tulloch 1976). The authors emphasize that severe sphincter disturbances, e.g. retention, loss of sensation, or incontinence are the result of bilateral lesions; thus hemisection of the spinal cord does not cause sphincter problems. Recovery is usually complete and the segmental distribution of any rash does not necessarily coincide with the level of myelopathy. Retention may occur with thoracic or lumbar lesions, and sacral involvement may be accompanied by sensory loss and a flaccid detrusor paralysis. Herpes zoster infections can be unpredictable, remaining dormant until another viral infection reduces the body's resistance; and myelopathy can be a feature of symptomatic herpes zoster infections, e.g. developing at the site of trauma, a metastatic deposit or a prolapsed intervertebral disc.

Acute necrotizing myelitis has been a frequent complication of herpes simiae infection in laboratory workers, less commonly with herpes simplex infection. It is particularly prone to occur in immune-compromised individuals. Clinically a rapidly progressive myelitis with necrotizing arteritis is found with Cowdray type A inclusions or HSV 2 antigens within the spinal cord (Wiley et al. 1987). Some cases have followed a viraemia provoking a severe inflammatory response to the viral infection and in others there is evidence of virus dissemination from intra-axonal spread into the spinal cord from the dorsal root ganglia.

Other Viruses

Immunosuppression in the recipients of renal transplants can lead to disseminated cytomegalovirus infection with acute transverse myelopathy (Spitzer et al. 1987). Rubella myelitis has been reported in conjunction with encephalitis in children and confirmed by MR imaging (Bitzen 1987). Rubella virus specific IgM has been detected in serum and spinal fluid using ELISA Rubazyme M. Likewise the Epstein–Barr virus has been identified by the direct fluorescent antibody test.

A syndrome primarily involving the bladder with acute but transient urinary retention can arise from sacral myeloradiculitis (Vanneste et al. 1980; Herbaut et al. 1987). It may be associated with anogenital herpes simplex infections, but non-herpetic causes include ECHO, cytomegaloviruses and Epstein–Barr viral infections. The differential diagnosis includes multiple sclerosis and disc protrusions.

Following Vaccination

Myelopathy may complicate smallpox vaccination (Shyamalan and Singh 1964), pertussis immunization, and rabies vaccination. The incidence of postvaccinal encephalomyelitis was between 1 in 5000 and 1 in 2000 000 vaccinations. Post-vaccinal encephalomyelitis was rare in infancy but more liable to occur with primary vaccination between the ages of 4–16 than with secondary vaccination. After an incubation period of 8–15 days the onset is abrupt or explosive with encephalitic symptoms. A flaccid paralysis from transverse myelitis was more frequently observed than hemiplegia. Survivors are said to make a complete recovery but Miller (1953) recognized numerous mild residual deficits.

Neuroparalytic accidents used to occur in 1 in 1000 to 1 in 4000 patients treated with anti-rabies vaccines. An acute disseminated encephalomyelitic reaction would occur because all three anti-rabies vaccines – Pasteur, Semple and even duck embryo vaccines – contain myelin (Behan and Currie 1978). Until vaccines were grown on duck embryos or tissue culture, patients received a lengthy course of repeated inoculations with an emulsion of animal nervous tissues containing dead or attenuated rabies virus. A monophasic illness would develop suddenly after an incubation period of 1–3 months and run a downhill course with a mortality of 30%. The condition could be almost indistinguishable from MS with dense plaques of demyelination scattered asymmetrically throughout the neuraxis (Matthews and Miller 1972). At other times the clinical picture resembled the Guillain–Barré syndrome with an ascending myelitis, transverse myelitis usually in the thoracic or lumbar segments, or a polyradiculitis with facial nerve involvement (Adaros and Held 1971; Toro et al. 1977). In no case are Negri bodies present.

Parasitic Infections

Schistosomiasis has been the most frequently reported cause of an acute tropical myelopathy (Kerr et al. 1987; Suchet et al. 1987) The eggs of *Schistosoma haematobium* and S. mansoni may lodge as emboli in the blood vessels of the cord and in infested areas there is probably much asymptomatic or unrecognized spinal cord involvement. However, symptoms may result from:

1. Vascular syndromes, e.g. anterior spinal artery occlusion
2. Granulomata around spinal roots or the cauda equina
3. Multiple small granulomata within the cord surrounding one or more eggs
4. Larger granulomata microscopically resembling gliomata

The lower lumbar and sacral regions of the spinal cord are most likely to be infected and widening of the conus has been reported radiologically (Kerr et al. 1987). Patients may present with wasting, fasciculation, back pain and distal weakness. The condition has been successfully treated with praziquantel, either given with steroids or in conjunction with oxamniquine and niridazole.

Another reported tropical cause of myelopathy is larva migrans (Weng et al. 1987). The diagnosis can be made on the clinical course of the disease and the finding of eosinophilia, serum IgE, raised CSF IgG and IgA and the presence of larvae in the CSF.

Collagen Vascular Disease

Spinal cord damage in collagen vascular diseases can occur as a result of thrombosed arteries or veins, or from microscopic haemorrhages. A true myelopathy can also result from a vasculopathy with proliferative changes involving small blood vessels. Transverse myelitis can occur in mixed connective tissue disease in the presence of antibodies to ribonucleoprotein (anti-RNP) (Pedersen et al. 1987) or, more commonly, in systemic lupus erythematosus (SLE). In SLE the vascular changes may be associated with demyelination or with areas of gliosis with associated perivascular collections of mononuclear cells and deposits of immune complexes and reactive (antineuronal) antibodies, also present in the CSF and plasma (Siebold et al. 1982; Kaye et al. 1987). Some cases, particularly in childhood, may be related to immune deficiency syndromes (Kaye et al. 1987).

Transverse myelitis may occasionally be the first manifestation of lupus erythematosus (Siekert and Clark 1955; Granger 1960) but the total number of reported cases does not exceed 40. The spinal cord is most vulnerable to damage in the event of an exacerbation of the underlying disease (Andrews et al. 1970). The most common neurological level is mid-thoracic in 60% (Hachen and Chantraine 1979–1980) and an abnormal signal may be obtained over a wide area by MR imaging (Kenik et al. 1987). In the vast majority of patients the paraplegia is complete and irreversible and multiple zones of myelomalacia in both grey and white matter with fibrinoid degeneration of arterioles may be present post mortem. Myelopathy at cervical (20%) or lumbar (20%) levels tends to be less severe with only partial motor and sensory loss (Piper 1953; Andrianakos et al. 1975).

In 3 of the 40 patients reported in the literature (April and VanSonnenberg 1976), systemic lupus sclerosis was combined with Devic's syndrome of neuromyelitis optica. Demyelination of white matter in SLE is a relatively rare finding. However, demyelinating plaques in MS display an outer ring of immune complexes and the overlapping condition of lupus sclerosis is well described where the levels of immunoglobulins in the CSF are particularly high.

The results of treatment of SLE myelopathy with high dosage corticosteroids have been disappointing. A slow recovery occurred in only three paraplegic patients and in one quadriplegic patient from a total of 26 (Andrianakos et al. 1975). Anecdotally, chloroquine has been successful in the treatment of one patient (Granger 1960). Slovick (1986) advocated the use of plasma exchange and immunosuppression and reported the successful treatment of one patient.

Transverse Myelopathy Related to Acute Disseminated Encephalomyelitis

Myelopathy occurring in conjunction with the Guillain–Barré syndrome of allergic, postinfective peripheral neuropathy or polyradiculopathy, confirms the hypothesis that many forms of transverse myelopathy can arise as a result of a cell-mediated response. The violence of this response may vary from perivenous demyelination to a severe necrotizing myelopathy. The clinical diagnosis of an accompanying myelopathy may not be easy but is suggested by the development of extensor plantar responses and severe sphincter disturbances.

In Devic's disease bilateral retrobulbar or optic neuritis with massive demyelination of the optic nerves may be followed after a few months by similar massive demyelination of the spinal cord. Thereafter the disease may be self-limiting or run a progressive downward course (Walton 1977). Demyelinating lesions, often with destruction of axis cylinders, are seen elsewhere in the neuraxis and there is a distinct tendency to necrosis and cavity formation within the spinal cord. Many remain unconvinced that Devic's disease is a distinct pathological entity (Hughes 1978).

In subacute myelo-optico-neuropathy (SMON) diarrhoea and abdominal pain are followed by the acute or subacute onset of an ascending sensory neuropathy spreading over the lower half of the body, accompanied in two-thirds of those affected by an ataxic gait. Half the patients also develop motor weakness in the lower limbs. Myelopathy or neuropathy with or without optic atrophy occurs in 26.2% of non-Japanese patients (Thomas 1984). The disease was originally thought to be a viral disorder but clioquinol toxicity is now incriminated as the causal agent. Yagi et al. (1978) found that the neurotoxicity of clioquinol depends on decomposition of the conjugated form and chelation with iron and other metals. When a concentration of free clioquinol in serum of 20 μg/ml has been maintained for several days (Tamura 1975) the drug is taken up in chelated form by neural tissue where it produces destructive peroxidases (Yagi et al. 1978). The simultaneous ingestion of drugs containing aluminium, calcium, magnesium, copper and bismuth will produce different chelates. Different combinations can affect the clinical severity of the disorder (Okada et al. 1984).

Myelopathy can also result from toxicity from other drugs: heavy metal poisoning, arsphenamine, paraquin, orthocresyl phosphate; drugs injected into the subarachnoid space, e.g. penicillin; or contrast agents used in aortography.

An allergic myelopathy can develop from scorpion stings, hymenoptera stings and spider bites (Rosenberg and Coull 1982). The venom of some scorpion species contains powerful neurotoxins capable of producing paralysis of the hind limbs and respiratory muscles of laboratory animals. Such findings fuel speculation that myelopathy in man may result from a direct neurotoxic effect as an alternative to a secondary immune-mediated response.

Ischaemic myelopathy is a recognized complication of anterior spinal artery occlusion, circulatory arrest as from clamping of the aorta, or Stokes–Adams attacks. Myelopathy following burns, heat stroke or trauma could be due to similar anoxic changes as a consequence of ischaemia, disseminated intravascular coagulopathy or electrolyte imbalance (Delgado et al. 1985). Alternatively, there may be an allergic response to the release of altered proteins into the circulation producing an autoimmune reaction within the spinal cord.

Opiates

Myelopathy has been described among heroin addicts. The circumstances of drug addiction, particularly when intravenous drugs are taken, favour both sepsis and thromboembolism. These factors require exclusion before a direct toxic effect on the spinal cord is accepted (Hughes 1978). Ell et al. (1981) list hypotension, toxic or hyper-sensitivity reactions, reactions to contaminants or to the heroin itself, vasculitis, embolism and hyperextension injury among the factors which may be involved and suggest that the most usual causative factor is an adulterant taken with the heroin. In favour of a hypersensitivity reaction is the fact that some cases have occurred after a period of abstinence (Ell et al. 1981). The chances of recovery are uniformly poor.

Treatment of Myelopathies

In many ways the least satisfactory aspect of acute transverse myelopathy is its treat-ment and the prevention of complications. A proportion of all types of myelopathy can improve spontaneously but an attempt should be made to determine the under-lying pathology and treat accordingly. Where specific agents can be given, e.g. acyclovir for herpes simplex or zoster, or praziquantel for myelopathy following schistosomiasis, there can be a reasonable expectation of improvement. Corticosteroids are potentially indicated where the cause of the myelopathy is unknown, where there is a possibility of a collagen disease, or an allergic reactive state (i.e. a hypersensitivity reaction). The results of steroid therapy remain uncer-tain and their efficacy has yet to be established. Early treatment with methyl-prednisolone has not been evaluated and should be tried as early as possible in the disease unless there is a clear alternative form of treatment available.

If the cord appears swollen it is advisable to perform a diagnostic decompression and biopsy and to follow this with dexamethasone. Acyclovir and similar drugs may be used in AIDS myelopathies where viruses other than HIV are implicated. Antibiotics, if necessary covered by steroids, should be used in myelopathy with meningovascular syphilis. In other situations, as with collagen vascular disease, Slovick's suggestion (1986) of a combination of plasma exchange and immuno suppression should be considered.

Spinal Multiple Sclerosis

Multiple sclerosis is a disease of the CNS and lesions are characteristically distrib-uted in time and space. In established disease it is rare for the spinal cord not to be involved. Among the manifestations recorded in patients with MS examined at autopsy, 98% will have developed paresis of the lower limbs, spasticity and hyperreflexia, 82% will have had urinary disturbances and 65% paraesthesiae such as episodes of numbness or a positive Lhermitte's phenomenon. The occurrence of MS limited to the spinal cord is probably rare but plaques seen only in the spinal cord are found occasionally in patients at autopsy. However, lesions of the spinal cord are the presenting feature in at least one-third of patients with MS (Shibasaki et al. 1981). In many it may be possible to confirm the diagnosis by finding evidence of silent lesions elsewhere, e.g. by visual evoked potentials or MR imaging. The finding of a lesion elsewhere merely increases the probability that the spinal cord manifestation is due to MS; it never constitutes absolute proof. The diagnosis of spinal MS depends upon the clinical presentation, the finding of confirmatory evidence and exclusion of alternative diagnoses, and increasingly upon supportive evidence from oligoclonal banding in the CSF, somatosensory evoked potentials and MR imaging of the cervical cord. At present none of these sophisticated investigations provide absolute proof of the diagnosis.

Among the highly characteristic presenting manifestations are:

1. Intermittent weakness of a leg occurring either on exertion with dragging of the foot after prolonged activity or as a paroxysmal symptom with sudden loss of power causing unexpected falls, locking of the knees or collapse of the legs.

2. About 10% of patients presenting with acute transverse myelopathy are found to have MS (Poser 1984). This may take one of three characteristic forms: as a partial Brown–Séquard syndrome, as a spastic paraplegia with negative myelography, or as numbness below the waist with sphincter disturbance and loss of vaginal sensation often improving spontaneously before myelography is possible.

3. As a chronic myelopathy or progressive spastic paraparesis. This may be the presenting form of the condition in middle age and in the elderly (Noseworthy et al. 1983). The differential diagnosis may include cord compression, cervical spondylosis or familial or sporadic forms of spastic paraparesis.

4. Paroxysmal phenomena such as Lhermitte's sign or unilateral spasms of limbs which are often painful with the limb "kicking out" or adopting a brief tetanic posture.

5. Isolated bladder disturbances, e.g. retention, urgency, or hesitancy of micturition; impairment of sex functions or, rarely, bowel dysfunction. Usually MS can only be diagnosed by exclusion.

6. Uncertain or bizarre paraesthesiae, hemianaesthesia or intermittent weakness or clumsiness. Some of these symptoms may have an allergic basis or even suggest hysteria. It is often wiser to regard them as due to an allergic neuritis unless there is positive proof of MS.

MR imaging of the cervical spinal cord to identify plaques is possible but difficult. Longitudinal (sagittal or coronal) cuts are more likely to be of value than axial cuts because of the longitudinal arrangement of plaques as seen post mortem. The cervical spinal cord is small compared to the brain stem or cerebrum and requires high imaging resolution but the signal to noise ratio can be improved by the use of surface coils (Maravilla et al. 1984). The thoracic and lumbar cord is almost impossible to image because of its smaller size and the presence of respiratory and cardiac movement artefact.

The differentiation of progressive spastic paraplegia due to MS from familial spastic paraparesis depends upon finding lesions at MR imaging, or delayed visual evoked potentials. A relative lymphocytosis in the CSF with a raised IgG, oligoclonal bands, or the presence of HLA DR2 antigen increases the likelihood of MS. Somatosensory evoked potentials from upper or lower limbs can be abnormal with either condition and although it is often worth trying the response to steroids over 4–6 weeks, this is an unreliable factor in making a differential diagnosis.

References

Adaros HL, Held JR (1971) Guillain–Barré syndrome associated with immunization against rabies: epidemiological aspects. In: Rowland LP (ed) Immunological disorders of the nervous system. Williams and Wilkins Co, Baltimore, pp 178–186

Addy DP (1987) When to do a lumbar puncture. Arch Dis Child 62:873–875

Al Deeb SM, Yaqub BA, Sharif HS, Phadke JG (1989) Neuro-brucellosis: clinical characteristics, diagnosis and outcome. Neurology 39:498–501

Amer MH, Al-Sarraf M, Baker LH, Vaitkevicius UK (1978) Malignant melanoma and central nervous system metastases. Incidence, diagnosis, treatment and survival. Cancer 42:660–668

Andrews JM, Cancilla PA, Kunin J (1970) Progressive spinal cord signs in a patient with disseminated lupus erythematosus. Bull Los Angeles Neurol Soc 35:78–85

Andrianakos AA, Duffy J, Suzuki M, Sharp JT (1975) Transverse myelopathy in systemic lupus erythematosus: report of 3 cases and a review of the literature. Ann Intern Med 83:616–625

April RS, VanSonnenberg E (1976) A case of neuromyelitis optica (Devic's syndrome) in systemic lupus erythematosus: clinicopathologic report and a review of the literature. Neurology 26:1066–1070

Behan PO, Currie S (1978) Clinical neurovirology. Saunders, London

Berman M, Feldman S, Alter M, Zilker N, Kahama E (1981) Acute transverse myelitis: incidence and etiologic considerations. Neurology 31:966–971

Bigner SH, Johnston WW (1981) Cytopathology of cerebrospinal fluid. Acta Cytol 25:461–479

Bitzen M (1987) Rubella myelitis and encephalitis in childhood: report of 2 cases with magnetic resonance imaging. Neuropaediatrics 18:84–87

Boiardi A, Ferrante E, Porta E, Sghirlanzoni A, Bussone G (1986) Herpes zoster myelitis: nervous system complications. Ital J Neurol Sci 7:617–622

Broadbent WW (1866) Zoster infections of the nervous system. Br Med J i:460

Brown K, Steer C (1986) Strategies in the management of children with acute encephalitis. In: Gordon N, McKinlay I (eds) Neurologically sick children, treatment and management. Blackwell, Oxford, pp 219–293

Critchley EMR (1988) Neurological emergencies. Saunders, London

Delgado G, Tundu T, Gallago J, Villenerva JA (1985) Spinal cord lesions in heat stroke. J Neurol Neurosurg Psychiatry 48:1065–1067

Ell JJ, Uttley D, Silver JR (1981) Acute myelopathy in association with heroin addiction. J Neurol Neurosurg Psychiatry 44:448–450

Foix C, Alajouanine T (1926) La myelite necrotique subaigue. Rev Neurol 2:1–42

Foley KM, Beresford HR (1974) Acute poliomyelitis beginning as transverse myelopathy. Arch Neurol 30:182–183

Granger DP (1960) Transverse myelitis with recovery: the only manifestation of systemic lupus erythematosus. Neurology 10:325–329

Hachen H, Chantraine A (1979–80) Spinal involvement in systemic lupus erythematosus. Paraplegia 17:337–346

Harriman DGF (1976) Infective diseases of the central nervous system. In: Blackwood W, Corseilles JAN (eds) Greenfield's neuropathology. Arnold, London, pp 238–268

Herbaut AG, Voordecker P, Monseu G, Germeau F (1987) Benign transient urinary retention. J Neurol Neurosurg Psychiatry 50:354–355

Hughes JT (1978) Pathology of the spinal cord, 2nd edn. Lloyd-Luke, London

Jellinek EH, Tulloch WS (1976) Herpes zoster with dysfunction of bladder and anus. Lancet 2:1219–1222

Kaye EM, Butler IJ, Conley S (1987) Myelopathy in neonatal and infantile lupus erythematosus. J Neurol Neurosurg Psychiatry 50:923–926

Kenik JG, Krohn K, Kelly RB, Bierman M, Hammeke MD (1987) Transverse myelitis and optic neuritis in systemic lupus erythematosus: a case report with magnetic resonance imaging findings. Arthritis Rheum 30:947–950

Kerr RSC, Marks SM, Sheldon PWE, Teddy PJ (1987) *Schistosomiasis mansoni* in the spinal cord: a correlation between operative and radiological findings. J Neurol Neurosurg Psychiatry 50:822–823

Lancet (1986) Acute transverse myelopathy. Lancet 1:20–21 (leading article)

Lipton HL, Teasdall RD (1973) Acute transverse myelitis in adults: a follow-up study. Arch Neurol 28:252–257

Maravilla KR, Wemret JC, Suss R, Nunnally R (1984) Magnetic resonance demonstration of multiple sclerosis plaques in the cervical cord. Am J Neuroradiol 5:685–689

Matthews WB, Miller H (1972) Diseases of the nervous system. Blackwell, Oxford

Miller HG (1953) Prognosis of neurologic illness following vaccination against smallpox. Arch Neurol 69:695–706

Moseley RP, Davies AG, Bourne SP, et al. (1989) Neoplastic meningitis in malignant melanoma: diagnosis with monoclonal antibodies. J Neurol Neurosurg Psychiatry 52:881–886

Newton RW (1987) Intracranial pressure and its monitoring in childhood: a review. J R Soc Med 80:566–570

Norris FH (1979) Neurological manifestations of systemic disease. In: Vinken PJ, Bruyn GW (eds) Handbook of clinical neurology, vol 38. North Holland, Amsterdam, pp 669–677

Noseworthy J, Paty DW, Wonnacott J, Feasby T, Ebergs G (1983) Multiple sclerosis after the age of 50. Neurology 33:1537–1544

Okada H, Aoki K, Ohno Y, Kitazawa S, Ohtani M (1984) Effects of metal containing drugs taken simultaneously with clioquinol upon clinical features of SMON. J Toxicol Sci 9:371–404

Olsen C, Chernik N, Posner J (1974) Infiltration of the leptomeninges by systemic cancer. A clinical and pathological study. Arch Neurol 30:122–137

Patel JK, Didolkar MS, Pickren JW, Moore RH (1978) Metastatic pattern of malignant melanoma. A study of 216 autopsy cases. Am J Surg 135:807–810

Pedersen C, Bonen H, Boesen F (1987) Transverse myelitis in mixed connective tissue disease. Clin Rheumatol 6:290–292

Piper PG (1953) Disseminated lupus erythematosus with involvement of the spinal cord. JAMA 153:215–217

Poser CM (1984) Taxonomy and diagnostic parameters in multiple sclerosis. Ann NY Acad Sci 436:233–245

Rich AR (1952) The pathogenesis of tuberculosis. Thomas, Springfield, Illinois

Roman GC (1987) Retrovirus associated myelopathies. Arch Neurol 44:659–663

Rosenberg NL, Coull BM (1982) Myelopathy after scorpion sting. Arch Neurol 39:127

Shibasaki H, McDonald WI, Kuroiwa Y (1981) Racial modification of clinical picture of multiple sclerosis: comparison between British and Japanese patients. J Neurol Sci 49:253–271

Shyamalan NC, Singh SS (1964) Transverse myelitis after vaccination. Br Med J i:434–435

Siebold JR, Buckingham RD, Medsger JA, Kelly RA (1982) Cerebrospinal immune complexes in systemic lupus erythematosus involving the central nervous system. Semin Arthritis Rheum 12:68–76

Siekert RG, Clark EC (1955) Neurologic signs and symptoms as early manifestations of systemic lupus erythematosus. Neurology 5:84–88

Slovick DI (1986) Treatment of acute myelopathy in systemic lupus erythematosus with plasma exchange and immunosuppression. J Neurol Neurosurg Psychiatry 49:103–105

Spitzer PG, Tarsy D, Eliopoulos GM (1987) Acute transverse myelitis during disseminated cytomegalovirus infection in a renal transplant recipient. Transplantation 44:151–153

Suchet I, Klein C, Horwitz T, Lalla S, Doodha M (1987) Spinal cord schistosomiasis: a case report and review of the literature. Paraplegia 25:491–496

Tamura Z (1975) Clinical chemistry of clioquinol. Jpn J Med Sci Biol 28:(suppl) 68–77

Tandon PN, Pathak SN (1973) Tuberculosis of the central nervous system. In: Spillane JD (ed) Tropical neurology, Oxford University Press, Oxford, pp 37–51

Thomas PK (1984) Neurotoxicity of halogenated hydroxyquinolones: non-Japanese cases. Acta Neurol Scand 70:(suppl 100) 155–158

Toro G, Vergara I, Roman G (1977) Neuroparalytic accidents of antirabies vaccination with suckling mouse brain vaccine. Arch Neurol 34:694–700

Tyler KL, Gross RA, Cascino GD (1986) Unusual viral causes of transverse myelitis: hepatitis A virus and cytomegalovirus. Neurology 36:855–858

Vannesse JAL, Karthaus PPM, Davies G (1980) Acute urinary retention due to sacral myeloradiculitis. J Neurol Neurosurg Psychiatry 43:954–956

Walton JN (1977) Brain's diseaes of the nervous system. Churchill Livingstone, London

Wells CEC (1971) Neurological complications of so-called "influenza": a winter study in south-east Wales. Br Med J i:369–373

Weng C, Huang CY, Chan PH, Preston P, Chen PY (1987) Transverse myelitis associated with larva migrans: finding of larvae in cerebrospinal fluid. Lancet 1:423

Wiley CA, Van Patten PD, Carpenter PM, Powell HC, Thal LJ (1987) Acute ascending necrotizing myelopathy caused by herpes simplex virus type 2. Neurology 37:1791–1794

Wood M, Anderson M (1988) Neurological infections. Saunders, London

Yagi K, Ohishi S, Ohtsuka K (1978) Effects of clioquinol on the cultured retinal nerve cells. Reports of SMON research commission, 94–96. (in Japanese, quoted by Okada et al. 1984)

Chapter 19

Myelopathies in HIV Infection

R.J. Guiloff

Myelopathies are seen clinically in about 7% of AIDS cases (McArthur 1987; Guiloff et al. 1988) and pathologically in 40%–50% of AIDS post mortems (Henin et al. 1992) but they are far less frequent in children (Sharer et al. 1990). The commonest is vacuolar myelopathy, an entity of unknown aetiology. Other myelopathies include infection by HIV-1, opportunistic infections, tumours, vascular lesions and myelopathies unrelated to HIV disease. Overall these other myelopathies are, as a group, as frequent as vacuolar myelopathy. Reasons for the lower clinical than pathological incidence include coexisting peripheral nerve or intracranial disease masking the signs of myelopathy, absence of clinical signs in cases with mild or moderate pathological change and failure to make the clinical diagnosis of vascular myelopathy in cases without weakness or spasticity or without the typical combination of pyramidal and posterior column signs.

Vacuolar Myelopathy

Initial reports (Snider et al. 1983; Goldstick et al. 1985) were followed by a definitive histological descriptions of 20 patients in a series of 89 AIDS post mortems (Petito et al. 1985). It usually occurs late in HIV infection when there is a CD4 count of less than $200/\mu$l. The presentation is with a slowly progressive spastic paraparesis or, less frequently, lower limb monoparesis or a tetraparesis, with brisk deep tendon reflexes, extensor plantar responses and impaired or absent vibration sense and position sense. A sensory ataxic gait, with a Romberg sign and symptoms of urgency, frequency of micturition and urinary incontinence are frequent. There was an associated dementia due to HIV-1 encephalopathy in 14 of the 20 patients in Petitio et al.'s (1985) series but there was no relation between the severities of the dementia and the myelopathy. Some patients have an associated distal sensory peripheral neuropathy also common in the late stages of HIV infection. In the initial stages of the myelopathy, there may be only exaggerated tendon jerks in the lower limbs or extensor plantar responses, without weakness or sensory signs. The patient may need a stick or become wheelchair bound after a few months, but in others the condition may arrest without leading to substantial disability.

The clinical picture resembles subacute combined degeneration of the cord due to vitamin B_{12} deficiency but there is no evidence that the myelopathy is due to a deficit of this vitamin. The differential diagnosis also includes cervical spondylotic myelopathy and rarer causes of cervical/dorsal cord compression, neurosyphilis and multiple sclerosis. The CSF is usually normal though the protein may be moderately elevated. Magnetic resonance imaging of the spinal cord is usually unremarkable.

Vacuolar myelopathy is characterized pathological by intramyelinic and periax-onal vacuoles (Petito et al. 1985; Maier et al. 1989). The white matter vacuolation and gliosis affects mostly the posterior and lateral columns, and less so the anterior columns, particularly in the middorsal region (Tan et al. 1995). The pathology and clinical features are not specific to HIV infection and have been described in other immunodeficiency states (Kamin and Petito 1991). Macrophages and microglia can be found in the vacuoles and may play a role in the pathogenesis by releasing cytokines, such as tumour necrosis factor alpha, that can damage the myelin (Tayor et al. 1993; Tan et al. 1996). The stimulus for such release may be infection or activa-tion by HIV-1 of microglia, multinucleated giant cells, macrophages, endothelial cells and glia. A toxic effect on myelin of the HIV-1 envelope protein gp120, which is expressed by macrophages, is also possible. A cellular deficiency of B_{12} due to increased demand might also operate (Tan et al. 1995). There is no good evidence of a direct role of HIV-1.The presence of HIV-1 antigen, RNA or DNA in the spinal cord does not correlate with the presence and severity of vacuolar myelopathy (Petito et al. 1994).

There is no effective treatment. Antispastic drugs such as baclofen, dantrolene and diazepam, and drugs for spastic bladder (oxybutinin) are helpful to control the symptoms.

Myelopathies Directly Related to HIV-1

Seroconversion

Denning et al. (1987) have described a case with a spastic paraparesis, lancinating back pain, and slow mentation that developed 22 days after a seroconversion illness due to primary HIV infection and that improved partially over about two months. The CSF showed mild mononuclear pleocytosis, slightly raised protein, intrathecal HIV IgG antibody and normal glucose. HIV was isolated from the CSF and serum but it is not clear whether the CSF HIV IgG antibody was the result of intrathecal production or was passively transferred from the serum.

HIV-1 Myelitis

In a number of patients, with or without vacuolar myelopathy, there is histopatho-logical evidence of multiple scattered foci of microglial nodules, multinucleated giant cells, macrophages, microglia and some lymphocytic infiltrates. Multi-nucleated giant cells, which are normally infected with HIV-1, are the hallmark of HIV-1 encephalitis and their presence also defines the above inflammatory abnormalities as HIV-1 myelitis (Budka et al. 1988; Grafe and Wiley 1989). There are as yet insufficient clinical descriptions for this well-established pathological picture. One patient is said to have had a flaccid paraparesis of subacute onset with urinary retention, depressed ankle jerks, extensor plantar responses and no sensory signs. The patient was confused and febrile. The CSF showed a protein of 0.63 g/l, normal glucose and 10 lymphocytes and a myelogram was normal. He had evidence of multiple small necrotic foci in both hemispheres and cerebellum due to toxoplasmosis. There were also necrotic foci and multinucleated giant cells in the cord, but *Toxoplasma gondii* was not identified in these. The authors felt that the changes were similar to those of "multifocal giant cell leukoencephalitis" (Geny et al. 1991).

Opportunistic Infections

The most frequent are viral, particularly cytomegalovirus.

Cytomegalovirus (CMV)

This usually causes an acute or subacute ascending radiculomyelitis but a pure myelopathy has also been described (Moskowitz et al. 1984; Vinters et al. 1989). The clinical and pathological incidence in AIDS cases is between 1% and 3%. It occurs in the late stages of the disease, with low CD4 counts but it can be the presentation of AIDS (Mahieux et al. 1989). Evidence of other CMV infections such as retinitis, pneumonitis, colitis, or oesophagitis may or may not be present. It normally starts with lumbosacral root involvement with early micturition difficulty or urinary retention, constipation, back pain often with radiation to the buttocks and thighs, reduced tone and weakness in the lower limbs with loss of tendon reflexes and sensory loss in sacral dermatomes. The upper limbs are initially spared but an ascending course usually follows, with spread of the CMV from the cauda equina to the substance of the cord producing a necrotic myelitis and subsequently an encephalitis with ventriculitis and brainstem and hemisphere involvement. A fatal outcome is likely within 4–8 weeks if untreated. The diagnosis is made by the characteristic clinical features and CSF, the latter typically shows a polymorphonuclear pleocytosis (up to 1500 cells), raised protein and low sugar. Cultures are usually negative but CMV may sometimes be found in CSF (Fuller et al. 1990; Miller et al. 1990) and blood. Imaging may be normal or show thickened or enhancing roots in the cauda equina (de Gans et al. 1990).

EMG and nerve studies may demonstrate delayed or absent F waves, loss of sensory nerve action potentials and acute partial denervation in the lower limbs.

A number of reports suggest that ganciclovir (10 mg/kg/day in the induction phase, 5 mg/kg twice a week as maintenance) may arrest disease progression and that improvement, usually partial, may occur after several weeks, particularly in those in whom treatment is initiated early (Fuller et al. 1990; Miller et al. 1990; Cohen et al. 1993).

Pathologically there is major involvement of the cauda equina and a myelitis more marked in the lumbosacral region with necrosis, Cowdry type inclusion-bearing cells, microglial nodules, inflammatory infiltrates with macrophages and lympho-cytes and microvascular thrombosis. In milder cases there may be no necrosis but only CMV inclusion-bearing cells and microglial nodules. There is usually dissemi-nation of the CMV infection with meningoencephalitis and ventriculitis. In treated patients with prolonged survival, there may be diffuse gliosis in the spinal cord (Fuller et al. 1990).

Herpes Zoster

Only a few cases of myelitis have been reported in AIDS patients though herpes zoster radiculopathy, particularly in the thoracic region, is quite frequent at all stages of HIV infection. Two fatal cases of an acute necrotizing ascending meningomyeloradiculitis without a preceding cutaneous eruption have been described (Vinters et al. 1988; Chretien et al. 1993). A flaccid paraplegia may develop slowly 5–21 days after the initial rash (Devinsky et al. 1991). The CSF may show xan-thochromia, a polymorphonuclear or mononuclear pleocytosis, often markedly raised protein and normal glucose. Imaging may show a swollen cord. Acyclovir has been tried as treatment but the reported anecdotal results have been disappointing. The spinal cords have shown haemorrhagic oedema and necrosis, vasculitis with fibrinoid necrosis in blood vessels and occasional Cowdry type inclusions.

Herpes Simplex

This is quite rare in HIV infection. HSV-2 has been implicated in a progressive asymmetrical myelopathy over two months with a previous history of perirectal herpes simplex and CMV retinitis and colitis (Britton et al. 1985). HSV-2 was also present in the cord of a patient who had a clinical and pathological picture consist-ent with CMV radiculomyeloencephalitis (Tucker et al. 1985).

Toxoplasmosis

This common opportunistic brain infection in AIDS can occasionally affect any level of the spinal cord (Harris et al. 1990; Fairley et al. 1992; Poon et al. 1992). Most patients have fever and present with back pain with radiation to the lower limbs and an acute or subacute paraparesis. If the conus medullaris is affected reflexes are absent or depressed in the legs and there is urinary retention, reduced anal tone and impaired sensation below L4 (Harris et al. 1990; Kayser et al. 1990; Overhage et al. 1990). A Brown–Séquard syndrome or a presentation with weakness and sensory loss in one upper limb are also on record. Untreated patients have progressed to a flaccid paraplegia.

The CSF may show a mononuclear pleocytosis, elevated protein and normal or slightly low glucose. Magnetic resonance scan may show a high intensity enhancing intramedullary mass and an enlarged cord with myelographic block (Mehren et al. 1988; Herskovitz et al. 1989). There may be concomitant cerebral toxoplasmosis. Treatment with pyrimethamine and sulphadiazine may result in clinical and radio-logical improvement if given early (Fairley et al. 1992; Poon et al. 1992). A biopsy of the cord lesion may be required. The differential diagnosis includes lymphoma, transverse myelitis, intrinsic cord tumours and CMV radiculomyelitis.

Mycobacteria

Cord abscesses due to mycobacteria are rare in AIDS. Two cases with involvement of the conus (Woolsey et al. 1988) and of the thoracic cord (Melhem and Wang 1992) have been described. In both the species of mycobacteria was not identified.

Syphilis

Syphilis can rarely give rise to a spinal cord or cauda equina syndrome in AIDS. A patient with an asymmetrical paraparesis, bladder involvement and a T8 sensory level progressing over four weeks (Berger 1992), another with an asymmetrical lumbosacral polyradiculopathy with wasting, weakness, leg pains, depressed reflexes and distal sensory loss (Lanska et al. 1988), and a further one with a spastic paraparesis, have been described.

Tumours

Epidural deposits from immunoblastic sarcoma and plasmacytoma were reported by Snider et al. (1983). Presentation of lymphoma as an acute myeloradiculopathy is on record (Klein et al. 1990; Leger et al. 1992) and it can be difficult to distinguish from the lumbosacral ascending CMV myeloradiculitis described above. The onset in the lumbosacral region with lymphoma infiltration of the cauda equina, the signs and the CSF findings can all be very similar to those of CMV myeloradicultis.

Miscellaneous

Aspergillus myelitis has been described in AIDS (Woods and Goldsmith 1990). A few cases of HTLV-1 *myelitis* or tropical spastic paraparesis (McArthur et al. 1990; Rosenblum et al. 1992) have been reported in HIV infected patients. Spinal cord involvement in AIDS related *progressive multifocal leucoencephalopathy* is quite rare; all four cases described also had cerebral involvement (Henin et al. 1992; von Einsiedel et al. 1993). An AIDS patient with a partial Brown–Séquard related to *disseminated intravascular coagulation* was described by Fenelon et al. (1991); he had multiple haemorrhagic infarcts in the cord. Rare abnormalities in the *long tracts* of the spinal cord include selective degeneration of the gracile tracts in AIDS patients with sensory neuropathy (Rance et al. 1988), degeneration of the posterior columns, corticospinal or multiple tracts (Rhodes and Ward 1989; Horoupian et al. 1984). Transverse myelitis of unknown aetiology has also been described (Dodson 1990).

In children Dickson et al. (1989) has reported delayed myelination of the lateral corticospinal tracts.

In a few patients the myelopathy may be only incidental to AIDS; we have seen, for example, cervical spondylotic myelopathy, spinal trauma and hysterical paraparesis in patients with HIV infection.

References

Berger JR (1992) Spinal cord syphilis associated with human immunodeficiency virus infection: a treatable myelopathy. Am J Med 92:101–103

Britton CB, Mesa-Tejada R, Fenoglio CM, Hays AP, Garvey GG, Miller JR (1985) A new complication of AIDS: thoracic myelitis caused by herpes simplex virus. Neurology 35:1071–1074

Budka H, Maier H, Pohl P (1988) Human immunodeficiency virus in vacuolar myelopathy of the acquired immunodeficiency syndrome. N Engl J Med 319:1667–1668

Chretien F, Gray F, Lescs MC et al. (1993) Acute varicella-zoster virus ventriculitis and meningo-myelo-radiculitis in acquired immunodeficiency syndrome. Acta Neuropathol 86:659–665

Cohen BA, McArthur JC, Grohman S, Patterson B, Glass JD (1993) Neurologic prognosis of cytomegalovirus polyradiculomyelopathy in AIDS. Neurology 43:493–499

de Gans J, Portegies P, Tiessens G, Troost D, Danner SA, Lange JM (1990) Therapy for cytomegalovirus polyradiculomyelitis in patients with AIDS: treatment with ganciclovir. Aids 4:421–425

Denning DW, Anderson J, Rudge P, Smith H (1987) Acute myelopathy associated with primary infection with human immunodeficiency virus. Br Med J 294:143–144

Devinsky O, Cho E-S, Petito CK, Price RW (1991) Herpes zoster myelitis. Brain 114:1181–1196

Dickson DW, Belman AL, Park YD et al. (1989) Central nervous system pathology in pediatric AIDS: an autopsy study. APMIS Suppl. 8:40–57

Dodson D (1990) Transverse myelitis and spastic paraparesis in a patient with HIV infection. N Engl J Med 322:1322

Fairley CK, Wodak J, Benson E (1992) Spinal cord toxoplasmosis in a patient with human immunodeficiency virus infection. Int J STD AIDS 3:366–368

Fenelon G, Gray F, Scaravilli F et al. (1991) Ischaemic myelopathy secondary to disseminated intravascular coagulation in AIDS. J Neurol 238:51–54

Fuller GN, Gill SK, Guiloff RJ et al. (1990) Ganciclovir for lumbosacral polyradiculopathy in AIDS. Lancet 335:48–49

Geny C, Gherardi R, Boudes P, Lionnet F, Cesaro P, Gray F (1991) Multifocal multinucleated giant cell myelitis in an AIDS patient. Neuropathol Appl Neurobiol 17:157–162

Goldstick L, Mandybur TI, Bode R (1985) Spinal cord degeneration in AIDS. Neurology 35:103–106

Grafe MJ, Wiley CA (1989) Spinal cord and peripheral nerve pathology in AIDS: the roles of cytomegalovirus and human immunodeficiency virus. Ann Neurol 25:561–566

Guiloff RJ, Fuller GN, Roberts A et al. (1988) Nature, incidence and prognosis of neurological involvement in the acquired immunodeficiency syndrome in central London. Postgrad Med J 64:919–925

Harris TM, Smith RR, Bognanno JR, Edwards MK (1990) Toxoplasmic myelitis in AIDS: gadolinium-enhanced MR. J Comput Assist Tomogr 14:809–811

Henin D, Smith TW, De Girolami U, Sughayer M, Hauw JJ (1992) Neuropathology of the spinal cord in the acquired immunodeficiency syndrome. Hum Pathol 23:1106–1114

Herskovitz S, Siegel SE, Schneider AT, Nelson SJ, Goodrich JT, Lantos G (1989) Spinal cord toxoplasmosis in AIDS. Neurology 39:1552–1553

Horoupian DS, Pick P, Spigland I et al. (1984) Acquired immune deficiency syndrome and multiple tract degeneration in a homosexual man. Ann Neurol 15:502–505

Kamin SS, Petito CK (1991) Idiopathic myelopathies with white matter vacuolation in non-acquired immunodeficiency syndrome patients. Hum Pathol 22:816–824

Kayser C, Campbell R, Sartorious C, Bartlett M (1990) Toxoplasmosis of the conus medullaris in a patient with hemophilia A-associated AIDS. Case report. J Neurosurg 73:951–953

Klein P, Zientek G, VandenBerg SR, Lothman E (1990) Primary CNS lymphoma: lymphomatous meningitis presenting as a cauda equina lesion in an AIDS patient. Can J Neurol Sci 17:329–331

Lanska MJ, Lanska DJ, Schmidley JW (1988) Syphilitic polyradiculopathy in an HIV-positive man. Neurology 38:1297–1301

Leger JM, Henin D, Belec L et al. (1992) Lymphoma-induced polyradiculopathy in AIDS: two cases. J Neurol 239:132–134

Mahieux F, Gray F, Fenclon G et al. (1989) Acute myeloradiculitis due to cytomegalovirus as the initial manifestation of AIDS. J Neurol Neurosurg Psychiatry 52:270–274

Maier H, Budka H, Lassmann H, Pohl P (1989) Vacuolar myelopathy with multinucleated giant cells in the acquired immune deficiency syndrome (AIDS). Light and electron microscopic distribution of human immunodeficiency virus (HIV) antigens. Acta Neuropathol 78:497–503

McArthur JC (1987) Neurologic manifestations of AIDS. Medicine 66:407–437

McArthur JC, Griffin JW, Cornblath DR et al. (1990) Steroid-responsive myeloneuropathy in a man dually infected with HIV-1 and HTLV-I. Neurology 40:938–944

Mehren M, Burnes PJ, Mamani F, Levy CS, Laureno R (1988) Toxoplasmic myelitis mimicking intramedullary spinal cord tumour. Neurology 38:1648–1650

Melhem ER, Wang H (1992) Intramedullary spinal cord tuberculoma in a patient with AIDS. Am J Neuroradiol 13:986–988

Miller RG, Storey JR, Greco CM (1990) Ganciclovir in the treatment of progressive AIDS-related polyradiculopathy. Neurology 40:569–574

Moskowitz LB, Hensley GT, Chan JC, Gregorios J, Conley FK (1984) The neuropathology of acquired immune deficiency syndrome. Arch Pathol Lab Med 108:867–872

Overhage JM, Greist A, Brown DR (1990) Conus medullaris syndrome resulting from Toxoplasma gondii infection in a patient with the acquired immunodeficiency syndrome. Am J Med 89:814–815

Petito CK, Navia BA, Cho ES, Jordan BD, George DC, Price RW (1985) Vacuolar myelopathy pathologically resembling subacute combined degeneration in patients with the acquired immunodeficiency syndrome. N Engl J Med 312:874–879

Petito CK, Vecchio D, Chen YT (1994) HIV antigen and DNA in AIDS spinal cords correlate with macrophage infiltration but not with vacuolar myelopathy. J Neuropathol Exp Neurol 53:86–94

Poon TP, Tchertkoff V, Pares GF, Masangkay AV, Daras M, Marc J (1992) Spinal cord toxoplasma lesion in AIDS: MR findings. J Comput Assist Tomogr 16:817–819

Rance NE, McArthur JC, Cornblath DR, Landstrom DL, Griffin JW, Price DL (1988) Gracile tract degeneration in patients with sensory neuropathy and AIDS. Neurology 38:265–271

Rhodes RH, Ward JM (1989) Immunohistochemistry of human immunodeficiency virus in the central nervous system and an hypothesis concerning the pathogenesis of AIDS meningoencephalomyelitis. Progr Aids Pathol 1:167–179

Rosenblum MK, Brew BJ, Hahn B et al. (1992) Human T-lymphotropic virus type I-associated myelopathy in patients with the acquired immunodeficiency syndrome. Hum Pathol 23:513–519

Sharer LR, Dowling PC, Michaels J et al. (1990) Spinal cord disease in children with HIV-1 infection: a combined molecular biological and neuropathological study. Neuropathol Appl Neurobiol 16:317–331

Snider WD, Simpson DM, Nielsen S, Gold JW, Metroka CE, Posner JB (1983) Neurological complications of the acquired immune deficiency syndrome: analysis of 50 patients. Ann Neurol 14:403–418

Tan SV, Guiloff RJ, Scaravilli F (1995) AIDS-associated vacuolar myelopathy. A morphometric study. Brain 118:1247–1261

Tan SV, Guiloff RJ, Henderson DC et al. (1996) AIDS-associated vacuolar myelopathy and tumor necrosis factor-alpha (TNFα). J Neurol Sci 138:134–144

Tucker T, Dix RD, Katzen C, Davis RL, Schmidley JW (1985) Cytomegalovirus and herpes simplex virus ascending myelitis in a patient with acquired immune deficiency syndrome. Ann Neurol 18:74–79

Tyor WR, Glass JD, Baumrind N et al. (1993) Cytokine expression of macrophages in HIV-1-associated vacuolar myelopathy. Neurology 43:1002–1009

Vinters HV, Guerra WF, Eppolito L, Keith PE (1988) Necrotizing vasculitis of the nervous system in a patient with AIDS-related complex. Neuropathol Appl Neurobiol 14:417–424

Vinters HV, Kwok MK, Ho HW et al. (1989) Cytomegalovirus in the nervous system of patients with the acquired immune deficiency syndrome. Brain 112:245–268

von Einsiedel RW, Fife TD, Aksamit AJ et al. (1993) Progressive multifocal leukoencephalopathy in AIDS: a clinicopathologic study and review of the literature. J Neurol 240:391–406

Woods GL, Goldsmith JC (1990) Aspergillus infection of the central nervous system in patients with acquired immunodeficiency syndrome. Arch Neurol 47:181–184

Woolsey RM, Chambers TJ, Chung HD, McGarry JD (1988) Mycobacterial meningomyelitis associated with human immunodeficiency virus infection [see comments]. Arch Neurol 45:691–693

Chapter 20

Disorders of the Anterior Horn Cell

J.D. Mitchell

Motor Neurone Disease (Amyotrophic Lateral Sclerosis)

In terms of the totality of disease, anterior horn cell disease is rare. Even in neurological practice spinal muscular atrophy is an uncommon condition. Motor neurone disease (MND) is the most common of the motor system diseases and, arguably, one of the most unpleasant diseases known to medical science. A large proportion of the work of neurological departments is devoted to the investigation of those suspected of having this disorder or in attempts to relieve the suffering of those in whom this diagnosis has been established.

Historical Background, Clinical Features and Diagnostic Criteria

Although the first report of MND is generally ascribed to Aran (1850) it is clear that others recognized the disease before him. Sir Charles Bell had described a patient with progressive weakness without sensory loss in 1836 who probably had progressive muscular atrophy (PMA) (Bell 1836). R.W.R. Robinson, a physician working in Preston in the early 19th century had previously written to Bell in 1825 describing a lady who almost certainly had progressive bulbar palsy and possibly MND. This was one of the patients described by Bell in his writings. Romberg also mentioned one of Bell's patients and also described three other probable cases of MND. One of these also had bulbar palsy and was probably the first report of what would today be recognized as the all too familiar clinical picture of MND in the terminal phase (Romberg 1851). These early authors were generally agreed on two points: first, that the clinical picture of the disease was similar to that associated with lead intoxication but without a history of exposure to lead and second that there was no effective treatment. This last point still rings true today over 150 years later and there is still no clear idea of the basic cause of MND

The crystallization of MND as a clinical syndrome encompassing upper and lower motor neurone features appeared in the writings of Charcot (1872, 1873) who realized that anterior horn cell degeneration could be associated with loss of pyramidal motor neurones and coined the term amyotrophic lateral sclerosis (ALS). It was not until even later that the relationship of bulbar palsy to ALS was fully recognized.

The concept of MND as a degenerative condition involving the motor system at all levels thus developed over a period of about 50 years.

By far the majority of patients (82%) show combined upper and lower motor neurone features and eventually develop bulbar palsy as described by Charcot. About 9% show a predominantly bulbar picture and a purely lower motor neurone form called progressive muscular atrophy (PMA) is seen in approximately 7% of patients. Although some patients presenting with PMA follow a clear progressive course and eventually develop the full clinical syndrome of ALS, others do not. The relationship of PMA to ALS is thus uncertain and controversial – many would regard PMA as being more akin to spinal muscular atrophy than MND. The existence of the pure upper motor neurone form of the disease, primary lateral sclerosis (PLS), is also controversial, but this probably accounts for no more than 2% of cases. MND most commonly presents with weakness which is often asymmetrical. Although the rate of progression varies greatly between patients, the disease tends to evolve at a uniform rate in any given sufferer. This rate of progression can be described as either a quadratic function or two discontinuous linear rates. Some patients report muscle twitchings as the subjective perception of the profuse fasciculation which is such a common clinical observation in MND. Many complain of muscle cramps, particularly in the lower limbs. The pathophysiology of this symptom is poorly understood. With very few exceptions the oculomotor nuclei are not affected. Sphincter control is also unaffected and because of the absence of sensory changes, pressure sores are very uncommon. The time from first symptom to death varies considerably in different series, but a median survival of 4.08 years was reported in one survival analysis of 397 patients (Caroscio 1986).

Although the clinical picture is usually unmistakable to the trained neurologist, it is important to exclude tandem cervical and lumbar spinal canal stenosis in patients suspected of suffering from MND. The advent of genetic linkage studies and the prospect of therapeutic trials in MND have both brought a need for clearly expressed diagnostic criteria. This has led to the Escorial Criteria for the Diagnosis of MND. According to these criteria, a diagnosis of *proven* MND requires histological evidence of anterior horn cell loss and can only be made after death. During life patients can be classified as *definite, probable or possible* MND. Although it is possible to make these classifications on clinical grounds alone, the results of laboratory investigations can be used according to the local availability and practice so that the criteria are sufficiently flexible to be used in any country in a reproducible way (Brooks 1994).

Pathology

Some pathological (Auerback and Crocker 1982) and physiological studies (Jamal et al. 1985) have suggested that MND is not entirely restricted to motor neurones as has traditionally been thought. It is difficult to be certain to what extent these findings are a result of the disease itself and to what extent they represent secondary phenomena or even variants of normal. The essential point to be remembered is that for practical clinical purposes MND is a degenerative disorder specifically affecting the motor system.

Pathologically, MND is characterized by atrophy and loss of cells at all levels of the motor system. Remaining motor cells show degenerative changes with shrinkage of the cell body which has traditionally been considered to contain an increased quantity of lipofuscin (Mann and Yates 1974). This has, however, been challenged. Nissl granules may be lost or form into large accumulations. The nucleus shrinks and loses its basophilia. Nuclear chromatin becomes more prominent and clumps may be seen (Mann and Yates 1974).

Neurofibrillary tangles have been reported in relation to Guamian MND but have only been described in one case of classical MND. Motor neurones from MND patients fail to show the usual central chromatolytic response which usually occurs in active axonal degeneration. It was suggested that this provides evidence of an impaired capacity of the cell to increase the rate of RNA synthesis in response to axonal disruption. This is of interest not only in relation to the work by Leigh et al. (1988) reporting ubiquitin inclusions in anterior horn cells from MND patients but also to the "DNA hypothesis" of MND (Bradley and Krasin 1982). Although ubiquitin inclusions have now been characterized at the light microscopic and ultrastructural levels, the molecular constitution of the inclusion remains poorly understood. There is accumulating evidence that these inclusions may be found in non-motor areas in MND patients with frontal lobe dementia (Lowe 1994).

Epidemiology

With the exception of the high incidence Pacific foci, the incidence of classical MND shows remarkable uniformity throughout the World and is between 1 and 2 new cases per 100 000 population per annum. The disease is consistently commoner in males than females (male to female ratio 1.6–1.8:1), and the most frequent age of onset is around 60 years. There is an increasing body of literature suggesting that the incidence of MND is increasing (Holloway and Mitchell 1986; Lilienfeld et al. 1989; Durrleman and Alprerovitch 1989). The reason for this apparent increase in the incidence of MND in recent years has been tantalizing and has culminated in a concept that there is a specific population of MND-susceptible individuals. Such is this susceptibility that if these individuals live long enough they will inevitably develop MND. With increasing preventive measures against ischaemic heart disease, hypertensive cerebrovascular disease and bronchial carcinoma these intrinsically susceptible individuals are more likely to survive to develop MND thus leading to the increased apparent incidence of MND which has been observed. Evidence to support this hypothesis has been advanced using Gompertzian analysis, an actuarial technique (Neilson et al. 1993, 1994) although this remains controversial.

Factors such as rural birthplace, extent of outdoor activity, history of military service in Guam or Japan, and consumption of sheep or calf brain do not confer an increased risk of developing MND. A case control study of 105 MND patients suggested that exposure to heavy metals was not likely to be important in the aetiology of the disease and no evidence to suggest excessive exposure to lead, mercury, aluminium, magnesium, manganese, nickel or selenium was found in another case control study of 66 MND patients.

An increased incidence of MND has been reported in those occupationally exposed to animal carcases and hides (Harnisch et al. 1976) and in leather workers (Hawkes and Fox 1981; Buckley et al. 1983) but not in a Scottish study where a possible excess of rubber workers was found (Holloway and Mitchell 1986). Another Scottish survey suggested that MND was more frequent among agricultural workers than might have been expected (Holloway and Emery 1982). An increased incidence of Parkinson's and Alzheimer's disease in relatives of MND patients has also been reported (Calne and Eisen 1989).

About 5% of cases of MND follow a familial pattern, usually with autosomal dominant inheritance (Emery and Holloway 1982). These do not show the usual male predominance and may present at any age from early adult life onwards. The existence of these familial cases is important as work attempting to understand mechanisms involved in the familial disease might enhance our knowledge of the pathogenesis of sporadic MND. Following work suggesting a linkage to chromosome 21 in some kindreds with familial MND (Siddique et al. 1991), a mutation in the chromosome 21 copper/zinc superoxide dismutase (Cu/ZnSOD, also known as SOD1) gene has been found (Rosen et al. 1993) and probably occurs in about 10%–20% of patients with familial MND. Several mutations exist and this finding has cast a new angle on previous work seeking a possible role for free radicals in the pathogenesis of MND (Mitchell and Jackson 1992). Cu/ZnSOD gene mutations do not, however, explain the other 80%–90% of patients with familial MND. It should also be noted that in patients with the SOD1 mutation the mutant enzyme is expressed in all tissues of the body and not solely the motor neurone. This raises fundamental questions regarding the selective vulnerability of the motor neurone. It is also note worthy in this context that affected individuals may be virtually asymptomatic for 20%–30% of their lifespan and then progress from disease onset to death in as little as 12–18 months.

Geographical clusters, though often discussed anecdotally, have only rarely been described in the literature. One report concerned three unrelated school teachers who taught in the same classroom over a period of 18 years and developed MND. A retrospective but systematic survey did not show any clear clusters but suggested that the geographical distribution of the disease is not entirely uniform (Mitchell et al. 1990). A cluster of four cases has been reported from an area with a very high soil selenium content (Kilness and Hochberg 1977). Although several examples of conjugal MND have now been reported (Chad et al. 1982) this is extremely rare and such instances may merely represent the chance affection of husband and wife. Their significance in terms of our attempts to understand the pathogenesis of MND is uncertain. The idea that space–time clustering might occur in MND remains a tantalizing possibility. This is currently being further investigated along similar lines as for multiple sclerosis in Western Norway (Riise et al. 1991). Such clustering could lead to the identification of one or more environmental factors in relation to the pathogenesis of sporadic MND.

Guamian MND and Lathyrism

Many epidemiological studies of MND have been particularly concerned with the Pacific Island of Guam, where, until recent years, a disorder resembling MND has been common among the native Chamorro population. Foci of a similar clinical syndrome also exist in the Kii Peninsula of Japan, the Kepi Region of New Guinea and among Hawaiian Filipinos. The incidence of Guamian MND (Lytico bodeg – MND and Parkinson-dementia forms) has been estimated to be about 100 times that of classical MND in continental USA. It is not surprising that attempts to learn about the aetiology of classical MND have been made from studies of Guamian MND. The important differences which exist between these two clinical entities should, however, be emphasized. Classical MND is characterized by purely motor features.

In general, intellect is preserved, even in the late stages of the disease. By contrast, Guamian MND is associated not only with dementia but also with features of extra pyramidal involvement.

Interest has principally been focused on the implication of environmental factors in the pathogenesis of Guamian MND. Manganese mining has been economically important on the island and the drinking water has been found to contain a high concentration of this element. The possibility that the mineral content of the public water supply might be related to the pathogenesis of the disease was to some extent supported by a report that the MND-like form of the disease has become much less common since improvements to the supply were made. The Parkinsonism/dementia complex has not declined in the same way and it has been noted that this bears a strong resemblance to the Steele–Richardson syndrome (progressive supranuclear palsy).

The possible importance of dietary factors should also be considered. The seed of the cycad, *Cycas circinalis* has been a staple source of carbohydrate on Guam, as well as the other islands of the Marianna Chain. The seed of *C. circinalis* contains β-*N*-methylamino-L-alanine (BMAA). Daily feeding of macaques with BMAA has been associated with degeneration of anterior horn and Betz cells. It is therefore possible that cycad consumption on the Island of Guam is implicated in the pathogenesis of Guamian MND and that reduced dependence on cycad as a staple in recent years has been a factor in the reduced incidence of this disease. This hypothesis has been supported by the finding that cycad has been important in folk medicine in both the Kii peninsula of Japan and the Irian peninsula of New Guinea. BMAA has, however, not been found in fasting plasma or CSF in sporadic MND. It is efficiently removed by the washing procedure used to prepare the cycad nut by the Chamorros. It is rapidly cleared from the circulation and only crosses the blood–brain barrier in small amounts. Although there is still considerable uncertainty whether BMAA is implicated in the pathogenesis of these clinical entities the current balance of opinion is that such involvement is unlikely.

Lathyrism is another progressive neurological disorder, the clinical features of which closely resemble primary lateral sclerosis and hereditary spastic paraparesis. It is related to the dietary consumption of the chickling pea (*Lathyrus sativa*) and occurs in the Indian subcontinent and Mediterranean regions. It is now rarely seen in Spain. β-*N*-oxalylamino-L-alanine (BOAA), a substance related to BMAA has been found in the Indian chickling pea. Daily feeding of macaques with BOAA has produced a primary lateral sclerosis-like syndrome. It has been postulated that BOAA might be the causative agent of lathyrism although like BMAA it only crosses the blood–brain barrier very poorly. Genetic factors may also be important in the development of the disease and it has also been suggested that the disease can be prevented by drinking milk.

Viruses and MND

Poliomyelitis is an example of a disease of known viral aetiology in which the motor system is selectively affected. This has prompted the suggestion that MND may have a viral aetiology. These ideas have been reinforced by slowly progressive, often highly localized, muscle wasting and weakness in patients who have previously had polio (Alter et al. 1982). Although polio-specific immunofluorescence has been reported in jejunal mucosa (Behan et al. 1977), this was subsequently found to be a non-specific reaction (Fraser et al. 1979) and further studies using nucleic acid probes have failed to reveal evidence that any material derived from polio virus is present within motor neurones in MND (Viola et al. 1982).

Interest in the relationship of viruses and MND has, however been reactivated by a number of recent contributions. The first was a report of a close geographical concordance between MND and past notification rates for poliomyelitis (Martyn et al. 1988). It is also possible that rates of polio vaccination may differ in patients developing MND and there may also be changes in the frequency of childhood varicella in MND patients. An association between enterovirus infection and MND has also been reported as well as an apparent geographical cluster of cases of MND in relation to epidemic of Coxsackie B infection. It is difficult to envisage how these various virological observations can be explained on the basis of a unitary hypothesis of the aetiology of MND and the significance of these apparently disparate reports remains uncertain in this context.

Amyotrophy resulting from anterior horn cell degeneration is sometimes seen in patients with Jacob–Creutzfeldt disease. This suggests that transmissible agents other than the polio virus may be involved in the pathogenesis of MND. Jacob–Creutzfeldt disease is thought to be prion related and is generally characterized by a subacute dementing process. In some patients amyotrophy is a particularly prominent feature such that the appearances might mimic motor neurone disease. This is sometimes associated with a longer survival than is usual in patients presenting with the non-amyotrophic form the disease. A course extending as long as six years has been recorded in the amyotrophic variant. Such patients show loss of anterior horn cells at post mortem with relatively little demyelination. In contrast to motor neurone disease, however, amyloid plaques are encountered. It is thought that these might contain the prions which are considered to be causative agent of this disease.

Immunology and MND

There is little to suggest an immunological abnormality in MND. The ESR and plasma proteins are normal and no abnormality of the CSF immunoglobulins has been reported (Antel et al. 1979). The significance of the increased CSF total protein seen in some cases (Blundell and Mitchell 1985) is uncertain, but this may reflect the degenerative process rather than damage to the blood–brain barrier. Renal glomerular basement membrane complement deposits (Oldstone et al. 1976) and abnormal circulating immune complexes (Noronha et al. 1981) have been described, but seem unlikely to yield an insight into the pathogenesis of MND. Impairment of the cellular inflammatory response has also been reported (Urbanek and Jansa 1974) but the abnormalities here are no different from changes observed in a wide range of other diseases. Others have made extensive studies of both humoral and cell-mediated immunity in MND without any abnormality being found (Bartfield et al. 1982).

Both blood group and HLA associations have been studied. Of 40 MND patients 25% were found to be of blood group B, the expected incidence having been 9% in a control population. A subsequent study in 346 patients and controls failed to reveal any significant association with the MNU, Rh, Kell, Duffy and Kidd systems. A significant association was, however, found with B secretor status and the P2 antigen. There have been several reports of HLA frequencies in MND (Pederson et al. 1977). One group reported a decreased incidence of HLA-A9 and an increase in

HLA-Bw35. More recent work suggests a reduced incidence of HLA-DR4 among Newcastle MND patients. This was not, however, found in patients from surrounding areas. A consistent HLA association in MND seems unlikely.

Physical Factors and MND

Patients developing MND often attempt to relate the onset of their condition to a particular event. The possibility that physical factors, including trauma, might be implicated in the pathogenesis of MND has been pursued by several authors. These range from a fall on the buttock to skeletal fracture (Campbell et al. 1970). The former relates to a single anecdotal case, the latter to a series of 74 MND patients in which skeletal fracture or disease of the axial skeleton was found in 25% compared with 9.4% of a control population. A recent case control study has not revealed any further evidence to suggest that there is an increased risk of skeletal fracture in MND. In considering these reports it is important to remember that patients with MND have a physical disability and are obviously more liable to fall than any non-disabled population. The immobility of MND patients and consequent osteoporosis further increases the risk of fracturing a bone.

Heavy Metals, Trace Elements, Nucleic Acids, Free Radicals, Excitotoxity and MND

The toxic effects of lead on the nervous system were known to the ancient Greeks. The possibility that lead might be implicated in the pathogenesis of sporadic MND has been extensively pursued despite the fact that most MND patients never receive significant exposure to lead. Attempts have been made to remove lead from the body by chelation therapy. Although a number of patients did seem to respond to this treatment, it seems likely that they had been excessively exposed and that their neurological disorder was the result of lead toxicity rather than MND. Nonetheless, much has since been done to study lead in MND. Lead has been measured in blood, CSF, muscle and spinal cord. With few exceptions no significant differences have been found between MND patients and control subjects. The positive findings have not been verified by others and their significance is difficult to assess. It does, however, seem clear that chelation therapy has nothing to offer in sporadic MND and that only patients with the MND-like syndrome that can undoubtedly occur in lead poisoning show a useful response.

There has also been a substantial interest in mercury in relation to anterior horn cell degeneration. A young male with clear clinical evidence of mercury poisoning and an MND-like illness was reported. He had been exposed to organic mercury, and although it was possible to remove mercury by chelation therapy, his neurological disease continued to progress and the classic changes of MND were seen at post mortem. Other patients have been reported who ingested material contaminated with organic mercury. They also failed to respond to chelating drugs. Other patients have developed PMA-like syndromes following exposure to both inorganic and elemental mercury. The neurological manifestations in these patients resolved spontaneously after withdrawal from the contaminated environment. In conclusion therefore it seems that mercury toxicity is sometimes associated with an MND-like syndrome. It is unlikely that mercury is implicated in the pathogenesis of sporadic MND (Mitchell 1987).

Many of the 92 naturally occurring elements have attracted interest in relation to the pathogenesis of MND. These include not only major elements such as calcium and magnesium but also elements which are ubiquitous in the environment but have no known essential biological function such as aluminium and trace elements which although by definition present only in minute amounts, have an essential biochemical role. Calcium and aluminium have been investigated in relation to the MND/Parkinson–Dementia complex which previously occurred on Guam. Disorders of mineral metabolism are sometimes associated with intraneuronal accumulation of aluminium (Mayor et al. 1980; Nakagawa et al. 1977) and it is suggested that this element may be concentrated intraneuronally in MND. Some work has been done in small numbers of patients with Guamian MND, and the suggestion is that calcium and aluminium levels are indeed increased in neurofibrillary tangle bearing neurones in the hippocampus (Garruto et al. 1985). This has, however, not yet been investigated to any great extent in MND as it occurs outside these high-incidence foci but an MND-like syndrome has occurred in a man who had excessive occupational aluminium exposure for many years in whom a parathyroid adenoma was also found at autopsy.

The essential trace elements have been investigated in MND with little clear evidence emerging. These elements are of crucial importance in many facets of intermediary metabolism and are also vital in maintaining the conformation of biological macromolecules. The role of selenium was investigated following a report of an apparent cluster of cases from a seleniferous area (Kilness and Hochberg 1977). Urinary levels were found to be normal in MND (Norris and U 1978) and there was little further interest until reports of increased levels in erythrocytes (Nagata et al. 1985), liver and spinal cord (Mitchell et al. 1986, 1991). Manganese has been previously mentioned in relation to the Guamian form of MND. This may also be important in MND as it occurs in other areas and there are now two independent reports of increased manganese levels in spinal cord tissue of patients dying of sporadic MND (Miyata et al. 1983; Mitchell et al. 1986, 1991). Both these elements are important in the inactivation of free radicals as constituents of free radical inactivating enzymes, selenium as a constituent of glutathione peroxidase (GSHPX) and manganese as a component of manganese containing superoxide dismutase (MnSOD).

It is now many years since the concept of abiotrophy was first applied to the degenerative neurological diseases (Gowers 1902). This centred on the possibility that a selective and premature ageing process might be implicated in the pathogenesis of neurodegenerative disease. Pathological investigations have led to the identification of certain histological features such as lipofuscin deposits (Mann and Yates 1974) which are to some extent common to all these disorders. Some support for the idea that MND might be the result of accentuated normal ageing processes in motor neurones came from motor unit counting (McComas et al. 1973). This led to the investigation of nucleic acid metabolism in MND. RNA levels were found to be reduced in surviving motor neurones, whereas the DNA content was preserved (Mann and Yates 1974; Davidson and Hartmann 1981). This has culminated in the DNA hypothesis of MND where it is proposed that there is a failure of enzymatic DNA repair mechanisms with the result that there is a progressive disruption of normal transcription. It is suggested that the defective enzyme is an isoenzyme unique to the motor system thus explaining the selectivity of the disease for motor neurones (Bradley and Krasin 1982). Although an attractive hypothesis, it was produced without direct experimental support and is a difficult hypothesis to test. Attempts to obtain collateral evidence have so far been unsuccessful (Vijayalaxmi et al. 1985).

It is possible that influences other than defective DNA repair mechanisms could explain these nucleic acid changes. They could also result from free-radical-mediated damage to the polynucleotide chain. In the light of the observed changes in trace element distribution it is possible that these changes might indicate altered concentrations or activities of the free radical inactivating enzymes GSHPX and MnSOD. The finding of an apparent serial decline in erythrocyte GSHPX activity with disease progression represents further evidence of a role for free radicals in the pathogenesis of sporadic MND (Mitchell et al. 1993). It will be recalled that 10%–20% of patients with the familial form of the disease have mutations of the Cu/ZnSOD gene on chromosome 21 resulting in reduced Cu/ZnSOD activities (Rosen et al. 1993). The link between free radicals in the familial and sporadic forms of the disease was heightened by a report of a Cu/ZnSOD gene mutation in three patients with apparent sporadic MND (Jones et al. 1993). Although Cu/ZnSOD is a cytosolic and MnSOD is a mitochondrial enzyme, MnSOD can be up-regulated if Cu/ZnSOD activity is insufficient to meet a free radical-mediated assault or injury. Possible evidence of increased anterior horn MnSOD activity in sporadic MND (Shaw et al. 1995) is particularly tantalizing in this context. If free radicals were shown to be important in the pathogenesis of MND, new opportunities for the experimental treatment of MND with free -radical modifying therapies would emerge. Although selegiline, a putative anti-oxidant drug, seems ineffective in MND (Mitchell et al. 1995) other possibilities for neuroprotective therapy are being actively pursued in other neurodegenerative diseases such as Parkinson's disease. Compounds such as polyethylene glycol conjugated SOD may even be used.

The possible role of excitotoxity in the pathogenesis of MND has also been exten-sively discussed. This has been reviewed by Shaw (1994). In this model, normal amino acid neurotransmitters such as glutamate are present at supraphysiological concentrations. By virtue of these increased concentrations, these physiological sub-stances become toxic (the phenomenon of excitotoxity) and cause neuronal death by allowing the influx of excessive amounts of calcium into the neurone. This process also raises possibilities for pharmacological manipulation as there are a number of drugs which affect gluatamate neurotransmission. Dextromethorphan is an antago-nist of the N-methyl-D-aspartate (NMDA) subpopulation of glutamate receptors and a constituent of several proprietary cough mixtures. Although there is no evidence that dextromethorphan modifies the clinical course of MND (Askmark et al. 1993), there is a suggestion that riluzole, a glutamate release inhibitor, may (Bensimon et al. 1994), although a definitive answer on this final point must await the outcome of large-scale multinational trials currently in progress.

The possible link between excitotoxicity and free radical mechanisms should be remembered. Excitotoxicity is essentially a membrane-related phenomenon and free-radical intermediates have been postulated in the cascade mechanism linking excitotoxicity at membrane level with calcium influx and the ultimate mechanisms determining neuronal death in the nucleus. Excitoxicity and free-radicals can there-fore be brought together into the "Free radical Hypothesis of MND" summarized in Fig. 20.1.

Thyrotrophin Releasing Hormone and MND

The differential diagnosis of MND and thyrotoxic myopathy has sometimes caused difficulty and has led to the study of thyroid hormones in relation to MND.

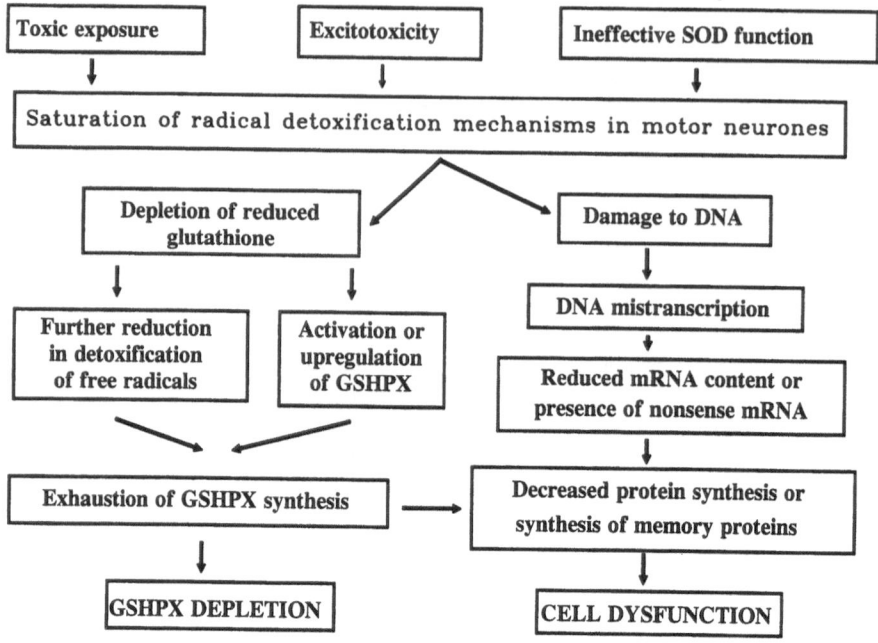

Fig. 20.1. The free radical hypothesis of motor neurone disease.

Receptors for hormones and trophic peptides are widely distributed in the spinal cord as well as in the brain and are the subject of increasing attention in MND research. Thyrotrophin releasing hormone (TRH) has been of particular interest following a report that its concentration in CSF was reduced in MND patients (Engel et al. 1983a). It has been tried as a therapeutic agent. It was reported that moderate intravenous doses resulted in a short-lived but definite improvement in motor power (Engel et al. 1983b). Truly blind clinical trials are unfortunately difficult because of the side effects associated with TRH administration but attempts to achieve this and substantiate the previous findings suggest that there is no objective evidence of a beneficial effect from either intravenous, intramuscular or subcutaneous injection of TRH. There is therefore no current indication for the therapeutic use of this substance in MND (Brooke et al. 1986; Caroscio et al. 1986; Mitsumoto et al. 1986). Although further work on the possible role of TRH analogues has been done it seems unlikely that these compounds will have a major role in the treatment of MND.

Spinal Muscular Atrophy

This rather heterogeneous group of disorders comprises a range of syndromes associated with patchy anterior horn cell degeneration. Although some forms, are progressive and life threatening, the degenerative process is not as generalized, nor as progressive, as that encountered in sporadic classical MND. This area has recently been reviewed (Morrison and Harding 1994). Adult forms are probably genetically distinct from childhood forms and this is reflected in the following treatment.

The Childhood Proximal Spinal Muscular Atrophies (Types I, II and III)

This category includes the rapidly progressive early (SMA type I), and more chronic, late (SMA type II and III) variants. Affected individuals tend to show a linkage to the long arm of chromosome 5 (5q11.2–13.3) and show autosomal recessive inheritance. The gene and thus the gene product have not yet been identified. It has been suggested that prenatal risk estimates are possible for couples who have had a severely affected child although this remains somewhat controversial. A dominantly inherited form has also been described in which sufferers may survive into adult life without major disability.

The early form (SMA I) is often apparent at birth and certainly before the age of six months. Affected individuals are never able to sit without support and the disease is almost always fatal before the age of three years. There are sometimes clues to the disease before birth in that fetal movements may be lost with retention of the fetal heart beat. The evidence suggests that this is inherited as an autosomal recessive with a recurrence rate for couples who have already produced an affected child of 1 in 4. The UK carrier frequency is 1 in 60–80.

The intermediate form (SMA II) presents before the age of 18 months and death rarely occurs before the age of two years. Affected individuals are unable to stand or walk without aid and complications such as scoliosis and pulmonary hypoventilation may occur. The incidence is similar to SMA I.

The mild form (SMA III) presents after the age of 18 months. Patients usually survive to adulthood and affected individuals have sometimes developed the ability to stand or walk. The incidence is similar to SMA I.

Arthrogryposis Multiplex

This disorder is characterized by multiple congenital articular deformities with associated muscle wasting. Although it has been categorized with the spinal muscular atrophies in the WHO classification of neuromuscular diseases, arthrogryposis multiplex as an entity associated with anterior horn disease and without other manifestations is a matter of controversy. It is usually seen in conjunction with pontocerebellar hypoplasia, congenital fractures, heart defects and respiratory insufficiency.

Pseudomyopathic Familial Form

First recognized by Kugelberg and Welander a little over 30 years ago, this is an adult disease which may be clinically confused with a dystrophic disorder. The proximal muscles are mainly affected. The observation of fasciculation and finding of neurogenic changes on electromyography are crucial in reaching this conclusion and avoiding the clinical pitfall of making an erroneous diagnosis of limb girdle dystrophy. Pseudohypertrophy of the calves may be present. The disease is compatible with a normal life expectancy and in many cases, the patient is still able to walk 10 years after the onset of symptoms. Some patients may have testicular failure. Autosomal recessive, X-linked and dominant patterns of inheritance have been reported in different kindreds (Kugelberg 1975). A disorder resembling this syndrome has been reported in a female patient who also had clinical signs of pyramidal and extrapyramidal involvement. The extrapyramidal features responded to levodopa and anterior horn cell loss was found in the spinal cord at post mortem with evidence of pallidonigral degeneration in the brain (Serratrice et al. 1983).

Scapuloperoneal Form

This form is associated with a particularly characteristic pattern of involvement whereby there is marked weakness and wasting around the shoulder girdle with distal changes in the lower limb. The clinical picture is similar to facio-scapulo-humeral dystrophy but the face is spared. Pedigrees showing an autosomal dominant inheritance pattern have been reported, and sporadic cases have also been recorded. In later years bulbar involvement and even ophthalmoplegia may be encountered (Kaeser 1965). Sporadic cases have been reported presenting in infancy (Feigenbaum and Munsat 1970).

This syndrome is sometimes associated with cardiac involvement in which the conducting system of the heart is usually predominantly affected. Such patients may be susceptible to paroxysmal cardiac dysrhythmias which may be life threatening and a permanent pacemaker may be required. This clinical pattern can be seen in kindreds showing both a dominant (Jennekens et al. 1975) and X-linked (Mawatari and Katayama 1973) pattern of inheritance.

Distal Form

These patients show considerable clinical and genetic heterogeneity. Symptoms may come on at widely varying ages and sporadic cases are also described. These are usually first noticed in the leg only later spreading to the arm. Pes cavus may be seen in patients presenting in younger life. Severe disability is uncommon and there may be confusion, on clinical grounds, with both the scapuloperoneal syndrome and the neuronal form of dominantly inherited hereditary motor and sensory neuropathy (McLeod and Prineas 1971).

Occasionally, the anterior horn cell degeneration may be associated with optic atrophy and nerve deafness (Iwashita et al. 1970; Chalmers and Mitchell 1987). Associated vocal cord paralysis has also been reported (Young and Harper 1980).

X-linked Bulbospinal Neuronopathy (Kennedy Syndrome)

This disease usually develops between the ages of 25 and 50 years. Muscle cramps may precede the weakness by several years. Proximal weakness in the lower limbs spreads to the shoulder girdle and then to the bulbar muscles. Fasciculation of the tongue may be a prominent feature and postcontraction fasciculation of the limbs is also frequently seen. A fine tremor is often present and 10–20 years may elapse between the first symptom and the onset of dysphagia or dysarthria. Patients may also have gynaecomastia, infertility and diabetes mellitus. Sporadic cases occur and, as far as is known, the disease always affects males (Harding et al. 1982). When the disease shows a familial incidence inheritance follows an X-linked recessive pattern (Harding 1984). This is linked with an abnormally long CAG repeat sequence in the first exon of the androgen receptor gene on the X chromosome. This trinucleotide repeat sequence results in an increased polyglutamine tract in the receptor but the number of repeats does not seem to correlate with neurological severity.

Monomelic Form

This is generally a sporadic disorder, tending to present in males between the ages of 15 and 25 years. The upper limb is usually mainly affected, the weakness often being first noted in the hand. The symptoms frequently spread proximally into the forearm but further progression rarely occurs after two years have elapsed since the first symptom (Hirayama et al. 1959).

In one series of 18 patients, a 2:1 male/female ratio was observed with a rather older mean age of onset of approximately 32 years. Two patients had close relatives who had had Werdnig–Hoffmann disease. It is important to distinguish patients with this disorder from those suffering from sporadic MND. The two conditions are clearly clinically distinct and the absence of bulbar involvement or pyramidal signs three years after the first symptom in the presence of depressed or absent deep tendon reflexes favours the diagnosis of chronic asymmetrical or monomelic spinal muscular atrophy. This syndrome tends to follow a particularly benign course (Harding et al. 1983) and its relationship to a particular form of MND occurring in the Madras region of India is uncertain.

Electrical Injury and the Anterior Horn Cell

The nature of any neurological sequelae of electrical injury depends on the path taken by the current and also the strength of the shock. If this is of moderate or high severity (0.025–5 A,> 1000 V), a motor and sensory syndrome affecting the limbs may occur which may improve after about 2 weeks. This may also follow a lightening strike. In some cases the myotomal pattern of muscle wasting corresponds to the dermatome in which the current has entered. Sometimes the amyotrophy may not develop until some months have elapsed after the injury and in only about half of these patients is the original shock of sufficient strength to cause loss of consciousness (Panse 1970). Reports of pyramidal signs and MND-like syndromes in this context are of uncertain clinical significance. A patient has, however, been described who developed amyotrophy of both upper limbs associated with a sensorimotor spastic paraparesis after accidentally severing a 33 000 V power line. The first neurological manifestations were noted on the 8th day and his condition was at its worst 21 days after the incident. Spontaneous recovery then followed and he was walking with two sticks after 160 days (Holbrook et al. 1970). Although delayed amyotrophy is clearly a frequent correlate of electrical injury, onset of muscle wasting with fasciculation two years after the shock is unusual in this context. This was, however, reported in a man who had received an 18 000 V AC (60Hz) shock. The symptoms and signs did not progress and it would thus seem unlikely that this represented an incidental case of MND (Farrell et al. 1968). A history of electrical injury should therefore be sought in patients with MND-like syndromes who do not pursue the usual rapidly progressive course.

Viruses and the Anterior Horn Cell

Poliomyelitis

Poliomyelitis is the example *par excellence* of a defined virus causing a disorder affecting a specific neuronal system, i.e. motor neurones at all levels including anterior horn cells. The causative virus is an RNA enterovirus which may be a gut commensal. The illness is initially systemic and related to viraemia. Although there may be some meningitic features at this stage, only 10% go on to the paralytic illness. The pattern of weakness is typically asymmetrical and patchy, usually reaching its peak within a few days. Recovery may begin within a week of the onset of the paralytic phase and fortunately most of the weak muscles eventually return to near normal power. Occasionally, patients develop a slowly progressive weakness (Dalakas et al. 1986), sometimes years after the initial illness, which may bear some clinical resemblance to progressive muscular atrophy, one of the variants of motor neurone disease. This is a subject of considerable interest in relation to the possibility that the polio virus might be implicated in the pathogenesis of MND. This is discussed further earlier in this chapter where the postpolio syndrome which can follow poliomyelitis is also described.

More recently other enteroviruses have occasionally been found to be associated with a polio-like illness. Enterovirus 70 is implicated in acute haemorrhagic conjunctivitis, a highly infectious disease. As the name suggests the main features are ocular but in some patients a paralytic illness, clinically indistinguishable from polio develops after 1–3 weeks (Kono et al. 1974). Enterovirus 71 was first reported from California and has since occurred in Bulgaria and Hungary. The paralysis in these patients has tended to follow a few days after the onset of an aseptic meningitis (Schmidt et al. 1974).

Rubella

Two patients were described in whom a diffuse myelopathy developed following live rubella vaccine. One developed symptoms after 4 days, the other after 2 weeks. A flaccid paraplegia was present in both cases with a sharp sensory level on the trunk. Only partial resolution of motor weakness was observed (Holt et al. 1976).

Mycoplasma

Man is the only known species for which this organism is pathogenic. It is most commonly encountered in relation to respiratory infections (atypical pneumonia). Neurological manifestations are the most common complication of *Mycoplasma* infection. These tend to develop about 10 days after the acute illness. Cord lesions occurring in this context tend to localize to a particular level ("transverse myelitis"). A clinical picture resembling the Guillain–Barré syndrome may also be seen (Levine and Lerner 1978; Decaux et al. 1980).

Non-metastatic Anterior Horn Cell Disease

A syndrome showing a strong clinical resemblance to MND has been described. The course of this disorder has been said to be less aggressive than that of sporadic MND (Brain et al. 1965). Thirteen patients with incidental carcinoma were reported in a series of 130 MND patients (Norris and Engel 1965) but no other reports of comparable or even larger series of MND patients have yielded such a high incidence of carcinoma. A single instance of an MND-like syndrome is reported in which the neurological features remitted when the large cell carcinoma of bronchus was resected (Mitchell and Olczak 1979). Despite these periodic contributions, however, the experience of routine neurological practice is that there is no relationship between anterior horn cell disease and occult neoplasia.

Paraproteinaemia and Anterior Horn Cell disease

The significance of the few cases described in which MND-like syndromes are associated with gammopathy (Parry et al. 1986) remains uncertain. A patient reported by Peters and Clatanoff (1968) with an MND-like syndrome associated with macroglobulinaemia responded to treatment with chlorambucil but had clear axillary lymphadenopathy on clinical examination at the time of presentation. A further patient has since been reported with a circulating IgM M paraprotein in which the abnormal protein was found to be bound presynaptically at the neuromuscular junction (Schluep and Steck 1988).

Anterior Horn Cell Involvement in Syringomyelia

The pattern of clinical signs in syringomyelia is variable, particularly in the early stages. In many cases the early findings can be related to a lesion at the cervicothoracic level. In other patients wasting of the intrinsic muscles of the hands is an important and prominent early sign. The clinicopathological correlates of this observation have been controversial. A series of 10 patients showed clear evidence of widespread neurogenic change in the upper limb using conventional EMG examination. On more quantitative testing using a single fibre EMG, the changes were found to affect the first dorsal interosseus muscle much more than either the biceps or extensor digitorum. This implied a relatively constant pattern of neurogenic change. The patterns seen on the single fibre studies closely resembled those associated with anterior horn cell degeneration. It was thus suggested that the distribution of anterior horn cell involvement in syringomyelia was consistent and that such changes could be demonstrated in most patients (Schwartz et al. 1980).

Stiff Person Syndrome

This curious condition shows some clinical similarity to tetanus. Females are only rarely affected and the disorder may persist for many years. Symptoms start in the truncal muscles and become progressively more generalized. Muscles may become board like. Sudden noise and attempts at passive movement may evoke painful spasms associated with manifestations of adrenergic discharge (Gordon et al. 1967) The muscles relax during sleep and general anaesthesia (Price and Allott 1958). Electromyography shows persistent tonic contraction which may be abolished by diazepam which has been used as well as clonazepam and baclofen in the treatment of this condition.

Its aetiology is obscure. Persistent α motor neurone activity has been postulated, possibly as a result of abnormal activity in the gamma motor system (Gordon et al. 1967).

References

Alter M, Kurland LT, Molgaard CA (1982) Late progressive muscular atrophy and antecedent poliomyelitis. In: Rowland LP (ed) Human motor neuron disease. Raven Press, New York, pp 303–309

Antel J, Medof M, Richman D et al. (1979) Immunological considerations in amyotrophic lateral sclerosis. In Rose FC (ed) Clinical neuroimmunology. Blackwell Scientific, Oxford, pp 227–244

Aran FA (1850) Recherches sur une maladie non encore d!ecrite du systeme musculaire. Arch Gén Méd (4me Sér) 24:1–35

Askmark H, Aquilonius S-M, Gillberg P-G et al. (1993) A pilot trial of dextromethorphan in amyotrophic lateral sclerosis. J Neurol Neurosurg Psychiatry 56:197–200

Auerback P, Crocker P (1982) Regular involvement of Clarke's nucleus in amyotrophic lateral sclerosis. Arch Neurol 39:155–156

Bartfield H, Dham C, Donnenfeld H et al. (1982) Immunological profile of amyotrophic lateral sclerosis patients and their cell-mediated responses to viral and CNS antigens. Clin Exp Immunol 48:137–147

Behan PO, Behan WM, Bell E et al. (1977) Possible persistent virus in motor neuron disease. Lancet ii:1176

Bell C (1836) The nervous system of the human body, 3rd edn. Longmans, London, pp 432–434

Bensimon G, Lacomblez L, Meininger V et al. (1994) A controlled trial of riluzole in amyotrophic lateral sclerosis. N Engl J Med 330:585–592

Blundell G, Mitchell JD (1985) The use of intrathecal IgG synthetic rates in diagnosis. In: Peeters H (ed) Protides of the biological fluids, Vol. 32. Pergamon Press, Oxford, pp 189–190

Bradley WG, Krasin F (1982) A new hypothesis of the etiology of amyotrophic lateral sclerosis – the DNA hypothesis. Arch Neurol 39:677–680.

Brain WR, Croft PB, Wilkinson M (1965) Motor neurone disease as an manifestation of neoplasm. Brain 88:479–500

Brooke MH, Florence JM, Heller SM et al. (1986) Controlled trial of thyrotropin releasing hormone in amyotrophic lateral sclerosis. Neurology 36:146–151

Brooks BR (1994) World Federation of Neurology Sub Committee on Neuromuscular Diseases. El Escorial Criteria for the diagnosis of amyotrophic lateral sclerosis. J Neurol Sci 124 (Suppl):96–108

Buckley J, Warlow C, Smith P et al. (1983) Motor neuron disease in England and Wales, 1959–1979. J Neurol Neurosurg Psychiatry 46:197–205

Calne DB, Eisen A (1989) The relationship between Alzheimer's disease, Parkinson's disease and motor neurone disease. Can J Neurol Sci 16:547–550

Campbell AMG, Williams ER, Barltrop D (1970) Motor neurone disease and exposure to lead. J Neurol Neurosurg Psychiatry 33:877–885

Caroscio, JT (1986) Amyotrophic lateral sclerosis: the disease. In: Caroscio JT (ed) Amyotrophic lateral sclerosis. Thieme, New York, pp 3–15

Caroscio JT, Cohen JA, Zawodiniak J et al. (1986) A double-blind, placebo-controlled trial of TRH in amyotrophic lateral sclerosis. Neurology 36:141–145

Chad D, Mitsumoto H, Adelman LS et al. (1982) Conjugal motor neurone disease. Neurology 32:306–307

Chalmers NC, Mitchell JD (1987) Optico-acoustic atrophy in distal spinal muscular atrophy. J Neurol Neurosurg Psychiatry 50, 238–239

Charcot JM (1872, 1873) Lecons sur les maladies du système nerveux fâites à la Salpetrière. Paris: Delahaye. Translated 1881, New Sydenham Society, London pp 180–191

Dalakas MC, Elder G, Hallett M et al. (1986) A long-term follow-up study of patients with post-poliomyelitis neuromuscular symptoms. N Engl J Med 314:959–963

Davidson TJ Hartmann HA (1981) RNA content and volume of motor neurones in amyotrophic lateral sclerosis. J Neuropathol Exp Neurol 40:187–192

Decaux G, Szyper M, Ectors M et al. (1980) Central nervous system complications of Mycoplasma pneumoniae. J Neurol Neurosurg Psychiatry 43:883–887

Durrleman S, Alprerovitch A (1989) Increasing trend of ALS in France and elsewhere: are the changes real. Neurology 39:768–773

Emery AEH, Holloway SM (1982) Familial motor neuron disease. In: Rowland LP (ed) Human motor neuron diseases. Raven Press, New York, pp. 139–147

Engel WK, Siddique T, Nicoloff JT et al. (1983a) TRH levels are reduced in CSF of amyotrophic lateral sclerosis and other spastic patients and rise with intravenous treatment. Neurology 33 (Suppl. 2):176

Engel WK, Siddique T, Nicoloff JT (1983b) Effect on weakness and spasticity in amyotrophic lateral sclerosis of thyrotropin releasing hormone. Lancet ii:73–75

Farrell DF, Starr A (1968) Delayed neurological sequelae of electrical injuries. Neurology 18:601–606

Feigenbaum JA, Munsat TL (1970) A neuromuscular syndrome of scapuloperoneal distribution. Bull Los Angeles Neurosurg Soc 35:47–57

Fraser KB, Shirodaria PV, Haire M (1979) Jejunal biopsy in multiple sclerosis. In: Behan PO, Rose FC (eds) Progress in neurological research. Pitman Medical, Tunbridge Wells, pp 73–78

Garruto RM, Swyt C, Fiori CE et al. (1985) Intraneuronal deposition of calcium and aluminium in amyotrophic lateral sclerosis of Guam. Lancet ii:1353

Gordon EE, Janusko DM, Kaufman L (1967) A critical survey of the stiff man syndrome. Am J Med 42:582

Gowers WR (1902) A lecture on abiotrophy: disease from defect of life. Lancet ii:1003–1007

Harding, AE (1984) The hereditary ataxias and related disorders. Churchill Livingstone, Edinburgh

Harding AE, Thomas PK, Baraitser M et al. (1982) X-linked bulbospinal neuronopathy: a report of ten cases. J Neurol Neurosurg Psychiatry 45:1012–1019

Harding AE, Bradbury PG, Murray NMF (1983) Chronic asymmetrical spinal muscular atrophy. J Neurol Sci 59:69–83

Harnisch R, Dworsky RL, Henderson BE (1976) A search for clues to the cause of amyotrophic lateral sclerosis. Arch Neurol 33:456–457

Hawkes CH, Fox J (1981) Motor neurone disease in leather workers. Lancet i:507

Hirayama K, Toyokura Y, Tsubaki T (1959) Juvenile muscular atrophy of unilateral upper extremity: a new clinical entity. Psychiatry Neurol Jpn 61:2190.

Holbrook LA, Beach FXM, Silver JR (1970) Delayed myelopathy: a rare complication of severe electrical burns. Br Med J 4:659–660.

Holloway SM, Emery AEH (1982) The epidemiology of motor neuron disease in Scotland. Muscle Nerve 5:131-133

Holloway SM, Mitchell JD (1986) Motor neurone disease in the Lothian Region of Scotland 1961-1981. J Epidemiol Community Health 40:344-350

Holt S, Hudgins D, Krishnan KR et al. (1976) Diffuse myelitis associated with rubella vaccination. Br Med J 2:1037-1038

Iwashira H, Inoue N, Araki S et al. (1970) Optic atrophy, neurol deafness and distal neurogenic atrophy. Arch Neurol 22:357-364

Jamal GA, Weir AI, Hansen S et al. (1985) Sensory involvement in motor neuron disease: further evidence from automated thermal threshold determination. J Neurol Neurosurg Psychiatry 48:906-910.

Jennekens FGI, Busch HFM, van Hemel NM et al. (1975) Inflammatory myopathy in scapulo-ilioperoneal atrophy with cardiopathy. A study of two families. Brain 98:709-722

Jones CT, Brock DJH, Chancellor AM et al. (1993) Cu/Zn superoxide dismutase (SOD1) mutations and sporadic amyotrophic lateral sclerosis. Lancet 342;1050-1051

Kaeser HE (1965) Scapuloperoneal muscular atrophy. Brain 88:407

Kilness AW, Hochberg FH (1977) Amyotrophic lateral sclerosis in a high selenium environment. JAMA 237:2843-2844

Kono R, Miyamura K, Tajiri E et al. (1974) Neurologic complications associated with acute haemorrhagic conjunctivitis virus infection and its serologic confirmation. J Infect Dis 129:590-593

Kugelberg E (1975) Chronic proximal (pseudomyopathic) spinal muscular atrophy. Kugelberg Welander syndrome. In: Vinken PJ, Bruyn GW (eds) Handbook of clinical neurology, Vol 22 (II). Elsevier, New York, pp 67-80

Leigh PN, Anderton BH, Dodson A et al. (1988) Ubiquitin deposits in anterior horn cells in motor neurone disease. Neurosci Lett 93:197-203

Levine DP, Lerner AM (1978) The clinical spectrum of Mycoplasma pneumoniae infections. Med Clin North Am 62:961-978

Lilienfeld DE, Chan E, Ehland J et al. (1989) Increasing mortality from motor neurone disease in the United States during the past two decades. Lancet i:710-713

Lowe J (1994) New pathological findings in amyotrophic lateral sclerosis. J Neurol Sci 124 (Suppl):38-51

Mann DMA, Yates PO (1974) Motor neuron disease - the nature of the pathogenic mechanism. J Neurol Neurosurg Psychiatry 37:1036-1046

Martyn CN, Barker DJP, Osmond C (1988) Motoneuron disease and past poliomyelitis in England and Wales. Lancet i:1319-1322

Mawatari S, Katayama K (1973) Scapuloperoneal muscular atrophy with cardiopathy. An X-linked recessive trait, Arch Neurol 28:55-59

Mayor GH, Remedi RF, Sprague SM et al. (1980) Central nervous system manifestations of aluminium: effect of parathyroid hormone. Neurotoxicology 1:33-42

McComas AJ, Upton ARM, Sica REP (1973) Motoneurone disease and ageing. Lancet ii:1477-1480

McLeod JG, Prineas JW (1971) Distal type of chronic spinal atrophy: clinical electro-physiological and pathological studies. Brain 94:703-714

Mitchell JD (1987) Heavy metals and trace elements in amyotrophic lateral sclerosis. Neurol Clin 5:43-60

Mitchell JD, Jackson MJ (1992) Free radicals, amyotrophic lateral sclerosis and neurodegenerative disease. In: Smith RA (ed) Handbook of amyotrophic lateral sclerosis. Marcel Dekker, New York, pp 533-541

Mitchell DM, Olczak SA (1979) Remission of a syndrome clinically indistinguishable from motor neurone disease after resection of bronchial carcinoma. B Med J 2:176-177

Mitchell JD, East BW, Harris IA et al. (1986) Trace elements in the spinal cord and other tissues in motor neuron disease. J Neurol Neurosurg Psychiatry 49:211-215

Mitchell JD, Gibson H, Gatrell AC (1990) Amyotrophic lateral sclerosis in Lancashire and South Cumbria 1976-1986: a geographic study. Arch Neurol 47:875-880

Mitchell JD, East BW, Harris IA, Pentland B (1991) Manganese, selenium and other trace elements in spinal cord, liver and bone in motor neurone disease. Eur Neurol 31:7-11

Mitchell JD, Gatt JA, Phillips TM et al. (1993) Cu/Zn superoxide dismutase, free radicals and motoneuron disease. Lancet 342;1051-1052

Mitchell JD, Houghton E, Rostron G et al. (1995) Serial studies of free radical and antioxidant activity in motor neurone disease and the effect of selegline. Neurodegeneration 4:233-235

Mitsumoto H, Salgado ED, Negroski D et al. (1986) Amyotrophic lateral sclerosis: effects of intravenous and subcutaneous administration of thyrotropin-releasing hormone in controlled trials. Neurology 36:152-159

Miyata S, Nakamura S, Nagata H et al. (1983) Increased manganese level in spinal cords of amyotrophic lateral sclerosis determined by radiochemical neutron activation analysis. J Neurol Sci 61:283-293

Morrison KE, Harding AE (1994) Disorders of the motor neurone. Baillieres Clin Neurol 3:431-445

Nagata H, Miyata S, Nakamura S et al. (1985) Heavy metal concentration in blood cells in patients with amyotrophic lateral sclerosis. J Neurol Sci 67:173–178

Nakagawa S, Yoshida S, Suematsu C et al. (1977) The calcium–magnesium deficient rat: a study on the distribution of calcium in the spinal cord using the electron probe microanalyser. Experientia 33:1225–1226

Neilson S, Robinson I, Clifford Rose F et al. (1993) Rising mortality from motor neurone disease: an explanation. Acta Neurol Scand 87:184–191

Neilson S, Gunnarsson L-G, Robinson I (1994) Rising mortality from motor neurone disease in Sweden 1961–1990: the relative role of increased population life expectancy and environmental factors. Acta Neurol Scand 90:150–159

Noronha ABC, Antel JP, Ross RP et al. (1981) Circulating immune complexes in neurologic disease. Neurology 31:1402–1407

Norris FH, Engel WK (1965) Carcinomatous amyotrophic lateral sclerosis. In: Brain WR, Norris FH (eds.) The remote effects of cancer on the nervous system. Grune & Stratton, New York, pp 81–82

Norris FH, U KS (1978) Amyotrophic lateral sclerosis and low urinary selenium levels. JAMA 239:404

Oldstone MBA, Wilson CB, Perrin LH et al. (1976) Evidence for immune-complex formation in amyotrophic lateral sclerosis. Lancet ii:169–172

Panse F (1970) Electrical lesions of the nervous system. In: Vinken PJ, Bruyn GW (eds) Handbook of clinical neurology, Vol 7. North Holland, Amsterdam, pp 344–387

Parry GJ, Holtz SJ, Ben-Zeev D et al. (1986) Gammopathy with proximal motor axonopathy simulating motor neuron disease. Neurology 36:273–276

Pederson L, Platz P, Jerseld C et al. (1977) HLA (SD and LD) in patients with amyotrophic lateral sclerosis. J Neurol Sci 31:313–318

Peters HA, Clatanoff DV (1968) Spinal muscular atrophy secondary to macroglobulinaemia. Neurology 18:101–118

Price TML, Allott EH (1958) The stiff man syndrome. B Med J 1:682

Riise T, Grønning M, Klauber MR et al. (1991) Clustering of residence of multiple sclerosis patients at age 13 to 20 years in Hordaland, Norway. Am J Epidemiol 133:932–939

Romberg MH (1851) Lehrbuch der Nervenkrankheiten des Menschen. 2nd edn. Dunker, Berlin. Translated and edited Sieveking (1853) Sydenham Society, London, pp 371–375

Rosen DR, Siddique T, Patterson D et al. (1993) Mutations in Cu/Zn superoxide gene are associated with familial amyotrophic lateral sclerosis. Nature 362:59–62

Schluep M, Steck AJ (1988) Immunostaining of motor nerve terminals by IgM M protein with activity against gangliosides GM1 and GD1b from a patient with motor neuron disease. Neurology 38:1890–18902

Schmidt NJ, Lennette EH, Ho HH (1974) An apparently new enterovirus isolated from patients with disease of the central nervous system. J Infect Dis 129:304–309

Schwartz MS, Stålberg E, Swash M (1980) Pattern of segmental motor involvement in syringomyelia: a single fibre EMG study. J Neurol Neurosurg Psychiatry 43:150–155

Serratrice GT, Toga M, Pellisier JF (1983) Chronic spinal muscular atrophy and pallidonigral degeneration: report of a case. Neurology 33:306–310

Shaw P (1994) Excitotoxicity and motor neurone disease: a review of the evidence. J Neurol Sci 124 (Suppl): 6–13

Shaw IC, Fitzmaurice PS, Mitchell JD et al. (1995) Studies on cellular free radical protection mechanisms in the anterior horn from patients with amyotrophic lateral sclerosis. Neurodegeneration 4:391–396

Siddique T, Figlewicz DA, Pericak-Vance JL et al. (1991) Linkage of a gene causing familial amyotrophic lateral sclerosis to chromosome 21 and evidence of genetic locus heterogeneity. N Engl J Med 324:1381–1384

Urbanek K, Jansa P (1974) Amyotrophic lateral sclerosis – abnormal cellular inflammatory response. Arch Neurol 30:186–187

Vijayalaxmi, Pentland B, Newton MS et al. (1985) Spontaneous and mutagen induced sister chromatid exchange in motor neurone disease. Mutat Res 150:355–358

Viola MV, Lazarus M, Antel J et al. (1982) Nucleic acid probes in the study of amyotrophic lateral sclerosis. In Rowland LP (ed) Human motor neuron diseases. Raven Press, New York, pp 317–329

Young ID, Harper PS (1980) Herditary distal spinal muscular atrophy with vocal cord paralysis. J Neurol Neurosurg Psychiatry 43:413–418

Chapter 21

Tropical Diseases of the Spinal Cord

K. Rajamani and C. Savant

Tropical Myeloneuropathies

The tropical myeloneuropathies are a heterogenous group of disorders affecting the spinal cord. They have been reported from various parts of the world – but within the tropical region extend from parts of Africa, Central and South America, the Caribbean islands, India and the Seychelles. These myeloneuropathic syndromes have been described under various headings and include Jamaican neuropathy. Tropical ataxic neuropathy, Konzo, Tropical spastic paraplegia, and Tropical myeloneuropathy. It is very likely that these are distinct and different disorders although some of the terms may have been used interchangeably. The causes are probably varied and include neurotoxicity due to cassava consumption, lathyrism, nutritional disorders due to malnutrition and malabsorption states and infections due to viruses and treponemes. The elucidation of the role of human T-cell lymphotropic virus (HTLV-1) in the aetiopathogenesis of Tropical spastic paraplegia in the mid-1980s has to some extent led to the clearer definition of these varied syndromes.

HTLV 1 Associated Myelopathy: Tropical Spastic Paraparesis

Probably the most common chronic non-compressive spastic paraplegia syndrome today in the tropics is Tropical Spastic Paraplegia (TSP). It is widely prevalent in the Caribbean islands (including Haiti, Jamaica, Dominican Republic, Martinique), parts of South America (Colombia, Brazil), India, South Africa and the Seychelles (Roman et al. 1986). For many years, neurologists in the tropics were aware of a non-compressive myelopathy with very distinct clinical features (Montgomerry et al. 1964). The cause of this condition remained unknown till Gessain et al. (1985) first showed the presence of antibodies to the human retrovirus, human T cell lymphotropic virus type 1 (HTLV-1) in the serum and cerebrospinal fluid (CSF) of patients with an unexplained myelopathy, in the island of Martinique. This virus had previously been isolated from certain aggressive forms of T-cell malignancies such as adult T-Cell leukaemia (ATL) (Posiesz et al. 1980). Based on the fact that the AIDS virus – another retrovirus – is neurotropic, they went on to postulate an aetiological role for this virus in TSP. Subsequently this observation has been confirmed

(Brew and Price 1988) and extended (Kira et al. 1992) and similar antibodies have been found in other countries, most notably Japan, where there is a high incidence of ATL as well as TSP. HTLV-1 proviral DNA has been found not only in the blood and CSF but also within the central nervous system (CNS) establishing the role of this retrovirus in the causation of this disorder. Osame et al. (1986b) described similar patients from Japan and coined the term HTLV-1 associated myelopathy (HAM). It is now widely believed that HTLV-1 associated myelopathy and tropical spastic paraplegia represents one and the same clinical entity, henceforth called HAM/TSP.

Clinical Features

The clinical features of HAM/TSP described from different parts of the world are uniform. The disease primarily affects adults in the third and fourth decades. With few exceptions it has been shown to have a slight female preponderance.

Carriers can remain asymptomatic for long periods of time. The exact incubation period is not known and could well be about 15–20 years. The onset is gradual and the disease progresses insidiously. Back pain may be a major presenting complaint before weakness begins in one or both legs. Upper limb involvement tends to be late and less severe. The neurological examination characteristically reveals a spastic paraparesis with exaggerated reflexes and extensor planter responses. Although numbness and dysaesthesiae may be present in the legs, a sensory level on the trunk is distinctly unusual. Posterior column loss as evidenced by distal vibration sense and proprioceptive sense loss may be seen in up to 58% of patients. Peripheral nervous system affection has been documented in up to 28% of patients with HAM/TSP (Bhagvati et al. 1988; Roman and Roman 1988). Cranial nerve involvement in the form of optic neuropathy and sensorineural deafness is also known to occur. Higher cognitive function is well maintained although frontal release reflexes may be present. Bladder involvement is characteristic and some patients may report impotence (Eardley et al. 1991). Other less common feature include a meningoencephalitis-like picture (Araga et al. 1989), predominant cerebellar involvement, cognitive decline, anterior horn cell disorder or a polymyositis like picture (Morgan et al. 1989; Kuroda and Sugihara 1991). The course of the disease is slowly progressive over months and years but only a minority become totally paraplegic. Patients acquiring the disease via contaminated blood transfusion tend to have a shorter incubation period and progress more rapidly.

Epidemiology and Modes of Transmission

Since the first report of HTLV-1 antibodies in patients of TSP by Gessain et al. from Martinique in 1985, many other pockets of HTLV-1 seropositivity have been identified in other islands of the Caribbean, in parts of Africa, including Kenya, Nigeria, Ghana and Zaire, Brazil, Colombia and in the Seychelles. HTLV-1 associated myelopathy has been described among West Indian born residents in the UK (Cruikshank et al. 1989), the immigrant black population in continental Europe and the USA (Newton et al. 1987). In Japan, a significant proportion of patients with a chronic myelopathy were detected to have antibodies to HTLV-1. Because Japan is geographically not within the tropics, Osame et al. (1986a) called this condition HTLV-1 associated myelopathy (HAM).

The modes of transmission of this condition seem to be varied (Ueda et al. 1988). Contaminated blood transfusion, intravenous drug abuse, vertical transmission from mother to child are all incrimininated. The seropositive mother can infect the child by the transplacental route due to uteroplacental bleeds, as well as by breast feeding. The breast milk contains large numbers of HTLV-1 positive lymphocytes which are responsible for the transmission of the infection. Prevention of breast feeding by seropositive mothers seems to reduce the risk of transmission from mother to child. Sexual transmission seems to be less important although conjugal cases have been described. Male to female sexual transmission seems to be more efficient than the other way around. Blood-sucking insect vectors like mosquitoes have been suggested as possible modes of transmission. The prevalence of HTLV-1 among homosexuals and intravenous drug abusers is said to be increasing (Robert-Guroff et al. 1986; Bartholomew et al. 1987).

Saxton et al. (1989) describe the detection of HTLV-1 virus in a white man who developed a myelopathy 15 months after intraoperative blood transfusion. Blood transfusion is not only very effective in the transmission of the disease, but the incubation period to the onset of the myelopathy seems to be significantly shortened and the progression of the disease seems to be more rapid. Cell-free serum does not lead to seroconversion in animals, highlighting the cellular association of the retrovirus (Anon 1988). With the introduction of screening for HTLV-1 antibodies among blood donors in Japan, the incidence of seroconversion fell to 0.15%, a marked decrease from the previously recorded 8.3%. It is, thus recommended that all donor blood in endemic areas be screened for HTLV-1 antibodies (Inaba et al. 1989).

Diagnosis

The diagnosis depends on the demonstration of a non-compressive myelopathy, either by a myelogram or an MRI scan of the spinal cord. Routine haematological and biochemical investigations are normal. Antibodies in the serum to HTLV-1 can be detected in 67%–94% by ELISA technique (Bhagvati et al. 1988). CSF examination reveals a mild to moderate increase in proteins and oligoclonal bands may be present in up to 75% of patients (Newton et al. 1987;415–417). Lymphocytic pleocytosis may be a feature but the elevation is seldom more than 100 cells/mm^3. Antibodies to HTLV-1 in the CSF may be seen in up to 75% of patients. Those who show the presence of these antibodies in the CSF are hardly ever seronegative (Rodgers–Johnson et al. 1985; Suehara et al. 1992). Japanese workers have shown, by the sensitive particle agglutination method, that these antibodies may also be found in asymptomatic carriers (Nakajima et al. 1989). Neopterin levels have been shown to be elevated in the CSF of HAM/TSP patients and is said to be useful to distinguish it from other chronic myelopathies. It is normal in asymptomatic carriers (Nomoto et al. 1991). It is an indicator of the activation of the immune system and is released by macrophages under stimulation by T lymphocytes. Visual evoked responses, somatosensory evoked responses as well as brainstem evoked responses may be abnormal in more than 50% of patients. MRI scan of the spinal cord may show diffuse swelling or a diffusely increased signal intensity within the spinal cord

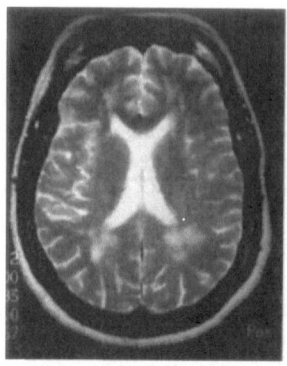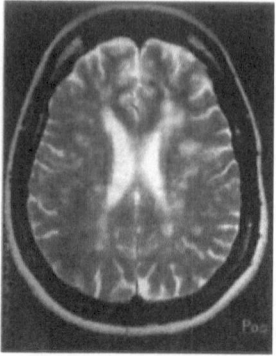

Fig. 21.1. MRI scan in a patient with HAM\TSP showing extensive periventricular white matter hyperintense signals on T2 weighted images.

on T2 weighted images. Brain MRI scan may be abnormal in a large number of patients and typically consists of multifocal white matter lesions (Fig. 21.1).

These changes are periventricular in distribution, appear as hyperintense lesions and tend to be less common in the brainstem and cerebellum compared to the supratentorial compartment. These changes have been reported even in asymptomatic HTLV-1 carriers. The MRI changes are quite similar to those seen in multiple sclerosis (MS) and although it has been claimed that the changes are not as profuse as that seen in MS, it can be difficult to distinguish between the two in a clinical setting (Miller et al. 1987; Mattson et al. 1987; Tournier–Lasserve et al. 1987). The diagnosis may not be difficult in tropical countries but in non-tropical countries, where MS is common, the difficulty is obvious. It has hence been suggested that in temperate regions, patients with unexplained chronic spastic paraparesis should have the blood and CSF tested for HTLV-1 antibodies.

Virology

The human T-cell lymphotropic virus type 1 belongs to a group of viruses called retroviruses – so called because of the characteristic presence of the enzyme, reverse transcriptase. This makes the virus capable of transcribing its own RNA into a DNA code which can be inserted into the host genome. HTLV-1 belong to the oncovirinae family, suggesting they are associated with tumours.

The human retroviruses include:

Human T-cell lymphotropic virus
   Type – 1   HTLV-1:   T cell leukaemia/TSP
   Type – 2   HTLV-2:   ? Hairy cell leukaemia
Human immunodeficiency virus
   HIV-1:   AIDS
   HIV-2:   mild AIDS

The HTLV-1 genome consists of three main genes:

1. The "gag" gene which codes for the core protein antigen of the virus.
2. The "pol" gene which codes for the reverse transcriptase enzyme.
3. The "env" gene which codes for the glycoprotien envelope protein of the virus.

In addition they have oncogenes which are associated with tumour production. Loss of the normally present regulatory mechanisms leads to the activation of the oncogenes and tumour production. More recently patients very similar to HAM/TSP have been described who had antibodies to HTLV-2 both in the serum as well as the CSF. HTLV-2 viral sequences have been identified in the peripheral lymphocytes as well (Jacobson et al. 1993; Harrington et al. 1993).

It has been conclusively shown by DNA blotting that the virus involved in HTLV-1 associated myelopathy and adult T-cell leukaemia are the same (Yoshida et al. 1987). It is intriguing, however, that some patients develop the neurological disease whereas others develop haematological manifestations. The two diseases seem to occur in the same individual very infrequently. Morgan et al. (1987) report a patient with HAM/TSP whose haematological picture was that of a preleukaemic state characterized by morphologically abnormal lymphocytes in the peripheral smear as well as an increase in the numbers of T-cells suggesting the emergence of a clone. Peripheral blood lymphocytes in patients with HAM/TSP seem to show an unusual increase in spontaneous proliferation, significantly higher than in controls or in asymptomatic HTLV-1 carriers. It is thought that this is possibly due to the increased expression of the interleukin-2 (IL-2) receptors on the lymphocytes of HAM/TSP patients (Itoyama et al. 1988a,b). Abnormal lymphocytes with lobulated nuclei called "flower cells" may be found in the peripheral blood and in the CSF of patients with HAM/TSP. The magnitude of the immune response to the virus is known to be regulated by immune response genes associated with the host's major histocompatibility complex (Usuku et al. 1988). Based on the magnitude of the response, carriers can be classified into "high" and "low" responders. The immune response to HTLV-1 may be an important factor in the development of the myelopathy and is genetically determined, (Vernant et al. 1987).

The "high" responders develop the neurological disease, and have high titres of HTLV-1 antibodies. In contrast, the "low" responders develop the haematological disease, and have relatively low titres of the antibody (Osame et al. 1989) Kayembe et al. (1990) describe a cluster of TSP patients associated with HTLV-1 antibodies in Zaire with striking familial and ethnic distribution suggesting again that susceptibility to TSP could be genetically determined. Familial cases of HTLV-1 associated myelopathy has been described from the Seychelles and the Kii peninsula of Japan. It is noteworthy that in some areas of the world like India and the Ivory Coast there seems to be a very low incidence of antibodies to HTLV-1 among patients with TSP (Hugon et al. 1990). The clinical and epidemiological features of "South Indian Paraplegia" (Mani 1973) seems to be similar to TSP described from the Caribbean and HAM from Japan, but none of the patients tested were positive for HTLV-1 antibodies (Richardson et al. 1989). No HTLV-1 antibodies were detected in a seroepidemiological study in India involving normal subjects and patients with various haematological malignancies (Advani et al. 1987). More recently Nishimura et al. (1993) have reported the presence of HTLV-1 viral sequences in the lymphocytes of an Indian patient with TSP who was HTLV-1 seronegative. This demonstrates that HTLV-1 infection can be present in the absence of HTLV-1 antibodies. Whether this is more widespread remains to be seen.

Pathology

The pathological changes are most striking in the spinal cord, the brunt of it being in the thoracic region. Both the grey matter and the white matter seem to be affected.

The long tracts in the lateral and anterior columns are affected. There is a loss of the axons as well as the myelin. There is a marked proliferation of astrocytes and infiltration by foamy macrophages. The blood vessels show perivascular cuffing with lymphocytes. The meninges show thickening with adhesions and lymphocytic infiltration. Perivascular cuffing may be evident in the medulla, pons, and the white matter of the cerebrum and the cerebellum (Akizuki et al. 1987).

Relationship Between Multiple Sclerosis and HAM/TSP

There seems to be an obvious overlap between the clinical, electrophysiological, and radiological features of these two conditions. This apparent similarity was strengthened with reports of HTLV-1 antibodies in patients with MS. Koprowski et al. (1985) reported a significantly higher incidence of HTLV-1 antibodies in Swedish MS patients compared with controls. They also reported detection of RNA homologous to HTLV-1 in CSF cells of MS patients. However, this initial report was not confirmed by subsequent workers (Ehrlich et al. 1991). Newton et al. (1987) did not find any evidence of HTLV-1 infection in 48 patients with MS in the UK. Although there is an isolated case report of a Japanese patient with MS with antibodies to HTLV-1 in the serum as well as the CSF (Kaji et al. 1989). Kuroda et al. (1987) based on a more extensive study, report that the incidence of antibodies to HTLV-1 in Japanese MS patients is not increased as compared to controls. Watanabe et al. (1989) report similar negative results using the more sensitive polymerase chain reaction in nine Japanese MS patients.

The treatment of HAM/TSP remains unsatisfactory. Osame et al. (1986b) reported a good response to steroids and other forms of immunosuppressive treatment, an observation which has not been confirmed by other workers. Antiviral therapy remains a possible avenue for exploration in the future, as has been the case for HIV disease. At the present time, prevention certainly seems to be better than cure!

Konzo

Konzo is a distinct clinical entity affecting the spinal cord. It has been reported from Zaire, Tanzania, Mozambique, Nigeria and the Central African Republic (Carton et al. 1986; Tylleskar et al. 1994). It occurs in epidemics although sporadic cases have also been described in between. An outbreak in 1981 in Mozambique is reported to have affected more than 1000 individuals (Ministry of Health, Mozambique 1984a,b)

The clinical features seem to be quite similar to those of lathyrism. The patients described have been children and adults, and both sexes are affected. The disease affects the individual quite suddenly and often presents as an inability to get up after a fall, or a weakness in the legs after a long walk. There is no preceding systemic illness like fever or malaise. A significant number of patients complain of backpain, pain in the knees, and dysaesthesias in the legs. The affection of the legs is characteristically symmetrical. The patients exhibit typically a scissor gait with marked spasticity, weakness and hyperreflexia in the lower limbs.

The upper limbs may show hyperreflexia but weakness is seldom present. Sensory signs, cerebellar involvement and bladder dysfunction are unusual. Visual symptoms and dysarthria may be present in the acute stages but tend to improve and are absent in the later stages. In fact, there tends to be an improvement in the overall clinical picture initially, but later the condition remains static. In a small number of patients, relapses with acute exacerbations of the residual symptoms and signs have been reported (Howlett et al. 1990).

Laboratory tests including CSF examination are normal. The CSF does not show the presence of oligoclonal bands. MRI of the brain and the spinal cord are normal in Konzo, in contrast to the diffuse white matter changes seen in T2 weighted images in HAM/TSP or MS. Nerve conduction studies, electromyography and brainstem evoked responses have all been normal. Transcranial magnetic stimulation of the motor cortex fails to evoke a motor response both in the lower limbs and the upper limbs, suggesting selective damage to the upper motor neurone. Responses may not be obtained in the upper limb inspite of relatively well preserved voluntary control of the arms (Tylleskar et al. 1993). Elevated levels of thiocyanate may be found in the serum especially in the acute stages.

There seems to be some debate about the exact aetiology of konzo. Clinically it seems to be quite similar to neurolathyrism, but *Lathyrus sativus*, or chick pea, which is incriminated in lathyrism is not cultivated in these parts of the world. Based on epidemiological factors, Carton et al. (1986) raise the possibility of an infectious agent like a virus. There is no evidence to link it to an HTLV-1 infection (Rosling et al. 1988). However, the more widely accepted explanation seems to be the consumption of inadequately prepared bitter cassava roots leading to cyanide toxicity. Bitter cassava is an important staple crop in these parts of Africa and its hardy nature makes it an important provider of calories especially during times of drought. Cassava is rich in cyanogenic glycosides which are normally removed by traditional cooking processes which involve soaking for an adequate length of time, followed by roasting and sun drying of the roots. The little cyanide left in the roots is detoxified in the body to thiocyanates by the sulphur-containing amino acids. Two things seem to occur during times of drought, leading to the disease. First, the processing time of the cassava roots is drastically reduced leaving the cyanide levels in the cassava roots at dangerously high levels. Secondly, these roots become the staple diet to the total exclusion of all other foods, leading to deficiency of notably the sulphur-containing amino acids, leucine and methionine. This causes an impairment in the individual's capacity to detoxify the ingested cyanide. The build up of cyanide by itself may be toxic to the nervous system (Tylleskar et al. 1992) and animal studies have confirmed this and have linked the cyanide to the aetiology of konzo. On the other hand, the diversion of the sulphur-containing amino acids to detoxify the cyanide may be contributing to the malfunction of the nervous system. Nutritional experts have also shown that the cyanide exposure can be reduced to negligible levels simply by encouraging traditional methods of cassava processing. As with beri-beri, simple measures like this can go a long way to preventing potentially devasting epidemics (Cliff et al. 1985). It is poverty, food shortage, and ignorance that are at the root of this dreadful disease.

Tropical Ataxic Neuropathy

Tropical ataxic neuropathy is another distinct spinal cord syndrome described from the tropics, in particular from Nigeria, Mozambique, Senegal, as well as the West

Indies. It is endemic particularly among the lower socioeconomic strata, where poor nutritional status is common (Anonymous, 1968).

Osuntokun (1973) has studied in detail 375 Nigerian patients who suffered from this condition. The sex distribution is roughly equal, and it can affect any age group, although the maximum incidence is in the fourth and fifth decades of life. The onset is usually insidious with an ataxia of gait, paraesthaesiae in the lower limbs or weakness. Very rarely the disease can begin with a sudden onset of retrobulbar neuropathy. In the majority of patients the disease follows a progressive course although a small minority may show fluctuations in the symptoms. Paraesthesiae or dysaesthesiae usually start in the lower limbs distally, and patients often complain of an inability to feel the ground. The paraesthesiae progressively ascends upwards and patients may complain of girdle pains in the lumbar region. Other symptoms include blurring of vision, deafness, and very rarely sphincter disturbances (Osuntokun 1968).

Physical examination often reveals evidence of malnutrition in the form of angular stomatitis and glossitis (Osuntokun et al. 1968). Up to 85% of patients have marked posterior column signs in the lower limbs as evidenced by joint position sense loss, loss of vibration sense, impaired coordination and a sensory ataxia. Ophthalmological findings include loss of visual acuity, with a concentric diminution of the visual fields. Fundoscopy commonly reveals temporal pallor of the optic discs, or even frank optic atrophy. Sensorineural deafness is seen in roughly half the patients. Weakness in the legs is seen in about 38% along with hypotonia and hyporeflexia. Spasticity is distinctly uncommon although extensor planter responses may be obtained. The upper limbs tend to be spared except in the advanced cases. The natural history is one of gradual progression although it may subsequently become static (Osuntokun 1968; Adesina 1991). CSF examination is usually normal. Myelographic examinations done on these patients have been normal. Electrophysiological studies show evidence of a symmetrical peripheral neuropathy, with slowing of motor conduction velocities as well as neurogenic changes of denervation (Osuntokun 1973).

Epidemiological studies have shown a high dietary intake of cyanide in patients with tropical ataxic neuropathy (Osuntokun et al. 1969; Makene and Wilson 1972). Cassava tubers are a rich source of cyanide and they form a staple diet for especially the lower socioeconomic strata. Many of these patients have glossitis and angular stomatitis, clinical signs classically attributed to nutritional deficiency states. It has been suggested that theoretically these represent only a depressed oxidative metabolism in the rapidly proliferating cells, something which can occur even in chronic cyanide intoxication. Moreover, field studies have shown vitamin deficiencies in Nigerians without neurological disease. Hence coexistent vitamin deficiencies probably play a relatively minor role, if any, in the pathogenesis of tropical ataxic neuropathy (Osuntokun et al. 1985). Studies have shown an absence or a diminution of the sulphur-containing amino acids, cysteine and methionine, in the serum of patients with this condition. This could represent either a low intake of proteins or its utilization in the detoxification of the excessive cyanide. Cassava tubers by themselves are a very poor source of protein (Monekosso and Wilson 1966).

What is intriguiging is why some people with cyanide intoxication from cassava consumption get konzo, whereas others get tropical ataxic neuropathy. The two diseases are quite distinct clinically and epidemiologically. It has been suggested that the cyanide exposure in cases of tropical ataxic neuropathy as reflected by the thiocyanate levels in the serum was considerably lower than that in patients with konzo. Exposure to high levels of cyanide for short periods of time probably results in pure upper motor neurone damage as in konzo, whereas in tropical ataxic neuropathy the exposure is said to be more prolonged at lower levels (Howlett et al. 1990).

Lathyrism

Lathyrism is a disease affecting the motor system, induced by prolonged primary consumption of the seeds of *Lathyrus sativus*.

Epidemiology

This disease has been known since the time of Hippocrates. It has also been mentioned in the ancient Ayurvedic treatise Bhav Prakash (Dastur 1962; Misra 1989). However, the first description of its clinical features and its relationship to the consumption of *Lathyrus sativus* was by Dr Francis Buchanan in 1811 (Sinha 1989). Cases of neurolathyrism have been reported from various parts of the world which include Bangladesh, northwest China, Ethiopia, Greece, Israel (survivors of World War II), India, Nepal, North Africa, Spain, Southern Eurasia and Germany. This disorder is now unknown in the western world. Endemic zones are India (Uttar Pradesh, Bihar, Madhya Pradesh), Nepal, Bangladesh and Ethiopia (Ludolph et al. 1987; Misra et al. 1993).

Lathyrism is more common in males than females, and the latter are usually less severely affected. Although cases have been reported between 2 and 70 years, men are usually affected between 5 and 40 years and women from ages 6 to 20 years. The legume *Lathyrus sativus* commonly known as chickling pea, is also known over the world by various names, grass pea (Africa), Khesari dal (India, Bangladesh), Matri dal (India). *Lathyrus sativus* is a hardy crop that needs no irrigation, fertilizers or pesticides. It survives natural calamities, such as floods, pestilence, famine and drought. Due to the scarcity of food this seed forms the staple diet of the poorer sections of the population, resulting in epidemics. This pulse is nutritious and is rich in protein (28%).

In India it is a winter crop, harvested in March. The disease therefore has seasonal occurrence, commonly seen from March to November with peak incidence in July. Several thousands of agricultural labourers in Central India have been living for decades on Khesari dal, given to them by landlords as payment (Jayaraman 1989).

Clinical Features

The clinical picture is essentially that of a spastic paraparesis which can appear acutely, subacutely or insidiously and is identical in its clinical presentation all over the world. Most often weakness is precipitated by a fall, following large consumption of the seed and exposure to cold. The patient often wakes up from sleep with weakness. The initial symptoms are cramping of the calves, tremulousness, sensation of heaviness in the legs, paraesthesiae, urgency and frequency of micturition, sphincter spasms, rarely abnormal thirst, nocturnal erections and ejaculations and impotence. These suggest some degree of diffuse and transient excitation of somatic, motor and autonomic nervous system functions. They usually reverse on cessation of *Lathyrus sativus* intake.

In 1922, H.W. Acton, while working in India, graded the disability according to the extent of walking difficulty and the need of physical support. The majority of cases could walk without support (no stick stage). A few needed to use a single stick, fashioned from a branch of a tree (one stick stage) or two sticks (two stick stage). Rarely, severely affected individuals would resort to crawling on their hands and feet for ambulation (crawler stage). There is a vast majority of people in the subclinical stage who do not seek medical attention.

Higher cortical functions and the cranial nerves are usually spared. The common findings are bilateral spastic weakness of the lower limbs with exaggerated reflexes with or without clonus and extensor plantars. The upper limbs are usually spared but increased tone, exaggerated reflexes with Hoffman's sign is noted in a few patients. Spasticity is out of proportion to the weakness in these individuals and is the main cause of disability. Tendon reflexes are difficult to elicit in a crawler stage due to severe contractures. Superficial reflexes are preserved in the majority. Due to the resistance of affected muscles to passive stretch most patients assume a characteristic posture with hip flexed, knee flexed and torso angled backwards to maintain the balance. The spasticity in hip adductors, quadriceps and gastrocnemius makes them walk with a characteristic weaving and jerking gait on the balls of their feet. Lower motor neurone signs and peripheral neuropathy is seen in a minority of the patients (Cohn and Striefler 1981; Ludolph et al. 1987; Misra et al. 1993).

Laboratory Findings

Neurophysiological assessment of central motor pathways showed delayed conduction predominantly in the lower limbs in some patients, whereas in others no response could be obtained. The upper limbs were less commonly affected (Hugon et al. 1993; Misra and Sharma 1994). Electrophysiological signs of lower motor neurones were seen in the lower limbs in patients with long-standing disease (Drory et al. 1992). The CSF was found to be normal.

Aetiology and Pathogenesis

β-N-Oxalylamino-L-alanine (BOAA), also known as Ox-Dapro and β-N-oxalyl-L-α, β-diaminopropionic acid (ODAP), is a potent neuroexcitatory amino acid present in the chickling pea and is probably responsible for lathyrism. This compound was first isolated and identified as a toxic principle in the seed by Rao and Murthy in 1964 (Rao et al. 1964; Wadia 1989).

This amino acid has a molecular structure similar to glutamate and is a potent glutamate agonist. Glutamate activates at least three types of receptors the NMDA, AMPA and kainic acid, BOAA is an AMPA receptor agonist (Krogsgaard and Hansen 1991). It produces seizures and acute neuronal degeneration when injected intraperitoneally in newborn Swiss albino mice (Olney et al. 1976). Macaques fed with *L. Sativus* seed, its extract and BOAA had fine tremors, myoclonus like jerks and hind-limb extension. Severely affected monkeys had exaggerated patellar reflexes with extensor plantars. Upper limbs were relatively spared. These changes were similar to macaques who had surgically induced pyramidal lesions (Spencer et al. 1986). Adult monkeys, when injected intrathecally with pure OX-Dapro, had transient weakness in both lower limbs on the smaller dose and partial, permanent spastic paraplegia on an increased dose (Rao et al. 1967).

Ludolph et al. (1987) showed an intake of 200–400 g of *L. sativus* per day for a period of 2–3 months to be sufficient to produce neurolathyrism in adequately nourished and malnourished individuals. They also noted that subjects who ingested high quantities of this seed had an acute onset of symptoms as compared to chronic onset in those who consumed less. Those who presented with acute onset were with few exceptions severely handicapped (Hugon et al. 1988).

Pathology

There are very few neuropathological reports on this disease, owing to the fact that it is crippling but not fatal. The most obvious changes are loss of axons and myelin in the anterior and dorsolateral corticospinal tracts predominantly at thoracic level. Retrograde secondary degeneration of Betz cells was seen. Striefler and Hirano in their single case report showed eosinophilic rod-like inclusions in the anterior horn cells. Some of the anterior horn cells showed degenerative changes, such as swelling, loss of Nissl substance and peripheral displacement of nuclei (Hirano 1976; Striefler et al. 1977). Nerve pathology has shown honeycombing of peripheral nerves with connective tissue proliferation and thickening along with degeneration of myelin (Dastur 1962; Striefler et al. 1977; Cohn and Striefler 1983).

The neuropathological involvement of the pyramidal tracts in the dorsal, lumbar and sacral regions shows predilection of this toxin for these regions and correlates well with the stereotyped clinical picture of spastic paraparesis.

The predominant involvement of the lower limbs suggests that the longer corticospinal tracts regulating motor function of the legs are affected first and to a greater extent than the shorter corticospinal tracts controlling the movements in the arm.

Course and Prognosis

The disease usually stabilizes after stopping consumption of *L. sativus*. In the initial stages of illness some improvement occurs allowing many individuals to be ambulant. Initial symptoms like cramping of the legs, heaviness and paresthesiae wane or reverse completely if consumption of the seed stops. In some, late deterioration occurs with the development of lower motor neurone signs in the form of atrophy of flexors and extensors of feet. Thus the whole clinical picture simulates motor neurone disease (Calne et al. 1986).

Prevention and Treatment

There is no known specific treatment. The disease is preventable by not consuming the pulse. Antispasmodics are helpful to some extent symptomatically, however they are prohibitively expensive in developing countries. Due to ignorance and unavailability of other food this seed is still consumed in the endemic areas. If the pulse must be eaten then the toxin can be detoxified by soaking the pulse in a large volume of hot water or by parboiling it before cooking. Efforts are being made to grow strains of *L. sativus* which are free of BOAA (Wadia 1989; Bharucha and Bharucha 1991, Haimanot et al. 1990).

Tuberculosis of Spine and Spinal Cord

The incidence of tuberculosis (TB) has declined sharply in the developed countries over recent decades. It still remains a major medical problem in developing countries particularly in Asia. In UK and USA, TB is on an upward trend in the immigrant population, in homeless elderly and with the advent of HIV infection (Medical Research Council TB and Chest Diseases Unit 1980).

Central nervous system (CNS) tuberculosis is always secondary to tuberculous infection elsewhere in the body, hence the incidence of CNS tuberculosis is in proportion to incidence of TB in a given community, which in turn depends on various factors like overcrowding, malnutrition, hygiene, socioeconomic conditions, and the availability of immunization programmes in that population.

It affects the spinal cord in various ways. It can be (a) a complication of tuberculous meningitis; (b) a complication of vertebral TB; (c) tuberculous radiculomyelitis as a first manifestation of tuberculosis of CNS.

Clinical Features

Various authors in the past have described the clinical picture under various headings like intradural spinal tuberculomas (Parsons and Pallis 1965), epidural spinal tuberculous granulomas (Kocen and Parsons 1970), intraspinal tuberculous granulomas (Tandon and Pathak 1973), tuberculous spinal arachnoiditis, spinal complication of tuberculous meningitis. Wadia coined the term tuberculous radiculomyelitis to describe these cases (Wadia and Dastur 1969).

In all patients irrespective of the cause, the clinical picture is that of various combinations of root and cord involvement. In the patients with known tuberculous meningitis, spinal cord complication follows the original event after a week to few years, especially following inadequate treatment. It can, however, be seen in patients undergoing treatment or having received full treatment in the past. The onset of illness can be subacute or insidious. In patients with subacute onset, the clinical picture develops to its maximum severity within a few days and then stabilizes. The patient appears ill and is febrile. Fever is low grade with malaise. Often an evening rise of temperature is noted and is associated with anorexia and weight loss. Very often clinical evidence of TB is seen elsewhere.

The symptoms include root pains, paraesthesiae, bladder disturbance, weakness and wasting of the muscles. Radicular pain is the commonest presenting symptom. These are severe, sharp lancinating and often do not respond to analgesics or hypnotics. A patient often presents with sciatica, usually bilateral. Vice-like girdle pains aggravated by breathing are common. The root pains ascend to involve the dorsal and subsequently the cervical region. In some patients they occur simultaneously over several segments. Patients with rapid progression have severe and multiple root pains. Pain and stiffness in the spine is seen over the involved segments. Paraesthesiae in the form of tingling sensations often follow the root pains. Numbness with loss of sensation is segmental, whereas a clearcut sensory level over the trunk suggests cord involvement. Posterior column sensation is affected in both lower limbs. Weakness in the lower limbs can vary in severity. Combination of upper and lower motor neurone involvement is a feature. Retention of urine usually accompanies weakness but can be a presenting symptom in some. This again depends on the rapidity with which the lesion has progressed. Those with chronic onset and progressive course clinically present like a spinal cord tumour. Scattered root pains makes one suspect the diagnosis.

Three distinct syndromes are observed. When the neurological deficit is confined to a single level the picture mimics transverse myelitis. Patients with multifocal radiculomyelopathy have cervical myelopathy with sciatica-like pains, lower motor neurone signs in the lower limbs and absent ankle jerks. The ascending variant can involve lumbar, thoracic and cervical roots extensively causing fatal diaphragmatic and intercostal paralysis and this can occasionally extend intracranially. The clinical syndrome simulates Guillain–Barré syndrome or ascending myelitis, but a careful history of extensive root pains gives a clue to the underlying pathology (Wadia and Dastur 1969). The diagnosis of tuberculous radiculomyelitis is clear when there is associated tuberculous meningitis or vertebral TB, but when it occurs as a first manifestation of CNS tuberculosis it can lead to a diagnostic problem.

Intramedullary tuberculomas are rare. They are evenly distributed along the whole length of the cord. Clinically they present like a spinal cord tumour. The onset of symptoms is insidious and slowly progressive. They may occasionally rupture into the subarachnoid space causing meningitis. Most often the patient has evidence of pulmonary TB (Lin 1960).

Vertebral Tuberculosis

Percival Pott in 1779 remarked on an association of palsy in the lower limbs to the curvature of the spine, but it was not until the TB bacillus was discovered by Koch in 1882, that the aetiology of this disease became clear.

The spine is the commonest site of bone TB accounting for more than half the cases (Gorse et al. 1983). The incidence of neural tissue involvement varies between 10% and 47% in different studies (Bailey et al. 1972; Tandon and Pathak 1973; Gorse et al. 1983; Omari et al. 1989). It is the commonest cause of compression of the spinal cord in developing countries. The commonest site of involvement is the lower dorsal followed by dorsolumbar, cervicodorsal and cervical in decreasing order of frequency. However, the incidence of paraplegia is higher in the cervicodorsal region than the lower dorsal region. Frequently more than one vertebra is involved.

In the developing countries with high rates of skeletal TB and infectivity, the affected population are predominantly children and young adults whereas in US and Europe it is the elderly population. The incidence of paraplegia is, however, higher in adults than in children (Gorse et al. 1983).

Pain locally is the commonest presenting symptom. This is associated with muscle spasms, tenderness and restriction of movements over the affected segments.

Kyphosis or gibbus formation occurs late in the disease. Patients with greater angulation of spine have higher incidence of neurological involvement. Scoliosis is rare. Flank or groin mass is seen in a few patients. Spasm or contracture of psoas muscle may lead to flexed deformity of the hip. Occasionally a psoas abscess can be felt in the thigh region due to trickling of the pus along the tendon. Spinal cord and root compression can occur due to extradural and paraspinal abscess extension intraspinally, granuloma encircling the cord, sequestered bone or intervertebral discs, pathological subluxation of vertebrae and stretching of the spinal cord over the bony and fibrous ridges. The last complication may cause paraplegia years after bony resolution of active tuberculous infection has occurred. Hence, it is essential that the patients with vertebral TB are followed-up. Paraplegia may be a presenting symptom, particularly in developing countries as earlier symptoms of pain and spasms are ignored by the patient. Frank meningitis is uncommon. Constitutional symptoms like fever and weight loss may be present. Draining sinuses are seen, which may or may not be in communication with the spinal canal. Non-compressive radiculomyelopathy as described earlier is seen as a direct spread of infection from the bone through dura with eventual involvement of the spinal cord. Radiculomyelitis may occur a few segments away from the vertebral lesion. Here vertebral involvement is purely coincidental (Freilich and Swash 1979). Thrombosis of the vessels supplying the spinal cord due to vasculitis may cause acute onset non-compressive paraplegia (Tandon and Pathak 1973).

TB of the cervical spine may present with torticollis and restriction of neck movements. The large abscesses particularly in children pushes the trachea onto the sternal notch causing difficulty in swallowing or respiratory stridor, whereas compression of the spinal cord is seen in adults causing tetraparesis (Hsu and Leong 1984). Tuberculous atlantoaxial dislocation is an infrequent entity and is one of the causes of cervicomedullary compression in developing countries. The clinical picture is similar to the TB of cervical spine (Lal et al. 1992).

Laboratory Findings

Peripheral blood smear, may show leucocytosis with relative lymphocytosis. ESR may be elevated. The Mantoux test is positive in most but may be negative in 20% (Tandon and Pathak 1973; Kocen 1977). It may be negative in patients with miliary tuberculosis and suppressed cellular immunity. With cases with tuberculous meningitis, the CSF is abnormal. The appearance may be clear to xanthochromatic. When allowed to stand at room temperature, it clots. Pleocytosis is common and is predominantly lymphocytic and mononuclear. In the acute stage of the disease, the response may be neutrophilic as seen in pyogenic meningitis (Kocen and Parsons 1970; Traub et al. 1984). Its protein content is elevated. CSF sugar is low but not to the extent seen in pyogenic meningitis. CSF may be completely normal in the initial stages but if the clinical picture strongly suggests the diagnosis, repeat CSF examination should be undertaken. A normal CSF should not exclude the possibility of tuberculous infection. In tuberculous arachnoiditis (radiculomyelitis) lumbar puncture may result in a genuine dry tap. In these patients a serial rise in the CSF protein content suggests impending spinal block, which is often followed by paralysis. Timely institution of steroids may prevent this (Wadia 1973). CSF protein content in a spinal block may be as high as 1–4 g/100 ml. Demonstration of tubercle bacilli in CSF is an absolutely confirmatory test, but depends on the experience of the observer and stage of infection. It can be as low as 15%–20% to as high as 87% (Kennedy and Fallon 1979; Molavi and Lefrock 1985). Examinations of serial CSF specimens may give a more positive yield. Very often CSF examination of patients who have been started on treatment will show tubercle bacilli (Kennedy and Fallon 1979). CSF should be cultured and sensitivity to antituberculous drugs must be checked. This is time consuming and an expensive procedure and again is positive in only 45%–90% of all patients (Molavi and Lefrock 1985; Omari et al. 1989). Often the clinical situation makes it necessary to start treatment without confirmatory evidence of TB. A good response to antituberculous drugs is diagnostic. In view of the difficulty in demonstrating the tuberculous bacilli in the CSF and the delay of 6–8 weeks in obtaining cultures, various other methods should be attempted to diagnose tuberculous meningitis as early as possible. CSF permeability to bromide is increased in tuberculous meningitis, so the plasma to CSF bromide ratio is less than 1.6:1 (normal 3:1). This test is useful in differentiating tuberculous meningitis from viral but not pyogenic meningitis (Mandal et al. 1972). It is also positive in various other lymphocytic infections (Weinberg and Coppack 1985). Other methods are demonstration of tuberculostearic acid by gas chromatography/mass spectroscopy (Mardh et al. 1983), tuberculous antigen detection in CSF by ELISA (Sada et al. 1983) and latex particle agglutination (Krambovitis et al. 1984), but these again lack specificity (Lancet 1983).

A chest X-ray must be done on all patients to look for evidence of pulmonary TB. Plain radiographs of the whole spine may be required to look for vertebral TB. This may show narrowing of the disc space adjacent to the affected vertebra. Erosion of the vertebral body with complete collapse may occur as the disease advances. If the anterior portion of the vertebral body is affected, it causes kyphosis. Lateral involvement results in scoliosis which is rare. Scalloping of the anterior vertebral margins is seen. Posterior neural arch involvement usually results in cavity formation which can be missed easily on plain radiographs. Loss of pedicle is rarely seen. Paravertebral abscess may appear as a fusiform or globular swelling with calcification in chronic cases. Psoas abscess is seen as a soft tissue shadow of increased density with or without calcification in that region. The cervical spine may show similar bony changes as mentioned above, with increased prevertebral shadow (Fig. 21.2).

Wadia and Dastur (1969) described the detailed myelographic findings in tuberculous radiculomyelitis. Total spinal block over several segments was demonstrated by both the cisternal and lumbar route in some patients. Partial block with multiple cystic filling defects occurred over several segments giving an appearance of candle guttering. The edge of the block was ragged. Thickening of the roots was noted in the cauda equina region. In a few cases large cystic filling defects were noted. Myelography in intramedullary tuberculoma may show complete block (Lin 1960).

The degree of bony destruction is best demonstrated on CT scan. Initially central lytic lesions are seen in the vertebral body which are confined. They subsequently coalesce and result in vertebral body collapse. The initial lesion affects the anterior and inferior portion of the vertebral body. CT scan is particularly useful in the thoracic region and for visualizing the rib involvement which can be difficult on plain radiographs. Posterior neural arch elements like pedicles are better defined on CT scan. The spinal thecal sac can be seen with a special window setting. Paraspinal abscesses which are occasionally missed on plain radiographs are noted on CT scan in about 10% of the patients.

MRI certainly has the advantage of showing the spinal cord and the effect of soft tissue elements on the cord. It is useful in distinguishing compressive from non-

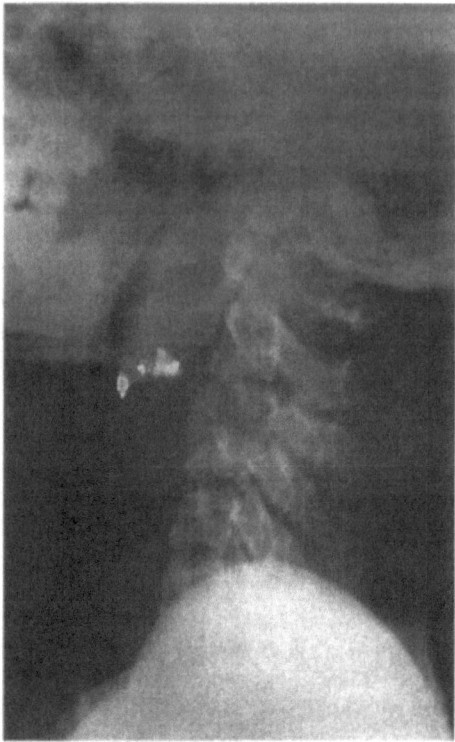

Fig. 21.2. Plain radiograph of the cervical spine. Note the destruction of C3 body as well as the end plate and C3–C4 disc space. Note also the soft tissue mass anterior to the bodies of vertebrae. (Photograph courtesy Professor S.N. Bhagwati, Bombay.)

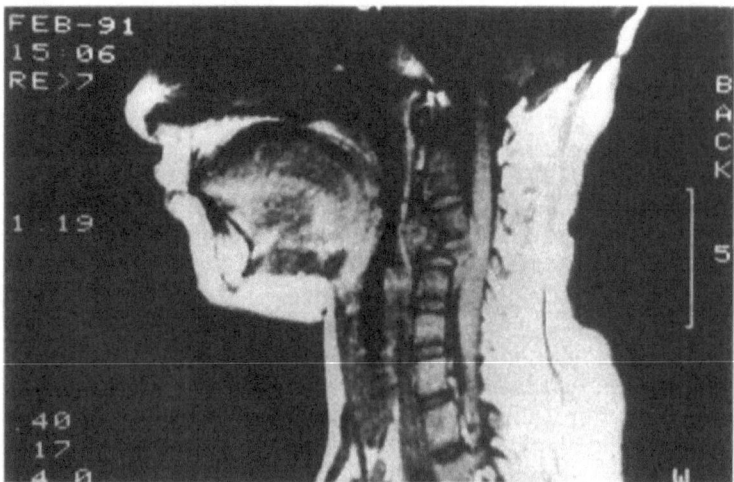

Fig. 21.3. MRI of the cervical spine (T1 weighted images). Note the destruction of the C3 and C4 vertebral bodies and the disc space, and the soft tissue pressing on the spinal cord. (Photograph courtesy Professor S.N. Bhagwati, Bombay.)

compressive neurological complications in vertebral TB. This helps to decide the choice between conservative and surgical management, or a combination of both. It helps to assess the response to therapy. The disadvantages are that it may miss a small bony fragment and calcification in the abscesses. Interventional procedures, however, are difficult with MRI imaging.

On MRI, lesions in the vertebral body have a low signal intensity on T1 weighted images (Fig. 21.3) with increase in intensity on T2 weighted images (Desai 1994). Gadolinium-enhanced images showed focal or rim enhancement within the vertebral bodies. At surgery this was found to be necrotic infected material. The extent of the lesion and spread of debris as well as pus under anterior and posterior longitudinal ligaments can be seen. Enhancement of anterior and posterior ligaments outlined paraspinal abscesses and their loculations which were not seen on unenhanced images. Liquid pus appears bright on T2 weighted images. Gadolinium enhancement is greater in fibrous tissue on T1 weighted images than pus. MRI thus helps to differentiate pus and granulation tissue from fibrosis. The fibrosis requires surgical decompression whereas pus and granulation tissue may respond to conservative treatment (Hoffman et al. 1993). The follow-up scans in patients receiving treatment showed reversal of the abnormal signal intensity on T1 weighted images, as well as a decrease in the signal intensity on T2 weighted images. The presence of paraspinal abscess with disc affection, associated spinal deformity, affection of posterior elements, extension of abscess and bony fragments all help to distinguish tuberculous vertebral involvement from other granulomatous lesions like brucellosis or fungal infection (Sharif et al. 1990).

The MRI appearance of intramedullary tuberculomas is identical to intracranial lesions. The two cases reported by Jena et al. (1991) showed a hypointense ring-like lesion with a hyperintense centre on T2 weighted images with a low to isointense signal on T1 weighted images in one of them, and in the other, multiple low intensity lesions with expansion of the cord on T2 weighted images. T1 weighted images here showed obliteration of the subarachnoid space with heterogeneous low intensity lesions in the cord. In contrast, Gupta et al. (1994), found that tuberculomas give normal to low signal on T1 weighted images and varied intensity on T2 weighted images. All these had rim or nodular enhancement on contrast injection. These changes depend on the stage of infection and size of the tuberculomas. Smaller lesions are hyperintense on T2 weighted images. As they grow, the signal becomes isointense and finally they give hypointense signal on T2 weighted images. Follow-up scans in both these studies showed regression of lesions on treatment.

MRI scan in tuberculous radiculomyelitis shows loculation of CSF, obliteration of the subarachnoid space with loss of the outline of the spinal cord in the thoracocervical region, where a CSF loculation with thickening and clumping of the roots is seen in the lumbar region. In addition cord oedema and cavitation may be seen. Contrast-enhanced scans show linear or plaque-like enhancement on the surface of the roots or cord or both in the leptomeninges (Gupta et al. 1994). MRI will obviate the need to use invasive techniques like myelography to diagnose tuberculous radiculomyelitis.

Pathogenesis

Mycobacterium tuberculosis is an acid-fast non-motile rod which does not stain well with conventional methods. The Ziehl–Nielson technique is used to visualize it. The bacterium grows slowly on egg-enriched media, when cultured over a period of 6–8 weeks. Niacin production characterizes *M. tuberculosis* and helps to distinguish it from other species. Radiometric techniques using highly selective media allow cultivation in 1–2 weeks, but confirmation of the identity of isolated organisms takes longer. Fluorescent stains like phenolic auramine or auramine rhodamine allow bacilli to be seen under low magnification and is a less laborious procedure.

The pathogenicity of TB bacilli depend on its ability to resist digestion by lysosomal enzymes and the ability of the host to mobilize effecive cell-mediated immunity. If the bacilli are not inactivated, they multiply within the cell and kill it. The lipid, protein and polysaccharide cell components of TB bacilli are immunogenic. They induce granuloma formation and macrophage activation. Some of the antigens can be immunosuppressive (Wood and Anderson 1988; Dunlop and Briles 1993). The human strain is responsible for the majority of the cases of CNS tuberculosis, but bovine, avian and atypical mycobacteria may cause CNS tuberculosis on rare occasions (Wood and Anderson 1988). The virulence of TB bacilli and the efficacy of defence mechanisms determine the nature and course of the illness. Patients with severe infection have rapid progression; here fever, retention of urine and arreflexic paralysis occurs within a few days. The cellular response and protein content of the CSF may be elevated, but TB bacilli are rarely isolated. Patients with less virulent infection have a slow progressive illness. They rarely develop cerebral meningitis. Infection is localized and organized (Kocen and Parsons 1970).

Rich (1951) postulated that CNS infection by TB bacilli occurs in two stages. A tubercular caseous focus is formed on the meninges through haematogenous spread from primary or rarely from chronic infection. The rupture of this focus into the subarachnoid space subsequently leads to CNS infection. In patients with tuberculous radiculomyelitis this focus is found on the meninges covering the spinal cord (Dastur and Wadia 1969).

Rich postulated this on the basis of the observations that all patients with miliary TB do not have CNS involvement. Experimental animals, when challenged haematogenously with a load of bacilli, developed miliary TB without simultaneous meningitis, whereas diffuse meningitis occurred when TB bacilli were introduced directly in the subarachnoid space of the susceptible animal. Vertebral involvement is always via haematogenous or lymphatic spread.

Pathology

Dastur and Wadia (1969) have given a detailed account of pathological changes in the spinal cord in patients with tuberculous radiculomyelitis. At surgery the extensive thickened exudate was seen to surround and squeeze the cord. Increased vascularity was observed. In chronic cases this granulomatous mass was adherent to dura and pia mater. Roots were compressed and atrophied. At autopsy dense exudate surrounded the spinal cord with discrete conglomerate tubercles which can be seen with naked eye. Exudate was densely adherent to the dura, and any attempt to remove it caused ragged margins. In the early stages the exudate was proliferative, becoming more organized and tenacious in the later stages. Arachnoid cysts were seen in the chronic stage.

Microscopically, the predominant changes observed were granulomatous reaction and vasculitis. Roots and spinal cord were surrounded by the exudate leaving a clear space around. Infiltration of roots and spinal cord was rarely seen. Frank tubercles were seen even on low magnification. Their appearance was similar to that seen intracranially or in TB of other organs. Central caseating necrosis was surrounded by giant cells and epitheloid cells, which in turn were surrounded by mononuclear cells. One may detect microcysts as the granulomatous state advances and becomes organized. Large arachnoid cysts within the fibrous matrix subsequently follow. The ensheathed roots were frequently intact. There was no loss of axons or demyelination in most. Spinal cord was compressed by spinal granulomatous exudate. The most frequent finding was border zone rarefaction. Axonal degeneration with demyelination was seen particularly affecting the lateral columns. Occasionally extensive atrophy of the cord with total disappearance of grey horns occured. This was thought to be vascular, as in one case thrombosed and occluded medium-sized arteries and veins particularly along the posterior meninges were observed. Sometimes there was total disappearance of spinal parenchymal architecture over a few segments. This was replaced by fat-filled gitter cells, a few mononuclear cells and early capillary proliferation. This was thought to be due to cord infarction resulting in ischaemic myelopathy.

Intramedullary tuberculomas appear round, smooth and are greyish in colour. They usually adhere to the cord. They may be associated with localized arachnoiditis. Microscopically, intramedullary tuberculomas have a central caseous material surrounded by Langhan's giant cells and epithelioid cells. Chronic tuberculomas have a thick fibrous capsule (Lin 1960; Tandon and Pathak 1973).

Vertebral TB occurs via haematogenous spread from the primary infection. In children it is usually pulmonary, whereas in adults the dissemination occurs via an extrapulmonary focus (gut, kidney, tonsil). It usually follows the primary pulmonary infection by a few days in children. The second mode of acquiring the infection is by direct spread of infection from the para-aortic lymph nodes or via lymphatic channels to the bone. The intercostal or lumbar arteries supply the adjacent parts of two vertebrae, that is the lower half of the upper vertebra and upper part of the lower vertebra. Dissemination of bacilli occurs via Batson's venous plexus which surrounds the vertebral column causing multiple vertebrae to be involved. The spread is non-contiguous and on occasion misses some vertebrae.

The infection begins in the subchondral area of the vertebral body adjacent to the disc, rarely in the lamina. It affects the cancellous bone followed by invasion of the cortex. Caseation necrosis occurs. Spread to the contiguous vertebra occurs through disc spaces and along the anterior and posterior longitudinal ligaments with pus formation beneath them, thus leading finally to paravertebral abscesses. Pus may track along the tissue planes producing a fascial abscess or track posterior to the vertebral body in the extradural space. In some, proliferation reaction leads to the formation of granulation tissue encircling the cord and compressing it and occluding its blood supply. Rarely breaching of the dura occurs causing meningitis. Healing of the vertebral body occurs with sclerosis and narrowing or disappearance of disc space. Bony fusion may occur subsequently and is desirable. Calcification is seen in the soft tissue as it heals (Gorse et al. 1983).

Treatment

Antituberculous chemotherapy is the mainstay of treatment in all cases including vertebral tuberculosis. Early initiation of the antituberculous drugs can significantly reduce morbidity and mortality. Difficulty in isolation of bacteria should not delay the treatment. The diagnosis must be considered in a patient from an immigrant population. Primary antituberculous drugs are isoniazid (INH), rifampicin(RMP), pyrazinamide(PZA), streptomycin(SM) and ethambutol(EMB). Second-line antituberculous drugs are para-aminosalicylic acid(PAS), ethionamide, cycloserine, kanamycin and capreomycin.

The duration of treatment in extrapulmonary TB is a matter of controversy. Prolonged treatment of 12–18 months results in non-compliance and high drug costs, whereas too short a duration results in frequent unacceptable relapses. Non-compliance results in secondary drug resistance. Primary drug resistance occurs in patients who have never received antituberculous therapy before. It is higher in the ethnic population (Medical Research Council Tuberculosis and Chest Diseases Unit 1980). Primary drug resistance is always to a single drug either SM or INH. Resistance to RMP or EMB is rarely seen (Glassroth et al. 1980), hence it is essential to have a knowledge of the pattern of resistance before initiating therapy. The usual two-drug regime may not work in these cases. The preferred choice is to initiate the therapy with three or four first-line drugs for a period of two months followed by two drugs that the patient is susceptible to on culture sensitivity for the period of eight months. In India the therapy for CNS tuberculosis is continued for 12–18 months (Bharucha and Bharucha 1991).

Isoniazid INH is a bactericidal drug, which is available in oral, intramuscular and intravenous form. It acts on rapidly growing TB bacilli. Penetration in all body fluids is good including the CSF. Common side effects are hepatitis in 1% which is age related affecting the elderly more than young. Rapid acetylators are genetically more susceptible. Peripheral neuropathy due to relative pyridoxine deficiency, is reversible on pyridoxine supplement. The dose of INH is 5 mg/kg/day upto 300 mg/day.

Rifampin RMP is bactericidal and is effective in both the rapid and slow phases of multiplication of bacilli. It is better absorbed on an empty stomach and is available in an oral and an intravenous form. It is well distrbuted in all body fluids including CSF. Common side effects are gastrointestinal upset with bleeding, cholestatic jaundice, thrombocytopenia. Hepatotoxicity increases in combination with INH. The dose is 10 mg/kg/day up to 600 mg/day.

Pyrazinamide PZA is active against TB bacilli in an acidic environment and is most effective intracellularly in the macrophages. The CSF penetration of this drug is good. Hepatotoxicity results from higher doses over long periods but is not a problem with short-course regimes. Uric acid levels are elevated, however gout is rarely seen. Arthralgias are seen but are unrelated to uric acid levels. The dose is 15–30 mg/kg/day.

Ethambutol is a bacteriostatic drug and does not penetrate normal meninges. Side effects are ocular toxicity with colour blindness, reduced visual acuity and central scotoma. The dose is 15–25 mg/kg/day

Streptomycin is a bactericidal drug effective in alkaline extracellular environment. It again does not penetrate normal meninges. Common side effects are ototoxicity, nausea and vertigo. The elderly are particularly susceptible. The dose is 15 mg/kg/day up to 1 g/day (Brausch and Bass 1993). RMP, INH and EMB are relatively safe in pregnancy. EMB and SM should be used with precaution in renal insufficiency.

The role of steroids in medical therapy of tuberculous radiculomyelitis is contro-versial. It helps in the impending spinal block as well as reducing tissue oedema (Ogawa et al. 1987).

Surgical treatment in tuberculous radiculomyelitis is not helpful. In patients with intramedullary tuberculoma surgery is only indicated if the size of the lesion does not regress on chemotherapy and the lesion is solitary. A large proportion of patients with vertebral TB improve on chemotherapy alone (Medical Research Council 1993). Surgical intervention is useful in patients who have a compressive lesion on radiological investigation and continue to deteriorate neurologically inspite of adequate chemotherapy and also in the situations where rapid neurologi-cal deterioration is evident. Occasionally surgical intervention may be necessary to obtain a tissue biopsy in both tuberculous radiculomyelitis and vertebral TB. Anterior excision of the diseased bone and immediate fusion by an autologous graft is thought to be best in the patient with vertebral body involvement at all spinal levels (Baily et al. 1972; Hsu and Leong 1984; Omari et al. 1989). However, this approach requires tremendous skill and experience. In the dorsal region posterolat-eral thoracotomy is required. Laminectomy is indicated in patients with posterior neural arch involvement.

Prevention

Bacillus Calmette–Guerin (BCG) vaccine is an attenuated strain of *M. bovis*. It is safe but its efficacy in prevention is controversial. The Joint Tuberculosis committee (1978) strongly recommend BCG vaccination in all those who are tuberculin nega-tive and all newborns of the immigrant population in UK. A trial from South India of BCG vaccination (Danish and French strain) failed to show any protective effect (Glassroth et al. 1980). INH prophylaxis at a daily dose of 5 mg/kg/day for a year has reduced the risk of developing clinical TB in patients with infection. Active sputum-positive pulmonary TB is the only contagious form. All contacts must be traced and treated. The effective control of TB infection in the population will automatically reduce the incidence of CNS tuberculosis.

Congenital Atlantoaxial Dislocation

The developmental anomalies that can be found at the level of the foramen magnum are varied, and can be related to both the bony skeleton and the neural tissues. Whereas some of these can be asymptomatic others can cause severe and sometimes life-threatening neurological problems. The various congenital anomalies, chiefly basilar invagination, Chiari malformation, atlantoaxial dislocation among others have been desribed from all over the world. Neurologists in India have been particu-larly impressed by the frequency of a distinct spinal syndrome due to congenital atlantoaxial dislocation (CAAD).

The atlas and the axis function as a unit because of the single median joint and the two lateral joints. The odontoid process of the axis (dens) interlocks with the ante-rior arch of the atlas in front, and is strapped posteriorly by the tough transverse ligament mantaining stability. The ring formed by the anterior arch of atlas and the tranverse ligament is called the annulus osseofibrosus. Dislocation of the atlas over the axis can occur partially or fully after violent injuries due to accidents or hanging. Tuberculosis, secondary deposits from malignancies and spread of infection from retropharyngeal and paravertebral spaces form the other causes. Today, rheumatoid arthritis deserves special mention as an important cause in the west. Other rarer causes include achondroplasia, ankylosing spondylitis, certain types of mucopolysaccharidoses, and Down's syndrome (Kopits et al. 1972).

Discussion in this chapter will be restricted to the congenital anomalies at the level of the craniovertebral junction leading to CAAD. Its particularly high incidence has been reported not only from India but also from Sri Lanka and Thailand (Wadia 1973; Bharucha and Dastur, 1964). To date more than 600 cases have been reported from the Indian subcontinent alone, although unreported cases are likely to be about two to three times more. In one study, CAAD formed 69% of a series of 82 cases of symptomatic craniovertebral anomalies (Chopra et al. 1988).

Symptoms

The presenting symptoms can be threefold (Wadia 1967).

1. *Cervical pain and stiffness.* Whereas pain and stiffness are a common presenting symptom of atlantoaxial dislocation due to acquired causes, neurological manifestations predominate in the congenital variety. Pain may be precipitated by sudden jerking or a manipulation of the neck. There is usually a limitation of lateral neck movements although remarkably the flexion extension movements are relatively free.

2. *Transitory attacks.* Although transient attacks of neurological dysfunction form a pathognomic feature of this condition not all patients may volunteer this symptom. These episodes occur due to intermittent compression of the spinal cord or the medulla. They are characterized by episodic paralysis of the limbs, paraesthaesiae, sudden unconsciousness and visual symptoms of blurring and blindness. These attacks are brought on by sudden flexion–extension movements occurring during everyday activities. They may last a few minutes to hours and sometimes may last for several weeks. These attcks may not be recognized for what they are and should be differentiated from multiple sclerosis, cerebrovascular disease and hysteria.

3. *Neurological symptoms and signs.* The neurological findings are those of a high cervical cord lesion. The signs of pyramidal tract dysfunction, including spasticity, and exaggerated deep tendon reflexes in the limbs may be asymmetrical. Bilateral extensor responses are seen consistently, but the abdominal reflexes are more often preserved than lost. Patients may complain of paraesthaesiae in the hands and clumsiness due to loss of position sense. The posterior column involvement may be more marked in the upper limbs as compared to the lower limbs. Cutaneous sensory loss occurs infrequently. Cerebellar signs may be present in the limbs, but dysarthria and nystagmus are not seen. Cranial nerve palsies are not a feature of this condition. A lower motor neurone type of paralysis with localized wasting and fasciculations may occasionally be seen. Even the wasted limbs exhibit exaggerated reflexes, distinguishing this from syringomyelia.

Males tend to be more commonly affected than females. The age at presentation can vary from 9 years to 70 years. General examination can often reveal various congenital anomalies including kyphoscoliosis, short neck with low hair line, webbing of the neck, dysmorphic facies and, uncommonly, radial agenesis of the forearm and Sprengle's shoulder.

Diagnosis

The diagnosis of CAAD is made entirely on radiology which should comprise plain X-rays and tomograms of the craniocervical junction, especially lateral views in flexion and extension and CT scan of the craniocervical junction with sagittal reconstuction images. The radiological examination should essentially be looking at two significant measurements. First, the distance between the posterior border of the anterior arch of atlas and the anterior border of the odontoid process is no more than 3 mm in adults and 4.5 mm in children. The increase in the distance may sometimes only be obvious in the flexion views. (Fig. 21.4) In cases where the odontoid is separate from the body of the axis, this measurement cannot be used. In these cases any gap between the inferior rim of the anterior arch of the atlas and the superior edge of the body of the axis is taken to be significant. Secondly, the spinal canal, which at this level is the distance between the the posterior surface of the odontoid and the posterior rim of the foramen magnum, usually measures 19–32 mm.

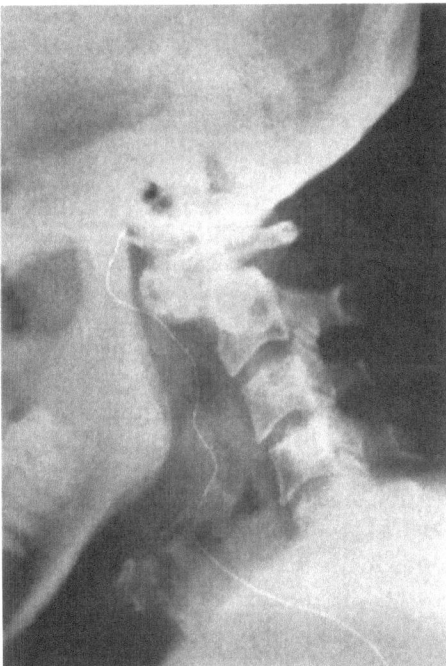

Fig. 21.4. Plain radiograph of craniocervical junction in a patient with atlantoaxial dislocation. Note the increased distance between the dens and the anterior arch of atlas. (Photograph courtesy Professor S.N. Bhagwati, Bombay.)

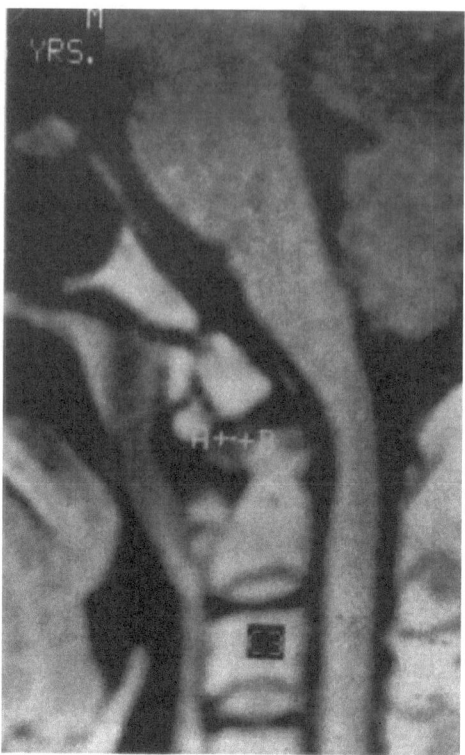

Fig. 21.5. MRI scan of the craniovertebral junction in a patient with atlantoaxial dislocation. Note the angulation of the cervicomedullary junction. (Photograph courtesy Professor S.N. Bhagwati, Bombay.)

Neurological signs are very likely if the spinal canal measures less than 19 mm. In a large number of patients in Wadia's series, the canal was less than 10 mm (Wadia 1967).

An accurate definition of the bony features of the associated anomalies at this site such as basilar impression, assimilation of the atlas, or os odontoideum can be obtained by conventional radiography. However, some features like congenital defects of the atlas and the axis are better demonstrated by CT scan. Intrathecal contrast (CT myelography) helps in better delineation of the position of the cerebellar tonsils. MRI scan provides an excellent delineation of the neural structures together with a satisfactory definition of the skull base and the cervical spine. Compression or distortion of the brainstem and spinal cord is well seen on T1 weighted images (Fig. 21.5). It has the added advantage of identifying associated cerebellar ectopia and syringomyelia.

Pathogenesis

The atlantoaxial articulation consists of four separate joints, two at the level of the odontoid, and the two lateral intervertebral joints. The odontoid joints are the anterior joint between the dens and the anterior arch of atlas, and the posterior joint between the dens and the transverse ligament. The unique position of the dens is the major factor in preventing dislocation of the atlas over the axis. The odontoid process is further strengthened by the paired alar ligaments extending from either side of the dens to the occipital condyles and the apical ligament from the tip of the dens to the anterior rim of the foramen magnum. The lateral intervertebral joints are perhaps not as important in maintaining stability. Abnormalities involving the following structures can lead to a tendency to dislocation (Greenberg 1968).

1. abnormalities of the transverse ligament is often a primary defect. The ligament is improperly formed. In autopsy studies, it has been shown that in place of the ligament, there is a mass of ill-defined fibrous tissue (Dastur et al. 1965).

2. maldevelopment of the odontoid is also an important factor in CAAD. Because of the complexity of its embryological development, the odontoid is susceptible to various types of malformations. Greenberg has classified these into five types;

Type 1: Os Odontoideum: the odontoid process develops normally but fails to fuse with the body of the axis.

Type 2: Ossiculum Terminale: there is failure of fusion of the odontoid and its base which is attached to the body of the axis.

Type 3: Agenesis of the odontoid base.

Type 4: Agenesis of the apical segment.

Type 5: Agenesis of the whole odontoid process.

3. Maldevelopment of the lateral articulating processes may contribute to the tendency to dislocate.

4. Occipitalization of the atlas: The nodding movement normally occurs at the atlanto-occipital joint. Fusion of the atlas to the occiput causes the movement to occur at the other joints including the atlantoaxial joint.

Stevens et al. (1994), however, stress that traumatic fractures of the odontoid process with subsequent remodelling of the distal fragment can radiographically be indistinguishable from os odontoideum. They also believe that in the os odontoideum deformity, the dens is formed normally, but it ossifies abnormally; that it is the result rather than the cause of the atlantoaxial instability.

Management

The treatment of congenital atlantoaxial dislocation is essentially surgical. Although over the years the management has evolved, most neurosurgeons believe that no single operation is universally suitable to all patients. The aims of surgery are three-fold: (a) to relieve compression on the neuraxis; (b) to achieve stabilization and (c) correct a disabling disability such as a fixed flexion or torticollis.

The pathological anatomy of the cervicomedullary region for treatment purposes can be categorized into reducible and irreducible pathology. The factors that are used to decide the treatment modality in individual cases are the mechanism of the compression and whether the bony abnormality can be reduced to its normal position. Routine preoperative use of skull traction is advised to try and achieve complete reduction (Nagashima 1970; Menezes et al. 1980). Where the reduction achieved is complete and the spinal canal is wide and roomy, a fusion procedure by itself may be adequate. This could be either a C1–C2 posterior fusion or could include C3 as well, if there is instability at the C2–C3 intervertebral joint. Others have used the lateral approach for fusion of the lateral masses of C1 and C2 (Schmidt et al. 1978; Chopra 1988).

In those cases where reduction cannot be achieved, or is achieved partially, a decompressive procedure is required. If the compression is predominantly dorsal, a posterior decompression is performed by a laminectomy at C1–C2 with or without a resection of the posterior margin of the foramen magnum. Compressive bands if any need to be divided. In ventral compression, the procedure of choice is transoral odontoidectomy. In either situation a stabilization procedure is required, which may be performed in the same or in a subsequent sitting. The posterior approach at best affords a partial decompression and leaves the deformity of the cord uncorrected. It does not make possible a direct attack on the pathologcal process. Furthermore, some degree of flexion is inevitable for adequate operative exposure, which causes further embarrassment to the cord. Intramedullary haemorrhages could be a danger with posterior decompression, with fatal results, although it is claimed that the danger can be minimized by preoperative skull traction for 2–3 weeks (Dastur et al. 1965). The anterior transoral approach on the other hand is performed in mild extension rather than flexion. This allows adequate decompression and removal of the offending element as well as correction of the spinal cord deformity (Greenberg 1968). In apparently irreducible cases, a bilateral approach to the lateral atlantoaxial joints can be used to achieve reduction.

Anterior Horn Cell Diseases in the Tropics

Motor Neurone Disease (MND) is a universal disease described from all parts of the world. In India the prevalence of MND has been estimated at 4 per 100 000 and matches the rest of the world. However, certain variants seem to occur more commonly in this part of the world and include the Madras pattern of motor neurone disease and the monomelic amyotrophy.

Madras Pattern of Motor Neurone Disease

As the name suggests, this variant of MND was reported from Madras, capital of the southern Indian state of Tamil Nadu, by Meenakshisundaram et al. in 1970. Classical MND is a progressive disorder usually affecting people in the sixth and seventh decades of life. Median survival for all sporadic MND has been estimated at about 3.5 years from the onset of symptoms. Bulbar onset of symptoms is associated with significantly reduced survival. The characteristic features which distinguish Madras MND from the classical variety are as follows (Jaganathan 1973; Gourie Devi and Suresh 1988):

1. Younger age of onset – The average age is 15 years and most patients present before the age of 30 years. The earliest age of onset recorded is 8 years.
2. All the cases described have been sporadic without a positive family history.

3. The disease follows an indolent slowly progressive course.

4. There is an early involvement of the cranial nerves, characterized by bilateral facial weakness, dysphagia, dysarthria and palatal weakness.

5. Deafness is another unique feature and has been shown to be sensorineural in origin. It is seen in up to a third of the patients. It is more often than not bilateral and the affection is moderate to severe. It usually accompanies the other symptoms, although it can be detected early by audiometry. Wadia et al. (1987) have shown that all the components of the brainstem auditory evoked responses are absent in these patients, but the electrocochleagram shows preservation of the cochlear microphonics, suggesting that the cause of the deafness in these patients is the degeneration of the cochlear nerve rather than a brainstem lesion, as was previously thought.

6. Persistent asymetry of involvement of the limbs in more than 50% of patients.

7. Sensory system involvement, cerebellar involvement, and cognitive impairment are characteristically absent.

8. Polymini-myoclonus is seen in up to a third of the patients.

9. Reduced plasma levels of citrate and elevated levels of pyruvate have been reported although its significance is not clear (Valmikinathan et al. 1973).

10. It has been described from only the southern part of the Indian subcontinent and is distinctly uncommon elsewhere.

The electrophysiological studies are similar to those described in classical MND. Nerve conduction studies are normal. Electromyographic studies show evidence of active degeneration with drop out motor units with giant and polyphasic potentials (Gourie Devi and Taly 1989).

Monomelic Amyotrophy

This is yet another type of anterior horn cell disorder reported from the tropics. It is characterized by muscular atrophy restricted to one limb. It seems to be slightly more common than the Madras pattern of MND, and has been described from various parts of India. There are in addition reports of this condition from places as far apart as Japan, Italy and Denmark (Hirayama et al. 1963; Pilgaard 1968; Uncini et al. 1992). Gourie Devi et al. (1984) working in Bangalore, India, report 212 patients with chronic anterior horn cell diseases seen over a 5-year period. Of these 23 (11%) had monomelic amyotrophy. Singh et al. (1980) from New Delhi, reported 24 patients seen over an unspecified period. The characteristic features include:

1. Clinical evidence of weakness and wasting of one extremity, usually the upper limb;

2. an insidious onset of the disease with very slow progression, followed by a stationary course;

3. absence of any sensory or long-tract signs.

The patients affected have usually been below 30 years of age. The most common initial symptom is weakness of the hand causing difficulty in holding a pen or in buttoning the shirt. The small muscles of the hand and the forearm muscles are commonly involved. The biceps and the triceps are involved to a lesser degree. Rarely both the upper limbs may be involved. Characteristically, the wasting is disproportionately severe as compared to the weakness. The deep tendon reflexes in the affected limb are depressed and there are no long tract signs either in the affected limb or in the other limbs.

Patients have been described with what has been called "Wasted Leg Syndrome". These patients had amyotrophy confined to one lower limb. Again the weakness is not as marked as the wasting, so much so that the patients themselves are not aware of the thinning of the leg until it is pointed out by another person (Wadia 1989).

Sensory and motor nerve conduction studies in patients with monomelic amyotrophy are normal. There is no significant difference as compared to the unaffected limb. Electromyography of the affected limb reveals changes of chronic partial denervation. Similar changes may sometimes be seen in the clinically uninvolved limbs. The combination of the presence of giant motor units, normal motor conduction velocity, and chronic partial denervation suggests a lesion at the level of the anterior horn cell.

There seems to be some debate as to whether monomelic amyotrophy and wasted leg syndrome are the same entity affecting different parts of the body. They certainly are different from the spinal muscular atrophies because of the asymetric affection of the limbs and the lack of a positive family history in any of them. Peiris et al. (1989) describe 102 patients from Sri Lanka with amyotrophy of both the upper limbs, without a positive family history in any of them, and claim it to be yet another distinct disorder. The aetiology of monomelic amyotrophy is unknown. It has been suggested that it may be a form of atypical poliomyelitis. However, its progressive nature and the lack of any serological evidence makes that possibility unlikely. In their patients Peiris et al. postulate a possible unknown toxin which could be absorbed transdermally and transported along the perineural lymphatic and vascular channels. Without a definitive aetiology, the differences between these conditions, at least clinically, remains arguably minimal.

Post-Acute Haemorrhagic Conjunctivitis Polio-Like Syndrome

In the early 1970s and subsequently in the 1980s, pandemics of acute haemorrhagic conjunctivitis (AHC) swept across south Asia, South America, USA, parts of Africa and the far East (Wadia 1989). The conjunctivitis seemed to be clinically similar in various parts of the world, but in the aftermath of these pandemics, neurologists in India started seeing patients with very characteristic neurological manifestations (Bharucha and Mondkar 1972; Thakur LC. 1981; Katiyar et al. 1981). Although the conjunctivitis affected millions of people, the neurological manifestations were seen in only a small number. It has been estimated that the nervous system was affected in about 1 in 10 000 to 1 in 15 000 patients (Anonymous 1982). Kono from Japan isolated the virus from the eyes of Japanese patients and designated it enterovirus 70(EV 70). It belongs to the same enterovirus subgroup as the polio virus. Although it is called an enterovirus, it is rarely found in the stools of patients. Isolation of the EV 70 from a patient in Florida (Hatth et al. 1981) and subsequent serological tests in patients in South America proved that the causative agent was the same all over the world (Anonymous 1982). Kono also innoculated the virus into the spinal cord of cynomolgus monkeys and reproduced the neurological complications.

Histopathological examination of the monkeys showed neuronal destruction and perivascular cuffing. (Kono et al. 1973).

Reports about the neurovirulence of the virus followed in quick succession predominantly from various parts of India as well as Japan, China, Taiwan and Thailand. The conjunctivitis typically lasts 3–7 days. It is characterized by pain, irritation, photophobia, conjunctival congestion and haemorrhages. In the vast majority of patients the disease is self-limiting, but in the unfortunate few the neurological illness strikes after a variable latent period. This can vary from 3 weeks to 3 months, the latent period being shorter in those presenting with cranial neuropathy as opposed to those presenting with symptoms in the limbs. Very rarely the neurological syndrome can present before the occurrence of the conjunctivitis. It can sometimes occur in close contacts who themselves did not suffer from the conjunctivitis. Young males tend to be commonly affected and children tend to be spared (Wadia et al. 1972, 1983) The neurological illness may begin with constitutional symptoms of fever, malaise and headaches. Weakness in the limbs follows and may be precipitated by an intramuscular injection or exhaustion, reminiscent of paralytic poliomyelitis. Weakness may be heralded by muscle pains and muscle tenderness. The weakness is commonly restricted to the limbs, the lower limbs more commonly involved than the upper limbs. The patient may describe a sudden buckling of his knees or an inability to rise from the floor. The paralysis is often severe, and it is assymetric with hypotonia and areflexia. Wasting in the limbs soon becomes evident. In the cranial form of the disease, one or more cranial nerves may be affected. Isolated lower motor neurone VIIth nerve palsy is the commonest and simulates Bell's palsy. There may be a variable affection of the V, VI, or the other lower cranial nerves. A combination of the cranial and the spinal form of the disease may also be seen. Although patients may have pain and paraesthesiae, objective sensory signs are extremely uncommon (Katiyar et al. 1983).

Diagnosis of a typical case in an epidemic can be relatively easy. The CSF in the acute stages shows elevation of the protein content and a mononuclear cellular response. Specific antibodies can be detected in the serum and the CSF making it a convenient diagnostic test. The antibodies can be found even in those patients without a history of AHC, suggesting a subclinical infection. Because the neurological illness occurs after a variable latent period after the AHC, the virus itself may be difficult to demonstrate (Wadia et al. 1983). Electromyographic studies characteristically indicate involvement of the anterior horn cells and the cranial nerve nuclei. The affected muscles show widespread fibrillation potentials and positive sharp waves (Chopra et al. 1986). Fasciculation potentials are uncommon. On maximal effort there is a fall out of motor units and a reduced interference pattern. Such evidence of denervation may also be seen in the clinically unaffected muscles. After a few weeks, the muscles start showing long duration polyphasic potentials as well as giant motor units suggestive of reinnervation. With the help of single fibre EMG studies, done over 5 years, Wadia and Ramamurthy (1987) have shown increased fibre density and abnormal jitter. Abnormally high amplitude potentials were seen on macro EMG. Based on this they postulate an unstable reinnervation process. Motor and sensory nerve conduction velocity in the peripheral nerves are normal. Katiyar et al. (1981) have done needle EMG studies even in the acute stage of the illness without inducing weakness in the muscles tested, and have shown it to be safe. Histopathological examination of the muscles show varying degrees of group atrophy along with normal or hypertrophied muscle fibres suggesting a neurogenic pattern of change.

Prognosis of the disease is usually unfavourable. Wasting in the muscles starts setting in as early as the second week. The weak and wasted muscles seldom recover fully. Poor recovery is similarly seen in the cranial nerves. Death has been reported due to bulbar palsy and consequent aspiration pneumonia. In the long term, orthopaedic input in the form of stabilization procedures is often required to mobilize the severely affected patients.

References

HTLV 1 Associated Myelopathy and Tropical Spastic Paraplegia

Advani SH, Fujishita M, Kitagawa T et al. (1987) Absence of HTLV-1 infection in India – a preliminary report. Indian J Medical Res 86:218–222

Akizuki S, Nakazato O, Higuchi Y et al. (1987) Necropsy findings in HTLV 1 associated myelopathy. Lancet ii:156–157

Anonymous (1988) HTLV-1 comes of age. Lancet i:217–219

Araga S, Takashashi K, Ooi S. (1989) Subacute meningoencephalitis associated with human T-cell lymphotropic virus 1, Report of a case. Acta Neurol Scand 79:361–365

Bartholomew C, Saxinger C, Clark JW et al. (1987) Transmission of HTLV 1 and HIV among homosexual men in Trinidad. JAMA 257:2604–2608

Bhagvati S, Ehrlich G, Kula R et al. (1988) Detection of human T-cell lymphoma/leukemia virus type 1 DNA and antigen in spinal fluid and blood of patients with chronic progressive myelopathy. N Engl J Med 318:1141–1147

Brew BJ, Price RW (1988) Another retroviral disease of the nervous system – chronic progressive myelopathy due to HTLV-1. N Engl J Med 318:1195–1197

Cruikshank JK, Rudge P, Dalgleish AG et al. (1989) Tropical spastic paraplegia and human T-cell lymphotropic virus type-1 in the United Kingdom. Brain 112:1057–1090

Eardley I, Fowler CJ, Nagendra K et al. (1991) The neurourology of tropical spastic paraparesis. Br J Urol 68:598–603

Ehrlich GD, Glaser JB, Bryz–Gornia V et al. (1991) Multiple sclerosis, retroviruses, and PCR. Neurology 37:156–158

Gessain A, Vernant JC, Maurs L et al. (1985) Antibodies to Human T cell lymphotropic virus type 1 in patients with tropical spastic paraplegia. Lancet ii:407–409.

Harrington WI, Sheremata W, Hjelle B et al. (1993) Spastic ataxia associated with human T cell lymphotropic virus type2 infection. Ann Neurol 33:411–414

Hugon J, Vollat JM, Dumas M et al. (1990) Low prevalence of HTLV 1 antibodies in the serum of patients with tropical spastic paraplegia fron the Ivory Coast. J Neurol Neurosurg Psychiatry 53:269

Inaba S, Sato H, Okochi K et al. (1989) Prevention of transmission of human T-lymphotropic virus type 1 through transfusion, by donor screening with antibody to the virus – one year's experience. Transfusion 29:7–11

Itoyama Y, Minato S, Kira J et al. (1988a) Spontaneous proliferation of peripheral blood lymphocytes is increased in patients with HTLV1 associated myelopathy. Neurology 38:1302–1307

Itoyama Y, Minato S, Kira J et al. (1988b) Altered subsets of peripheral blood lymphocytes in patients with HTLV-1 associated myelopathy. Neurology 38:816–818

Jacobson S, Lehky T, Nishimura M et al. (1993) Isolation of HTLV-2 from a patient with chronic progressive neurological disease clinically indistinguishable from HTLV1 myelopathy/tropical spastic paraplegia. Ann Neurol 33:392–396

Kaji M, Joujima H, Kaji Y et al. (1989) A case of multiple sclerosis with high CSF antibody titre to HTLV-1. Rinsho Shinkeigaku 29:219–221

Kayembe K, Goubau P, Desmyter J et al. (1990) A cluster of HTLV-1 associated tropical spastic paraplegia in Equateur (Zaire): ethnic and familial distribution. J Neurol Neurosurg Psychiatry 53:4–10

Kira J, Itoyama Y, Koyanagi Y et al. (1992) Presence of HTLV 1 proviral DNA in the central nervous system of patients with HTLV 1 associated myelopathy. Ann Neurol 31:39–45

Koprowski H, DeFreitas EC, Harper ME et al. (1985) Multiple sclerosis and human T cell lymphotropic retrovirus. Nature 318:154–160

Kuroda Y, Sugihara H (1991) Autopsy report of HTLV 1 associated myelopathy presenting with ALS-like manisfestations. J Neurol Sci 106:199–205

Kuroda Y, Shibashaki H, Sato H et al. (1987) Incidence of antibody to HTLV 1 is not increased in Japanese MS patients. Neurology 37:156–158

Mani KS (1973) Neurological disease in South India. In: Spillane JD (ed) Tropical Neurology, Oxford University Press, Oxford, pp 81–85

Mattson DH, MacFarlin D, Mora C et al. (1987) Central nervous system lesions detected by magnetic resonance imaging in an HTLV-1 antibody positive symptomless individual. Lancet ii:49

Miller DH, Newton MR, Rudge P et al. (1987) Magnetic resonance imaging in HTLV-1 antibody positive patients. Lancet ii:514

Montgomerry RD, Cruikshank EK, Robertson WB et al. (1964) Clinical and pathological observations on Jamaican neuropathy. A report of 206 cases. Brain 87:425–462

Morgan St CO, Rodgers-Johnson PE, Nigel–Gibbs W et al. (1987) Abnormal peripheral lymphocytes in tropical spastic paraplegia. Lancet ii:403–404

Morgan St CO, Rodgers-Johnson P, Mora C et al. (1989) HTLV-1 and polymyositis in Jamaica. Lancet ii:1184–1187

Nakajima O, Horna T, Ueno J et al. (1989) Measurement of anti HTLV 1 antibody titre in cerebrospinal fluid. (in Japanese) Rinsho Byori (Jpn J Clin Pathol) 37:1029–1032

Newton M, Cruickshank K, Miller D et al. (1987) Antibodies to human T-cell lymphotropic virus type 1 in West Indian-born UK residents with spastic paraparesis. Lancet i:415–416

Nishimura M, Mingioli E, McFarlin D et al. (1993) Demonstration of human T-cell lymphotropic virus type 1 (HTLV-1) from an HTLV-1 seronegative south Indian patient with chronic progressive spastic paraparesis. Ann Neurol 34:867–870

Nomoto M, Yasuhiko U, Soejima Y, Osame M (1991) Neopterin in cerebrospinal fluid: a useful marker for diagnosis of HTLV 1 associated myelopathy/tropical spastic paraparesis. Neurology 41:457

Osame M, Izumo S, Igata A et al. (1986a) Blood transfusion and HTLV-1 associated myelopathy. Lancet ii:104

Osame M, Usuku K, Izumo et al. (1986b) HTLV-1 associated myelopathy, a new clinical entity. Lancet i:1031–1032

Osame M, Igata A, Matsumoto M (1989) HTLV 1 associated myelopathy (HAM) revisited. In: Roman GC, Vernant JC, Osame M (eds) HTLV 1 and the nervous system. Alan R. Liss, New York, pp 213–223

Posiecz BJ, Ruscetti FW, Gazdar AF et al. (1980) Detection and isolation of Type C retrovirus particles from fresh and cultured lymphocytes of a patient with cutaneous T cell lymphoma. Proc Natl Acad Sci USA 77:7415–7419

Richardson JH, Newell AL, Newman PK et al. (1989) HTLV-1 and neurological disease in South India. Lancet i:1079

Robert–Guroff M, Weiss SH, Giron JA et al. (1986) Prevalence of antibodies to HTLV 1, –2, –3, in intravenous drug abusers from an AIDS endemic region. JAMA 255:3133–3137

Rodgers–Johnson P, Gajdushek C, St C Morgan O et al. (1985) HTLV-1 and HTLV-3 antibodies and tropical spastic paraparesis. Lancet ii:1247–1248

Roman GC, Roman LN (1988) Tropical spastic paraparesis, A clinical study of 50 patients from Tumaco (Colombia) and review of the worldwide features of the syndrome. J Neurol Sci 87:121–138

Roman GC, Lubbock T, Schoenberg BS et al. (1986) Tropical spastic paraparesis in the Seychelles Islands of the Indian Ocean. Neurology 36(suppl):106

Saxton EH, Lee H, Swanson P et al. (1989) Detection of human T-cell leukemia/lymphoma virus type 1 in a transfusion recepient with chronic myelopathy. Neurology 39:841–844

Suehara M, Izumo S, Kumamoto I, Osame M (1991) Significance of anti HTLV 1 antibody in cerebrospinal fluid in the diagnosis of HTLV 1-associated myelopathy (HAM) (in Japanese). Rinsho Byori (Jpn J Clin Pathol) 40:311–316

Tournier–Lasserve E, Gout O, Gessain A et al. (1987) HTLV-1, Brain abnormalities on magnetic resonance imaging, and relations with multiple sclerosis. Lancet ii:49–50

Ueda K, Kusuhara K, Togukawa K et al. (1988) Transmission of HTLV-1. Lancet i:1163–1164

Usuku K, Sonoda S, Osame M et al. (1988) HLA Haplotype-linked high immune responsiveness against HTLV-1 in HTLV-1 associated myelopathy: comparison with adult T-cell leukemia/lymphoma. Ann Neurol 23(suppl):S143–S150

Vernant JC, Bruisson GC, Sobesky G et al. (1987) Can HTLV-1 lead to immunological disease? Lancet ii:404

Yoshida M, Osame M, Usuku K et al. (1987) Viruses detected in HTLV-1 associated myelopathy and adult T-cell leukemia are identical on DNA blotting. Lancet ii:1085–1086

Watanabe T, Iwasaki Y, Tashiro K, Yoshida M et al. (1989) No evidence of HTLV 1 infection in Japanese MS patients with polymerase chain reaction. Jpn J Cancer Res 80:1017–1020

Konzo

Carton H, Kayembe K, Kabeya et al. (1986) Epidemic spastic paraparesis in Bandundu(Zaire). J Neurol Neurosurg Psychiatry 49:620–627

Cliff J, Lundquist P, Martensson J et al. (1985) Association of high cyanide and low sulphur intake in cassava-induced spastic paraparesis. Lancet ii:1211–1212

Howlett WP, Brubaker GR, Mlingi N, Rosling H (1990) Konzo: an epidemic upper motor neuron disease studied in Tanzania. Brain 113:223–235

Ministry of Health, Mozambique. (1984a) Mantakassa: an epidemic of spastic paraparesis associated with chronic cyanide intoxication in a cassava staple area of Mozambique. 2. Nutritional factors and hydrocyanic acid content of cassava products. Bull WHO 62:485–492

Ministry of Health, Mozambique. (1984b) Mantakassa: an epidemic of spastic paraparesis associated with chronic cyanide intoxication in a cassava staple area in Mozambique. 1. Epidemiology and clinical and laboratory findings in patients. Bull WHO 62: 477–484

Rosling H, Gessain A, De The G et al. (1988) Tropical and endemic spastic paraparesis are different. Lancet i:1222–1223

Tylleskar T, Banea M, Bikangi N et al. (1992) Cassava cyanogens and konzo, an upper motor neuron disease found in Africa. Lancet 339:208–211

Tylleskar T, Howlett WP, Rwiza HT et al. (1993) Konzo: a distinct disease with selective upper motor neuron damage. J Neurol Neurosurg Psychiatry 56:638–643

Tylleskar T, Legue FD, Peterson S et al. (1994) Konzo in the Central African Republic. Neurology 44:959–961

Tropical Ataxic Neuropathy

Adesina AM (1991) Neurology in Africa. In: Bradley W, Marsden CD, Fenichel G, and Daroff RB (eds) Neurology in clinical practice Butterworth–Heinemann, Boston, pp 1914–1924

Anonymous (1968) Tropical ataxic neuropathy. Br Med J iii:632–633

Howlett WP, Brubaker GR, Mlingi N, Rosling H (1990) Konzo: an epidemic upper motor neuron disease studied in Tanzania. Brain 113:223–235

Makene WJ, Wilson J (1972) Biochemical studies in Tanzanian patients with tropical ataxic neuropathy. J Neurol Neurosurg Psychiatry 35:31–32

Osuntokun BO (1968) An ataxic neuropathy in Nigeria – a clinical biochemical and electrophysiological study. Brain 91:215–248

Osuntokun BO (1973) Neurological disorders in Nigeria. In: Spillane JD (ed) Tropical neurology, Oxford University Press, Oxford, pp 173–187

Osuontokun BO, Durowoju JE, Macfarlane H et al. (1968) Plasma amino acids in the Nigerian patients with degenerative neurological diseases. Br Med J iii:647–649

Osuntokun BO, Monekosso GL, Wilson J (1969) Relationship of a degenerative tropical neuropathy to diet – report of a field survey. Br Med J i:547–550

Osuntokun BO, Aladetoyinbo A, Bademosi O (1985) Vitamin B nutrition in the Nigerian tropical ataxic neuropathy. J Neurol Neurosurg Psychiartry 48:154–156

Monekosso GL, Wilson J (1966) Plasma thiocyanate and vitamins in Nigerian patients with degenerative neurological diseases. Lancet i:1062–1064

Lathyrism

Bharucha NE, Bharucha EP (1991) Regional neurology. In: Bradley WG, Daroff RB, Fenichel GM, Marsden CD (eds) Neurology in clinical practice. Butterworth–Heinemann, Boston, pp 1925–1941

Calne DB, McGeer E, Eisen A, Spencer P (1986) Alzeimer's disease, Parkinson's disease and motor neurone disease: aging and environment. Lancet ii:1067–1070

Cohn DF, Striefler M (1981) Human lathyrism: a follow up study of 200 patients. Part I Clinical investigations. Arch Suisses Neurol Neurochir Psychiatrie 128:151–156

Cohn DF, Striefler M (1983) Intoxication by the chickling pea (Lathyrus sativus): nervous system and skeletal findings. Arch Toxicol Suppl 6: 190–193

Dastur DK (1962) Lathyrism: some aspects of the disease in man and animals. World Neurol 3:721–730

Drory VE, Rabey MJ, Cohn DF (1992) Electrophysiologic features in patients with chronic neurolathyrism. Acta Neurol Scand 85:401–403

Haimanot RT, Kidane Y, Wuhib E et al. (1990) Lathyrism in rural northwestern Ethiopia: a highly prevalent neurotoxic disorder. Int J Epidemiol 19:664–672

Hirano A (1976) Anterior horn cell changes in a case of neurolathyrism. Acta Neuropathol 35:277–283

Hugon J, Ludolph A, Roy DN, Schaumberg HH, Spencer PS (1988) Study on aetiology and pathogenesis of motor neurone disease. II. Clinical and electrophysiological features of pyramidal dysfunction in macaques fed *Lathyrus sativus* and IDPN. Neurology 38:435–442

Hugon J, Ludolph AC, Spencer PS, Gimenez RS, Dumas JL (1993)
Studies of the aetiology and pathogenesis of motor neurone diseases, III. Magnetic cortical stimulation in patients with lathyrism. Acta Neurol Scand 88:412–416

Jayaraman KS (1989) Neurolathyrism remains a threat in India. Nature 339:

Krogsgaard LP, Hansen JJ (1991) Naturally occurring excitatory amino acids as neurotoxins and leads in drug design. Toxicol Lett special issue 64–65:409–416

Ludolph AC, Hugon J, Dwiwedi MP, Spencer PS (1987) Studies on the aetiology and pathogenesis of motor neurone disease. I. Clinical findings in established cases of lathyrism. Brain 110:149–165

Misra UK (1989) Neurotoxicology. In: Pandya SK (ed) Neurosciences in India, retrospect and prospect. Neurological Society of India, Medical College and Hospital, Trivandrum, Council of Scientific and Industrial Research, New Delhi, pp 297–315

Misra UK, Sharma VP, Singh VP (1993) Clinical aspects of neurolathyrism in Unnao, India. Paraplegia 31:249–254

Misra UK, Sharma VP (1994) Peripheral and central conduction studies in neurolathyrism. J Neurol Neurosurg Psychiatry 57:572–577

Olney JW, Misra CH, Rhee V (1976) Brain and retinal damage from lathyrus excitotoxin, β-N-oxalyl-L-a, b-diaminopropionic acid. Nature 264:659–661

Rao SLN, Adiga PR, Sarma PS (1964) Isolation and the characterisation of Beta-N-oxalyl-L-α, β-diaminopropionic acid. A neurotoxin from seeds of *Lathyrus sativus*. Biochemistry 3:432–436

Rao SLN, Sarma PS, Mani KS, Rao TRR, Sriramchari S (1967) Experimental neurolathyrism in monkeys. Nature 214:610–611

Sinha KK (1989) A historical account of lathyriasis. In: Pandya SK (ed) Neurosciences in India, retrospect and prospect. Neurological Society of India, Medical College and Hospital, Trivandrum, Council of Scientific and Industrial Research, New Delhi, pp 41–43

Spencer PS, Roy DN, Ludolph A, Hugon J, Dwiwedi MP, Schaumburg HH (1986) Lathyrism: evidence for role of neuroexcitatory amino acid BOAA. Lancet ii:1066–1067

Striefler M, Cohn DF, Hirano A, Schujman E (1977) The central nervous system in a case of neurolathyrism. Neurology 27:1176–1178

Wadia NH (1989) Clinical neurology, In: Pandya SK (ed) Neurosciences in India, retrospect and prospect, Neurological Society of India, Medical College and Hospital, Trivandrum, Council of Scientific and Industrial Research, New Delhi, pp 437–508

Tuberculosis of Spine and Spinal Cord

Bailey HL, Gabriel M, Hodgeson AR, Shin JS (1972) Tuberculosis of the spine in children. Operative findings and results in 100 consecutive patients treated by removal of the lesion and anterior grafting. J Bone Joint Surg 54A:1633–1657

Bharucha NE, Bharucha EP (1991) Regional neurology. In: Bradley W, Marsden CD, Fenichel G Daroff RB (eds) Neurology in Clinical Practice, Butterworth–Heinemann, Boston, pp 1925–1941

Brausch LM, Bass JB Jr (1993) The treatment of tuberculosis, Med Clin North Am 77:1277–1288

Dastur DK, Wadia NH (1969) Spinal meningitides with radiculomyelopathy. Part 2: Pathology and pathogenesis. J Neurol Sci 8:261–297

Desai SS (1994) Early diagnosis of spinal tuberculosis by MRI, J Bone Joint Surg 76B:863–869

Dunlop NE, Briles DE (1993) Immunology of tuberculosis, Med Clin North Am 77:1235–1252

Freilich D, Swash M (1979) Diagnosis and management of tuberculous paraplegia, J Neurol Neurosurg Pschiatry 42:12

Glassroth J, Robins AG, Snider DE (1980) Tuberculosis in the 1980s, N Engl J Med 302:1441–1450

Gorse GJ, Pais MJ, Kusske JA, Cesario TC (1983) Tuberculous spondylitis. A report of 6 cases and a review of the literature. Medicine 62:178–193

Gupta RK, Gupta S, Kumar S, Kohli A, Misra UK, Gujral RB (1994) MRI in intraspinal tuberculosis. Neuroradiology 36:39–43

Hoffman EB, Crosier JH, Cremin BJ (1993) Imaging in children with spinal tuberculosis. A comparison of radiography, computed tomography and magnetic resonance imaging. J Bone Joint Surg 75B:233–239

Hsu LCS, Leong JCY (1984) Tuberculosis of the lower cervical spine (C2 to C7). J Bone Joint Surg 66B:1–5

Jena A, Banerji AK, Tripathi RP et al. (1991) Demonstration of intramedullary tuberculomas by magnetic resonance imaging: a report of two cases. Br J Radiol 64:555–556

Kennedy DM, Fallon RJ (1979) Tuberculous meningitis. JAMA 241:264–268

Kocen RS (1977) Tuberculous meningitis. Br J Hosp Med 18:436–444

Kocen RS, Parsons M (1970) Neurological complication of tuberculosis. Some unusual manifestations. Q J Med 39:17–30

Krambovitis E, McIlmurray MB, LockPE, Hendrickse W, Holzel H (1984) Rapid diagnosis of tuberculous meningitis by latex particle agglutination. Lancet 11:1229–1231

Lancet (1983) Immunological tests for tuberculosis. Lancet 1:1024–1025

Lal AP, Rajshekhar V, Chandy MJ (1992) Management strategies in tuberculous atlanto-axial dislocation. Br J Neurosurg 6:529–535

Lin TH (1960) Intramedullary tuberculoma of the spinal cord. J Neurosurg 17:497–499

Mandal BK, Evans DIK, Ironside AG, Pullan BR (1972) Radioactive bromide partition test in differential diagnosis of tuberculous meningitis. Br Med J iv:413–415

Mardh PA, Larsson L, Hoiby N, Engbaek HC, Oldham G (1983) Tuberculostearic acid as a diagnostic marker in tuberculous meningitis. Lancet 1:367

Medical Research Council Tuberculosis and Chest Diseases Unit (1980) National survey of tuberculosis notifications in England and Wales, 1978–79. Br Med J 281:895–898

Medical Research Council Working Party on Tuberculosis of the Spine (1993) Controlled trial of short-course regimens of chemotherapy in the ambulatory treatment of spinal tuberculosis: results at three years of a study in Korea. J Bone Joint Surg 75B:240–248

Molavi A, LeFrock JL (1985) Tuberculous meningitis. Med Clin North Am 69:315–332

Ogawa SK, Smith MA, Brennessel DJ, Lowy FD (1987) Tuberculous meningitis in an Urban Medical Center. Medicine 66:317–326

Omari B, Robertson JM, Nelson RJ, Lee CC (1989) Potts disease. A resurgent challenge to the thoracic surgeon. Chest 95:145–150

Parsons M, Pallis CA (1965) Intradural spinal tuberculomas. Neurology 15:1018–1022

Rich AR (1951) The pathogenesis of tuberculosis, 4th edn. Blackwell, Oxford

Sada E, Ruiz-Palacios GM, Lopez-Vidal Y, Ponce de Leon S (1983) Detection of mycobacterial antigen in CSF of patients with tuberculous meningitis by enzyme linked immunosorbent assay. Lancet 11:651–652

Sharif HS, Clark DC, Aabed MY et al. (1990) Granulomatous spinal infections: MR imaging. Radiology 177:101–108

Tandon PN, Pathak SN (1973) Tuberculosis of central nervous system. In: Spillane JD (ed) Tropical neurology, 1st edn, Oxford University Press, London, pp 37–62

Traub M, Colchester ACF, Kingsley DPE, Swash M (1984) Tuberculosis of central nervous system. Q J Med 53:81–100

Wadia NH (1973) Radiculomyelopathy associated with spinal meningitides (arachnoiditis) with special reference to the spinal tuberculous variety. In: Spillane JD (ed) Tropical Neurology, 1st edn. Oxford University Press, London, pp 63–72.

Wadia NH, Dastur DK (1969) Spinal meningitides with radiculomyelopathy. Part 1. Clinical and radiological features. J Neurol Sci 8:239–260

Weinberg JR, Coppack SP (1985) Positive bromide partition test in the absence of tuberculous meningitis. J Neurol Neurosurg Psychiatry 48:278–280

Wood M, Anderson M (1988) Chronic meningitis. In: Walton J (ed) Neurological infections, 1st edn, WB Saunders, London, pp 169–248

Congenital Atlantoaxial Dislocation

Bharucha EP, Dastur HM (1964) Craniovertebral anomalies. Brain 87:469–480

Chopra JS, Sawhney IMS, Kak VK, Khosla VK (1988) Craniocervical anomalies; a study of 82 cases. Br J Neurosurg 2:455–464

Dastur DK, Wadia NH, Desai AD, Sinh G (1965) Medullospinal compression due to atlantoaxial dislocation and sudden haematomyelia during decompression. Brain 91:655–683

Greenberg AD (1968) Atlantoaxial dislocations. Brain 91:655–683

Greenberg AD, Scoville WB, Davey LM (1968) Transoral decompression of atlantoaxial dislocation due to odontoid hypoplasia - report of 2 cases. J Neurosurg 28:266-269

Kopits SE, Perovic MN, McKusick V et al. (1972) Congenital atlanto axial dislocation in various forms of dwarfism. J Bone Joint Surg 54A:1349-1350 (abstract)

Menezes AH, Van Gilder JC, Graf CJ, et al. (1980) Craniocervical abnormalities: a comprehensive surgical approach. J Neurosurg 53:444-455

Nagashima C (1970) Atlantoaxial dislocation due to agenesis of the os odontoideum or odontoid. J Neurosurg 33:270-280

Schmidt H, Sartor K, Heckl RW (1978) Bony malformations of the craniocervical region. In: Vinken PJ, Bruyn GW (eds) Handbook of clinical neurology, Vol 32. North Holland, Amsterdam, pp 1-120

Stevens JM, Chong WK, Barber C et al. (1994) A new appraisal of abnormalities of the odontoid process associated with atlantoaxial subluxation and neurological disability. Brain 117:133-148

Wadia NH (1967) Myelopathy complicating congenital atlanto axial dislocation. Brain 90:449-472

Wadia NH (1973) Congenital atlantoaxial dislocation and it's manifestations due to spinal cord compression. In: Spillane JD (ed) Tropical neurology, Oxford University Press, Oxford, pp 99-107

Madras Pattern of Motor Neurone Disease

Gourie Devi M, Suresh TG (1988) Madras pattern of motor neuron disease in South India. J Neurol Neurosurg Psychiatry 51:773-777

Gourie Devi M, Taly AB (1989) Clinical neurophysiology, In: Pandya SK (ed) Neurosciences in India, retrospect and prospect. Neurological Society of India, Medical College and Hospital, Trivandrum, Council of Scientific and Industrial Research, New Delhi, pp 405-436

Jaganathan K (1973) Juvenile motor neuron disease. In: Spillane JD (ed) Tropical neurology. Oxford University Press, Oxford, pp 127-130

Meenakshisundaram E, Jaganathan K, Ramamurthy B (1970) Clinical pattern of MND in the younger age group in Madras. Neurology (India) 18:109-112

Valmikinathan K, Mascreen M, Meenakshisundaram E et al. (1973) Biochemical aspects of MND - Madras Pattern. J Neurol Neurosurg Psychiatry 36:753-756

Wadia PN, Bhatt MN, Misra VP (1987) Clinical neurophysiological examination of deafness associated with juvenile MND. J Neurol Sci 78:29-33

Monomelic Amyotrophy

Gourie Devi M, Suresh TG, Shankar SK (1984) Monomelic amyotrophy. Arch Neurol 41:388-394

Hirayama K, Tsubaki T, Toyokura Y, Okinaka S (1963) Juvenile muscular atrophy of the unilateral upper extremity. Neurology 13:373-380

Peiris JB, Seneviratne KN, Wickremasinghe HR et al. (1989) Non-familial juvenile distal spinal muscular atrophy. J Neurol Neurosurg Psychiatry 52:314-319

Pilgaard S (1968) Unilateral muscular atrophy of upper limbs. Acta Orthop Scand 39:327-331

Singh N, Sachdev KK, Susheela AK (1980) Juvenile muscular atrophy localized to the arms. Arch Neurol 37:297-299

Uncini A, Servedei S, Delli Pizzi C et al. (1992) Benign monomelic amyotrophy of the lower limb, report of 3 cases. Acta Neurol Scand 85:397-400

Wadia NH (1989) In: Pandya SK (ed) Neurosciences in India, retrospect and prospect. Neurological Society of India, Medical College and Hospital, Trivandrum, and Council of Scientific and Industrial Research, New Delhi, pp 437-508

Post-Haemorrhagic Conjunctivitis Polio-like Syndrome

Anonymous (1982) Neurovirulence of enterovirus 70. Lancet ii:373-374

Bharucha EP, Mondkar VP (1972) Neurological complications of a new conjunctivitis. Lancet ii;970

Chopra JS, Sawhney IMS, Dhand UK, et al. (1986) Neurological complications of acute haemorrhagic conjunctivitis. J Neurol Sci 76:177-191

Hatth MH, Mallinson MD, Palmer ER et al. (1981) Isolation of enterovirus 70 from the acute haemorrhagic conjunctivitis in key West, Florida. N Engl J Med 305:1648–1649

Katiyar BC, Misra S, Singh RB, Singh AK (1981) Neurological syndromes after acute haemorrhagic conjunctivitis. Lancet ii:866–867

Katiyar BC, Misra S, Singh RB et al. (1983) Adult polio like syndrome following enterovirus 70 conjunctivitis (natural history of the disease). Acta Neurol Scand 67:263–274

Kono R, Sasagawa A, Kodama H et al. (1973) Neurovirulence of acute haemorrhagic conjunctivitis virus in monkeys. Lancet ii:970

Thakur LC (1981) Cranial nerve palsies associated with acute haemorrhagic conjunctivitis. Lancet ii:584

Wadia NH, Irani PF, Katrak SM (1972) Neurological complications of a new conjunctivitis. Lancet ii:970

Wadia NH, Wadia PN, Katrak SM, Misra VP (1983) A study of the neurological disorders associated with acute haemorrhagic conjunctivitis due to enterovirus 70. J Neurol Neurosurg Psychiatry 46:599–610

Wadia NH (1989) Clinical neurology. In: Pandya SK (ed) Neurosciences in India, retrospect and prospect. Neurological Society of India, Medical College and Hospital, Trivandrum, Council of Scientific and Industrial Research, New Delhi, 437–508

Wadia PN, Ramamurthy S (1987) Electrophysiological study of ongoing reinnervation in acute poliomyelitis causedby EV 70 – a 5 year follow up. Electroencephalogr Clin Neurophysiol 66:s110

Chapter 22

The Conus Medullaris and Sphincter Control

M. Swash

The anal and urinary sphincters are responsive to filling of the anorectum and urinary bladder respectively. The normal storage and voiding functions of these organ systems reflect their pressure/volume relationships, and the ability of the detrusor mechanisms to overcome the passive and active resistance to the passage of faeces and urine offered by the anal canal and urethra. In both systems voiding may occur in response to the activity of the smooth muscle of the anorectum and colon, and of the urinary bladder, or it may be assisted by the additional contraction of the abdominal wall. In both systems, voiding depends on the orderly relationship between detrusor mechanisms and relaxation of the smooth and striated muscular sphincters that guard the exits of the bladder and anal canal. In this review, the anatomical arrangements responsible for continence and voiding will be described, and the role of the conus region of the spinal cord will be considered in relation to disorders of its function.

Innervation of the Anorectum

The rectal mucosa receives sensory innervation from non-myelinated, beaded nerve fibres terminating in free axonal swellings. This type of innervation resembles that found elsewhere in the gut (Duthie and Gairns 1960). More distally, from a region 10–15 cm above the anal valves to the hairy skin of the anal canal itself the innervation of the mucosa is richer, consisting of free and specialized nerve endings. The latter consist of Meissner corpuscles, Golgi–Mazzoni bodies, Krause end-bulbs, genital corpuscles, and other less well-classified endings. Pacinian corpuscles are also found in the deeper layers of the anal canal close to the internal anal sphincter. Pacinian corpuscles are found in large number in the mesentery of the gut, including that of the rectum. Duthie and Gairns (1960) pointed out that the innervation of the lower rectum and anal canal resembled that of the skin elsewhere in the body, a feature that is perhaps not surprising in view of the developmental origin of the anal canal from the ectodermal anal pit. Free and encapsulated nerve endings are probably more numerous in the region of the anal valves than more distally (Duthie and Gairns 1960; Gould 1960). Duthie and Gairns (1960) noted that touch, pin-prick and thermal stimuli were all readily perceived in the anal canal in a zone corresponding to the distribution of this extensive sensory innervation, an observation that has since been confirmed by others (Roe et al. 1986; Rogers et al. 1988). However, it must be noted that there is no immediate physiological basis for temperature sensation in the rectum or upper anal canal and this sensory experience appears to be relatively limited to the lower part of the anal canal.

The rectum contains motor and sensory neurones of the enteric nervous system in its myenteric and submucosal plexuses. These have the same function in the regulation of contraction of the smooth muscle components of the rectal wall as in other parts of the gut (Furness and Costa 1987; Gershon 1990). No detailed studies are available of the anatomy and function of the rectal enteric nervous system, and there is no information as to whether the interstitial cells of Cajal, the pacemaker cells for smooth muscle cell activity elsewhere in the gut, are present in the rectum (Thuneberg 1982). It is assumed that there is some regulation of the activity of the enteric nervous system of the rectum from its parasympathetic and sympathetic input, as there is in other parts of the gut.

In the human the internal anal sphincter (IAS) is relatively sparsely innervated. It is virtually devoid of ganglia of the enteric nervous system, perhaps simply because there is no further enteric tissue caudad to the IAS to which enteric ganglia could project, rather than from some particular specialization of the IAS with respect to other gut smooth muscle. Ultrastructural studies of the IAS disclose the presence of sparse, unmyelinated nerve fibres, some containing dense-core vesicles that come into close apposition to smooth muscle cells without making synaptic contact with this syncitium of cells (Swash et al. 1986). Visceral innervation to the IAS is derived from the same projections of the autonomic nervous system as the rectum.

Afferent projections from the rectum consist of thinly myelinated, slowly conducting parasympathetic and sympathetic nerve fibres that enter the dorsal horn of the spinal cord through the posterior roots, and either project rostrally through the spinal cord to the hypothalamus or participate in segmental reflex pathways. The sensory innervation of the anal canal, unlike that of the rectum, is of somatic origin; the afferent projections from sensory receptors in the anal canal enter the dorsal horn through thickly myelinated, fast-conducting fibres and project rostrally to the thalamus and sensory cortex in the posterior columns of the cord. Visceral sensations from the rectum also reach consciousness, probably as a result of projections from the hypothalamus rather than from direct projections of the visceral nervous system itself. The efferent projections of the autonomic nervous system to the rectum and anal canal are also derived both from the sympathetic and parasympathetic nervous systems.

Parasympathetic nerve fibres reach the rectum in the sacral nerves. These fibres arise in the intermediolateral cell columns of the sacral spinal cord at the S2–4 levels. They emerge from the cord with the ventral spinal nerve roots and give rise to the pelvic nerve plexus. Their second order neurones lie in this plexus or in the walls of the anorectum. Sympathetic innervation to the anorectum is derived from the thoracolumbar chain of ganglia, and is carried in the hypogastric nerves. Stimulation of the sympathetic nerve fibres in the hypogastric nerves in the human has yielded controversial results. Carlstedt et al. (1988) found that the IAS contracted in response to pelvic sympathetic nerve stimulation, but others have recorded sphincter relaxation in similar experiments (Shepherd and Wright 1968; Lubowski et al. 1987). These differences may relate to different experimental conditions, such as depth of anaesthesia, or to differences in the resting state of the muscle. For example, there is doubt also as to whether the parasympathetic innervation of the IAS contributes to its resting tone (Frenckner and Ihre 1976; Meunier and Mollard 1977). The resting anal pressure, representing tonic contraction of the IAS, decreases during high but not during low spinal anaesthesia, indicating a tonic effect of excitatory sympathetic activity, but no effect of any tonic parasympathetic activity on the sphincter muscle (Burnstock 1990). On the other hand, damage to the sacral outflow seems to cause a lower resting anal tone, suggesting that resting parasympathetic tone may play a role in the maintenance of IAS contraction. Burnstock and colleagues (1990) have concluded that, in general, smooth muscle sphincters are controlled independently from non-sphincteric smooth muscle. Stimulation of the parasympathetic nerves supplying the internal anal sphincter muscle inhibits the spontaneous resting tone of this muscle, by an effect mediated by non-adrenergic, non-cholinergic nerves (NANC) (Burnstock 1990). The neurotransmitter for this effect is likely to be purinergic. The possible role of neuropeptides in increasing or decreasing resting anal tone is uncertain, but neuropeptide Y is thought to be active at this location. Acetylcholine contracts the internal anal sphincter. Whatever the role of the visceral innervation, it is certainly less important than that of the enteric nervous system, as shown by the large relaxation of the IAS that occurs in response to dilatation of a balloon in the rectum – the recto-anal reflex.

The identification of the receptors subserving the sensation of rectal distension has proved difficult. Although it was for long thought that these receptors must be located in the wall of the rectum, experiments in patients after rectal excision and colo-anal anastomosis showed that this sensation was often preserved postoperatively, suggesting that the receptors for this sensation must lie outside the rectum and presumably, therefore, must be located in the pelvic floor musculature or in the pelvic fascia. The muscles of the pelvic floor contain muscle spindles as well as Pacinian corpuscles, and it is possible that this sensation of rectal filling is mediated by these receptors, together with the "sampling" function of the anorectal mucosal receptors themselves.

Innervation of the Bladder

The bladder receives parasympathetic innervation that induces contraction of the smooth muscle of the detrusor. This is partly acetylcholinergic, but the response of the detrusor muscle to pelvic (parasympathetic) nerve stimulation is only partially blocked by atropine (Langley and Anderson 1895), a phenomenon now recognized as due to the presence of a NANC transmitter acting at this site (Moss and Burnstock 1985). This NANC transmitter is ATP (Burnstock 1990). There is thus a clear implication that acetylcholine and ATP may be co-transmitters in the bladder wall, and perhaps also in the intrinsic neurones of the bladder wall (Burnstock 1990). Speakman et al. (1989) have confirmed the presence of this NANC component of neurotransmission in the trigonal area of the human bladder and have shown that this is probably purinergic. Such responses are virtually absent from the dome of the bladder.

The sympathetic innervation to the bladder is derived from the hypogastric nerves and these nerve endings contain both noradrenaline and neuropeptide Y (Crowe and Burnstock 1989). In addition, substance P and calcitonin gene-related peptide have been located in the abundant sensory-motor nerves of the trigone region of the bladder, and vasoactive intestinal peptide and leuencephalin have been located in parasympathetic nerves, and also in the intrinsic ganglia (Burnstock 1990). Both 5-hydroxytryptamine and prostaglandins have also been shown to be capable of eliciting contractile responses in the bladder wall musculature; the latter may form part of the normal response to noxious stimuli in the bladder, e.g. infection. The degree of homology of the neurotransmitters found in the intrinsic innervation of the bladder with that of the enteric nervous system is uncertain but is unlikely to be close in view of the differing embryological origins of these two tissues. However, it has recently become apparent that the intrinsic neurones and ganglia of the bladder wall and urethra (Burnstock 1990) contain circuitry that supports integrative activity of the bladder smooth muscle, and that may also subserve a sensory function.

The innervation of the urethra differs from that of the body of the bladder. Its adrenergic nerves are excitatory, inducing powerful contractile responses, and there is an additional innervation from cholinergic fibres, together with a non-purinergic NANC component (Ito and Kimoto 1985; Burnstock 1990). The latter may serve to relax the urethral smooth muscle.

Innervation of Pelvic Floor Muscles

The innervation of the pelvic floor muscles is derived from the S2, S3 and S4 sacral segments. The afferent and efferent nerve fibres providing sensory and motor innervation to these muscles travel in the pelvic nerves and in the pudendal nerves. The pelvic nerves enter the levator ani and puborectalis (PR) muscles from their peritoneal surface (Stelzner 1960; Duthie and Gairns 1960), and the pudendal nerves innervate the external anal sphincter (EAS) muscle through its inferior rectal branches that approach the muscle through Alcock's canal and the ischiorectal fossa. Perineal branches of the pudendal nerves pass forward through the perineum to innervate the periurethral striated urinary sphincter muscles, and thus to control urinary continence. The direct pelvic route for the somatic innervation of the PR muscle has been shown by two related electrophysiological investigations (Percy et al. 1981; Snooks and Swash 1986), and this is strong evidence for a separate developmental origin for the EAS and PR muscles (see above).

The external urethral sphincter muscle (EUS) may be a site in which there is a functional interaction between somatic efferent innervation and the autonomic nervous system, since close proximity relationships between the striated muscle fibres of this muscle and nor-adrenergic and VIP-ergic nerves have been observed (Crowe et al. 1989). The conventional somatic innervation of the EUS is derived from the paired perineal branches of the pudendal nerves and the intrinsic component of the striated urethral sphincter muscle, located in the urethral wall itself, seems to be derived, like the innervation of the puborectalis muscle, from direct somatic innervation given off from pelvic branches of the sacral plexus (S3 and S4) (Snooks and Swash 1986).

Central Connections of the Sphincter Innervation

The motor nerve fibres innervating the EUS, EAS and PR muscles, but probably not those innervating the levator ani muscle, arise in the ventral grey matter of the sacral cord. The lower motor neurones innervating these muscles lie in the S2 and S3 segments, forming a discrete motor nucleus named after Onuf, who described it in 1899 (Onuf 1900). These neurones differ from other somatic efferent motor neurones in that they are smaller and more densely packed, and show architectonic features resembling parasympathetic neurones, which lie nearby in the lateral cell columns of the sacral cord. Other characteristics that suggest a functional interrelationship with parasympathetic neurones include the presence of direct afferent connections with paraventricular hypothalamic neurones, and a rich peptidergic input. Leuencephalin, VIP and somatostatin are found in and around the Onuf nucleus, but not on the adjacent somatic efferent neurones (Roppolo et al. 1985). In addition, clinicopathological studies have shown that these neurones are lost in primary autonomic failure, and in Shy-Drager syndrome (Sung et al. 1979), but not in amyotrophic lateral sclerosis or spinal muscular atrophy (Mannen et al. 1977). The Onuf nucleus cells have connections mainly orientated in the rostrocaudal plane, a feature that may be related to the tonic output of the cells of this nucleus, since a similar anatomical pattern is found in the cells of the phrenic nucleus in the cervical spinal cord (Kuzuhara et al. 1980). Lateral dendritic branches probably establish connections with the parasympathetic neurones in the adjacent cell columns of the lateral grey matter, with primary afferents from the pudendal nerves and with descending fibres from brainstem and cortical centres.

The upper motor neurones for the voluntary sphincter muscles lie close to those innervating the lower limb muscles in the parasagittal motor cortex, adjacent to the sensory representation of the genitalia and perineum in the sensory cortex. Corticospinal fibres project from the motor cortex direct to the motor cells of the contralateral Onuf nucleus; some fibres recross in the sacral cord to project to the ipsilateral nucleus, so that there is bilateral cortical input to the two halves of this nucleus, and so to the two sides of the somatic sphincter muscles in the anorectum (Nakagawa 1980). Using transcutaneous electrical stimulation of the motor pathways in alert human subjects at the level of the cortex and cauda equina, Merton et al. (1982) showed that these upper motor neurone pathways form a fast-conducting oligosynaptic pathway. This pathway consists of a narrow strip of fibres in the lateral corticospinal tract in which the efferent fibres are situated medial to the afferent fibres (Nathan and Smith 1953). The frontal lobes are important in defaecation, straining and micturition (Andrews and Nathan 1964) and direct projections from the paraventricular hypothalamic nuclei and from the pontine reticular formation may also be important in the central integration of visceral and somatic muscle function required for defaecation and micturition, and for continence (Swash and Mathers 1989). In dogs, defaecatory behaviour can be induced by distension of the rectum, and this reflex response was shown by Fukuda and Fukai (1986) to be dependent on reflex straining centres in the pons and medulla.

De Groat and Kawatani (1985) have constructed a diagram of the central reflex connections and encephalinergic mechanisms that regulate micturition in the cat. It is reasonable to suppose that a similar system of neuronal connections is involved in the control of defaecation. In their micturition model (Fig. 22.1)

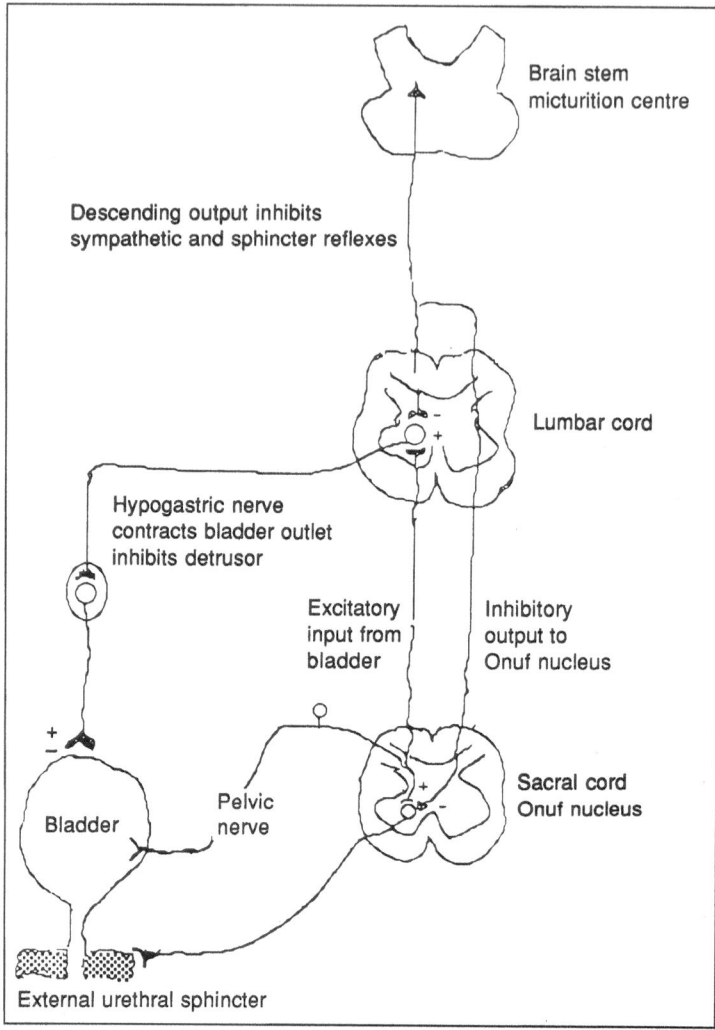

Brain stem
micturition centre

Descending output inhibits
sympathetic and sphincter reflexes

Lumbar cord

Hypogastric nerve
contracts bladder outlet
inhibits detrusor

Excitatory   Inhibitory
input from   output to
bladder   Onuf nucleus

Bladder   Pelvic   Sacral cord
               nerve   Onuf nucleus

External urethral sphincter

Fig. 22.1. Diagram to show the reciprocal excitatory and inhibitory innervation of detrusor and striated urethral sphincter muscles in the control of urine storage and of micturition. Note that the descending projection from the pontine micturition centre to the Onuf nucleus at the S2 level in the conus medullaris is inhibitory to the striated sphincter, thus acting as a "switching off" mechanism in relation to the normal continuous activity of that muscle. (Diagram from work of De Groat 1985, 1990.)

micturition is initiated by a supraspinal reflex pathway passing through a "micturition centre" in the brainstem. This pathway is excited by input from small unmyelinated afferents originating in tension receptors in the bladder wall, that project to the brainstem centre. A spinal reflex mechanism, that becomes evident in spinal man, is inhibited in the intact nervous system. De Groat (1990) has suggested that the micturition reflex is inhibited by descending brainstem activity, directed onto the Onuf nucleus in the sacral cord, and it is likely that defaecation is similarly inhibited by this pathway. The descending pathway that initiates voiding therefore acts as a switch, burning off the tonic activity of the sphincter muscles that maintains continence in the resting state. The diagram clearly indicates the importance of the functional interrelationship between the autonomic and somatic components of the sphincter mechanisms.

Conus Medullaris and Cauda Equina Disorders

The separation of cauda equina and conus lesions in clinical practice is difficult, mainly because the clinical features of lesions at these two sites overlap. Pure lesions of the conus medullaris are rare and perhaps occur most frequently in multiple sclerosis. However in *multiple sclerosis*, lesions of the conus are usually accompanied by lesions elsewhere in the central nervous system. *Vascular disorders*, e.g. spinal cord infarction, rarely involve the conus medullaris in isolation, and intermittent claudication of the cauda equina produces symptoms and signs that are, at least in part, due to a combination of ischaemia both of the cauda equina and of the conus medullaris. *Trauma* to the lumbosacral spine, similarly, is more likely to produce either a combination syndrome or a pure cauda equina lesion because of the vulnerability of the spinal roots to traumatic damage as they exit from the spinal canal through the intervertebral foramina. *Intrinsic tumours* of the conus medullaris, especially astrocytomas and ependymomas, selectively damage the conus medullaris, and produce the best demonstration of the typical features of this syndrome. Unfortunately, because there are few.abnormalities on conventional neurological examination in the early stages of the disorder, the diagnosis is often missed until the syndrome is relatively advanced.

The typical features of a conus lesion, illustrated by the slowly progressive course of a patient with an *intrinsic tumour* in this region, derive from damage to the middle and lower sacral segments (Brodal 1981). The clinical signs, largely confined to the pelvic floor, may be missed by the inexperienced examiner, since routine neurological examination of the legs, and even of the lateral buttocks, may reveal no abnormality, and the plantar responses may be flexor. There is weakness and loss of tone in the pelvic floor musculature, including the muscles of the perineum and perianal region. The anal reflex is absent, and there is loss of sensation in the perianal and perivulval or scrotal region. This sensory disturbance may extend onto the posterior aspect of the upper thigh if it extends rostral to the S2 level. This is "saddle anaesthesia". In low conus lesions, the S1 segment is not involved and, therefore, the ankle jerks are normal, a finding accounting for most instances of failure to make the diagnosis. The preganglionic parasympathetic connections in the cord are interrupted leading to paralysis of the bladder detrusor, retention of urine and, sometimes, especially in women, to the development of incontinence with overflow. There is no reflex contraction of the bladder as occurs with cord transection syndromes at higher levels, in which the inhibitory outflow from the pontine micturition centres to the Onuf nucleus is interrupted, leading to an "automatic bladder". There is also incontinence of faeces, with a patulous anus, together with impaired motility of the descending colon and rectum, due to the preganglionic parasympathetic lesion, resulting in impaction of faeces. In men there is failure of penile erection and ejaculation, although seminal emission can occur since the sympathetic innervation of the seminal vesicles and ductus deferens is intact. In some patients with progressive conus lesions, and rarely in acute demyelination of the conus region, priapism occurs, and there are often various components of the complete syndrome developing separately during the course of the onset of the syndrome. If the lesion extends rostrally a few segments, there may be associated wasting of the gluteal and posterior thigh muscles but this feature is often absent or difficult to recognize. Both plantar responses are flexor unless the lesion extends rostrally to about the level of S1. The spine itself is normal. In intrinsic lesions of this type there is usually a greal deal of spontaneous pain in the perineal area, that has a characteristic spinothalamic persistence. This pain may be burning or lancinating and is often made worse by movement or by defaecation. It persists despite rest, and may be debilitating, being unrelieved by analgesics, except perhaps to some extent by carbamazepine or Dolobid. When the conus lesion is due to *extrinsic compression*, usually by a *central disc prolapse*, or by a *spinal fracture*, the onset is abrupt, with pain, incontinence, numbness in the perineum, and severe low back pain. The prognosis for functional recovery, even with urgent surgical decompression, is poor. *Secondary tumours* in this region usually present with local pain from bony invasion before features of cauda equina or conus involvement develop. Other localized tumours, e.g. *chordoma*, may be large before they involve the conus or cauda equina roots, so that a major and wide excision is required with a difficult postoperative course.

Lesions restricted to the *cauda equina* are usually painful, with pain experienced in the distribution of the affected nerve roots. Most cauda equina lesions, except central disc prolapse syndromes, involve the whole cauda equina, for example, chronic adhesive arachnoiditis syndromes, so producing pain radiating down the backs of both legs, perhaps asymmetrically, toward the soles of the feet, as well in the buttocks. Sensory loss is often extensive affecting the L5 and S1–5 distributions, and there is extensive wasting of the buttocks, posterior thighs and lateral lower leg muscles, with foot drop and absent ankle jerks but preserved knee jerks. The plantar responses, if elicitable, are flexor. There is painful restriction of straight leg raising depending on the degree of mechanical tethering of the affected nerve roots. The bladder and bowel are paralysed, and there is denervation of the perineal muscles resembling that seen in conus lesions.

Sacral spinal dysraphism may be associated with conus and cauda equina lesions, and despite the congenital nature of the disorder the clinical features may progress, probably because the cord is tethered at its insertion into the abnormal sacral spinal sac, leading to repeated stretch injury during movement. The patient usually shows loss of spinal height as part of the malformation, and there is an abnormal gibbus at the site of the dysraphism. If the lesion extends to the lumbar cord the plantar responses will be extensor (provided that there is sufficient muscle acting around the foot to allow the reflex to be tested). Saddle sensory loss is usually present and this may have extended in distribution as part of the clinical progression of the syndrome before presentation.

In *multiple sclerosis* incontinence of urine (Miller et al. 1965) and faeces (Swash et al. 1987) is common, and there may also be constipation (Glick et al. 1982) or urinary retention. These apparently conflicting features are the expected result of conus involvement but proof that they result from a single lesion in this site is invariably lacking (Mathers et al. 1990). Indeed, most patients with multiple sclerosis have multiple lesions in different parts of the nervous system and the pathways for bladder and bowel control are so long and extend through so many vulnerable parts of the nervous system that it is hardly surprising that bladder and bowel dysfunction form so conspicuous a part of the clinical features of the disease. Many patients with multiple sclerosis and incontinence have electrophysiological evidence of lower motor neurone lesion involving the striated sphincter muscles (Miller et al. 1965; Glick et al. 1982). There is evidence that this may often be associated with childbirth, thus relating denervation of these muscles to damage to the pelvic floor innervation of the type found in the common variety of stress incontinence that is so common in women who have borne children (Swash 1990), rather than demyelination-induced damage to the central component of the lower motor neurone pathways in the cord.

Pure efferent lesions of the bladder innervation in the pelvis, and pure afferent lesions in the cord, such as tabes dorsalis, also lead to a large flaccid bladder without reflex micturition. These conditions can be diagnosed by the absence of the other features of cauda equina or conus lesion. However, infiltrative lesions in the pelvis can also involve the somatic innervation of the perineum, and may thus mimic in all respects the features of a conus lesion. Most infiltrative lesions in the pelvis are asymmetrical, a finding that is also a feature of cauda equina disease, but which is less marked in conus lesions. A finding of extensor plantar response, only present if the conus lesion is rostral to the S1/L5 level, is also important in raising the suspicion of a conus lesion. The advent of CT and MR scanning in the investigation of suspected pelvic infiltration, and its parallel use in patients investigated by myelography, has made this otherwise difficult clinical diagnosis much more secure.

Investigation and Diagnosis

Modern imaging techniques have greatly enhanced the capability of the clinician in the diagnosis of these difficult problems, and in the planning of appropriate medical, surgical and oncological therapies. However although relatively non-invasive, the technology of modern medical imaging is expensive and furthermore it cannot provide a guide to functional assessment of the pelvic floor or viscera. There is therefore a place in clinical investigation for functional tests of bladder and bowel, and for neurophysiological assessment of the striated pelvic floor musculature and its central connections.

Cystometry and Anal Manometry

These tests are useful in assessing functional capacity, but a description of their methodologies is beyond the scope of this chapter. Modern reviews are available elsewhere (Drife et al. 1990; Henry and Swash 1991). They are useful in providing objective measurement of the processes of storage and voiding of urine and of faeces, for example of measuring flow rate during micturition as an index of detrusor function, in measuring maximal tolerated storage volumes of urine or faeces as an index of the integrity of the central neural processes subserving the relation between storage and initiation of the micturition response, in imaging the processes of micturition or defaecation, and in assessing the first perceived volume of urine or faeces as a measure of sensory function. These assessments can be carried out simultaneously with electromyography of the external urinary and anal sphincter muscles in order to provide timing of the relationship of detrusor activity and relaxation of the voluntary, striated sphincter musculature. These tests measure the functional competence of the pelvic sphincters, and of the smooth muscle of the bowel and anorectum.

Electrophysiological Tests of the Lower Motor Neurone Pathway to the Pelvic Floor Muscles

Motor conduction in the terminal part of the pudendal nerves can be studied using commercially available surface electrodes mounted on a disposable examination glove. The pudendal nerve is stimulated transrectally at the level of the sciatic notch by bipolar electrodes located at the tip of the examiner's index finger, and the evoked motor response recorded from the external anal sphincter muscle by surface electrodes mounted at the base of the finger attachment (Kiff and Swash 1984). A catheter-mounted, bipolar ring electrode placed in the urethra at the level of the striated urinary sphincter muscle allows simultaneous recording of the perineal nerve terminal motor latency (Snooks and Swash 1984). Transcutaneous electrical or magnetic stimulation over the lumbar spine at two levels (T12 and L5) can be used to detect cauda equina lesions by measuring the latency of the motor response to the striated urinary or anal sphincter muscles (Swash and Snooks 1986; Chokroverty et al. 1989).

EMG, or single fibre EMG, has been used extensively in clinical research and in routine clinical management for assessing the presence of chronic partial denervation (reinnervation) in the striated pelvic floor sphincter muscles (Neill and Swash 1980; Fowler et al. 1984; Henry and Swash 1991). Polyphasic motor unit potentials are found when the lower motor neurone is damaged at any site, whether distally in the pelvis, or in the cauda equina or conus medullaris. The nerve conduction studies can more precisely localize the abnormality to these levels.

Sensory pathways in the nervous system relevant to the problem of conus lesions can be assessed using somatosensory evoked potentials following stimulation of the skin of the anus, the dorsal nerve of the penis or clitoris, and of the lower urinary tract (Mathers and Swash 1990). However, these methods are not often used in routine clinical practice. Attempts to use measurements of short- or long-latency components of the cutaneous anal reflex in clinical diagnosis have not proved reliable because of the complexity of the response and the variability in the latency of the various components recorded (Swash 1982; Vodusek et al. 1983).

References

Andrews J, Nathan P (1964) Lesions of the anterior frontal lobes and disturbances of micturition and defaecation. Brain 87:233–262

Brodal A (1981) Neurological anatomy in relation to clinical medicine, 3rd edn. Oxford University Press, p 779

Burnstock G (1990) Innervation of bladder and bowel. In: Bock G, Whelan J (eds) Neurobiology of incontinence. CIBA Foundation symposium 151. Wiley, Chichester, pp 2–43

Carlstedt A, Nordgren S, Fasth S, Appelgren L, Hulten L (1988) Sympathetic influence on the internal anal sphincter and rectum in man. Int J Colorectal Dis 3:90–95

Chokroverty S, Sachdeo R, Dilullo J, Duvoisin RC (1989) Magnetic stimulation in the diagnosis of lumbosacral radiculopathy. J Neurol Neurosurg Psychiatry 52:767–772

Crowe R, Burnstock G (1989) A histochemical and immunohistochemical study of the autonomic innervation of the lower urinary tract of the female pig. Is the pig a good model for the human bladder and urethra? J Urol 141:414–422

Crowe R, Burnstock G, Light JK (1989) Adrenergic innervation of the striated muscle of the intrinsic external urethral sphincter from patients with lower motor spinal cord lesion. J Urol 141:47–49

De Groat WC (1990) Central neural control of the lower urinary tract. In: Bock G, Whelan J (eds) Neurobiology of incontinence. CIBA Foundation symposium 151. Wiley, Chichester, pp 27–56

De Groat WC, Kawatani M (1985) Neural control of the urinary bladder: possible relationship between peptidergic inhibitory mechanisms and detrusor instability. Neurourol Urodyn 4:285–300

Drife JO, Hilton P, Stanton SL (eds) (1990) Micturition. Springer-Verlag, London

Duthie HL, Gairns FW (1960) Sensory nerve endings and sensation in the anal region of man. Br J Surg 47:585–590

Fowler CJ, Kirby RS, Harrison WJG, Milroy ELJ, Turner-Warwick R (1984) Individual motor unit analysis in the diagnosis of disorders of urethral sphincter innervation. J Neurol Neurosurg Psychiatry 47:637–641

Frenckner B, Ihre T (1976) Influence of autonomic nerves on the internal anal sphincter of man. Gut 17:306–312

Fukuda H, Fukai K (1986) Location of the reflex centre for straining elicited by activation of pelvic afferent fibres of decerebrate dogs. Brain Res 380:287–296

Furness JB, Costa M (1987) The enteric nervous system. Churchill Livingstone, Edinburgh

Gershon MD (1990) The enteric nervous system: neurotransmitters and neuromodulators. Curr Opin Neurol Neurosurg 3:517–522

Glick ME, Meshkinpour H, Haldeman S, Bhatia NN, Bradley WE (1982) Colonic dysfunction in multiple sclerosis. Gastroenterology 83:1002–1007

Gould RP (1960) Sensory innervation of the anal canal. Nature 187:337–338

Henry MM, Swash M (1991) Coloproctology and the pelvic floor, 2nd edn. Butterworth–Heinemann, London

Ito Y, Kimoto Y (1985) The neural and non-neural mechanisms involved in urethral activity in rabbits. J Physiol (Lond) 367:57–72

Kiff ES, Swash M (1984) Slowed motor conduction in the pudendal nerves in idiopathic (neurogenic) anorectal incontinence. Br J Surg 71:614–616

Kuzuhara S, Kanazawa I, Nakanishi T (1980) Topographical localization of the Onuf's nuclear neurons innervating the rectal and vesical striated sphincter muscles: a retrograde fluorescent double labelling study in cat and dog. Neurosci Lett 16:125

Langley JN, Anderson HK (1895) The innervation of the pelvic and adjoining viscera. IV: the internal generative organs. J Physiol (Lond) 19:122–130

Lubowski DZ, Nicholls RJ, Swash M, Jordan MJ (1987) Neurol control of internal anal sphincter function. Br J Surg 74:668–670

Mannen T, Iwata AR, Toyokura Y, et al. (1977) Preservation of a certain motoneuron group of the sacral cord in amyotrophic lateral sclerosis: its clinical significance. J Neurol Neurosurg Psychiatry 40:464–469

Mathers SE, Swash M (1990) The neurology of sphincter control mechanisms. In: Kennard C (ed) Recent advances in clinical neurology 6. Churchill Livingstone, Edinburgh, pp 157–186

Mathers SE, Ingram DA, Swash M (1990) Electrophysiology of motor pathways for sphincter control in multiple sclerosis. J Neurol Neurosurg Psychiatry 53:955–960

Merton PA, Morton HB, Hill DK, et al. (1982) Scope for a technique for electrical stimulation of human brain, spinal cord and muscle. Lancet ii:597–600

Meunier P, Mollard P (1977) Control of the internal anal sphincter (manometric study with human subjects). Pflugers Archivs 370:233–239

Miller H, Simpson CA, Yeates WK (1965) Bladder dysfunction in multiple sclerosis. Br Med J i:1265

Moss HE, Burnstock G (1985) A comparative study of electrical field stimulation of the guinea pig, ferret and marmoset bladder. Eur J Pharmacol 114:311–316

Nakagawa S (1980) Onuf's nucleus of the sacral cord in the South American monkey (Saimiri); its location and bilateral cortical input from area 4. Brain Res 191:337–344

Nathan PW, Smith MC (1953) Spinal pathways subserving defaecation. J Neurol Neurosurg Psychiatry 16:245–256

Neill ME, Swash M (1980) Increased motor unit fibre density in the external anal sphincter muscle in anorectal incontinence: a single fibre EMG study. J Neurol Neurosurg Psychiatry 43:343–347

Onuf (Onufrowicz) B (1900) On the arrangement and function of the cell groups of the sacral region of the spinal cord in man. Arch Neurol Psychopathol 3:387–412

Percy JP, Neill ME, Swash M, Parks AG (1981) Electrophysiological study of motor nerve supply of pelvic floor. Lancet i:16–17

Roe AM, Bartolo DCC, Mortensen NJM (1986) A new method for assessment of anal sensation in various anorectal disorders. Br J Surg 73:310–312

Rogers J, Henry MM, Misiewicz JJ (1988) Combined sensory and motor deficit in primary neuropathic faecal incontinence. Gut 29:5–9

Roppolo JR, Nadelhaft I, De Groat WC (1985) The organization of pudendal motoneurons and primary afferent projections in the spinal cord of the rhesus monkey revealed by horseradish peroxidase. J Comp Neurol 234:475–488

Shepherd JJ, Wright PG (1968) The response of the internal anal sphincter in man to stimulation of the presacral nerve. Am J Digestive Dis 13:421–427

Snooks SJ, Swash M (1984) Perineal nerve and transcutaneous spinal stimulation: new methods for investigation of the urethral striated sphincter musculature. Br J Urol 56:407–411

Snooks SJ, Swash M (1986) The innervation of the muscles of continence. Ann R Coll Surg Engl 68:406–409

Speakman MJ, Walmsley D, Brading AF (1989) An in vitro pharmacological study of the human trigone – a site of non-adrenergic, non-cholinergic neurotransmission. Br J Urol 61:304–309

Stelzner F (1960) Uber die Anatomie des analen Sphincterorgans wie sie der Chirurg sieht. Z Anat Entwicklung 121:525–535

Sung JH, Mastri AR, Segal E (1979) Pathology of the Shy-Drager syndrome. J Neuropathol Exp Neurol 38:353–367

Swash M (1982) Early and late components in the human anal reflex. J Neurol Neurosurg Psychiatry 45:767–769

Swash M (1990) The neurogenic hypothesis of stress incontinence. In: Bock G, Whelan J (eds) Neurobiology of incontinence. CIBA Foundation symposium 151. Wiley, Chichester, pp 156–169

Swash M, Mathers S (1989) Sphincter disorders and the nervous system. In: Aminoff M (ed) Neurology and general medicine. Churchill Livingstone, New York, pp 449–470

Swash M, Snooks SJ (1986) Slowed motor conduction in lumbo-sacral nerve roots in cauda equina lesions; a new diagnostic technique. J Neurol Neurosurg Psychiatry 46:808–816

Swash M, Gray A, Lubowski DZ, Nicholls RJ (1986) Ultrastructural changes in internal anal sphincter in neurogenic faecal incontinence. Gut 29:1692–1698

Swash M, Snooks SJ, Chalmers DHK (1987) Parity as a factor in incontinence in multiple sclerosis. Arch Neurol 44:504–508

Thuneberg L (1982) Interstitial cells of Cajal: intestinal pacemaker? Adv Anat Embryol Cell Biol 71:1–130

Vodusek DB, Janko M, Lokar J (1983) Direct and reflex responses in perineal muscles on electrical stimulation. J Neurol Neurosurg Psychiatry 46:67–71

Chapter 23

Psychosexual and Psychosocial Aspects of Spinal Cord Disease

M.T. Isaac

We do not have to follow Freud's insistence that sex is at the bottom of everything to recognize the centrality of sexuality to our emotional and psychological well-being. Sexual function may form the foundation of one's self-esteem and perception of one's proper role in society. The importance and symbolic meaning of the voluntary renunciation of sexual activity in many religious traditions underlies the pivotal position of sex in Man. Moreover, the characteristic human ability, and inclination, to perform sexually at all times, without being bound by the constraints of an oestrus cycle, has allowed sexual activity to transcend the requirements of reproduction alone – itself, of course, a powerful emotional and social imperative – and take on a more pervasive role in pair bonding, both homo- and heterosexual, and aesthetic pleasure. On the other side of the coin, sexual difficulties are the source of profound anxiety and unhappiness. The sense of loss and damage suffered by those who have spinal cord dysfunction is compounded by such problems.

In view of this, it is perhaps surprising that the literature on psychosocial and psychosexual sequelae of spinal cord dysfunction is relative sparse. Most studies focus on the problems of men after traumatic spinal cord injury, with relatively few authors giving serious consideration to the problems of women, or to spinal cord dysfunction following neurodegenerative disease. This chapter necessarily reflects this bias.

Trieschmann (1992) argued that the historic view of spinal cord injury as a psychological (and physical) catastrophe, with which only some people could deal, is unduly pessimistic. Many would support the contention that normal life is indeed possible after spinal cord injury; but many would also agree that the process of emotional and psychological adjustment to disability may be a long and arduous matter, where the process of mourning for loss, and anticipatory loss, of function must be worked through. It is also an emergent observation that these emotional issues are seldom discussed adequately with the patient and those who are close to him or her. The teaching or facilitation of coping skills in new patients is also perceived as important.

It should not be forgotten that most spinal cord dysfunction is far less dramatic, more common and less studied than the more severe injuries implied above. Bigos et al. (1986) suggested that some 85% of the population suffer injury to the lower back at some point in life. The social, psychological and economic consequences of this are difficult to overestimate.

In an admittedly small scale Australian study (50 men who had been medically retired from work following lower back injury and their spouses), Coates and Ferroni (1991) noted that all respondents had reduced their sexual activity. More than one in three had ceased sexual activity entirely. This, coupled with chronic pain and loss of self-esteem due to unemployment, contributed markedly to an observed increase in marital disharmony. Erectile difficulties, not attributable to significant segmental lesions in the spinal cord, were also common, together with premature ejaculation. Many respondents reported intense testicular pain that forced curtailment of intercourse that in any case had lost much of its enjoyment and was seen more as a duty.

Adjustment to Spinal Cord Dysfunction

The themes of adjustment to loss are, in principle, closely similar almost regardless of the severity, or even the abruptness, of the spinal cord dysfunction. Most formulations have followed the classic paradigm of Kubler-Ross (1975), who depicted normal bereavement as a sequence of denial ("I'm not going to die"), anger ("It's your [the doctor, the family, etc.] fault; Why me?), bargaining ("If I get better, I'll do anything"), depression and acceptance. It is not necessary to follow these stages in precise sequence, or even to display all of them, but the paradigm has been of great heuristic value in the management of grief and of the dying. It is commonplace to think of adjustment to spinal cord dysfunction in similar terms, although the stages vary. Stewart (1977) and Hohmann (1975) stress the initial denial phase, followed by externally directed hostility as a reaction to the realization of (physical) dependence.

The presence of "depression" in Kubler-Ross's paradigm is important. It should probably be taken to mean subjective and objective sadness, albeit sometimes quite profound, rather than a clinical depression according to, for example, the World Health Organization's ICD-10 Classification of Mental and Behavioral Disorders. By no means all patients with spinal cord injury become clinically depressed; a commonly quoted range is 25%–30% (Howell et al. 1981; Richards 1986). However, one should not be led into complacency by these figures. Although the data on suicide among people with spinal cord dysfunction are very incomplete, the presence of chronic pain and disability is an undoubted risk factor for suicide, among men particularly, compounded by the social consequences of unemployment and isolation that commonly occur.

It is essential to be alert to features of clinical depression, such as social withdrawal (especially from family, friends and visitors), loss of concentration, tearfulness, pessimism, irritability and disproportionate guilt. Suicidal ideation should be asked about directly and explicitly. The so-called "biological", or "vegetative", features of depression (diurnal variation in mood, sleeplessness, poor appetite and loss of enjoyment) are less clinically important in the physically ill, since such persons may often be uncomfortable and, deprived of exercise, may display the lassitude that may mimic "biological" depression. Unfortunately, many of the commonly used diagnostic instruments (rating scales) used to study depression give prominence to these "biological" features, and we suggest that scales which focus on more "psychic" aspects of depression (e.g. the Montgomery–Åsberg Depression Rating Scale: Montgomery and Åsberg 1979) are probably of more use in those with spinal cord dysfunction.

There is a danger that, in the quest for depression, one may overlook the more adaptive ways in which a patient adjusts to his or her loss (Dijkers and Cushman 1990), and that the actual nature and severity of psychological disturbance may similarly be overestimated (Richards 1986). What is important is the distinction between "normal" and "pathological" adjustment. This is largely an arbitrary judgment, based on operational criteria.

A "normal" bereavement or adjustment reaction should last about six months or so, perhaps a little longer. Over that time, the emotional intensity surrounding the loss diminishes as the person "comes to terms" with it. The reaction becomes "pathological" if the intensity of the affective disturbance persists beyond six to nine months, certainly beyond a year, with little or no diminution. However, an adjustment reaction may be construed as "pathological" even earlier. The presence of psychotic symptoms – a sustained loss of touch with reality – typically of guilt, one's own evil, a sense of punishment and the experience of perceptual disturbances such as mood congruent auditory (derogatory voices, etc.) and visual (coffins, blood, graves, etc.) hallucinations clearly go beyond "normal" whenever they are found in the process of loss.

Individual factors

The foregoing may be all very well in the description of populations, but says relatively little about factors in the individual that determine the response to spinal cord dysfunction. Most of the studies that examine personality variables have done so using Rotter's (1966) concept of locus of control. In essence this describes an individual's attribution of the causes of what happens to him in terms of either having little or no sense of personal control of, or responsibility for, events (external locus of control); or having a sense of personal control of the same events (internal locus of control). Those who have a predominately internal locus of control are said to be better able to adapt to the vicissitudes of life and be less susceptible to depressive illness. Standardized measures of locus of control, of which the Multidimensional Health Locus of Control Scale (Wallston and Wallston 1981) is a well-tried example, have a potential use in the identification of those individuals who may simultaneously require more intensive support after the onset of spinal cord dysfunction and need to be directed away from undue dependence on professional help, particularly in hospital.

There is commonly a shift in the dynamic of a sexual partnership after spinal cord injury. The injured partner may no longer be able to fulfill his or her role in the home. Again, this has been more studied in men who frequently report that loss of a traditional male role, especially as economic provider, but also in ways such as household repairs, carrying heavy shopping and assuming the dominant position sexually, is demeaning and strongly contributory to a pervasive sense of low self esteem.

The Sexual Response in Spinal Cord Dysfunction

The anatomical location of the spinal lesion is of crucial importance in any effect on sexuality, as indicated by a consideration of the anatomy of the sexual response.

Libido (sexual interest) is a function of the cerebral cortex, and, in the absence of affective disturbance, is largely unaffected after spinal cord injury (Talbot 1991). It is worth remembering that the premorbid level of libido is the most valid object of comparison, rather than an arbitrarily assigned standard of interest.

In the male, the sequence of erection, penetration (intromission) and ejaculation (Masters and Johnson 1966) is mediated by the spinal cord. Erection is mediated by the thoracolumbar sympathetic outflow, with the sensory part of the loop supplied by somatic sensory nerves from the skin and bulb of the penis. As in the case of libido, erection depends on cortically integrated sensory information in all modalities, especially visual and tactile, but also involving olfaction and hearing. Sporadic, ill-sustained, erections are common after spinal cord injury, but unaided, penetrative, intercourse is difficult and anorgasmia is the rule, especially in more central spinal lesions.

Ejaculation is mediated by both limbs of the autonomic system, with emission of semen stimulated by sympathetic efferents to the prostate, seminal vesicles and vas. However, the contraction of the bulb of the penis, forming the pulsatile ejaculation, is mediated by the sacral parasympathetic outflow, while sensory information is transmitted by the pudendal nerve (S2,3). The sensation of orgasm is usually impaired after spinal cord injury, often by referral of a distorted sensation to the lower abdomen or to the thigh. It is frequently abolished altogether. In addition, the sperm count after spinal cord injury is greatly reduced, perhaps in part due to the greater scrotal temperatures found in the wheelchair bound (Brindley 1982, 1984).

In women, the sexual sequence moves from the resting state through excitation (lubrication), the plateau, orgasm and relaxation (Masters and Johnson 1966).

Excitation is mediated by somatic sensation which is lost in lesions above T10, and diminished in those below that level to a greater or lesser degree. Control of the pelvic musculature is similarly affected. Moreover, lubrication is abolished by lesions above the lower thoracic levels, resulting in vaginal dryness and increased vulnerability to infection. Lesions in the lumbar or sacral cord regions are not associated with impairment of this phase, or the plateau and orgasm phases, although the latter is perceived as a rather frustrating pseudo-orgasm where the lesion is below T10. The relaxation phase is an activity mainly of the cerebral cortex, being the crucible of sexual fantasies. It is unaffected by spinal cord dysfunction, and is of great importance in conveying a sense of sexual fulfilment. After an initial three- to nine-month period of amenorrhoea following injury, female fertility is unimpaired by spinal cord dysfunction, and pregnancy and normal delivery are possible if intensive obstetric management is available. Parturition is affected by spinal cord dysfunction inasmuch as lesions in the region of T10 impair the quality of uterine contractions.

Treatment

Treatment of sexual problems following spinal cord dysfunction falls crudely into three main categories: psychological ("talking") therapy, mechanical aids and drugs.

Psychological therapy may take the form of counselling, which revolves around sensitive listening, provision of information, practical advice, reassurance and the facilitation of communication, and specific sex therapy, a specialized combination of psychotherapeutic, behavioural and educational techniques. Although special training and supervision are advisable for sex therapy, most professionals involved with those who have spinal cord dysfunction should be able to counsel their patients. Indeed, counselling is probably all that most patients need, but perceive also that, too often, they do not receive it.

Sexual behaviour is difficult to discuss openly in our society, even among people who have no spinal cord dysfunction. It is much more so in those who have, since there is a popular belief that sexual behaviour in disabled people is such a distasteful idea that it is not acknowledged or talked about. To be able sensitively, without shock or revulsion, to listen to people with spinal cord dysfunction may in itself help the patient feel less unusual or stigmatized. To extend this by discussing how spinal cord dysfunction may interfere with "normal" sexual practices, and how to substitute other sexual techniques, may prevent many problems later on, especially if the matter is tackled earlier rather than later.

Sexuality in spinal cord dysfunction depends on social factors such as support from spouse or partner, if any, and the quality of the sexual life before the injury, as well as on the site of the lesion. A major contributory factor is whether these issues have been openly and explicitly discussed with the individuals concerned. In Coates and Ferroni's (1991) series, many of the psychosexual difficulties encountered could probably have been prevented, or at least alleviated, by advice on matters such as alternative sexual positions (the so-called "missionary" position may be too painful, but other positions may not be considered or may be deemed "perverted" or "abnormal") and means of sexual stimulation other than penile penetration. This lesson, that frank advice on sexual aspects after spinal cord dysfunction, is still applied too seldom. A similar point is made by Gardner and Rainsbury (1992), who identify the first weekend home and the first weeks after discharge from hospital as important "sexual milestones" in the rehabilitation of those with spinal cord injury.

To be able to facilitate communication between sexual partners who may be too inhibited or inarticulate to discuss their sexual needs and expectations with each other should be well within the scope of most professionals, who are also in a position to offer specific advice on alternative techniques. Last, but far from least, a counsellor may be able to advance the idea that sexual fulfilment and true intimacy do not entirely depend on sheer performance. For a man whose notions of sexuality rely on his personal potency, this idea may be difficult to implant, but a sensitive and matter-of-fact approach may help to dispel some prejudices.

Sex therapy was developed to help people with often deep-seated sexual difficulties, where psychological problems impinge on sexual activity. The chief aims of sex therapy are:

1. Emphasizing that sexual success and sexual performance are not necessarily equated, and that other forms of sexual stimulation exist beyond standard penetrative intercourse;
2. maximizing the partner's pleasure by attention to, for example, erogenous zones ("sensate focus") ands other non-genital contacts;
3. identifying and working through obstacles to mutual understanding and pleasure;
4. education on sexual anatomy and physiology;
5. giving specific help to adjust to a partner's pain or disability, allowing the ventilation of attendant anxieties.

Most of the literature on sex therapy has concentrated on the problems encountered in people without spinal cord dysfunction. But the principles are the same, and referral for sex therapy is often well worth considering.

For some men, the loss of potency following spinal cord dysfunction requires at least the illusion of restoration. Mechanical aids may then be employed, although all have significant disadvantages and none is free of complications. There are two main categories of mechanical aid. Penile implants (prostheses) may be semirigid, "string" or inflatable systems (Leyson 1991). All are expensive, prone to act as foci of infection or immunological rejection, and are often disliked by the sexual partner. The most frequently used device, in carefully selected patients, is the semirigid implant (Stien 1992). A penile ring placed around the base of the penis, thus blocking venous drainage and prolonging the erection, is also in common use. This may have aesthetic drawbacks, but seems to be reasonably safe if well made. The use of locally applied vibrators or rectal probe stimulation (Halstead et al. 1987) to promote ejaculation falls into the category of mechanical aids.

The use of drugs in the attempted restoration or enhancement of sexual function has a long and chequered history. Drugs such as yohimbine (α-adrenergic blocker) and L-DOPA (dopamine agonist) have been used orally, but without much effect. Intracavernous injections of similar drugs, as well as prostaglandin E_1 (PGE_1) and vasoactive intestinal peptide (VIP), have been used, with mixed results. The chief drawbacks are expense, the present inability to inject the drug in a smoothly controlled way, the possibility of priapism (where the happy novelty of the condition soon wears off) and local fibrosis and infection. Intrathecal administration of the choline esterase inhibitor neostigmine has been used to induce ejaculation after spinal cord injury. The risks of infection, intracranial haemorrhage and abrupt hypertension militate against the use of such methods.

In the end, no great improvement on talking to the patient, allowing the ventilation of anxieties and being available to give sensitive advice and education, has yet evolved. Early intervention seems to pay off, and its delivery is not confined to those with special training. To be able to acknowledge the psychosocial an psychosexual implications of spinal cord dysfunction, and to look for further ways to alleviate an important and common source of unhappiness or worse, does our patients a great service.

References

Bigos J, Spengler D, Martin N, Zeh, J, Fisher L, Nachemson A (1986) Back injuries in industry: a retrospective study – employee-related factors. Spine 11:246–251

Brindley GS (1982) Deep scrotal temperature and the effect on it of clothing, air temperature, activity, posture and paraplegia. Br J Urol 54:49–55

Brindley GS (1984) The fertility of men with spinal injuries. Paraplegia 22:337–348

Coates R, Ferroni PA (1991) Sexual dysfunction and marital disharmony as a consequence of chronic lumbar spinal pain. Sexual Marital Ther 6:65–69

Dijkers M, Cushman LA (1990) Differences between rehabilitation disciplines in views of depression in spinal cord injury patients. Paraplegia 28:380–391

Gardner BP, Rainsbury P (1992) Sexual function following spinal cord injury In: Illis LS (ed) Spinal cord dysfunction, vol 2, Oxford University Press, Oxford, pp 167–184

Halstead LS, VerVoort S, Seager SWJ (1987) Rectal probe electro-stimulation in the treatment of anejaculatory spinal cord injured men. Paraplegia 25:120–129

Hohmann G (1975) Psychological aspects of treatment and rehabilitation of the spinal cord injured person. Clin Orthop 112:81–88

Howell T, Fullerton DT, Harvey RF Klein M (1981) Depression in spinal cord injured patients. Paraplegia 19:284–288

Kubler-Ross E (1975) Death, the final stage of growth. Prentice Hall, Englewood Cliffs, NJ

Leyson JFJ (1991) Sexual rehabilitation of the spinal cord injured. Humana Press, Clifton, NJ

Masters WH, Johnson VE (1966) Human sexual response. Churchill, London

Montgomery SA, Åsberg M (1979) A new depression scale designed to be sensitive to change. Br J Psychiatry 134:382–389

Morris J (1992) Psychological and sociological aspects of patients with spinal injuries. In: Frankel HF (ed) Handbook of neurology, vol 17 Elsevier Science, Amsterdam

Richards JS (1986) Psychological adjustment to spinal cord injury in the first postdischarge year. Arch Phys Med Rehabil 67:362–365

Rotter JB (1966) Generalized expectancies for internal versus external control of reinforcement. Psychol Monogr 80 (609)

Stewart TD (1977) Coping behavior and moratorium following spinal cord injury. Paraplegia 15:338–342

Stein R (1992) Sexual dysfunctions in the spinal cord injured. Paraplegia 30:54–57

Talbot H (1971) Psychosocial aspects of sexuality in spinal cord injured patients. Int J Paraplegia 9:37–39

Trieschmann RB (1992) Psychological research in spinal cord injury: the state of the art. Paraplegia 30:58–60

Wallston KA, Wallston BS (1981) Health locus of control scales. In: Leftcourt H (ed) Research with the locus of control construct. Academic Press, New York.

Chapter 24

Spinal Vascular Disease

M.J. Aminoff

Vascular disorders of the spinal cord are a rare but important cause of disability. They merit consideration particularly because disability can often be prevented by a rational approach to the treatment of certain of these disorders.

Vascular Anatomy

Three sorts of artery enter the spinal canal with the anterior and posterior nerve roots. The radicular arteries supply just the nerve roots, whereas the radiculopial arteries also feed the pial–leptomeningeal arterial plexus. Only the radiculomedullary arteries contribute to the blood supply of the spinal cord, and these are present only at certain segmental levels.

The spinal cord is supplied by the anterior and posterior spinal arteries. The posterior spinal arteries are paired vessels that arise intracranially from the vertebral arteries. They interconnect with an anastomotic arterial plexus and, as they descend the length of the spinal cord, are fed at different levels by a variable number of posterior radiculomedullary vessels.

The anterior spinal artery, which also arises from the intracranial vertebral arteries, is a single vessel that descends the length of the spinal cord overlying the anterior longitudinal fissure. It is supplied by a variable number of vessels, usually between four and seven, as it descends. For descriptive purposes, the supply to the anterior spinal artery is best considered in three longitudinal territories. In the cervical and upper thoracic region, the anterior spinal artery receives contributions from usually three or more segmental vessels, including one vessel arising from the costocervical trunk. In the midthoracic region (between T4 and T8) the anterior spinal artery is often fed by only a single vessel, and it has its smallest diameter in this region, sometimes being discontinuous. In the region below T8, the anterior spinal artery receives its blood supply mainly from a single large vessel, the artery of Adamkiewicz, which commonly arises from a segmental vessel between about T9 and L2 on the left side.

Branches of the anterior and posterior spinal arteries form a fine plexus around the cord from which radially oriented branches are given off. Blood flow through these vessels supplies much of the white matter and the posterior horns of grey

423

matter. The largest branches of the anterior spinal artery are the central or sul-cocommissural arteries, which arise (in varying number) at each segmental level in the anterior longitudinal fissure and turn to one or other side of the cord. The central arteries are larger and more numerous in the cervical and lumbar cord than in the thoracic. Blood passes through them to supply the grey matter (except the posterior horns) and the innermost portion of the white matter.

An anterior median group of intrinsic veins drains the capillaries of the grey and white commissures, the medial cell columns of the anterior horns, and the anterior funiculi, emptying through the central veins into the anterior median spinal vein which runs in the anterior longitudinal fissure. The rest of the cord drains through radial veins to the coronal plexus of venous channels that runs longitudinally over the posterior and lateral surfaces of the cord. The superficial veins around the cord drain by the medullary veins which accompany the nerve roots to the intervertebral foramina, where radicular veins draining the nerve roots and communications from the anterior and posterior epidural and paravertebral plexuses also converge.

Ischaemic Myelopathies

An ischaemic myelopathy may occur when space-occupying lesions cause vascular compression, may contribute to post-traumatic cord dysfunction, and may occur as a sequel to irradiation. Thus, neoplastic or granulomatous epidural or extravertebral lesions may cause a rapidly progressive paraparesis by obstruction of an entering artery. In some instances there may be an apparent discrepancy between the level of the lesion and the clinical deficit. For example, a sensory disturbance may extend for several segments above the level of a cord lesion, because the territory supplied by a radicular vessel contributing to the cord circulation extends beyond the vessel's level of origin. Again, wasting of the intrinsic muscles of the hand in patients with a foramen magnum lesion may occur if the anterior spinal artery is compressed (Symonds and Meadows 1937; Henson and Parsons 1967).

Pathology may involve the aorta and those of its branches (i.e. the intercostal, lumbar or vertebral arteries) supplying the spinal circulation. Pathological involvement of the spinal arteries and their branches may also occur. When this leads to cord infarction, treatment is symptomatic. Care of the skin, bladder and bowels is important, as is active rehabilitation of the patient.

Disorders of Vessels Supplying the Spinal Circulation

Paraplegia may follow occlusion of the abdominal aorta when the blood supply to the artery of Adamkiewicz is interrupted, and sometimes occurs despite a seemingly normal peripheral circulation (Cook 1959). An ischaemic myelopathy may similarly occur with dissecting or non-dissecting aortic aneurysms (Goodin 1989), inflammatory aortitis (Goodin 1989), and infective and non-infective emboli involving the aorta (Dickson et al. 1984; Syrjanen et al. 1986), and after aortic surgery (Ross 1985; Shaw 1986; Skillman 1986). The most critical aortic region encompasses the site of origin of the artery of Adamkiewicz, and thus is between the eighth thoracic and second lumbar segments. Abdominal aortography may also cause an acute ischaemic myelopathy (Killen and Foster 1960), the occurrence of which probably depends on such factors as the concentration of and duration of exposure to the contrast agent, the injection pressure, and injury to the artery of Adamkiewicz. Cervical myelopathy may result from imaging studies such as mediastinal angiography (DiChiro and Wener 1973), aortography (Brust et al. 1959), and injection of contrast material into the thyrocervical trunk during cerebral angiography, as well as from vertebral artery thrombosis (Boudin et al. 1966).

Adult-type coarctation of the aorta may cause ischaemia and hypotension of segments of the cord supplied from the aorta below the narrowed segment, leading to weakness and sensory disturbances in the legs, and a sphincter disturbance. Neurogenic intermittent claudication (p. 428) may also occur, due to diversion of blood away from the cord by retrograde flow in the anterior spinal artery to bypass the narrowed aortic segment (Kendall and Andrew 1972). In classic coarctation, a collateral circulation involving the anterior spinal artery may be visualized radiologically or at autopsy, lying usually between the C6 and T4 segments. Flow is from enlarged vertebral, thyrocervical and costocervical spinal arteries, via a distended anterior spinal artery, to dilated radicular branches of the intercostal vessels below the coarctation, thereby by-passing the stenosed aortic segment. A cervicothoracic myelopathy may result, relating either to cord compression by the enlarged collateral vessels or to a steal phenomenon (Weenink and Smilde 1964; Herron et al. 1958). Aneurysmal distension of the anterior spinal artery or a segmental feeder may occur, and subsequent rupture will then lead to subarachnoid haemorrhage (Wyburn-Mason 1943; Blackwood 1958). Treatment is of the underlying coarctation.

Marked hypotension, regardless of aetiology, may cause an ischaemic myelopathy. Some authors have reported an especial vulnerability of the watershed regions between the three longitudinal territories of the anterior spinal artery, or of the midthoracic region, where the anterior spinal artery is usually supplied by only a single, small feeder. The regional extent of such vulnerable areas is unclear, and whether they are truly at increased risk of ischaemic damage is uncertain (Goodin 1989). In any given segment of the cord, a reduction in blood flow sometimes involves predominantly the central area between the territories of the anterior and posterior spinal arteries, with particular involvement of grey matter (Zulch 1962; Kepes 1965; Garland et al. 1966).

Acute ischaemic total transverse myelopathy is characterized by the rapid development of a flaccid areflexic paraplegia or quadriplegia, with analgesia and anaesthesia below the lesion, and urinary and faecal retention. Severe back pain may occur initially at the level of the lesion. The cerebrospinal fluid (CSF) is usually normal, but in the acute phase sometimes exhibits a mild pleocytosis and increased protein concentration. With occlusion of the named spinal arteries, certain distinctive clinical features may be found.

Disease of the Spinal Arteries

Occlusion of the spinal arteries or their intramedullary branches may result from thrombus, atherosclerosis (Gruner and Lapresle 1962), or an inflammatory process such as syphilis (Williamson 1894; Spiller 1909), polyarteritis nodosa (Roger et al. 1955), systemic lupus erythematosus (Andrianakos et al. 1975), Sjögren's syndrome (Alexander et al. 1981), rheumatoid arthritis (Watson et al. 1977), and sarcoidosis

(Matthews 1965). Cardiogenic emboli are rare causes of spinal artery occlusion (Madow and Alpers 1949; Wolman and Bradshaw 1967), as also are embolic fragments of nucleus pulposus (see p. 427). Rapid decompression of divers may lead to nitrogen embolism (the "bends"), and a similar disorder may follow rapid exposure to high altitude, with haemorrhagic or ischaemic necrosis of the cord, especially in the thoracic region, and resulting paraplegia. A transverse myelitis or Brown–Séquard syndrome has been reported as a sequel to injection of heroin or quinine adulterant, and may relate to a vasculitis, hypersensitivity reaction, hypotension or embolization (Richter and Rosenberg 1968; Krause 1983).

The territory supplied by the anterior spinal artery is more vulnerable to ischaemia than that supplied by the posterior spinal circulation. This is because there are fewer vessels feeding the anterior than the posterior spinal arteries, and because the anterior spinal artery is a single – sometimes discontinuous – vessel whereas the posterior spinal arteries are in reality an anastomotic network.

Anterior Spinal Artery Occlusion

This results in infarction of the anterior two-thirds of the cord. Many cases attributed to occlusion of the anterior spinal artery are probably due to occlusion of a major radicular feeder or the vessel from which such a feeder originates (Garland et al. 1966). Sudden back pain, sometimes having a girdle or radicular distribution, may occur at the onset, and a flaccid paraplegia or quadriplegia then develops over several minutes or hours, depending on the involved level of the cord, accompanied by retention of urine. Pyramidal signs ultimately develop below the level of the lesion as "spinal shock" wears off, while wasting occurs of muscles supplied from the infarcted region. Typically, pain and temperature appreciation are impaired, with relative sparing of light touch and proprioceptive sensation. A Brown–Séquard syndrome may result from occlusion of a central or sulcocommissural artery, which supplies only one side of the cord, or from occlusion of one anterior spinal artery when this vessel is duplicated (Wells 1966). Swelling of the cord may be visualized by imaging studies. There is a poor prognosis for recovery except when definite improvement occurs within the first 48 h.

Posterior Spinal Artery Syndrome

This is characterized clinically by impaired vibration and joint position sense below the level of the lesion due to ipsilateral posterior column involvement, with segmental anaesthesia and areflexia. A pyramidal deficit may also be present if the lateral funiculus is affected, but is usually transient and mild compared to the sensory disturbance. Because of the many feeders to these vessels, infarction in the territory of the posterior spinal arteries is rare, but described (Gruner and Lapresle 1962; Garland et al. 1966; Hughes 1970).

Ischaemia Affecting Predominantly the Anterior Horns

This causes a lower motor neurone deficit, sometimes combined with minor pyramidal signs but with sensory sparing. This presentation may simulate progressive spinal muscular atrophy or amyotrophic lateral sclerosis but sphincter dysfunction is an occasional accompaniment, and autopsy reveals haemorrhagic necrosis in the anterior horns (Gruner and Lapresle 1962; Jellinger and Neumayer 1962). The clinical disorder usually has an insidious onset and a gradually progressive course, but occasionally it begins abruptly (Jellinger and Neumayer 1962; Herrick and Mills 1971). Cases have been ascribed to spinal arteriosclerosis (Skinhoj 1954; Gruner and Lapresle 1962), and to aortic disease or surgery (Beattie et al. 1953; Kepes 1965; Herrick and Mills 1971). The selective grey matter involvement probably results from its increased vulnerability to hypoxia (Gelfan and Tarlov 1955) or to its location in the watershed area between the anterior and posterior spinal circulations.

Venous Infarction of the Cord

Venous infarction of the cord is rare except in the context of an associated arteriovenous malformation (AVM). When it does occur, spinal venous stasis and thrombosis are usually associated with malignant disease, sepsis, vertebral disorders, or a generalized thrombotic syndrome. Sudden pain in the back is followed within a few hours or so by weakness and sensory loss that develop in the legs, accompanied by urinary and faecal retention. Progression commonly occurs over the next few days, leading to a clinical picture of cord transection, and often ultimately to a fatal outcome from pulmonary embolism or the underlying disease associated with the infarction. The CSF is often normal, but a pleocytosis and increased protein concentration are not uncommon. Imaging studies may reveal a swollen cord. Postmortem examination reveals distended, thrombosed spinal veins, and there may be haemorrhagic necrosis of the cord itself, especially centrally.

Intervertebral Disc Embolism

A number of cases of nucleus pulposus embolism of the spinal cord have been recognized. There is a preponderance of women among the reported cases, and ages have ranged between 15 and 77 years (Bots et al. 1981). Presentation is typically with acute pain in the back or neck, followed after a few minutes by rapidly progressive limb weakness and sensory impairment, usually to all modalities. The neurological deficit is fully established within a few hours. The cervical cord is the region affected most often, but involvement may initially be in the lumbosacral area (Jurcovic and Eiben 1970). Death eventually follows, usually due to infective complications. The correct diagnosis is generally not made until autopsy, when emboli histochemically identical to the fibrocartilage of the nucleus pulposus are found in the spinal arteries or veins, and sometimes in the vertebral marrow interstitial spaces and sinusoids (Srigley et al. 1981). The manner that such material enters the vascular system is not known. It may be that fragments of nucleus pulposus enter the arterial circulation through a tear in an adjacent radicular artery after lateral rupture of degenerated disc material, that an increase in disc pressure is responsible for injecting disc material into small blood vessels (which are said to be present in degenerate but unruptured annulus fibrosus), or that anomalous vascularity next to or within the vertebral disc is responsible (Naiman et al. 1961; Hayes et al. 1978). Material may also be extruded directly into an overlying venous sinus.

Neurogenic Intermittent Claudication

Neurogenic intermittent claudication has been used to designate symptoms that develop after a predictable amount of exercise and disappear with rest, and that result from disorders of the spinal cord and cauda equina.

Intermittent Claudication of the Cauda Equina

Pain, numbness and paraesthesias that develop with exercise, and are relieved by rest characterize this syndrome, which is more common in men than women. Symptoms may begin in the feet and spread up to involve the buttocks, or conversely begin proximally and spread down the legs. Similar symptoms typically occur with the adoption of certain postures. Clinical examination is usually normal unless performed while the patient is symptomatic, when there may be motor and sensory abnormalities. Imaging studies are diagnostic in showing compression of the cauda equina (Blau and Logue 1961; Wilson 1969), as by a central disc protrusion. Treatment is surgical.

Sagittal narrowing of the lumbar spinal canal, with compression of nerve roots at one or more levels, predisposes to the disorder. Reported associations include developmental or spondylotic narrowing of the vertebral canal, spina bifida, disc protrusion and achondroplasia. In patients with a mildly narrowed lumbar canal, any additional encroachment, such as by a small disc protrusion, may result in the development of symptoms. Actions or postures that involve extension of the lumbar spine usually precipitate symptoms, which are relieved when the patient leans forward or squats. Hyperextension of the lumbar spine displaces the cauda equina roots posteriorly and causes the roots to thicken because their course is shortened, and this results in increased compression and hence the production of symptoms. Only occasionally are symptoms precipitated by exercise of the extremities, presumably because of relative ischaemia of active cauda equina roots during exercise (Blau and Logue 1961; Evans 1964). Experimental studies in the mouse (Blau and Rushworth 1958) showed that after exercise of the hind limb, vessels of the regional spinal nerve roots dilate widely. When symptoms of cauda equina claudication are precipitated specifically by exercise, it is probable that they relate not only to compression of nerve roots but also to a limitation of the extent to which the blood supply can increase with activity because of impaired blood flow through radicular arteries at points of constriction (Blau and Logue 1961).

Clinical evaluation must distinguish between a neurogenic basis for intermittent claudication and peripheral vascular disease. In peripheral vascular disease, intermittent claudication is characterized by pain in exercised muscles, without spread such as typically occurs in neurogenic intermittent claudication. Other sensory disturbances are rare, and apart from some tightening of ischaemic muscles with activity there is no motor deficit. Examination generally reveals cutaneous evidence of peripheral vascular disease, diminished or absent peripheral pulses and a proximal arterial bruit; arteriography is diagnostic.

Intermittent Claudication of the Spinal Cord

This rare disorder may occur in patients with syphilitic arteritis, atherosclerosis (Henson and Parsons 1967), terminal aortic thrombosis (Ratinov and Jimenez-

Pabon 1961), and pronounced lumbar spondylosis or lower thoracic disc protrusion (Bergmark 1950; Garcin et al. 1959), but the most common cause nowadays is probably a spinal AVM (Wyburn-Mason 1943; Aminoff 1976). When it occurs in coarctation of the aorta, the reduced blood supply to the cord below the narrowed aortic segment (Tyler and Clark 1958) or aortic steal from the anterior spinal artery (Kendall and Andrew 1972) may be responsible.

Initial symptoms may consist of a heaviness in one or both legs that comes on with activity and is relieved by rest, or of sensory symptoms, pain or sphincter disturbances that show a similar relationship to activity (Garcin et al. 1962; Aminoff 1976). Examination at rest is generally normal or reveals only minor abnormalities. After exercise, however, there is weakness of one or both legs, with hyper-reflexia and extensor plantar responses; there may also be a sensory deficit, sometimes severe enough to cause gait ataxia. The syndrome is occasionally the prelude to infarction (Garcin et al. 1959, 1962; Henson and Parsons 1967), but frequently there is no change or only gradual progression over a long period of time, with reduction in exercise tolerance until a lasting deficit is present.

The regional blood flow in the cord (and appropriate nerve roots) increases with leg exercise (Blau and Rushworth 1958), presumably to meet increased metabolic requirements. In patients with intermittent claudication of the cord, it seems likely that the underlying lesion prevents the increased circulatory requirements of activity from being met.

Haemorrhage

Haematomyelia and Spinal Subarachnoid Haemorrhage

Haematomyelia or spontaneous spinal subarachnoid haemorrhage occurs most commonly from AVMs (Wyburn-Mason 1943; Aminoff 1976), which are discussed on p. 433. It may also occur from other types of spinal hamartoma, such as telangiectases, and following trauma (Fig. 24.1). Subarachnoid haemorrhage may be associated with intradural spinal neoplasms located particularly about the conus or cauda equina, such as ependymomas, neurofibromas, meningiomas and meningeal sarcomas. It may occur with coarctation of the aorta (Wyburn-Mason 1943; Blackwood, 1958); with rupture of mycotic or other spinal aneurysms; in certain connective tissue diseases, such as polyarteritis nodosa (Henson and Croft 1956), systemic lupus erythematosus (Fody et al. 1980) and Sjögren's syndrome (Alexander et al. 1982); in association with blood dyscrasias or anticoagulant drug therapy; in such toxic-infectious conditions as typhoid fever; and in relation to lumbar puncture (King and Glas 1960). In some cases, no specific cause can be recognized.

The onset of spinal subarachnoid haemorrhage is typically with sudden severe back pain overlying the site of bleeding, spreading rapidly to the rest of the back. Radicular pain, particularly bilateral sciatica, may occur as blood passes into the lumbar sac. With small and purely intramedullary haemorrhages, however, pain may not be conspicuous. When subarachnoid haemorrhage arises in the cervical region, distinction from intracranial haemorrhage may be impossible clinically. Symptoms of cerebral dysfunction may ultimately develop, and include vomiting, photophobia, a disturbance of consciousness, and seizures. Such symptoms tend to

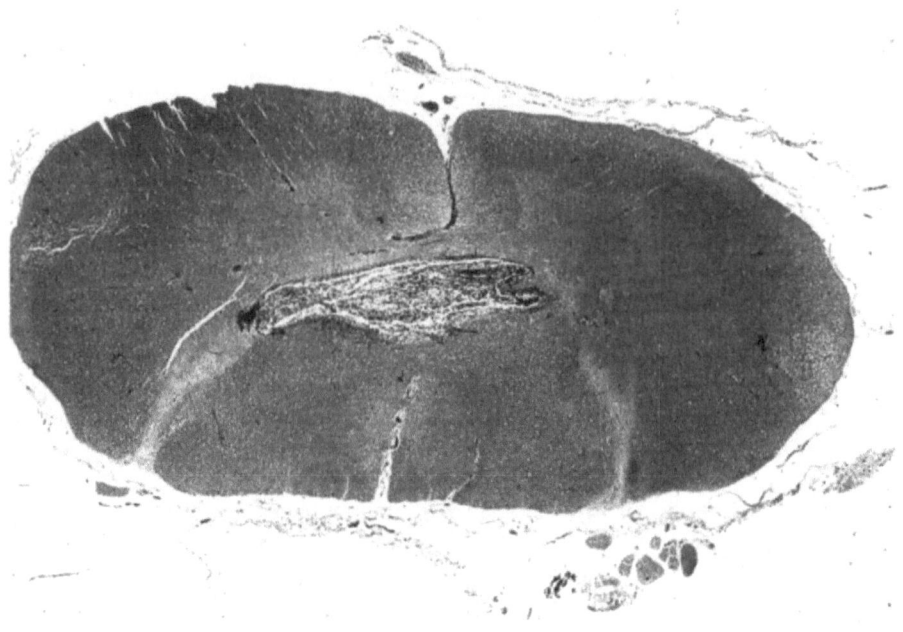

Fig. 24.1. Low power photomicrograph showing a traumatic haematomyelia of recent onset. (Courtesy of R.L. Davis, MD, Pathology Department, UCSF.)

be milder and more short-lived than symptoms of cord dysfunction, which result from haematomyelia or compression of the cord or nerve roots by blood or blood clot. The cord dysfunction may lead to flaccid limb weakness, sensory disturbances, and impaired sphincter function.

Signs of meningeal irritation are usually conspicuous. Cranial nerve palsies, nystagmus and a depressed level of consciousness reflect cerebral involvement, whereas motor, sensory or reflex abnormalities in the limbs usually relate to spinal cord or root disturbances. The presence of a cutaneous angioma or spinal bruit suggests an underlying spinal vascular malformation, and careful inspection and auscultation of the spine is therefore important in patients with subarachnoid haemorrhage of uncertain cause.

The diagnosis of subarachnoid haemorrhage is confirmed by the presence of blood in the CSF or by the findings on CT scanning. Recognition of a spinal vascular malformation or neoplasm will generally depend on the findings at myelography or with other imaging techniques such as MRI and CT scanning.

Prognosis depends on the severity of the haemorrhage and on its cause. Surgical treatment may be necessary if the spinal lesion is neoplastic, or there are signs of cord compression by blood or blood clot. If the myelogram suggests a spinal vascular malformation, angiographic delineation and operative treatment may be necessary, as discussed on p. 436. Collagenoses, blood dyscrasias, and anticoagulant-induced haemorrhage require appropriate medical management.

Spinal Subdural Haematoma

Spinal subdural haematomas are rare. They may occur spontaneously or after lumbar puncture (Fig. 24.2) in patients with blood dyscrasias that predispose to bleeding, such as haemophilia or thrombocytopenia, or in patients taking anticoagulant drugs. They may also occur spontaneously or after trauma of varying severity in patients without a bleeding diathesis, and are said to be an important cause of perinatal paraplegia (Towbin 1969).

Symptoms characteristically begin with sudden severe back pain, often accompanied by root pain. The clinical features of a spinal cord or cauda equina syndrome, due to compression by the haematoma, may then develop. When haemorrhage follows lumbar puncture, the clinical deficit usually develops within about 24 hours.

Myelography reveals a filling defect or a block at the site of the haematoma, or fixed displacement of the contrast material to one side. CT scan or MRI is also helpful in visualizing the lesion and in suggesting its nature, but experience with it in this context is limited. Complete recovery may follow early evacuation of the haematoma, whereas any delay in surgical intervention often leads to an irreversible neurological deficit. Patients with blood dyscrasias require appropriate therapy; if anticoagulant drugs are being taken, they should be discontinued and their effect reversed.

In order to reduce the chances of haemorrhage, lumbar puncture must be undertaken with particular care in patients with a haematological disorder that predisposes to bleeding, being performed by a skilled physician and only when really necessary, using a small needle; consideration must also be given to correcting the

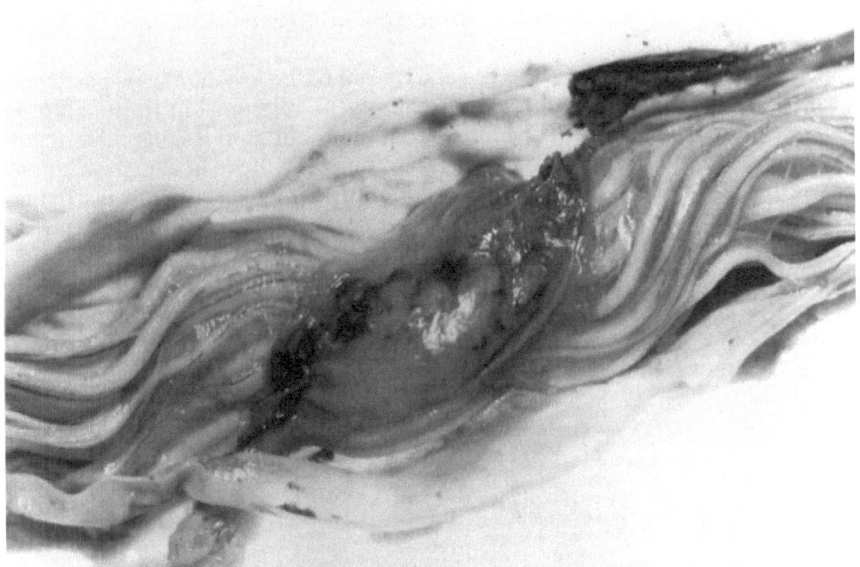

Fig. 24.2. Subdural haematoma of several weeks duration involving the cauda equina in a patient with systemic lupus erythematosus, who had undergone several lumbar punctures. (Courtesy of R.L. Davis, MD, Pathology Department, UCSF.)

haematological disorder by transfusion if feasible. In thrombocytopenic patients, spinal haematoma may be more likely to complicate lumbar puncture as the platelet count declines, and in patients with a rapidly dropping platelet count (Edelson et al. 1974); platelet transfusion just before lumbar puncture should be considered if the platelet count is below 20 000/mm³ or dropping rapidly.

Spinal Epidural Haematoma

Spinal epidural haematoma may occur at any age, but in children the haematoma is most often in the lower cervical region, whereas in adults the lower thoracic or thoracolumbar region is also a common site for haematomas.

Epidural haemorrhage may relate to trauma, particularly in neonates (Towbin 1969). In adults it may follow minor injuries without accompanying vertebral fracture or dislocation, symptoms of a progressive cord lesion commencing within a few hours or days of the trauma. It may also occur in patients with epidural vascular malformations (Cube 1962; Dawson 1963) or tumours, and in patients with blood dyscrasias or an iatrogenic predisposition to bleeding. Spinal epidural haemorrhage may occur spontaneously (Markham et al. 1967; Posnikoff 1968), occasionally in relation to pregnancy (Bidzinski 1966), and after lumbar puncture or epidural anaesthesia (Gingrich 1968), especially in anticoagulated patients (De Angelis 1972).

Clinical presentation is usually with a sudden, severe, constant back pain that may begin in relation to minor straining, overlies the site of haemorrhage, and is enhanced by percussion over the back, movements of the spine, or manoeuvres that increase the pressure in the vertebral venous plexus. Girdle pain, or radicular or diffuse pain in the extremities may also be present. After an interval of several hours (but, rarely, up to a few weeks), a cord or cauda equina syndrome develops. It may be impossible to distinguish epidural from subdural haematoma save by imaging studies or at operation.

Imaging studies demonstrate the site and nature of the lesion. MRI is particularly helpful for detecting a haematoma and defining its relationship to the cord and thecal sac, as well as for distinguishing it from other epidural lesions. Treatment is by urgent evacuation of the haematoma at laminectomy. Rebello and Dastur (1966) reported that 29 of 59 patients coming to operation recovered satisfactorily, 16 made a partial recovery and 14 failed to benefit, whereas of 11 treated conservatively only one recovered completely. Most of those who recovered were operated on within 72 hours of the onset of symptoms, emphasizing the importance of early diagnosis and prompt surgical treatment. The prognosis for functional recovery is generally worse in patients with a severe or rapidly progressive deficit. In patients on anticoagulant therapy, treatment should be stopped and vitamin K or fresh frozen plasma provided.

Spinal Aneurysms

Isolated arterial aneurysms of the spinal vasculature are rare. They usually lead to subarachnoid haemorrhage or a focal cord lesion (Henson and Croft 1956; Leech et al. 1976), but are rarely the cause of patients presenting in such a way. Marked aneurysmal distension of spinal arteries may occur in coarctation of the aorta (Wyburn-Mason 1943; Blackwood 1958), and in association with spinal AVMs (Herdt et al. 1971; Vogelsang and Dietz 1975; Caroscio et al. 1980). In the latter circumstance the aneurysm may be a more frequent source of haemorrhage than the AVM. Thus, in one series of 50 cases of spinal AVM, all patients with a history of spinal subarachnoid haemorrhage had a coexistent aneurysm intimately associated with their AVM (Herdt et al. 1971).

Dural and Intradural Spinal Arteriovenous Malformations

AVMs, which are the most common kind of hamartoma related to the spinal cord, consist of an abnormal nidus of vessels between the arterial and venous systems, without intervening capillaries. In rare instances there may be a true fistula rather than a nidus of abnormal vessels between the main artery and vein involved in the malformation (Gueguen et al. 1987; Aminoff et al. 1988). Telangiectasias and cavernous angiomas uncommonly involve the spinal cord and are usually a-symptomatic, although they occasionally bleed or lead to a focal neurological deficit.

Spinal AVMs may be associated with other vascular anomalies, including cutaneous, vertebral, paraspinal and epidural angiomas, cerebral or cerebellar angiomas, Osler–Weber–Rendu syndrome, and lymphatic anomalies (Aminoff 1976). The association with spinal aneurysms has already been discussed.

Most spinal AVMs are located below the T3 cord segment. These are usually wholly or partially extramedullary, lie behind the cord, and are fed by one or more arteries that either do not supply the cord at all or only supply the posterior spinal circulation. In many instances the site of the arteriovenous shunt is actually on the dura rather than intradural (Oldfield et al. 1983; Symon et al. 1984), but it is not possible to distinguish between these lesions either clinically, by CT scan or MRI, or myelographically.

Spinal AVMs have been classified into four basic types depending on their angiographic features, and especially on their arterial supply and venous drainage. Type I lesions are AVMs in which the abnormal arteriovenous fistula is dural in location, and these are the most common variety. In Type II lesions the AVM is intramedullary, with the nidus containing the fistulous portion of the malformation actually located within the spinal cord itself. Type III AVMs, which are also referred to as juvenile AVMs, are extensive lesions that may be both intra- and extramedullary; The Type IV malformations are located within the dura but are extramedullary; they are fed by either the anterior or the posterior spinal artery rather than by a dural vessel such as is involved with Type I lesions, and they drain directly into an enlarged vein. There is a marked male preponderance among reported cases, particularly when the AVM is dural (Type I), and patients may present at any age.

The 20% of AVMs located in the cervical or upper thoracic segments have an approximately equal sex incidence, and are usually diagnosed earlier than more caudal lesions because they are more likely to bleed. Most of these lesions are wholly or partially intramedullary, are anteriorly situated, and are supplied by vessels contributing also to the anterior spinal circulation. Multiple feeders are common, and the arteriovenous shunt is usually of large volume.

Clinical Features

Spinal AVMs may present with subarachnoid haemorrhage or with a myeloradiculopathy. The most common cause of non-traumatic spinal subarachnoid haemorrhage is an AVM. About 10% of all spinal AVMs and over 40% of cervical AVMs will cause subarachnoid haemorrhage, at least once (Aminoff 1976). The features of such haemorrhage were described on p.429. The overall mortality of the initial bleed is at least 15%, and approximately half the survivors will have a second haemorrhage. Half of the subsequent survivors have further haemorrhages unless the underlying lesion is treated. The second bleed occurs within one year of the first in about 40% of cases with recurrent haemorrhage.

The myeloradiculopathy resulting from spinal AVMs may have an insidious onset and progression or, less commonly, follows a relapsing and remitting course, sometimes with long intervals between relapses. Aminoff and Logue (1974a) reported initial symptoms to consist of pain in 25 of 60 patients (42%), other sensory symptoms in 20 (33%), leg weakness in 19 (32%), disturbed sphincter or sexual function in 6 (10%), and subarachnoid haemorrhage in 3 (5%); most (two-thirds) had developed weakness, sensory symptoms, pain and a disturbance of bladder function by the time of diagnosis, and 6 (10%) had experienced a subarachnoid haemorrhage.

In 19 of the 60 patients there were symptoms suggestive of neurogenic claudication of the cord or cauda equina, and in 14 symptoms were precipitated or aggravated by certain postures. Exercise tolerance varied among these patients, but tended to diminish with time. Less common precipitants of symptoms include pregnancy, trauma, increased body temperature, non-specific infective illnesses, straining at stool, the menstrual cycle and a heavy meal.

Although examination sometimes reveals no abnormalities, even after exercise, most patients with thoracolumbar AVMs have a mixed upper and lower motor neurone deficit in the legs, with an accompanying sensory disturbance, by the time of diagnosis. Occasionally a purely motor deficit is present, simulating motor neurone disease (except for the restricted distribution). With cervical AVMs, abnormal findings may be present in the arms as well as the legs. Although sensory deficits may have an upper level on the trunk, this sometimes correlates poorly with the angiographic level of the lesion. Occasional patients have coexisting cutaneous vascular lesions, which may relate segmentally to the spinal anomaly and which are more easy to recognize while patients perform the Valsalva manoeuvre. The presence of a spinal or paraspinal bruit is helpful in suggesting the underlying diagnosis, but its absence does not exclude an AVM.

The myeloradiculopathy is often rapidly progressive. Thus, within 6 months of the onset of any leg weakness or gait distrubance, 10 of the 60 patients reported by Aminoff and Logue (1974b) required two sticks or crutches to get about, or had become unable to walk at all, and 28 were so disabled within 3 years. Among the remaining patients, the disability was often sufficient to interfere with normal daily activities.

Pathophysiology

The myeloradiculopathy is not due to cord compression as judged by the radiological, operative or autopsy findings. Intravascular thrombosis may contribute to the clinical deficit, but this would not account for the marked fluctuations in symptoms that sometimes occur spontaneously or in relation to exercise, posture or the other factors mentioned earlier. Moreover, thrombotic vascular occlusion is conspicuously absent in some autopsied cases. A common belief is that cord ischaemia results from diversion or "steal" of blood from the normal spinal circulation by the AVM. However, except in the cervical region, the supply to the AVM is usually distinct from that to the cord and does not even arise from the same segmental stem as a vessel supplying the anterior spinal artery, so that steal cannot normally occur by this route. Steal might occur via connections between the intramedullary circulation and the AVM, but such interconnections are usually inconspicuous at operation; further, if steal occurred by this route, ligation of the AVM's main feeders should enhance it (by reducing the pressure in the AVM) rather than producing clinical benefit.

The most likely explanation for the myeloradiculopathy is that the anomalous arteriovenous shunt increases the pressure in veins draining the cord, and intramedullary venous pressure therefore rises. This, in turn, reduces the intramedullary arteriovenous pressure gradient, diminishes intramedullary blood flow, and thus produces cord ischaemia beyond the territory of any individual spinal artery (Aminoff et al. 1974). This sequence of events would account for the cord syndrome described by Logue (1979) in a patient with an epidural AVM lying in the hollow of the sacrum; a large vein passed intradurally to ascend on the cord's surface, and division of this vessel reversed the patient's symptomatology.

Bederson and Spetzler (as cited by Anson and Spetzler 1993) have recently calculated the perfusion pressure across the spinal cord by measuring intraluminal venous pressure before and after closure of the dural arteriovenous fistula. They found that mean perfusion pressure increased from 38.9 mmHg to 57.5 mmHg after closure of the fistula in 10 patients. When the spinal cord perfusion pressure is less than 50 mmHg, spinal cord blood flow is reduced (Griffiths et al. 1978).

An acute onset or exacerbation of symptoms probably relates to intramedullary haemorrhage or thrombotic occlusion of a major extramedullary vessel, whereas a steady progression of symptoms relates to increasing cord ischaemia resulting from the reduced intramedullary arteriovenous pressure gradient (Fig. 24.3). Transient spontaneous fluctuation of symptoms probably reflects minor variations in cord blood flow (for example, by posture) or requirements (which are increased by activity). Intramedullary malformations may also cause symptoms by displacement of adjacent structures. Radicular symptoms presumably relate to ischaemia of nerve roots or to compression of roots by enlarged vessels.

Radiological Investigations

Plain radiographs of the spine are usually of little help. In most cases, the diagnosis is suggested by myelography, the length of the cord being visualized in both the prone and supine positions. The characteristic myelographic appearance is of localized or extensive vermiform defects due to vascular impressions in the column of

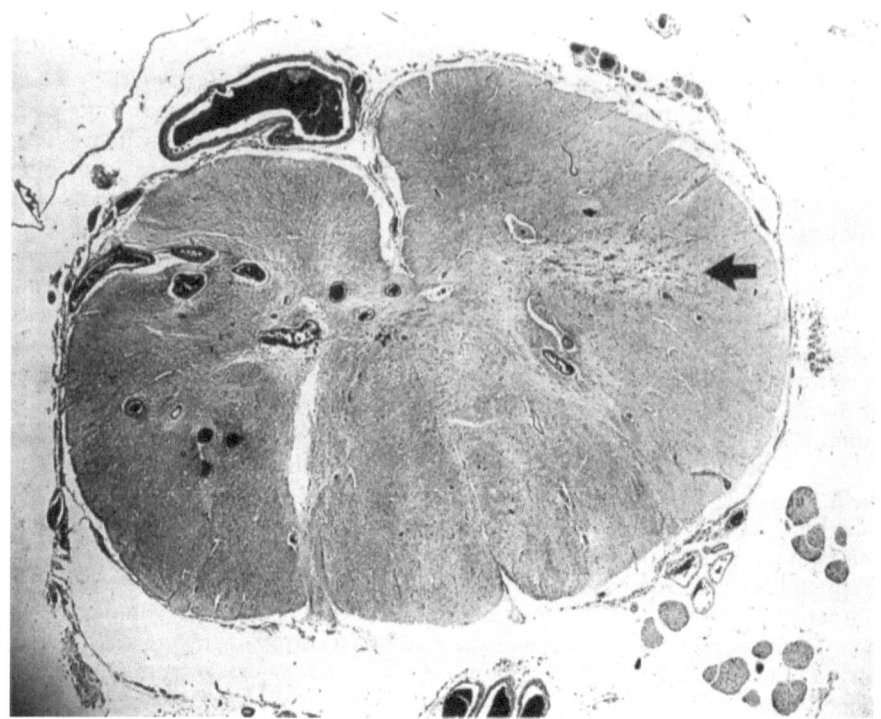

Fig. 24.3. Subacute necrotic myelopathy due to a spinal AVM. Low power photomicrograph showing large abnormal vascular channels in the subarachnoid space and spinal cord parenchyma. An incomplete infarct (*arrow*) is also seen. Original magnification × 5. (Courtesy of R.L. Davis, MD, Pathology Department, UCSF.)

contrast material (Fig. 24.4). In the thoracic region they are usually most conspicuous on the posterior aspect of the cord, and may not be seen except on supine films.

When the myelographic appearance suggests the presence of an AVM, selective spinal arteriography is undertaken to confirm its presence and to determine the level and extent of the vascular anomaly, its position in relation to the spinal cord, and the vessels feeding the AVM and the anterior spinal artery in the region of the malformation. Spinal angiography is usually unrewarding when a technically satisfactory myelogram, with both prone and supine views, fails to suggest an AVM.

The angiographic appearances of AVMs depend in considerable part upon their location. Cervical malformations usually lie in front of the cord and may be partly intramedullary. Such malformations are often fed by several different vessels, which may also supply the cord itself. More caudal AVMs usually lie more posteriorly and are supplied by only one or two vessels that generally do not contribute to the cord circulation (Fig. 24.4). Many of these caudal lesions are actually dural in location. The site of the fistula is usually projected lateral to the spinal cord, generally outside the plane of the dura and often encroaching into an intervertebral foramen (Kendall and Logue 1977). Surgical treatment of the latter malformations is thus simple in most instances.

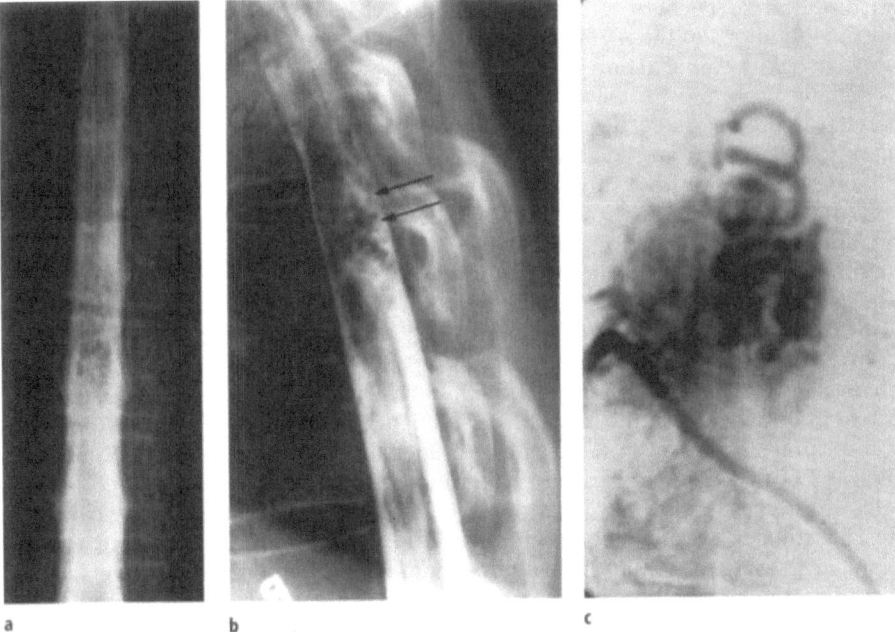

a   b   c

Fig. 24.4.   A 65-year-old woman with a dural spinal AVM causing a spastic paraparesis. **a**, myelogram showing serpiginous defects in the column of contrast material in the lower thoracic region, suggestive of an AVM. **b**, myelogram, lateral view, showing serpiginous filling defects (*arrows*) mainly behind the cord, at about T9 level. **c**, arteriogram following injection of the right T9 intercostal artery, which is supplying an extramedullary spinal AVM. (Courtesy of Grant Hieshima, MD, Radiology Department, UCSF.)

Spinal AVMs can sometimes be visualized with contrast-enhanced CT scans and magnetic resonance imaging, but a normal study does not exclude the possibility of an underlying AVM.

Indications for Treatment

Surgical excision of the AVM or the embolic occlusion of its feeding vessels may arrest a rapidly progressive myeloradiculopathy and may also prevent recurrence of bleeding in patients with subarachnoid haemorrhage. Whether patients with mild symptoms and no incapacity should undergo surgery or an embolization procedure can only be decided on an individual basis, with the general condition of the patient, the available angiographic and surgical facilities, and the risks of intervention in mind. The potential benefits of obliteration of the AVM are greater at this stage, but must be balanced against the involved risks.

An asymptomatic malformation discovered incidentally is best left undisturbed until it becomes clinically evident.

Treatment

Surgical treatment of dural or intradural extramedullary malformations situated posteriorly and fed by vessels not contributing to the cord circulation is usually uncomplicated. Feeders to the malformation can be ligated, and the fistulous portion ("nidus") of the AVM removed if desired. Alternatively, feeding vessels can be occluded by embolization.

Embolization, most often with either polyvinyl alcohol particles or with cyano-acrylate liquid polymers, has now been widely used (Merland and Reizine 1987; Hall et al. 1989; Morgan and Marsh, 1989) especially in the treatment of dural AVMs. Because these lesions are supplied by vessels that fail to supply the spinal cord, the risks to the cord are low. Embolized AVMs occasionally become revascularized by the enlargement of small feeders that were not recognized in the original angiographic studies because their contribution to the blood supply of the malformations was so insignificant. However, recanalization of vessels after embolic obliteration also occurs not uncommonly (Hall et al. 1989; Morgan and Marsh 1989; Biondi et al. 1990). Recanalization is especially likely to occur when polyvinyl alcohol particles are used, rather than a cyanoacrylate liquid polymer. With the liquid polymers the extent of obstruction in the injected vessels depends on the injection rate, polymerization time and blood flow (Anson and Spetzler 1993); one major problem with their use is that the polymerized material forms a hard mass that may complicate later surgical excision. Moreover, embolization may be followed by neurological deterioration as a result of obstruction of the blood supply to the cord.

In considering the feasibility of embolization, attention is directed at the anatomy of the malformation in relation to the normal spinal circulation. For example, embolization is hazardous when the same arterial vessel supplies both the AVM and the anterior spinal artery. Similarly, inability to catheterize selectively the feeder to the AVM contraindicates treatment by embolization.

Surgical treatment is indicated either as the primary approach or as treatment for those AVMs that are not successfully obliterated by embolization. The optimal surgical approach involves ligation of feeding vessels within the spinal canal, and all of the feeding vessels must be occluded. The procedure is best combined with excision of the fistulous portion of the malformation in case small feeding vessels are unrecognized at angiography or operation and are left intact. If the AVM is actually dural in location, the draining vessels on the surface of the cord can be left undisturbed, thereby reducing the risk of neurological complications. Mourier et al. (1989) compared the benefits of embolization to surgery in a series of 70 patients with dural AVMs. Among 63 patients in whom embolization was undertaken, it successfully obliterated the AVM in 40 but was unsuccessful in 23 patients, whose clinical disturbance progressed and who had angiographic persistence of the lesion. These 23 patients underwent surgery, as did an additional seven patients in whom embolization was not feasible. Of these 30 patients treated operatively, approximately one-half improved and the remainder stabilized, suggesting that surgical treatment is more effective than embolization. One patient who underwent surgery worsened following the procedure, but this same patient had also shown a deterioration after previous embolization.

Therefore, surgical obliteration of the nidus of the AVM is generally very worthwhile. A review by Anson and Spetzler (1993) showed that among 131 patients in several different series, 87 patients improved after surgery, 27 showed clinical stabilization and only two deteriorated.

It may not be possible to excise malformations in front of or within the cord and fed by the anterior spinal artery or vessels supplying it. Many such AVMs are cervical. However, accessible feeders can be ligated or embolized, and inaccessible ones sometimes occluded by embolization. Because the anterior spinal artery is fed by several vessels in the cervical region, a multistaged procedure, with occlusion of only one or two feeding vessels at any one time, is often well tolerated. The occasional thoracolumbar malformation supplied directly by the anterior spinal artery or one of its feeders is also difficult to treat. However, advances in radiological techniques have permitted better delineation of such lesions, and in some centres the operative treatment of intramedullary or mixed AVMs supplied by long sulcocommissural arteries is feasible (Riche et al. 1982). Inoperable AVMs supplied by short, sulcocommissural arteries feeding directly into them may sometimes be treated successfully by embolization (Riche et al. 1982).

In rare instances there is a direct arteriovenous fistula involving the anterior spinal artery and a draining vein, without an intervening nidus of abnormal vessels. Depending on the angiographic appearance, a direct surgical approach is sometimes feasible, whereas in other instances embolization or treatment with detachable balloons may be possible (Riche et al. 1983; Gueguen et al. 1987; Aminoff et al. 1988).

References

Alexander EL, Craft C, Dorsch C, Moser RL, Provost TT, Alexander GE (1982) Necrotizing arteritis and spinal subarachnoid hemorrhage in Sjogren syndrome. Ann Neurol 11:632–635

Alexander GE, Provost TT, Stevens MB, Alexander EL (1981) Sjogren syndrome: central nervous system manifestations. Neurology 31:1391–1396

Aminoff MJ (1976) Spinal angiomas. Blackwell, Oxford

Aminoff MJ, Logue V (1974a) Clinical features of spinal vascular malformations. Brain 97:197–210

Aminoff MJ, Logue V (1974b) The prognosis of patients with spinal vascular malformations. Brain 97:211–218

Aminoff MJ, Barnard RO, Logue V (1974) The pathophysiology of spinal vascular malformations. J Neurol Sci 23:255–263

Aminoff MJ, Gutin PH, Norman D (1988) Unusual type of spinal arteriovenous malformation. Neurosurgery 22:589–591

Andrianakos AA, Duffy J, Suzuki M, Sharp JT (1975) Transverse myelopathy in systemic lupus erythematosus. Report of three cases and review of the literature. Ann Intern Med 83:616–624

Anson JA, Spetzler RF (1993) Spinal dural arteriovenous malformations. In: Awad IA, Barrow DL (eds) Dural arteriovenous malformations. American Association of Neurological Surgeons, Illinois, pp 175–191

Beattie EJ, Nolan J, Howe JS (1953) Paralysis following surgical correction of coarctation of the aorta. Case report with autopsy findings. Surgery 33:754–760

Bergmark G (1950) Intermittent spinal claudication. Acta Med Scand Suppl 246:30–36

Bidzinski J (1966) Spontaneous spinal epidural hematoma during pregnancy. Case report. J Neurosurg 24:1017

Biondi A, Merland J-J, Reizine D et al. (1990) Embolization with particles in thoracic intramedullary arteriovenous malformations: long-term angiographic and clinical results. Radiology 177:651–658

Blackwood W (1958) Discussion on vascular disease of the spinal cord. Proc R Soc Med 51:543–547

Blau JN, Logue V (1961) Intermittent claudication of the cauda equina. An unusual syndrome resulting from central protrusion of a lumbar intervertebral disc. Lancet i:1081–1086

Blau JN, Rushworth G (1958) Observations on the blood vessels of the spinal cord and their responses to motor activity. Brain 81:354–363

Bots GTAM, Wattendorff AR, Buruma OJS, Roos RAC, Endtz LJ (1981) Acute myelopathy caused by fibrocartilaginous emboli. Neurology 31:1250–1256

Boudin G, Pepin B, Cassan J-L, Vernant J-C, Gazengel J (1966) Le retentissement medullaire des thromboses ou stenoses de l'artere vertebrale. (A propos de 3 observations). Rev Neurol (Paris) 114:263–270

Brust AA, Howard JM, Bryant MR, Godwin JT (1959) Coarctation of the abdominal aorta with stenosis of the renal arteries and hypertension. Clinical and pathologic study of two cases and review of the literature. Am J Med 27:793–802

Caroscio JT, Brannan T, Budabin M, Huang YP, Yahr MD (1980) Subarachnoid hemorrhage secondary to spinal arteriovenous malformation and aneurysm. Arch Neurol 37:101–103

Cook AW (1959) Occlusion of the abdominal aorta and dysfunction of the spinal cord. A clinical syndrome. Bull NY Acad Med 35:477–489

Cube HM (1962) Spinal extradural hemorrhage. J Neurosurg 19:171–172

Dawson BH (1963) Paraplegia due to spinal epidural haematoma. J Neurol Neurosurg Psychiatry 26:171–173

De Angelis J (1972) Hazards of subdural and epidural anesthesia during anticoagulant therapy: a case report and review. Anesth Analg 51:676–679

DiChiro G, Wener L (1973) Angiography of the spinal cord: a review of contemporary techniques and applications. J Neurosurg 39:1–29

Dickson AP, Lum SK, Whyte AS (1984) Paraplegia following saddle embolism. Br J Surg 71:321

Edelson RN, Chernik NL, Posner JB (1974) Spinal subdural hematomas complicating lumbar puncture. Occurrence in thrombocytopenic patients. Arch Neurol 31:134–137

Evans JG (1964) Neurogenic intermittent claudication. Br Med J 2:985–987

Fody EP, Netsky MG, Mrak RE (1980) Subarachnoid spinal hemorrhage in a case of systemic lupus erythematosus. Arch Neurol 37:173–174

Garcin R, Godlewski S, Lapresle J, Fardeau M (1959) Syndromes vasculaires aigus probables de la partie inférieure de la moelle chez des sujets porteurs de lesions discarthrosiques du rachis dorso-lombaire. Rev Neurol (Paris) 100:212–229

Garcin R, Godlewski S, Rondot P (1962) Etude clinique des médullopathies d'origine vasculaire. Rev Neurol (Paris) 106:558–591

Garland H, Greenberg J, Harriman DGF (1966) Infarction of the spinal cord. Brain 89:645–662

Gelfan S, Tarlov IM (1955) Differential vulnerability of spinal cord structures to anoxia. J Neurophysiol 18:170–188

Gingrich TF (1968) Spinal epidural hematoma following continuous epidural anesthesia. Anesthesiology 29:162–163

Goodin DS (1989) Neurological sequelae of aortic disease and surgery. In: Aminoff MJ (ed) Neurology and general medicine. Churchill Livingstone, New York, pp 23–48

Griffiths IR, Pitts LH, Crawford RA, Trench JG (1978) Spinal cord compression and blood flow. I: The effect of raised cerebrospinal fluid pressure on spinal cord blood flow. Neurology 28:1145–1151

Gruner J, Lapresle J (1962) Etude anatomo-pathologique des medullopathies d'origine vasculaire. Rev Neurol (Paris) 106:592–631

Gueguen B, Merland JJ, Riche MC, Rey A (1987) Vascular malformations of the spinal cord: intrathecal perimedullary arteriovenous fistulas fed by medullary arteries. Neurology 37:969–979

Hall WA, Oldfield EH, Doppman JL (1989) Recanalization of spinal arteriovenous malformations following embolization. J Neurosurg 70:714–720

Hayes MA, Creighton SR, Boysen BG, Holfeld N (1978) Acute necrotizing myelopathy from nucleus pulposus embolism in dogs with intervertebral disk degeneration. J Am Vet Med Assoc 173:289–295

Henson RA, Croft PB (1956) Spontaneous spinal subarachnoid haemorrhage. Q J Med 25:53–66

Henson RA, Parsons M (1967) Ischaemic lesions of the spinal cord: an illustrated review. Q J Med 36:205–222

Herdt JR, DiChiro G, Doppman JL (1971) Combined arterial and arteriovenous aneurysms of the spinal cord. Radiology 99:589–593

Herrick MK, Mills PE (1971) Infarction of spinal cord. Two cases of selective gray matter involvement secondary to asymptomatic aortic disease. Arch Neurol 24:228–241

Herron PW, Foltz EL, Plum F, Bruce RA, Merendino KA (1958) Partial Brown–Séquard syndrome associated with coarctation of the aorta: review of literature and report of a surgically treated case. Am Heart J 55:129–134

Hughes JT (1970) Thrombosis of the posterior spinal arteries. A complication of an intrathecal injection of phenol. Neurology 20:659–664

Jellinger K, Neumayer E (1962) Myelopathies progressives d'origine vasculaire. Rev Neurol (Paris) 106:666–669

Jurcovic I, Eiben E (1970) Fatal myelomalacia caused by massive fibrocartilaginous venous emboli from nucleus pulposus. Acta Neuropathol (Berl) 15:284–287

Kendall BE, Andrew J (1972) Neurogenic intermittent claudication associated with aortic steal from the anterior spinal artery complicating coarctation of the aorta. Case report. J Neurosurg 37:89–94

Kendall BE, Logue V (1977) Spinal epidural angiomatous malformations draining into intrathecal veins. Neuroradiology 13:181–189

Kepes JJ (1965) Selective necrosis of spinal cord gray matter. A complication of dissecting aneurysm of the aorta. Acta Neuropathol (Berl) 4:293–298

Killen DA, Foster JH (1960) Spinal cord injury as a complication of aortography. Ann Surg 152:211–230

King OJ, Glas WW (1960) Spinal subarachnoid hemorrhage following lumbar puncture. Arch Surg 80:574–577

Krause GS (1983) Brown–Séquard syndrome following heroin addiction. Ann Emerg Med 12:581–583

Leech PJ, Stokes BAR, ApSimon T, Harper C (1976) Unruptured aneurysm of the anterior spinal artery presenting as paraparesis. Case report. J Neurosurg 45:331–333

Logue V (1979) Angiomas of the spinal cord: review of the pathogenesis, clinical features, and results of surgery. J Neurol Neurosurg Psychiatry 42:1–11

Madow L, Alpers BJ (1949) Involvement of the spinal cord in occlusion of the coronary vessels. Arch Neurol Psychiatry 61:430–440

Markham JW, Lynge HN, Stahlman GEB (1967) The syndrome of spontaneous spinal epidural hematoma. Report of three cases. J Neurosurg 26:334–342

Matthews WB (1965) Sarcoidosis of the nervous system. J Neurol Neurosurg Psychiatry 28:23–29

Merland J-J, Reizine D. (1987) Treatment of arteriovenous spinal-cord malformations. Semin Interventional Radiol 4:281–290

Morgan MK, Marsh WR (1989) Management of spinal dural arteriovenous malformations. J Neurosurg 70:832–836

Mourier KL, Gelbert F, Rey A et al. (1989) Spinal dural arteriovenous malformations with perimedullary drainage: indications and results of surgery in 30 cases. Acta Neurochir (Wien) 100:136–141

Naiman JL, Donohue WL, Prichard JS (1961) Fatal nucleus pulposus embolism of spinal cord after trauma. Neurology 11:83–87

Oldfield EH, DiChiro G, Quindlen EA, Rieth KG, Doppman JL (1983) Successful treatment of a group of cord arteriovenous malformations by interruption of dural fistula. J Neurosurg 59:1019–1030

Posnikoff J (1968) Spontaneous spinal epidural hematoma of childhood. J Pediatr 73:178–183

Ratinov G, Jimenez-Pabon E (1961) Intermittent spinal ischemia. Neurology 11:546–549

Rebello MD, Dastur HM (1966) Spinal epidural hemorrhage. (A review and two case reports). Neurol India 14:135–145

Riche MC, Modenesi-Freitas J, Djindjian M, Merland JJ (1982) Arteriovenous malformations of the spinal cord in children. A review of 38 cases. Neuroradiology 22:171–180

Riche MC, Scialfa G, Gueguen B, Merland JJ (1983) Giant extramedullary arteriovenous fistula supplied by the anterior spinal artery: treatment by detachable balloons. AJNR 4:391–394

Richter RW, Rosenberg RN (1968) Transverse myelitis associated with heroin addiction. JAMA 206:1255–1257

Roger H, Poursines Y, Roger J (1955) Les aspects neurologiques de la periarterite noueuse. Rev Neurol (Paris) 92:430–464

Ross RT (1985) Spinal cord infarction in disease and surgery of the aorta. Can J Neurol Sci 12:289–295

Shaw PJ (1986) Neurological complications of cardiovascular surgery. II. Procedures involving the heart and thoracic aorta. Int Anesthesiol Clin 24:159–200

Skillman JJ (1986) Neurological complications of cardio-vascular surgery. I. Procedures involving the carotid arteries and abdominal aorta. Int Anesthesiol Clin 24:135–157

Skinhoj E (1954) Arteriosclerosis of the spinal cord. Three cases of pure "syndrome of the anterior spinal artery". Acta Psychiatr Neurol Scand 29:139–143

Spiller WG (1909) Thrombosis of the cervical anterior median spinal artery; syphilitic acute anterior poliomyelitis. J Nerv Ment Dis 36:601–613

Srigley JR, Lambert CD, Bilbao JM, Pritzker KPH (1981) Spinal cord infarction secondary to intervertebral disc embolism. Ann Neurol 9:296–301

Symon L, Kuyama H, Kendall B (1984) Dural arteriovenous malformations of the spine: clinical features and surgical results in 55 cases. J Neurosurg 60:238–247

Symonds CP, Meadows SP (1937) Compression of the spinal cord in the neighbourhood of the foramen magnum. Brain 60:52–84

Syrjanen J, Iivanainen M, Kallio M, Somer H, Valtonen VV (1986) Three different pathogenic mechanisms for paraparesis in association with bacterial infections. Ann Clin Res 18:191–194

Towbin A (1969) Latent spinal cord and brain stem injury in newborn infants. Dev Med Child Neurol 11:54–68

Tyler HR, Clark DB (1958) Neurologic complications in patients with coarctation of aorta. Neurology 8:712–718

Vogelsang H, Dietz H (1975) Cervical spinal angioma combined with arterial aneurysm. Neuroradiology 8:223–228

Watson P, Fekete J, Deck J (1977) Central nervous system vasculitis in rheumatoid arthritis. Can J Neurol Sci 4:269–272

Weenink HR, Smilde J (1964) Spinal cord lesions due to coarctatio aortae. Psychiatr Neurol Neurochir 67:259–269

Wells CEC (1966) Clinical aspects of spinovascular disease. Proc R Soc Med 59:790–796

Williamson RT (1894) Spinal thrombosis and haemorrhage due to syphilitic disease of the vessels. Lancet ii:14–16

Wilson CB (1969) Significance of the small lumbar spinal canal: cauda equina compression syndromes due to spondylosis. Part 3: intermittent claudication. J Neurosurg 31:499–506

Wolman L, Bradshaw P (1967) Spinal cord embolism. J Neurol Neurosurg Psychiatry 30:446–454

Wyburn–Mason R (1943) The vascular abnormalities and tumours of the spinal cord and its membranes. Kimpton, London

Zulch KJ (1962) Réflexions sur la physiopathologie des troubles vasculaires médullaires. Rev Neurol (Paris) 106:632–645

Chapter 25

Decompression Illnesses and the Spinal Cord

R.R. Pearson

Introduction

Although diving as a purposeful activity has been going on since at least 5000 BC and almost certainly predates any recorded history, the decompression illnesses which can result from diving are a comparatively recent phenomenon and were not even described in detail until well into the 19th century. The reason for this is that despite many attempts to produce a practical means of breathing underwater, most of which were positively dangerously with little or no understanding of the physics and physiology involved, breath-hold diving from the surface or from submerged diving bells was the only way of venturing underwater. However, the advent of an effective and relatively safe underwater breathing capability came with the 1819 introduction of Augustus Siebe's diving helmet, a device which allowed the diver to be provided with compressed air from a pump on the surface. Apart from the much greater freedom given to the diver by this equipment, divers were provided with a much easier means of achieving depth-time limits underwater which were capable of causing what came to be known as decompression sickness (DCS) which, in its more acute forms, involves the central nervous system (CNS). Indeed, it is said that when Greek sponge divers began to use the 1839 version of Siebe's helmet, which by now was combined with a suit and heavy boots, 50% of them died within the first year! Equally, the very fact that it was now possible to breathe underwater made divers vulnerable to decompression pulmonary barotrauma, the second decompression illness capable of damaging the CNS. Developments of Siebe's helmet, which remained remarkably close to the original design, were used almost exclusively by military and commercial divers up to World War II when, as is so often the case, accelerated technological development for military purposes led to the first effective self-contained underwater breathing apparatus (SCUBA) and, with it, a further dramatic increase in underwater freedom and flexibility. The initial use of this equipment was by the so-called "frogmen" who used closed-circuit breathing apparatus with pure oxygen as a breathing mixture. Similar closed-circuit apparatus using oxygen or nitrogen–oxygen breathing mixtures is still much used by specialist military divers for a variety of offensive and defensive purposes. The advent of recreational diving as a popular pastime dates mainly from the 1946 invention of the "demand valve" by Cousteau and Gagnan. The demand valve is a self-regulating device which automatically provides the diver with a breathing mixture at the same pressure as the surrounding water. This simple and cheap device, combined with diver-borne compressed air cylinders, led to a dramatic change in routine commercial and military diving practice but, even more importantly, also provided the impetus for what was to become a veritable explosion in recreational or "sports" diving. It is in this population of recreational divers that the decompression illnesses and their sequelae are now most commonly seen and, in the United Kingdom where approximately 50 000 active "sports" divers give rise to approximately 150 decompression illnesses each year which require recompression therapy. About 90% of these cases exhibit evidence of CNS involvement. This high incidence of CNS involvement in decompression illnesses has risen from a 1985 level of approximately 50% and is undoubtedly the result of the deeper, repetitive and generally more adventurous diving allowed by advances in breathing equipment, thermal protection and an increasing reliance on diver-borne computers to control dives. A similar trend has occurred in the United States where the Divers Accident Network (DAN), a central reporting agency, deals with 250–300 decompression illnesses each year from an estimated diver population of about 2 million. However, it has been estimated that these accidents represent only about one half of the decompression illnesses treated each year in the United States and the Caribbean. In contrast, commercial diving has been the subject of increasingly stringent safety requirements and serious DCS is now rare in commercial diving activities in British waters. Further, legislation requires that all commercial diving activities have on-site recompression facilities or rapid access to such facilities to ensure that decompression illnesses are treated as quickly as possible. Such support is clearly impossible for recreational diving.

Regrettably, the world over, there is an all too common failure in the timely diagnosis of decompression illnesses and, with it, inevitable delays in definitive treatment. These delays can result in permanent neurological sequelae and there is nothing more true concerning the treatment of decompression illnesses than the simple fact that the sooner specific therapy is initiated, the better the prognosis is for full recovery.

Decompression Illnesses

The two decompression illnesses which may involve the CNS and, more specifically, cause spinal cord damage, are DCS and decompression pulmonary barotrauma (DPB). In DPB, alveolar gas may enter the pulmonary venous return to give the condition known as arterial gas embolism (AGE) whereas the various manifestations of DCS are due to the direct and indirect effects of bubbles of inert gas which can result from decompression after exposure to hyperbaric pressure. Although for comparative data collection, diagnostic and therapeutic purposes, it is increasingly fashionable to use the generic term "decompression illness" without qualification to describe collectively these phenomena (Smith et al. 1993), it is intended here to retain the identity of the two components to allow fuller understanding of the processes involved.

Decompression Sickness

DCS may occur in divers or compressed air workers on decompression from hyperbaric environments such as those used in tunnelling and caisson work. It may also result from decompression to altitude from normal ambient pressure at ground level. The latter situation may arise in altitude chambers or unpressurized aircraft. In the case of individuals who breathe compressed air during their hyperbaric exposure and those who are decompressed to altitude, the inert gas responsible for DCS will be nitrogen but other inert gases such as helium and, more rarely, neon and hydrogen, are used in deep diving, by definition diving in excess of 165 feet of sea water (fsw), as carrier gases or diluents for the essential oxygen component of the breathing mixture. The use of these inert gases is mainly confined to commercial and military diving and they avoid the problems of nitrogen narcosis and gas density which effectively limit air as a breathing mixture. In the UK, legislation forbids diving on compressed air deeper than 165 fsw, (50 metres of sea water (msw)). The toxic effects on the CNS of oxygen breathed at increased pressure limit the use of pure oxygen as a breathing mixture to depths shallower than 26 fsw/8 msw.

In general, the rate at which inert gases are taken up and released by body tissues during hyperbaric exposure and subsequent decompression is controlled by both perfusion and diffusion, the former being the more important. For practical purposes, the process of uptake and elimination of inert gas may be regarded as exponential and, quite simply, well perfused tissues will take up inert gas more rapidly than relatively poorly perfused tissues. A further controlling factor in the actual amount of inert gas taken up by any tissue is the solubility of inert gases in that particular type of tissue and, in this respect, it is unfortunate that nitrogen is much more soluble in fatty tissue than helium, which is expensive and reserved for breathing mixtures used in deep diving. It is generally accepted that this is the reason for the well-established fact that DCS involving the CNS in divers breathing helium–oxygen (heliox) mixtures is quite rare. When it does occur, it is largely similar to CNS involvement in DCS arising from compressed air diving. All further comment will, therefore, relate to DCS arising from breathing air or oxygen–nitrogen mixtures and, therefore, the result of nitrogen bubbles. This is, in any case, the type of DCS seen in recreational divers who generally use compressed air. Also, apart from a difference in the incidence of cases with neurological involvement, DCS arising from work in compressed air or altitude exposure has no other major difference from that seen in divers and these groups will not be considered separately.

The decompression phase of any hyperbaric exposure is, at least in theory, capable of causing nucleation of inert gas with bubble formation as tissues and blood release gas taken up during compression and the time spent at pressure. However, decompression tables exist to allow divers either to limit their depth/time exposure to enable a direct return to the surface or, if this limit is exceeded, to carry out a controlled decompression with stops at various depths during the ascent. Formal tables for air diving were first designed by Haldane in 1908 for use by the Royal Navy, although the relatively simple concepts of the factors involved in elimination of inert gas during decompression which were used in the design of these tables have since been shown to be inappropriate for the more extreme exposures in air diving. However, a wholly reliable mathematical model of the complex processes involved in single or multiple dives to a wide range of depths and time exposures has yet to be developed despite numerous and continuing attempts. Apart from those which are evolved stochastically from experience, many of these models are based on notional tissues which take up and release inert gas at different rates. These rates are expressed as "half-times", a term which refers to the time taken for the notional tissue to become half-saturated with inert gas. Saturation occurs when the partial pressure of the inert gas in solution in any given tissue is in equilibrium with the partial pressure of that gas in the breathing mixture. It is a process which may take as long as 24 h or more to occur in very poorly perfused tissues but may occur in minutes in well-perfused tissues such as the cerebral cortex. However, a largely empirical evolution of decompression tables and techniques for air diving has been going on for long enough to have evolved suitably safe decompression rules for air diving and the great majority of cases of DCS occur when these rules are ignored.

Inert Gas Bubbles

Inert gas bubbles are generally categorized as being either extra- or intravascular and although firm evidence does not, as yet, exist to suggest that they may also be intracellular, the smallest "bubble" is two molecules of gas and there is no theoretical reason why bubbles should not be intracellular. The effects of these bubbles may be direct and mechanical, or indirect by activation of various inflammatory responses with all their complexities.

Although it is essential to consider DCS as a particularly complex disease process with the potential to have a multi-organ and multisystem impact, the classification Golding et al. 1960 is still widely used. It is based on organ or system-related signs and symptoms, particularly those associated with onset and presentation. Most treatment regimes are based on this classification but it is increasingly seen as limited and even potentially dangerous in that it tends to disguise the widespread impact of the disorder. The classification divides DCS into Type 1 (Mild) and Type 2 (Serious) and Table 25.1 details the various manifestations of these categories, including the descriptive names that have, over the years, become associated with various presentations ("staggers", "chokes" etc.). The term "bends" originated in the 19th century as a descriptive term for the musculoskeletal manifestations of DCS but is now widely used to indicate any form of DCS.

Extravascular Inert Gas Bubbles

Before discussing the potential of DCS to damage the spinal cord, it is necessary to outline the respective role of extra- and intravascular inert gas bubbles. Without doubt, extravascular gas bubbles do occur and have been visualized both macro- and microscopically in a variety of tisues in man and experimental animals. It is fashionable to refer to such bubbles as "autochthonous" which literally means

Table 25.1.   Classification of decompression sickness (after Golding et al. 1960)

Type 1 (mild)	–	Joint pain ("niggles" to severe pain)
	–	Cutaneous (pruritus, erythema, lividity)
	–	Lymphoedema
	–	Constitutional (fatigue, malaise)
Type 2 (serious)	–	CNS (spinal cord and/or brain)
	–	Audiovestibular ("staggers")
	–	Respiratory ("chokes")
	–	Cardiovascular (hypovolaemia)

"formed in the region where found". If they arise in subcutaneous tissues, they can result in histamine and other vasoactive substance release and it is logical to attribute the cutaneous manifestations of itching and erythema to such substances. Inert gas bubbles may also block cutaneous lymphatic drainage channels and cause localized swelling and oedema. Equally, expansion of autochthonous bubbles occurring in poorly perfused tissues such as cartilage and ligamentous tissues associated with joints is assumed to produce direct pressure on sensitive nerve endings (Nims 1951) and cause the varying degrees of pain in, or adjacent to, joints which are a characteristic feature of Type 1 DCS. Although no incontrovertible evidence exists to support this concept, and it has been suggested that such pain may be centrally mediated as a consequence of spinal cord or nerve root involvement, the great majority of such cases respond so rapidly to recompression and, where it can be applied, local pressure, that it is difficult to attribute the pain to anything other than some local phenomenon involving autochthonous bubbles. The role of autochthonous bubbles in the CNS will be discussed later.

Intravascular Bubbles

As with extravascular bubbles, intravascular inert gas bubbles have been seen and recorded by a variety of methods on numerous occasions, commencing with Sir Robert Boyle (1670) whose experiments in subjecting a variety of animals to a vacuum resulted in visible intravascular bubbles which he described as "… choking up some passages and vitiating the figure of others …". Paul Bert (1878), the famous French physiologist, also described intravascular bubbles in his famous treatise and not only correctly attributed these bubbles to release of nitrogen during decompression, but indicated them as the cause of DCS.

It is generally accepted that, during decompression, the first intravascular gas emboli to occur are venous and pass to the microcirculation of the lungs which acts as a filter, allowing the inert gas to diffuse into the alveoli. The size of detectable decompression-induced venous gas emboli (VGE) probably ranges from 15 to 200 μm (Hills and Butler 1981) and ultrasonic doppler tranducers can detect VGE as they transit the right heart (Spencer and Clarke 1972; Powell and Johanson 1978). It is evident from numerous studies of divers during decompression that a certain degree of venous bubbling is tolerable and equally numerous animal experiments show that surprising amounts of venous gas can be tolerated, particularly if they are given as an infusion of bubbles. VGE have been recorded on many occasions in asymptomatic divers but they can, in sufficient quantity, lead to rises in pulmonary artery and right ventricular pressures, both factors which assist the migration of VGE through the pulmonary microcirculation (Butler and Hills 1985) or a patent foramen ovale (Moon and Camponesi 1989; Wilmshurst et al. 1989) to give arterial gas emboli (AGE) which are a much less tolerable form of intravascular gas.

Notwithstanding the embolic potential of intravascular gas, it is also a particularly potent initiator of the acute inflammatory response. Powerful electrochemical forces at the blood–gas interface of bubbles can result in denaturation of proteins with formation of globules of free fats and fat emboli may result from release of fatty acids from cell membranes. Platelet and leucocytes also adhere to bubbles (Philip et al. 1972) and the net effect is a cascade of events commencing with Hageman Factor activation which, in turn, leads to kinin, complement, clotting and fibrinolytic system activation. At worst, these reactions can add to the embolic potential of bubbles as well as having an adverse effect on vascular endothelial permeablity. Further, the stability of bubbles may be enhanced by the formation of a very thin (20 nm) "shell" of precipitated protein on their surface and this shell may also fragment to form circulating microemboli. In its most acute form, DCS may result in disseminated intravascular coagulation although this requires major decompression stress and is a rare outcome. A number of sources are available for a more comprehensive description of these events (Bove 1982; Francis et al. 1990) and it is sufficient to note that intravascular gas may not only cause ischaemia but that this ischaemia will adversely affect perfusion and thereby further hinder the elimination of inert gas from tissues.

Decompression Pulmonary Barotrauma (DPB)

If gas trapping occurs in the lungs or exhalation is inadequate during decompression, DPB, sometimes called the "pulmonary overinflation syndrome" may occur. The gas in the lungs must expand in accordance with Boyle's Law and overpressures necessary to cause alveolar rupture, be they localized or general, are surprisingly modest. Experiments with cadavers (Malhotra and Wright 1961) and animal models (Schaefer et al. 1958) suggest that as little as 100 mmHg overpressure can cause alveolar rupture. This degree of overpressure will be generated if gas trapping occurs during an ascent from depths as shallow as 4 fsw, a fact confirmed by a number of recorded cases of DPB occurring after ascents from shallow depths in swimming baths when SCUBA divers have not exhaled during the ascent. Once alveolar rupture has occurred, the gas may track to the lungs along the perivascular sheaths to give mediastinal emphysema or, much more frequently, it will go to the left heart via the pulmonary veins and become arterialized to give AGE. By far the most frequent destination of AGE is via the carotid arteries to give cerebral arterial gas embolism (CAGE), a dramatic event with potentially lethal consequences. The gas emboli usually end up in the areas of brain served by the anterior and middle cerebral arteries, particularly the "watershed" areas between the two circulations. Occasionally, the brainstem will be involved by gas emboli that have entered the vertebrobasilar ateries and it has been postulated that sudden death, a not uncommon outcome of CAGE, may be due to cardiac arrest or arrhythmias following brainstem involvement (Greene 1978). Once in the cerebral circulation, AGE tend to arrest in the precapillary arteriolar circulation to give ischaemia and the exposure of the endothelium to gas leads to a very rapid loss of integrity of the blood–brain barrier. Once the circulation is restored, either spontaneously or as a result of recompression therapy, oedema of the "vasogenic" type may occur (Pearson 1984). It is difficult to believe that AGE arresting in the microcirculation of the spinal cord will behave any differently.

Animal models have been used to show that the distribution of bubbles in the arterial circulation is influenced strongly by their buoyancy (Van Allen and Hrdina 1929). However, the bubbles used by Van Allen and Hrdina were relatively large and small bubbles (<100 μm) are much less buoyant indicating that more widespread systemic arterial embolization is possible, particularly if the victim is not erect when the embolic gas reaches the aorta. Coronary artery embolization is a possibility but remarkably few such cases are recorded of which only one fatal case had undeniable evidence of such an outcome (Harveyson et al. 1956). Evidence of other organ involvement by AGE is even more rare and only three cases of spinal cord involvement which were undeniably due to DPB are known to the author. Although it will be evident that the embolizing gas in DPB is whatever gas is being breathed, which contrasts with the inert gas emboli of DCS, the effect of different embolizing gases is qualitatively virtually identical with the exception of carbon dioxide which is sufficiently soluble to effectively preclude it as a potentially embolic gas. Also, whereas DCS requires a sufficiently stressful depth/time profile and decompression to initiate a critical degree of bubbling, and this will be evident in most cases, DPB can occur after minimal time at equally minimal depths. That said, emergency ascents often occur after submerged times that would also give DCS and an accurate differential diagnosis may be almost impossible; indeed, the two conditions may frequently coexist. If the apparent frequency with which venous inert gas emboli become arterialized is also taken into account, the need to distinguish between the two decompression illnesses becomes almost academic, more especially when the recommended recompression therapy for both is identical in a number of commonly used therapeutic regimes.

Presentation of the Decompression Illnesses

Decompression Sickness

Historically, the first descriptions of DCS appear to be by Triger, a French engineer, whose 1839 description of joint pain in caisson workers is cited by Bert (1878) and Pol and Watelle (1854), the latter authors describing a variety of more serious manifestations in caisson workers during the 1839 use of a caisson to sink a mineshaft. Pol and Watelle must also take the credit for recommending recompression as "the most certain way of easing" the symptoms of DCS. The building of a bridge across the Mississippi at St Louis, in 1867–74, involved much use of caissons and led to 19 deaths from DCS as well as 91 other cases, some severe and permanently disabling. These events were recorded in detail by Clark (1870–71) and Jaminet (1871), the two physicians who treated these cases. Jaminet was successful in reducing both morbidity and mortality by empirically adjusting the length and frequency of the hyperbaric exposures and also provided a graphic account of his own episode of DCS which involved transient quadriplegia and aphasia for which he was given Jamaica rum and beef tea. The value of alcohol in the treatment of DCS is a myth which, unfortunately, persists and it is all too frequently the first choice of recreational divers. Neither Jaminet nor Clark seem to have been aware of the use of recompression to treat DCS. Numerous accounts of DCS in compressed air workers then began to appear but some years elapsed before the problem was described as a specific hazard of diving (Khrabrostin 1888). Further accounts of DCS in divers then began to appear at regular intervals including one particularly graphic account of the short- and long-term sequelae of DCS (Blick 1909). Blick described over 200 cases of "divers palsy" in Australian pearl divers. Many of these divers had long-standing bladder paralysis and a urethral catheter was regarded as a standard item of their equipment. Since then, a truly vast amount of literature has accumulated concerning DCS in individuals and groups of divers and compressed air workers.

The symptoms and signs of DCS may appear singly or in combination and CNS involvement may be accompanied by any or all of the other categories listed in

Table 25.1. However, CNS involvement is always regarded as a form of Type 2 DCS and qualifies for the designation of "serious". Symptoms and signs of CNS involvement tend to appear shortly after surfacing from the causative decompression, occasionally even occurring during decompression. Francis et al. (1988a) analysed the latency of 1070 cases of CNS DCS occurring in divers and compressed air workers and showed that 66% presented within 10 min of surfacing and 84% within 1 h. Of those cases exhibiting unequivocal evidence of cerebral involvement, either on its own or associated with spinal cord DCS, 76% had presented within 10 min and 96% within 1 h. In contrast, the onset of joint pain and other less serious manifestations tended to be more delayed. This study confirmed that 99% of all DCS occurs within 24 h of the causative dive and that anything over 48 h is extremely rare. It reinforces the belief that any unusual symptom or sign occurring within 48 h of a dive should be regarded as a decompression illness unless there is compelling evidence to the contrary.

The neurological manifestations of DCS range from minor, localized sensory disturbances and weakness in one or more limbs to profound quadriplegia. Often, the symptoms and signs occur in seemingly bizarre combinations which are difficult to explain on a rational basis but must be seen as evidence of the very widepread involvement of the nervous system which may occur with DCS. Bladder paresis with retention is common in more acute cases. Localized disturbances of sensation in limbs are also common and the term "peripheral nerve decompression sickness" is sometimes used. However, there is no basis for the belief that peripheral nerves are ever directly involved and no pathological changes have ever been seen in the peripheral nerves of decompressed animals. It used to be thought that, in the absence of clear evidence of cerebral involvement, virtually all such symptoms and signs were indicative of spinal cord involvement and no doubt many neurological examinations of divers have been carried out with the tacit assumption that the spinal cord was the target organ for decompression sickness.

The most common symptoms and signs of cerebral involvement are usually described as visual disturbances, headaches and alterations in levels of consciousness but a number of studies show that a much wider variety of indications of cerebral involvement occurs. Table 25.2 lists the incidence of symptoms and signs in the study by Rivera (1963) of 935 cases of DCS.

Although the reported incidence of obvious cerebral involvement in DCS is about 20% (Pearson 1981, Francis et al. 1988a), one study which used radioisotopes to study cerebral perfusion deficits after decompression illnesses (Adkisson et al. 1989), suggested that some degree of cerebral involvement may be much more common, perhaps even universal, in DCS where there is any evidence whatsoever of CNS involvement. Although this study is continuing, there is no doubt that every case of DCS deserves the most detailed neurological examination that time will allow before treatment and expert neurological assessment as soon as possible after treatment.

One especially sinister, fortunately relatively rare, presentation of serious DCS is so-called "girdle pain" which is characteristic of severe spinal cord involvement. Such pain may be lower thoracic or upper abdominal and invariably comes on within 5 min of surfacing. It is a presentation requiring the most urgent recourse to recompression therapy and the response to therapy is often incomplete and disappointing.

If the spinal cord is involved in DPB, it can only be as a result of systemic AGE. In the only three cases known to the author, sudden uncontrolled decompression from relatively shallow depths resulted in a very rapid onset of profound paraplegia with a sharply demarcated upper level of symptoms and signs. Although all these cases were treated promptly, the response was universally poor and significant residual

Table 25.2. Distribution and percentage incidence of presenting symptoms and signs in 935 cases of DCS with CNS involvement

	Incidence (%)		Incidence (%)
Numbness/paraesthesia	21.2	Unconsciousness	2.7
Motor weakness	20.6	Personality change	1.6
Paralysis	6.1	Agitation/restlessness	1.3
Urinary disturbance	2.5	Convulsion	1.1
Muscular twitching	1.2	Equilibrium disturbance	0.7
Incoordination	0.9	Auditory disturbance	0.3
Dizziness/vertigo	8.5	Cranial nerve deficits	0.2
Nausea/vomiting	7.9	Aphasia	0.2
Visual disturbance	6.8	Dyspnoea	2.0
Headache	3.9	Fatigue	1.2

After Rivera (1963).

disability resulted. In each case, it was presumed that a gas embolus had occluded a major nutrient artery to the cord resulting in an acute ischaemic insult which, despite the probable restoration of perfusion on recompression, was sufficient to cause a considerable degree of irreversible damage. The presentation of cerebral AGE (CAGE) may be equally dramatic and always occurs within 10 min of surfacing, often immediately on reaching the surface. Table 25.3 gives an analysis of the presentation of 188 cases of CAGE arising from submarine escape training and diving accidents.

Table 25.3 shows that the presentation of CAGE is characterized by the high incidence of alterations of levels of consciousness, with or without convulsions, as well as a predominance of unilateral motor and/or sensory deficits. This is in contrast to DCS affecting the spinal cord where bilateral involvement is more common.

Table 25.3. Presentation of 188 cases of cerebral arterial gas embolism arising in submarine escape training and diving

Symptoms and signs	Incidence (%)
Coma with convulsions	14
Coma without convulsions	29
Stupor and confusion	21
Acute vertigo	12
Visual disturbances	8
Headache	8
Unilateral paresis	17
Unilateral sensory deficit	10
Unilateral motor and sensory deficits	4
Bilateral paresis	4
Bilateral sensory deficit	1

Pathogenesis and Pathology of Decompression Illness

Decompression Sickness

It is most surprising that the precise way in which inert gas bubbles give rise to spinal cord DCS still remains a matter of controversy and even what is known about the associated pathology is, in some respects, not too helpful in providing an explanation. The arguments are largely concerned with the respective roles of embolic and autochthonous gas bubbles.

Gas Embolism

The possible contribution of VGE was first proposed by Haymaker and Johnston (1955) and supported by Hallenbeck (1976) who, using a laminectomy to view the spinovertebral epidural venous plexus in decompressed dogs, recorded a dramatic accumulation of VGE in this system with the development of complete stasis in a few minutes. It was argued that the degree of stasis was such that venous infarction could ensue and, in turn, result in the characteristic lesions in the white matter of the cord (see below) which have been described as the most prominent feature of spinal cord DCS by numerous authors over the past 100 years. Other studies in animals and humans (Kitano et al. 1977; Wolkiewiez et al. 1979) have tended to support this theory but Hills and James (1982) argued that it has some fundamental limitations and that the stasis in the spinovertebral epidural venous plexus may be the result rather than the cause of DCS. They also challenged the concept that the stasis in the epidural venous plexus would selectively affect the white matter. Indeed, it is difficult to explain the well-described vulnerability of certain levels and elements of the spinal cord on such a basis. Dutka et al. (1990) have repeated Hallenbeck's experiment using somatosensory evoked potential (SEP) monitoring to correlate observed intravascular events with spinal cord function. They found that occlusion of the epidural venous plexus by a foam of bubbles did not, in itself, seem to cause any dramatic loss of SEP amplitude but the appearance of AGE in the small arteries on the surface of the cord usually led to a rapid and profound loss of SEP amplitude and electrophysiological function. The source of the observed AGE could not be determined in that, over a short period of time following their initial appearance, they were seen to travel in different directions in the same vessel. This suggests that the gas emboli might be arising from within the cord and moving in retrograde fashion back along the arteries. However, it is also possible that the vessels studied were in a "watershed area" where alternating flow is normal.

Arterialization of VGE

This, or de novo origin of AGE within the lungs, has also been proposed as an important factor in the pathogenesis of spinal cord DCS (Gersh and Catchpole 1951; Hempleman 1972). One fundamental objection to this theory was voiced by Hallenbeck et al. (1976) who pointed out that the brain is almost universally involved in all other embolic conditions and this did not seem to be the case in DCS, although this latter observation is less tenable as evidence grows that cerebral involvement in DCS is much more common than previously thought. A more fundamental objection to the role of arterialized VGE is that, despite the previously mentioned AGE seen by Dutka, other experiments involving the injection of representative inert gas emboli (50–200 μm) into the thoracic aorta of dogs (Francis et al. 1989; Pearson et al. 1990), with consequent profound loss of electrophysiological function in the cord, produced pathology typical of acute anoxic–ischaemic damage to the grey matter of the cord with complete sparing of the white matter. Fig. 25.1 shows the severe degree of grey matter damage resulting from such an experiment. These experiments confirm the relative vulnerability of grey matter to ischaemia and the sparing of the the white matter is in sharp contrast to the effects of DCS on the cord already described. However, there is no reason to believe that the pathology in the very few recorded cases of spinal cord involvement resulting from DPB would be any different from the lesions produced in this animal model.

Autochthonous Bubbles

The concept of the role of the autochthonous bubbles of inert gas arising in the tissues of the cord and causing mechanical damage as they expand in response to decompression, has long been popular. Bert (1878) discussed such a possibility but Hills and James (1982) were perhaps the first to attempt to describe and model the

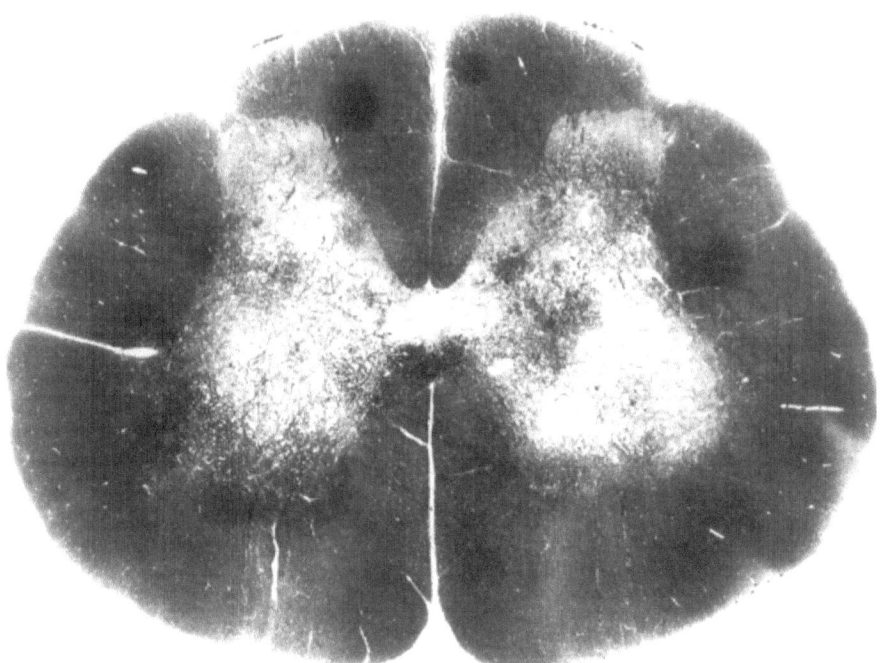

Fig. 25.1. Low power cross-section of cord (L1) following introduction of inert gas microemboli (50–200 μm) into thoracic aorta. Note severe disruption of grey matter with sparing of white matter.

process in a scientific manner. Certainly, bubbles of what was assumed to be inert gas have been described from time to time in autopsy reports in humans following fatal decompression accidents. Some of these reports describe "lacerations" of the cord tissue in association with the bubbles. Sykes and Yaffee (1985) described decompression-induced myelin sheath abnormalities seen with electron microscopy in the cord of dogs and presumed these were evidence of gas bubbles. Francis et al. (1988b) used the same model, admittedly one producing acute DCS with an early onset, to demonstrate numerous non-staining space-occupying lesions, presumably bubbles, in the white matter of the cord. The lesions were clearly extravascular and caused either displacement or frank disruption of axonal sheaths. Such lesions were also shown to be transient and had largely disappeared within 6 hours to be replaced by discrete haemorrhagic areas with leucocytic infiltration and early organization. On the assumption that these lesions were bubbles, it was suggested they had three potentially injurious effects: mechanical disruption of conducting tissues, pressure on adjacent axons and pressure on the adjacent microcirculation to give ischaemia, the last having the effect of hampering inert gas elimination. The transient nature of these lesions no doubt explains why they have not been described more often. Broome et al. (1994) have shown that, in decompressed pigs, the degree of multifocal haemorrhage in the white matter of the cord, which was also associated with underlying spongiform changes, correlates well with a failure to respond to recompression therapy. It is impossible to attribute such changes to any direct effect of an embolic process. It may well be that the "girdle pain" described previously is the result of a degree of haemorrhage and tissue disruption so severe that the resulting damage is irreversible and unresponsive to recompression therapy.

To sum up, convincing evidence now exists to implicate autochthonous bubbles in the pathogenesis of acute, early onset DCS of the cord. The precise role of VGE and AGE remains less clear but it is quite probable that their ability to limit perfusion by blocking the arterial and venous sides of the cord microcirculation has a crucial part to play in limiting the ability of the tissues of the cord to get rid of accumulated inert gas during decompression. This could, in turn, produce the dynamic conditions necessary for inert gas nucleation and extravascular bubble formation. The less acute and delayed presentations of DCS may be the result of ischaemia secondary to embolic phenomena.

Because of the frequency with which cerebral manifestations of DCS occur in conjunction with spinal cord involvement, comment on the accompanying cerebral pathology is appropriate. Cerebral involvement is almost certainly due to arterialized VGE. The luxurious nature of the cerebral circulation would seem to preclude the formation of autochthonous bubbles of inert gas in all but the most extreme situations and they have never been described. Using a cranial window to study the effects of decompression on the cerebral circulation of dogs, Pearson et al. (1992) found that the initial appearance of AGE in the pial arterial circulation led to an almost immediate loss of cortical somatosensory evoked potentials (SEPs). Complete occlusion of the pial arteries by bubbles then occurred rapidly with complete stasis ensuing unless recompression was undertaken. Recompression led to an equally rapid clearing of the bubbles with restoration of perfusion. These events were accompanied by cerebral pathological changes compatible with an embolic insult. These changes were discrete infarcts concentrated in the grey–white matter marginal areas supplied by the anterior and middle cerebral arteries. Small perivascular haemorrhages were also seen in the white matter but were a less prominent feature. These lesions were identical to the numerous descriptions of the pathology of CAGE secondary to DPB and a wide variety of iatrogenic accidents even though the extent and severity of these latter lesions was dependent on the amount and, to some extent, size of embolic bubbles. It is this similarity that leads to the previous comment that the distinction between the cerebral manifestations of DCS and CAGE secondary to DPB is, to a large extent, academic. A final point of interest in these experiments, admittedly involving severe decompression challenges, was that loss of cortical SEPs almost always preceded loss of spinal cord SEPs.

The distribution of the pathological changes in the cord due to compressed air-induced DCS may be a function of the varying amounts of fatty tissue in different levels of the cord and the greater solubility of nitrogen in fatty, as opposed to other, tissue. The lower thoracic and upper lumbar sections of the cord seem especially vulnerable (Kidd and Elliott 1969; Desola and San Pedro 1984).

Pathological material relevant to the acute process of DCS in the human cord is surpisingly scanty and little autopsy evidence is available. Fig. 25.2 shows the presence of autochthonous bubbles in the white matter of the cord of a diver who died of fulminating DCS within 2 hours of surfacing. There is remarkably little reaction to the bubbles at this stage. The overall appearance of the white matter in Fig. 25.2 is remarkably similar to that described by Francis et al. (1988b) in an animal model. The grey matter of the cord shown in Fig. 25.2 was described as essentially normal. Later stages in the development of the white matter lesions begin to show punctate haemorrhages and demyelination of axons both distally and proximally (Calder 1986).

The chronic changes associated with DCS of the cord have been described more frequently and reinforce the evidence for the relative sparing of the grey matter in this process as well as showing that the dorsal and lateral columns of the white matter seem to be most often affected (Palmer 1986). Cases have been described where the degree of scarring in the white matter was very extensive and seemingly out of proportion to the degree of functional disability and clinical signs (Palmer et al. 1981). Of

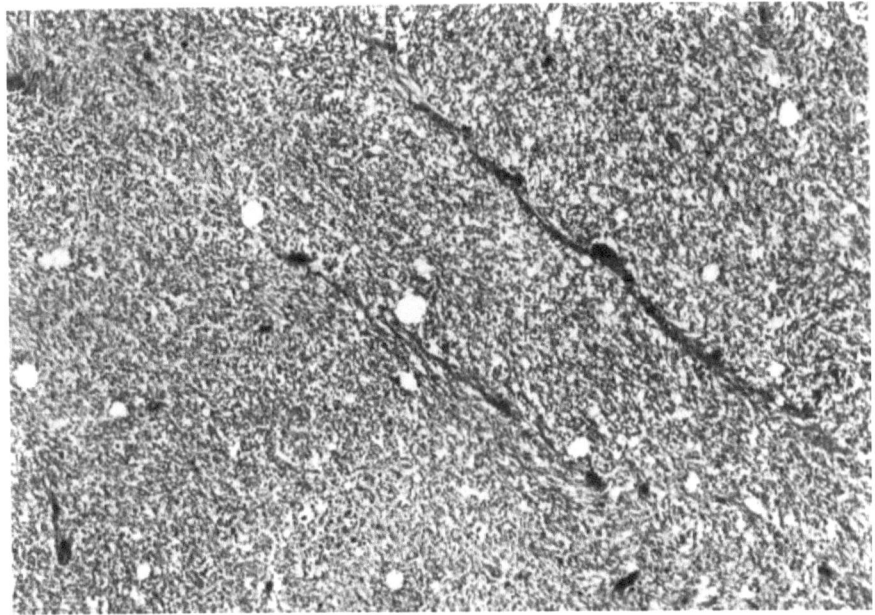

Fig. 25.2. Acute DCS. Autochthonous bubbles in white matter (×125).

some concern is the dicovery of less specific degenerative changes in the cords of a number of divers who died from non-diving related causes and who had no history of overt decompression illnesses (Palmer et al. 1988) although Mork et al. (1992), using staining techniques different from those used by Palmer, could not identify similar pathological changes in the cords of divers without a history of decompression illness. These changes described by Palmer were mainly in the posterior, lateral and anterior columns of the white matter and, in the posterior columns, suggested a degree of damage to the afferent fibres from the nerve roots. In support of Palmer's observations are those by Dick and Broome (1994) who found significant white matter pathology (multifocal areas of spongy change with axonal disruption and demyelination) in the white matter of pigs which had not exhibited any overt signs of DCS after decompression. Whatever the significance of these changes, they add to the growing concern that diving may result in hitherto unrecognized chronic damage to the CNS. The pathogenesis of these changes can only be speculative but it has been proposed that they result from chronic asymptomatic arterialization of VGE although the relative sparing of the grey matter in such a process remains difficult to understand.

Treatment of Decompression Illnesses

The treatment of decompression illnesses is a specialist subject in itself but it is important to re-state that the earliest possible recompression remains the definitive treatment for any decompression illness where there is CNS involvement. Expert advice and treatment is available from a number of centres in the United Kingdom (vide infra) and they should always be consulted when decompression illnesses are suspected. Any delay can adversely affect the chances of successful treatment.

A number of regimes exist for the conduct of recompression therapy and recommend varying combinations of pressure, time under pressure and amount of oxygen breathed by the patient. However, all aim to "crush" the inert gas bubbles which are considered to be fundamental to all decompression illnesses and thereby allow relief from their space-occupying effects and restoration of perfusion where intravascular embolic gas is a factor. In the case of AGE, it is hoped that recompression will diminish bubble size to such a degree that they will be able to transit the capillary bed and return to the pulmonary venous circulation where gas exchange into the alveoli will eliminate them. The breathing of pure oxygen or oxygen-inert gas mixtures is also fundamental to most regimes and is aimed at enhanced oxygenation of tissues prejudiced by hypoxia/anoxia. Another theoretical benefit of hyperoxic breathing mixtures is their ability to enhance elimination of inert gas from bubbles although this factor can have little effect in situations where circulation in blood vessels is static due to gas emboli. The majority of regimes use "treatment tables" which detail the time/pressure profiles and breathing mixtures to be used. The most commonly used tables are those which require an intitial recompression to an equivalent 60 fsw (9 msw) breathing pure oxygen. Higher pressures may be used or the tables extended depending on the response to this initial recompression. While some regimes make no distinction between the various forms of decompression illness in terms of this initial recompression, others allow for initial recompression to 165 fsw (50 msw) if the diagnosis is thought to be CAGE. At this higher pressure, breathing pure oxygen is impractical due to the toxicity of oxygen on the CNS and respiratory system at such a pressure and oxygen–nitrogen mixtures are commonly used. As yet, there is no evidence to allow comparison of the various regimes, particularly in the case of acute presentations and it is sufficent to repeat the absolute requirement for early recompression. Fortunately, timely recognition and early treatment will achieve a high cure rate for all forms of decompression illness. Also, any response to recompression is a powerful argument in favour of a decompression illness.

A number of forms of first-aid and adjuvant therapy are frequently advocated although good scientific evidence for the efficacy of most does not exist. There is, however, increasing evidence that breathing of pure oxygen is an effective first-aid measure until recompression therapy can be given and there is also good reason to initiate intravenous fluid replacement therapy with crystalloid solutions in all cases of serious decompression illness. Similarly, for serious cases, a reasonable argument exists for adjuvant therapy with intravenous glucocorticoids such as dexamethasone which may protect vascular endothelium from the effects of arrested gas emboli, thereby reducing the complicating effects of vasogenic oedema. Initial loading doses of dexamethasone in the order of 16 mg are recommended. A rational approach to the use of adjuvant therapy in decompression illnesses is that recommended by Bove (1982). Diuretics, anticoagulants, vitamins and even ethyl alcohol all have their advocates but none are of proven value.

Relapses may occur during or after recompression treatment, particularly where it has been delayed or the choice of initial treatment has been inadequate. Secondary deterioration is relatively common and, in the case of CAGE, may be life-threatening (Pearson and Goad 1982). All promulgated treatment regimes give guidance on the management of such cases and usually recommend extension of the time spent under pressure with additional periods of oxygen breathing. However, such relapses are notoriously difficult to treat and an incomplete response frequently ensues. The most common approach to an incomplete response after completion of the initial recompression therapy is to carry on with shorter hyperbaric oxygen (HBO) sessions on a daily or twice daily basis (Pearson and Leitch 1979). The risks of cerebral and pulmonary oxygen toxicity limit the amount of oxygen which may be given under pressure and must always be respected when treatment is prolonged or repetitive. In general, it is customary to continue HBO therapy until a plateau of response has been reached and no sustained objective improvement can be elicited after two consecutive sessions.

With appropriate support and remedial therapy, the long-term prognosis for residual neurological deficits after decompression illnesses involving the cord is much the same as for other types of injury to the cord. Truly surprising degrees of recovery may continue for as long as two years or more. This improvement is probably attributable to processes of adaptation and the degree of redundacy available within the CNS. However, a number of serious cases treated by the author eventually began to deteriorate again and one interesting feature of some of these cases is the emergence of severe limb pain where it had not featured in previous symtomatology.

One of the most vexed questions which follows CNS involvement in decompression illnesses is whether a return to diving can be recommended. Increasing use is being made of a number of specialized investigations such as evoked potential testing (Sedgewick 1987), CAT and MRI scanning (Moon et al. 1987), and radioisotope imaging to demonstrate perfusion deficits (Adkisson et al. 1989). There is a good deal of controversy about the ability of these techniques to detect subtle abnormalities in the CNS that are not evident from a thorough clinical examination of the CNS and their relevance to recommendations about a return to diving is equally controversial. It still seems prudent to advise against a return to diving where there is any symptomatic or clinically detectable evidence of lasting neurological sequelae. This advice should be extended to all cases where evidence of CNS involvement has not responded rapidly and completely to the initial recompression therapy.

Finally, there is increasing concern about the long-term health effects of diving, particularly on the central nervous system. In addition to those already cited, a number of studies, using a variety of techniques, have looked at healthy divers with and without a history of decompression illness as well as divers who have carried out deep experimental saturation dives. Although many of these studies have failed to provide convincing evidence of unsuspected permanent neurological sequelae, there is a continuing worry that subtle adverse effects may be developing in divers who have never experienced overt decompression illnesses. Details of the the majority of these studies are contained in reviews by Evans and Shields (1992) and Moon and Elliott (1993). Additionally, a cross-sectional study of 282 professional divers (Morris et al. 1991) suggested that there was a cognitive impairment in some apparently healthy divers who had experienced decompression illnesses. In those divers who had no history of decompression illnesses, such cognitive changes as were identified were attributed to age rather than diving. The net result of these various concerns is that proposals at present being studied by the United Kingdom Health and Safety Executive which would amend the obligatory routine medical examinations of professional divers to allow for intermittent detailed assessment of the CNS to identify and monitor those areas of concern.

References

Adkisson GH, Hodgson M, Smith F et al. (1989) Cerebral perfusion deficits in dysbaric illness. Lancet ii:119–122

Behnke AR (1955) Decompression sickness. Milit Med 117:257–271

Bert P (1878) La pression barometrique. Recherches de physiologie experimentale. Masson, Paris. (Translated by MA and FA Hitchcock, 1943, Columbus, Ohio: College Book Co and reprinted Bethesda, MD: Undersea and Hyperbaric Med Soc 1978)

Blick G (1909) Notes on divers paralysis. Br Med J ii:1796–1798

Bove AA (1982) The basis for drug therapy in decompression sickness. Undersea Biomed Res 9:91–111

Boyle R (1670) New pneumatical observations about respiration. Phil Trans R Soc 5:2011–2056

Broome JR, Dick Jr EJ, Dutka AJ (1994) Multifocal CNS haemorrhage as a cause of recompression treatment failure in a pig model of neurological decompression illness. Undersea Biomed Res 21 (suppl):69–70

Butler BD, Hills BA (1985) Transpulmonary passage of venous air emboli. J Appl Physiol 59:543–547

Calder IM (1986) Dysbarism: a review. Forensic Sci Int 30:237–266

Clark EA (1870–1871) Effects of increased atmospheric pressure on the human body. A report of thirty five cases brought to the City Hospital from the St Louis and Illinois Bridge. Med Arch St Louis 5:1–30

Desola AJ, San Pedro AG (1984) Epidemiological study of 146 dysbaric diving accidents. In Desola AJ (ed) Diving and hyperbaric medicine. Proc IX Congress of Eur Undersea Biomed Soc, Barcelona

Dick Jr EJ, Broome JR (1994) Occult spinal cord damage in clinically normal pigs following diving. Undersea Biomed Res 21 (suppl):68

Dutka AJ, Knightly J, Collins J, Pearson RR, Mink RB, Hallenbeck JM (1990) The presence of bubbles in vessels surrounding the spinal cord correlates with changes in the spinal somatosensory evoked potential (SSEP) amplitude. Undersea Biomed Res 17 (suppl):137

Evans SA, Shields TG (1992) A critical review of the literature on the potential neurological consequences of diving. Robert Gordon Institute of Technology, Aberdeen.

Francis TJR, Pearson RR, Robertson AG, Hodgson M, Dutka AJ, Flynn ET (1988a) Central nervous system decompression sickness: latency of 1070 human cases. Undersea Biomed Res 15:402–411

Francis TJR, Pezeshkpour GH, Dutka AJ, Hallenbeck JM, Flynn ET (1988b) Is there a role for the autochthonous bubble in the pathogenesis of spinal cord decompression sickness? J Neuropathol Exp Neurol 47:475–487

Francis TJR, Pezeshkpour GH, Dutka AJ (1989) Arterial gas embolism as a pathophysiologic cause for spinal cord decompression sickness. Undersea Biomed Res 16:439–451

Francis TJR, Dutka AJ, Hallenbeck JM (1990) Pathophysiology of decompression sickness. In: Bove AA, Davis JC (eds) Diving medicine, WB Saunders, Philadelphia, pp 170–187

Gersh I, Catchpole HR (1951) Decompression sickness: physical factors and pathologic consequences. In: Fulton JF (ed) Decompression sickness. WB Saunders, Philadelphia, pp 165–181

Golding FC, Griffiths P, Hempleman HV et al. (1960) Decompression sickness during the construction of the Dartford Tunnel. Br J Ind Med 17:167–180

Greene KM (1978) Causes of death in submarine escape training casualties: analysis of cases and review of the literature. AMTE(E) Report R78-402, Alverstoke, Hampshire

Hallenbeck JM (1976) Cinematography of dog spinal vessels during cord-damaging decompression sickness. Neurology 26:190–199

Hallenbeck JM, Bove AA, Elliott DH (1976) Decompression sickness studies. In: Lambertsen CJ (ed) Underwater physiology V. FASEB, Betheseda, MD, pp 273–286

Harveyson KB, Hirschfield BEE, Tonge J (1956) Fatal air embolism from use of compressed air diving unit. Med J Aust 1:658–660

Haymaker W, Johnston AD (1955) Pathology of decompression sickness: a comparison of lesions in airmen with those in caisson workers and divers. Milit Med 117:285–306

Hempleman HV (1972) The site of origin of gaseous emboli produced by decompression from raised pressure of air and other gases. In: Fructus X (ed) Proc 3rd Int Conference on Hyperbaric Med Underwater Physiol, Doin, Paris, pp 160–162

Hills BA, Butler BD (1981) Size distribution of intravascular air emboli produced by decompression. Undersea Biomed Res 8:163–174

Hills BA, James PB (1982) Spinal decompression sickness; mechanical studies and a model. Undersea Biomed Res 9:185–210

Jaminet A (1871) Physical effects of compressed air. (Privately printed), St Louis, MO, pp 1–7

Khrabrostin MN (1888) Work under water and diseases of divers. Medits Pribavl 68:68–84

Kidd DJ, Elliott DH (1969) Clinical manifestations and treatment of decompression sickness in divers. In: Bennett PB, Elliott DH (eds) The physiology and medicine of diving and compressed air work. Balliere-Tindall and Cassell, London, pp 464–490

Kitano M, Hayashi K, Kawashima M (1977) Three autopsy cases of acute decompression sickness. Consideration of pathogenesis about spinal cord damage in acute decompression sickness. Jpn Orthop Traum 26:402–408

Malhotra MS, Wright HC (1961) The effects of raised intrapulmonary pressure on the lungs of fresh unchilled cadavers. J Path Bact 82:198–202

Moon RE, Camporesi EM, Massey EW, Erwin CW, Djang WG (1987) Functional imaging of the central nervous system (CT, MRI, xenon blood-flow) and use of evoked potential during therapy of decompression sickness and arterial gas embolism. In: Bove AA, Bachrach AJ, Greenbaum LJ (eds) Proc 9th International Symp. Underwater and Hyperbaric Physiology. Undersea and Hyperbaric Medical Society, Betheda MD

Moon RE, Camporesi EM (1989) Patent foramen ovale and decompression sickness. Lancet i:513–514

Moon RE, Elliott DH (1993) Long term health effects in divers. In: Bennett PB, Elliott DH (eds) The physiology and medicine of diving, 4th edn. Saunders, London.

Mork SSJ, Eidsvik S, Nyland H, Brubakk AO, Giertsen J (1992) Does diving damage the spinal cord? A study of 20 professional and amateur divers. Undersea Biomed Res 19 (suppl):111

Morris PE, Leach J, King JD, Rawlins JSPR (1991) Psychological and neurological impairment in professional divers. Report 2050, Department of Energy, London

Nims LF (1951) Environmental factors affecting decompression sickness. In: Fulton JF (ed) Decompression sickness. Saunders, Philadelphia, pp 264–278

Palmer AC (1986) The neuropathology of decompression sickness. In: Cavanagh JB (ed) recent advances in neuropathology, 3rd edn. Churchill Livingstone, New York, pp 141–162

Palmer AC, Calder IM, McCallum RI, Mastaglia FL (1981) Spinal cord degeneration in "recovered" spinal decompression sickness. Br Med J 283:288

Palmer AC, Calder IM, Hughes JT (1988) Spinal cord damage in active divers. Undersea Biomed Res 15 (suppl):70

Pearson RR (1981) The aetiology, pathophysiology, presentation and therapy of pulmonary barotrauma and arterial gas embolism arising from submarine escape training and diving. MD Thesis, Newcastle University

Pearson RR (1984) Diagnosis and treatment of gas embolism. In: Shilling CW, Carlston CB, Mathias RA (eds) The physicians guide to diving medicine. Plenum Press, London, pp 333–367

Pearson RR, Goad RF (1982) Delayed cerebral edema complicating cerebral arterial gas embolism: case histories. Undersea Biomed Res 9:823–296

Pearson RR, Leitch DR (1979) Treatment of air or oxygen/nitrogen mixture decompression illnesses in the Royal Navy. J R Nav Med Serv 65(2):53–62

Pearson RR, Francis TJR, Pezeshkpour GH, Dutka AJ (1990) Spinal cord dysfunction and pathology following arterial gas embolism. Undersea Biomed Res 17 (suppl):32–33

Pearson RR, Pezeshkpour, Dutka AJ (1992) Cerebral involvement in decompression sickness. Undersea Biomed Res 19 (suppl):39–40

Philp RB, Ackles KN, Inwood MJ et al. (1972) Changes in the hemostatic system and in blood and urine chemistry of human subjects following decompression from a hyperbaric environment. Aerospace Med 43:498–505

Pol B, Watelle T (1854) Memoire sur les effets de la compression de l'air applique au creusement des puits a houille. Ann Hyg Publ et med legh, Paris

Powell MR, Johanson DC (1978) Ultrasound monitoring and decompression sickness. In: Shilling CW, Beckett MW (eds) Underwater physiology IX. Undersea and Hyperbaric Med Soc, Bethesda, MD, pp 503–510

Rivera JC (1963) Decompression sickness amongst divers: an analysis of 935 cases. Milit Med 129:314–334

Schaefer KE, McNulty WP, Carey CR, Liebow AA (1958) Mechanisms in development of interstitial emphysema and air embolism in decompression from depth. J Appl Physiol 13:15–29

Sedgewick EM (1987) Somatosensory evoked potentials in a case of decompression sickness. In: Elliott DH, Halsey MJ (eds) Workshop on diagnostic techniques in diving neurology. Medical Research Council, London, pp 74–76

Smith DJ, Francis TJR, Pethybridge RJ, Wright JM, Sykes JJW (1993) An evaluation of the classification of decompression disorders. Undersea Biomed Res 20 (Suppl):17–18

Spencer MP, Clarke HF (1972) Precordial monitoring of pulmonary gas embolism and decompression bubbles. Aerospace Med 47:762–767

Sykes JJW, Yaffee LJ (1985) Light and electron microscopic alterations in spinal cord myelin sheaths after decompression sickness. Undersea Biomed Res 12:251–258

Van Allen CM, Hrdina LS (1929) Air embolism from the pulmonary vein. Arch Surg 19:567–599

Wilmshurst PT, Byrne JC, Webb-Peploe MM (1989) Neurological decompression sickness. Lancet i:731

Wolkiewiez J, Martin PJ, Lapoussiere JM, Kermarec J (1979) Spinal cord decompression sickness. Med Aeronaut Spat Med Subaquat Hyp 18:313–317

Chapter 26

Inherited Diseases of the Spinal Cord

L.A. Bindoff and R.A. Shakir

Inherited diseases that affect just the spinal cord are few in number, but of great importance medically and socially. The following section will deal with the clinical and pathological features of these conditions and consider what is known about the genetics, an extremely exciting area where there have been major developments in the last few years. Details of other conditions in which spinal cord involvement is a key feature will also be included, but it is not the intention to embark on a detailed review of all the diseases that may involve the spinal cord. The reader is referred to more specialized texts.

Diseases of the Motor Neurone

This is an heterogeneous group of disorders that includes the spinal muscular atrophies (SMA), familial motor neurone disease and less common conditions such as X-linked bulbospinal neuronopathy (Kennedy's syndrome) and neurogenic arthrogryposis. An overview of the diseases which arbitrarily divides them into categories based on age of onset is given in Table 26.1. The pathological hallmark of these diseases is degeneration of the anterior horn cells in the spinal cord or motor nuclei of the brainstem (covered elsewhere).

Spinal Muscular Atrophy (SMA)

Debate surrounds the classification of the SMAs and clearly this area will change as more information regarding the genetic basis of the different conditions becomes available. Early onset SMA is one of the commonest autosomal recessive disorders recognized in the UK (Bundey 1985; Lewin 1995). The other SMAs are much more uncommon and can follow dominant, recessive or X-linked patterns of inheritance (Bundey 1985; Morrison and Harding 1994).

Table 26.1. Review of the inherited disorders of motor neurones. Not all are covered in the text. AR = autosomal recessive; AD = autosomal dominant (Based on Morrison and Harding 1994)

Condition	Inheritance	Gene identified
Spinal muscular atrophies **In infancy/childhood**		
• Type I/Werdnig–Hoffmann	AR	Chromosome 5 site mapped (5q11.2–13.3). Gene not characterized
• Type II/intermediate	AR	As for type I; conditions appear allelic
• Type III/Kugelberg–Welander	AR	As for types I and II; conditions appear allelic
• Chronic proximal SMA	AD	Identical to type III, but dominantly inherited. Estimated 2% of all chronic proximal SMA
• Distal SMA	AD/AR	Estimated 10% all cases of SMA. Severity varies. Both dominant and recessive pedigrees (Pearn and Hudgson 1979). May occur with Type I in same family. No linkage to the 5q. locus found in types I–III
• Bulbar SMA	AR	With deafness (Vialetto–Van Laere) without deafness (Fazio–Londe). Also seen with mental retardation ± ataxia & external ophthalmoplegia
In adolescence/adult life		
• With calf hypertophy	X-linked	
• Scapuloperoneal	AD	
• Fascioscapulohumeral	AD	
• Monomelic forms	Sporadic	
• Chronic proximal SMA	AR/AD	Appears genetically distinct from proximal childhood form. Both dominant (Pearn 1978a) and recessive forms (Pearn 1978b)
Arthrogryposis		
• Arthrogryposis multiplex congenita	AR	Clinically hetrogeneous; recessive inheritance suggested
Motor neurone diseases		
• Inherited ALS	AD	Most dominant; candidate genes include super-oxide dismutase and neurofilament proteins
• Juvenile ALS	AR	3 groups defined (see text) all seem recessive and candidate region (2q33–35) identified
• Bulbospinal neuronopathy	X-linked	Caused by trinucleotide repeat (CAG) in androgen receptor

SMA with Onset in Infancy and Childhood

The diagnostic criteria of early onset SMA have been reviewed and the following clinical features accepted (Munsat 1991): weakness should be symmetrical, proximal more than distal and involve the arms more than the legs; the trunk should be involved and denervation must be present on EMG and muscle biopsy. Features against the diagnosis are: CNS involvement, arthrogryposis, eye muscle or marked facial muscle weakness and involvement of other neurological sites (visual or auditory systems, sensory loss) or other organs (cardiac). The commonest clinical entities recognized are – SMA type I, also termed Werdnig–Hoffmann disease, acute infantile or severe SMA (Osawa and Keiko 1991); SMA type II, intermediate SMA;

and SMA type III, also called mild SMA or Kugelberg–Welander disease (Zierz and Zerres 1991). These are all autosomal recessive disorders.

Patients with SMA type I have severe hypotonia, generalized limb weakness, respiratory and bulbar weakness and commonly have tongue fasciculations. Tendon reflexes are absent and skeletal deformities present in 5–10% at birth. Onset of symptoms is always before 6 months and often they are present from birth. These infants never gain motor control sufficient to sit unaided and die before the age of two years.

Patients with SMA type II develop symptoms (weakness) before the age of 18 months, but may, in that time, have been able to sit or even crawl, but never to stand. Survival can be into adult life, but respiratory weakness develops and, as in SMA type I, this is the major factor in determining life expectancy.

In the mildest forms of SMA, type III, symptoms begin after the age of 18 months and these individuals are always able to walk. The first symptom is usually weakness (proximal) and this progresses slowly although more dramatic decline can be associated with immobilization. Calf hypertrophy and muscle fasciculation may be present (estimated present in >25%) and tendon reflexes are depressed or absent.

Autosomal dominant early onset SMA resembles type III, but may produce minimal disability and affect the legs more than the arms.

The incidence of all three types of early onset, autosomal recessive SMA is estimated to be around 1 in 24 000 with a carrier frequency for SMA type I of approximately 1 in 60–80 (Pearn 1973) and 1 in 100 for types II and III (Pearn 1978). Physical mapping by linkage analysis first assigned types II and III (Brzustowicz et al. 1990; Melki et al. 1990a) to chromosome 5 (region 5q 11.2–13.3) and subsequently type I (Gilliam et al. 1990; Melki et al. 1990b). Recent work published by two independent groups has established the precise region involved in the causation of these diseases, however, each group identified apparently different genes; one is termed survival motor neurone (SMN) gene (Lefebvre et al. 1995) and the other neuronal apoptosis inhibitory protein (NAIP) gene (Roy et al. 1995). Explanation of these conflicting results is difficult and resolution of the problem compounded by the unstable nature of the region involved (Lewin 1995). Nevertheless, each group identified abnormalities of their candidate region in all three types of SMA confirming the suspicion that the disorders are indeed allelic. The function of neither gene product is known although both have been ascribed putative functions compatible with current understanding of the neuronal degeneration seen in SMA.

Other Forms of Early Onset SMA

These are a mixture of conditions with mainly recessive inheritance (Table 26.1). SMA has been described together with mental retardation, vocal cord paralysis, external ophthalmoplegia and cerebellar ataxia (see Bundey (1985) and Morrison and Harding (1994) for reviews). Bulbar SMA with deafness (syndrome of Vialetto-Van Laere) or without (Fazio–Londe disease) or with other cranial nerve palsies has also been described (Baraitser 1989). An autosomal dominant chronic proximal SMA has also been described which is clinically similar to SMA type III, Kugelberg–Welander disease. The precise genetic nature of these disorders is not yet known. In most cases, however, linkage to chromosome 5 seems to have been excluded.

The SMA phenotype has also been described in association with a metabolic disorder due to hexosaminidase A deficiency (reviewed by Troost 1991). Several mutations (Navon et al. 1995) involving this enzyme have been identified in patients with this disease which may also present with cerebellar ataxia, dysarthria and/or upper and lower motor neurone signs in the limbs.

SMA in Adolescence and Adulthood

Distal SMA may be inherited as a dominant or recessive trait. Symptoms can start in childhood or early adult life and the clinical features consist of weakness and wasting mainly affecting the lower limbs. In most patients ankle reflexes are lost, but knee and upper limb reflexes usually preserved. Motor nerve conduction velocities are normal or near normal and sensory nerve conduction is normal distinguishing the condition from hereditary sensory motor neuropathy. The degree of disability varies from minor to the need for mechanical assistance for walking (Harding and Thomas 1980; Bundey 1985).

X-linked Bulbospinal Neuronopathy

This condition, which also bears the eponym Kennedy's disease (Kennedy et al. 1968), was first described in the 1950s. It affects men from the age of 15, but usually after the age of 25. The first symptom is often muscle cramps which may predate the onset of weakness by many years. Weakness is predominantly proximal and there is bulbar involvement causing dysarthria and dysphagia. Fasciculation of the lower face and tongue may be marked and, unlike the conditions described above, there is sensory impairment. Additional features include postural tremor, the features of hypogonadism – gynaecomastia, testicular atrophy and infertility – and diabetes mellitus. Examination shows areflexia and sensory loss which can be confirmed electrophysiologically as an axonal neuropathy. Mild EMG abnormalities may be found in female carriers.

This condition is the only motor neurone disease so far linked with an unstable trinucleotide repeat. Initial linkage studies (Brown et al. 1989) mapped the disorder to the same region of the X-chromosome as the androgen receptor (Xq11–12) and subsequent studies showed that the disease was due to an expanded CAG repeat (CAG encodes the amino acid glutamine) in the first open reading frame of this gene (La Spada et al. 1991). Other disorders caused by unstable trinucleotide repeats include Huntington's chorea, myotonic dystrophy, Fragile X and spinocerebellar ataxia type I. Several unique features are associated with these so-called dynamic mutations (Willems 1994). First, the size of expansion may increase from one generation to the next leading to an earlier and more severe manifestation. This explains the phenomenon of anticipation seen classically in Huntington's chorea and myotonic dystrophy. Second, the size of expansion correlates with disease severity and age of onset. Normal individuals have a variable number of CAG repeats (glutamine residues) in the androgen receptor gene ranging from 15 to 31, affected men have 40–62 (La Spada et al. 1992). Lastly, disease severity may differ depending on whether the affected allele is inherited from the mother (as in myotonic dystrophy) or father (as in Huntington's). This is not relevant to X-linked bulbospinal neuronopathy since the disease can only be inherited from one parent. Unlike the candidate genes in SMA, the function of the gene causing Kennedy's syndrome is known. The androgen receptor is a DNA binding protein involved in the regulation of transcription in tissues responsive to androgens (La Spada et al. 1991).

Inherited Amyotrophic Lateral Sclerosis (ALS)

It is estimated that between 5% and 10% of patients with ALS have an inherited disorder (Mulder et al. 1986; Strong et al. 1991). The clinical and neuropathological features of this condition do not differ substantially from the sporadic disease (reviewed elsewhere).

Unlike sporadic ALS, in which there is an increasing incidence with age, mean age of onset of the inherited form is between 45 and 48 years. Moreover, there can be wide clinical variability between family members. Clear autosomal dominant inheritance is present in some families and males and females are affected equally. Median survival is around 2 years but can vary between 4 months to 36 years (Mulder et al. 1986). Survival is thought to be affected by age of onset with the earlier onset associated with decreased survival (Strong et al. 1991).

Several candidates have been identified in the search for genes causing inherited ALS. Copper/zinc superoxide dismutase (SOD1) was identified after tight linkage was established, in some families, between the disease and a site on chromosome 21 (21q22.1–22.1) (Siddique et al. 1991; Rosen 1993). SOD1 is involved in the removal of the superoxide (O^-) anion converting it to hydrogen peroxide. Although oxygen free radicals are highly destructive species, damaging cellular proteins, DNA and lipids, debate surrounds the mechanism whereby SOD1 mutations might act at a cellular level – whether this simply relates to a loss of function or whether the mutations induce a novel function which is cytotoxic (reviewed by Brown 1995). In addition, it remains to be explained why a defect in a ubiquitously expressed enzyme leads specifically to neuronal damage. Studies looking at other enzymes involved in detoxifying free radicals have not identified any further defects.

The finding, in both sporadic and inherited ALS, of neurofilament accumulation in cell bodies and axons has led to another exciting avenue of research. Mutations in the heavy chains of neurofilament have been found in three patients with ALS (Figlewicz et al. 1994). Also, transgenic mice overexpressing either normal or mutant neurofilament develop a motor neurone disease phenotype (Cote et al. 1993). Interestingly, transgenic mice that express a mutant light chain neurofilament also develop a disease that, pathologically, resembles ALS (Xu et al. 1993). The role of trophic factors in the survival of motor neurones has also been explored and there is evidence to suggest that loss of ciliary neurotrophic factor leads to motor neurone degeneration in transgenic mice.

Research in to the cause of motor neurone degeneration is at a very exciting stage and there are bound to be major developments in the next five years some of which may confirm the findings discussed above, others may point to new areas.

Chronic Juvenile ALS

The combination of distal amyotrophy and upper motor neurone signs occurring in infants or adolescents has provoked the use of the term juvenile ALS. Sporadic reports documented a number of families, but the study by Ben Hamida in 1990 is by far the largest (Ben Hamida et al. 1990). This work defines three groups: Group 1 is characterized by wasting and fasciculation of the small hand muscles, spastic paraparesis and gradually progressive bulbar weakness. Average age of onset varied between 10.6 years (inherited form) and 17.6 (sporadic). No bladder dysfunction or sensory abnormality was found. In familial cases, inheritance was autosomal recessive: Group 2 is characterized by spastic paraplegia, wasting of the lower limb muscles and frequent loss of ankle jerks. No sensory or bladder dysfunction occurs. Average age of onset was 14.2 years and inheritance was autosomal recessive: Group 3 is characterized by spasticity of facial muscles, a spastic dysarthria and uncontrolled laughter and weeping. Severe muscle atrophy and fasciculation were absent and as for groups 1 and 2 there was no bladder or sensory disturbance. Average age of onset was 6.5 years and inheritance was autosomal recessive. Recently, linkage studies have mapped a gene in the large family with group 3 features to chromosome 2q33–35 (Hentati et al. 1994a).

Neurogenic Arthrogryposis

Arthrogryposis multiplex congenita (AMC) is a heterogeneous group of conditions whose major manifestation is congenital limb contractures. AMC may be due to disease in the infant or the mother (Bundey 1985) and different patterns of inheritance have been identified. Inherited AMC has been reported in association with anterior horn cell disease and an autosomal recessive mode of inheritance suggested (Vuopala et al. 1995).

Diagnosis and Treatment of Motor Neurone Diseases

Diagnosis of spinal muscular atrophy is essentially clinical although electrophysiological studies and muscle biopsy are important to confirm the central neurogenic aetiology. Similarly, with all forms of ALS, the diagnosis depends on clinical recognition with laboratory evidence for central denervation. Investigations to exclude, for example, sensory nerve involvement, lysosomal enzyme deficiencies and heavy metal intoxication will all be applicable to individual patients.

No specific treatment exists for disorders of the motor neurone. For patients with spinal muscular atrophy, management involves mechanical support for walking and daily living activities. Awareness of respiratory muscle involvement is crucial and some patients may require ventilatory support often in the form of nocturnal positive pressure ventilation. Appropriate genetic counselling is also essential. Several drugs have been evaluated in the treatment of adult motor neurone disease. These include branch-chain amino acids, TRH analogue and an antagonist of the N-methyl-D-aspartate (NMDA) receptor, riluzole. Generally results have been disappointing (Rowland 1994).

Hereditary Spastic Paraplegias

Hereditary spastic paraplegias (HSP) are characterized by predominantly lower limb spasticity and to a lesser degree weakness. This may occur in isolation – the so-called "pure" phenotype – or in association with a variety of other features (Harding 1993). Whether these complicated forms are part of the same disorder is, however, questionable. HSP may manifest differently in the same family with severely affected and asymptomatic individuals both being present.

The pathological findings in HSP consist of degeneration of the lateral corticospinal tracts mainly in the lumbar cord, but also involving the cervical region and to a lesser extent the uncrossed pyramidal tracts. Spinocerebellar tracts are reported to be involved in >50% (Bruyn 1992) and clinically silent dorsal column dysfunction detected by evoked potential studies is also recorded (Bruyn et al. 1994). The pathological findings appear similar in all forms of pure HSP.

Pure HSP is inherited most commonly as an autosomal dominant condition (Boustany et al. 1987; Polo et al. 1993; Durr et al. 1994; Fink et al. 1995a), but autosomal recessive or X-linked inheritance also occurs. Harding (1993) divides dominant HSP into early and late onset depending on whether symptoms develop before (early, type I) or after 35 years (late, type II). The use of this age to define the two types is questioned and some prefer an earlier cut off point (Polo et al. 1993). Symptoms may present at any age; initially this can be a tendency to trip or a feeling of stiffness although delay in first walking and poor athletic ability are also frequent complaints. Upper limb symptoms are unusual whilst sphincter disturbance, urgency and frequency of micturition and occasionally defaecation, occur in 50%, mostly in those with later onset disease. Examination shows marked spasticity of the lower limbs with hyperreflexia and extensor plantar responses. Weakness is not usually marked. Additional features may include sensory impairment and wasting of the small hand muscles, both of which occur late in the disease, pes cavus and diminished vibration sense in the lower limbs. Patients usually remain ambulant and life expectancy is normal.

Type II dominant HSP presents later, but displays more severe weakness and has a more rapid progression than type I with most patients losing the ability to walk independently by the sixth or seventh decade. Sensory loss and sphincter disturbance are also more common. Autosomal recessive HSP is similar clinically to the dominant phenotype showing early and late onset forms and the X-linked phenotype is similar to autosomal type I HSP.

Complicated forms of HSP are rare and heterogeneous. Spastic paraplegia is a major feature but associated with such a variety of other features that it is difficult to believe there is any genetic congruity. These are reviewed by Harding (1993) and Bruyn (1991).

Prevalence figures for pure HSP varied; studies from Northern Spain have suggested a figure of 9.6 per 100 000 (Polo et al. 1991) and this may also be true for other European countries (Harding 1993). Currently, no biochemical abnormality has been identified in HSP. From linkage studies it is clear that autosomal dominant HSP is genetically heterogeneous. Three different loci have been identified thus far: chromosome 14q (Gispert et al. 1995; Hazan et al. 1993), the centromeric region of chromosome 15 (Fink et al. 1995b) and chromosome 2p (Hentati et al. 1994c). The first two loci were identified in families with an early onset of symptoms (type I) whereas the marker on chromosome 2 was found in families with both early and late onset disease. No significant differences in clinical expression were shown although the family linked to chromosome 15 had a milder disease compared with those linked to 14q. Autosomal recessive HSP has been linked to chromosome 8 (Hentati et al. 1994b), but importantly these studies show that the recessive disease is also genetically heterogeneous.

Diagnosis and Treatment of HSP

In pure HSP, the combination of clinical findings and family history should establish the diagnosis. Perhaps the most important differential diagnosis is the syndrome of progressive dystonia with diurnal variation (Segawa's disease). In cases of clinical doubt a trial of dopa may be advisable. Interestingly, this syndrome of dopa-responsive dystonia has also been linked to chromosome 14. Other disorders that may enter the differential diagnosis include inherited ALS and adult onset adrenomyeloneuropathy, the first should be excluded by EMG studies and the latter by measurement of very long chain fatty acids. Diagnosis of the early onset recessive form may be more difficult and conditions such as lysosomal storage diseases (Krabbe's and metachromatic leukodystrophy) may need to be excluded.

Treatment of HSP is symptomatic. Spasmolytic drugs such as baclofen and danrolene sodium are often helpful in relieving spasticity and the associated discomfort it generates. Surgical correction of foot deformity is often attempted especially in the young. Continence advice and mobility appliances, including wheelchairs, are also important.

X-linked Adrenoleukodystrophy

Adrenoleukodystrophy is a peroxisomal disorder. Peroxisomes are subcellular organelles whose function is to degrade very long chain fatty acids (VLCFA – that is fatty acids with a chain length greater than 22 carbon atoms) (Fournier et al. 1994). X-linked adrenoleukodystrophy may manifest in neonatal life or early childhood, as a rapidly progressive fatal cerebral leukodystrophy with adrenal insufficiency, or in adulthood with a slowly progressive myelopathy (called adrenomyeloneuropathy) (Moser et al. 1995). This section will concentrate on the latter although the genetic and biochemical defect appears to be the same in both.

Adrenomyeloneuropathy (AMN) was first described in 1976 (Budka et al. 1976). Presentation is characteristically with a slowly progressive paraparesis often on a background of recurrent episodes of nausea and vomiting. Sphincter disturbance and impotence develop. Examination shows a spastic paraparesis usually with normal upper limbs. Abnormal vibration sense may be found in the legs plus neurophysiological evidence of a mild peripheral neuropathy. Pigmentation, nausea and vomiting and blood biochemical changes can establish the adrenal insufficiency which is present in approximately two thirds of young men with AMN. Mean age of onset of the neurological symptoms is around 27 and whilst progression is slow most are wheelchair bound within 10–15 years (Moser et al. 1995). Cerebral involvement appears in up to 50% and can be associated with MRI abnormalities and cognitive impairment. This group tend to do less well than those without evidence of cerebral disease. Interestingly, adrenal insufficiency may precede neurological dysfunction by many years and there also appears to be a group who develop adrenal dysfunction without neurological features.

Investigation of patients shows abnormal brainstem and somatosensory evoked potentials in >98%; visual evoked potentials are abnormal in only 24%. Motor conduction velocities may be reduced in the lower limbs and in those with cerebral involvement, MRI may show white matter changes. About 61% of women who are heterozygous for the condition also have neurological abnormalities, some severe. Features range from mild sensory impairment to a severe paraparesis. Laboratory findings in these women include abnormal somatosensory (90%) and brainstem (42%) potentials and cognitive impairment (39%). Most women that develop signs have been diagnosed as having multiple sclerosis (Moser et al. 1995).

The pathological features of AMN are dissimilar to the early onset cerebral form. The latter shows marked inflammatory changes whereas in AMN there is loss of myelinated axons in the long ascending and descending tracts of the spinal cord. These changes are maximal in the lumbar corticospinal, cervical gracile and dorsal spinocerebellar tracts suggesting that they represent a dying back process. Spinal grey matter appears unaffected. Brainstem tracts may also be affected and ultrastructurally the lesions show segmental demyelination and axonal degeneration (Powers 1985). Changes in the adrenal gland and testes are due to the accumulation of VLCFA.

Moser et al. (1995) have calculated an incidence of approximately 1 in 100 000 for X-linked adrenoleukodystrophy. Because many cases are not correctly identified they suggest, however, that the incidence is higher. The gene causing AMN (and adrenoleukodystrophy) has been identified. Mosser et al. (1994) showed that the gene encoded a protein that was an integral peroxisomal membrane protein and together with subsequent studies (Kobayashi et al. 1994; Sarde et al. 1994) have shown the protein to belong to the ATP cassette transporter family of proteins which includes the cystic fibrosis gene (Moser 1995).

Diagnosis and Treatment

The diagnosis of adrenomyeloneuropathy is confirmed by measuring the VLCFA concentration is serum. It is important that the C_{26} level as well as the ratios between C_{26}:C_{24} and C_{24}:C_{22} are established since in AMN the values may not be as strikingly abnormal as in other peroxisomal disorders and only one or two of the parameters may be abnormal. Patients with the clinical features, but normal plasma levels, have been reported and these cases must be diagnosed using cultured skin fibroblasts (Wanders et al. 1992). The differential diagnosis of AMN includes multiple sclerosis as well as other spinocerebellar degenerations (with little cerebellar dysfunction) and HSP.

Treatment of AMN must include steroid replacement where necessary. Specific treatments are not yet available but much interest has centred on the use of dietary manipulation especially the mixture of glycerol trioleate and glycerol triucate that has been popularized by the title "Lorenzo's oil" named after the son of Mr and Mrs Odone who had the cerebral form of X-linked adrenoleukodystrophy. Bone marrow transplantation has been used in ALD as have a variety of drugs that modify the inflammatory response, but perhaps the most promising avenue, that of gene therapy, comes with the precise identification of the gene and gene-product. Until that becomes a reality, symptomatic treatment continues to be the mainstay with spasmolytic drugs, rehabilitation and counselling all important factors.

Friedreich's Ataxia

This is the commonest and perhaps most well-known inherited ataxia. The clinical features of Friedreich's ataxia (FA) have been extensively reviewed (Harding 1984) and will only briefly be documented here. The cardinal features of FA are a progressive ataxia, dysarthria, dorsal column sensory loss, areflexia, extensor plantar responses, scoliosis and pes cavus (see Table 26.2). Much debate surrounds the diagnosis of FA mainly because of the overlap between the various spinocerebellar ataxias. This confusion will gradually diminish as molecular genetic analysis identifies the different genes responsible. The criteria established by Harding (1981, 1984) are given in Table 26.2. Age of onset is (by definition) early with all cases beginning before 20 and most before the age of 15. Most patients are chairbound by age 30 and it is the associated cardiomyopathy, respiratory disease and diabetes mellitus that are important causes of mortality.

Pathological findings consist of degeneration of the posterior columns throughout the length of the cord; loss of anterior horn cells is seen and mainly affects the cervical and upper thoracic cord and there is demyelination of the anterior roots (Harding 1984). The lateral columns are also affected and the damage is most severe in the lateral spinocerebellar tracts. In the peripheral nervous system, demyelination of the large fibres is documented. Involvement of the brainstem tracts and nuclei, loss of Purkinje cells and loss of the large pyramidal cells of the motor cortex are all recorded.

Table 26.2. The features of FA are divided into several categories based on (Harding 1984) and Geoffroy et al. 1976). The first category signs are found in the vast majority (100% except extensor plantar responses >96%) and are essential features for diagnosis. Harding also adds the neurophysiological parameters as an essential criterion. Features in category 2 are found in large numbers of patients ranging from over 90% for pes cavus, scoliosis and cardiomyopathy to over 50% for the remainder. To these features should be added linkage to chromosome 9.

Category 1
Onset of symptoms < age 25
Progressive ataxia of limb/gait
Lower limb areflexia
Dysarthria
Dorsal column sensory loss in legs
Extensor plantar responses
Pyramidal muscle weakness
Motor nerve conduction velocity >40 m/sec in arms but with absent/small sensory nerve action potentials

Category 2
Scoliosis
Cardiomyopathy + abnormal ECG
Pes cavus
Optic atrophy/reduced acuity
Nystagmus
Essential tremor
Deafness
Diabetes mellitus

Although considerable detail has been recorded about the clinical manifestations, little is known about the biochemical or genetic nature of FA. The condition is inherited in an autosomal recessive manner with equal numbers of affected males and females. The gene has been linked to the centromeric region of chromosome 9 (Chamberlain et al. 1988) and this linkage is sufficiently good for it to be useful in prenatal testing (Wallis et al. 1989). Neither the precise localization nor the function of the putative gene product is known, however.

Diagnosis and Treatment

There are no diagnostic tests for FA. Diagnosis is clinical and based on the features outlined in Table 26.2. Symptomatic treatment and rehabilitation are essential in the management of this condition as in any other chronic spinocerebellar disorder. Optimizing mobility with physiotherapy and appropriate aids and appliances helps the well-being of patients. Prolonged immobility must be avoided. Identification and prompt treatment of chest infections and the cardiac failure that commonly occurs are vital as is awareness of the risks of diabetes mellitus.

Disorders of Vitamin E Metabolism

Vitamin E deficiency can result directly from fat malabsorption or because of an inherited defect in the transport or uptake of the vitamin. This section will deal with the latter where two different inherited diseases have been recognized, abetalipoproteinaemia or Bassen–Kornzweig disease and familial isolated vitamin E deficiency. Although vitamin E is a powerful antioxidant and free-radical scavenger, the precise reason why lack of vitamin E results in neurological dysfunction is unknown.

Abetalipoproteinaemia

This is a systemic disorder with haematological, gastrointestinal, hepatic and ophthalmological manifestations in addition to the neurological features (Rader and Brewer 1993). Usually, failure to thrive first attracts medical attention and as these patients have malabsorption they were often diagnosed as having coeliac disease. Structurally abnormal red blood cells, called acanthocytes, are typical (but not exclusive to this condition) and are the cause of a mild haemolytic anaemia (Bassen and Kornzweig 1950). A coagulation defect due to the associated malabsorption of the fat-soluble vitamin K may also be found.

The neurological features include ataxia, areflexia, proprioceptive sensory loss and dysarthria; scoliosis and pes cavus are also seen, so this condition resembles Friedreich's ataxia. Pigmentary retinopathy occurs (unlike Friedreich's) and can lead to blindness. Muscle weakness, if present, tends to be generalized and external ophthalmoplegia and ptosis can also develop. The onset of symptoms is usually before the age of 20 with a significant number presenting before the age of 10. Loss of deep tendon reflexes can precede other signs and symptoms, but progressive ataxia and peripheral neuropathy are the clinical hallmarks of the disorder (Kane and Havel 1995; Rader and Brewer 1993). Pathological changes, consisting of demyelination, have been found in the spinocerebellar tracts, anterior horns and cerebellum (molecular layer) (Sobrevilla et al. 1964).

Abetalipoproteinaemia is caused by the failure to absorb and transport fat-soluble vitamins (A, D, E and K) due to the absence of apolipoprotein B (apo B), an obligatory component of triglyceride-rich lipoproteins (Kane and Havel 1995). This absence is, in turn, due to the loss of a protein, microsomal triglyceride transfer protein (MTTP), which catalyses the transport of triglyceride, cholesterol ester and phospholipid between phospholipid surfaces. Although all fat-soluble vitamins are affected, it is the loss of vitamin E that results in significant neurological dysfunction. Abetalipoproteinaemia is an autosomal recessive condition, but with a slight predominance in men (6:4). There is a high incidence of parental consanguinity and the disorder is common amongst the Ashkenazi Jews. Recently, the gene for MTTP has been cloned and sequenced (Sharp et al. 1993) and mutations identified in patients with this disease.

Diagnosis and Treatment of Abetalipoproteinaemia

The presence of acanthocytes, very low concentrations of cholesterol, triglyceride and absence of chylomicrons, low and very low density lipoproteins (VLDL and LDL) are diagnostic in the appropriate clinical setting. The main differential diagnosis is with patients homozygous for the condition of familial hypobetalipoproteinaemia (Kane and Havel 1995). These individuals can have an identical clinical disease (said to be milder), but the condition is dominantly inherited and heterozygotes have detectable levels of LDL, cholesterol and apo B.

Treatment consists of fat avoidance to minimize the steatorrhoea. Vitamins K and A can be replaced easily, but very large doses of vitamin E (>100 mg/kg/day) are required to overcome the deficiency.

Familial Isolated Vitamin E Deficiency

This condition was identified in the early 1980s (Burck et al. 1981; Muller et al. 1983) and is also called ataxia with vitamin E deficiency (AVED). Individuals have a phenotype that closely mimics Friedreich's ataxia with severe and progressive ataxia, dysarthria, loss of reflexes, extensor plantar responses and skeletal abnormalities – kyphoscoliosis and pes cavus. Cardiomyopathy also occurs. There is no malabsorption or abnormality of plasma lipoproteins, but vitamin E levels are very low. AVED is inherited as an autosomal recessive disorder and, as in abetalipoproteinaemia, there is a high incidence of consanguinity.

Studies by Ben Hamida et al. (1993b) showed no linkage to the chromosome 9 region associated with Friedreich's ataxia, but linked it to chromosome 8 (Ben Hamida et al. 1993a). Using the candidate gene approach, Ouahchi et al. (1995) have found the gene responsible. This encodes the α-tocopherol transfer protein which is essential for the incorporation of α-tocopherol (vitamin E) into nascent VLDL. Treatment with moderate amounts (5–10 mg/kg/day) of vitamin E are thought beneficial.

Note in Proof

Since this chapter was written the gene responsible for Friedreich's ataxia has been identified. Campuzano V et al, Science, Vol 271, pp 1423–1427 showed that the locus on 9q13 encodes a gene of 210 aminoacids and that the major abnormality was a homozygous unstable GAA trionucleotide expansion in the first intron.

References

Baraitser M (1989) The genetics of the spinal muscular atrophies. Progr Clin Biol Res 306:75–84

Bassen FA, Kornzweig AL (1950) Malformation of the erythrocytes in a case of atypical retinitis pigmentosa. Blood 5:381–387

Ben Hamida M, Hentati F, Ben Hamida C (1990) Hereditary motor system diseases (chronic juvenile amyotrophic lateral sclerosis). Brain 113:347–363

Ben Hamida C, Doerflinger N, Belal S et al. (1993a) Localization of Friedreich ataxia phenotype with selective vitamin E deficiency to chromosome 8q by homozygosity mapping. Nat Genet 5:195–200

Ben Hamida M, Belal S, Sirugo G et al. (1993b) Friedreich's ataxia phenotype not linked to chromosome 9 and associated with selective autosomal recessive vitamin E deficiency in two inbred Tunisian families. Neurology 43:2179–2183

Boustany RM, Fleischnick E, Alper CA et al. (1987) The autosomal dominant form of "pure" familial spastic paraplegia: clinical findings and linkage analysis of a large pedigree. Neurology 37:910–915

Brown CJ, Goss SJ, Lubahn DB et al. (1989) Androgen receptor locus on the human X chromosome: regional localization to Xq11-12 and description of a DNA polymorphism. Am J Hum Genet 44:264–269

Brown RHJ (1995) Amyotrophic lateral sclerosis: recent insights from genetics and transgenic mice. Cell 80:687–692

Bruyn RPM (1991) Differential diagnostic work-up of spastic paratetraplegia. In: PJ V, Bruyn GW Klawans HL (eds) Handbook of clinical neurology. vol 15 Elsevier Science Publishers, Amsterdam, pp 425–445

Bruyn RPM (1992) The neuropathology of hereditary spastic paraparesis. Clin Neurol Neurosurg 94:S16–S18

Bruyn RPM, van Dijk JG, Scheltens P, Boezeman EH, Ongerboer de Visser BW (1994) Clinically silent dysfunction of dorsal columns and dorsal spinocerebellar tracts in hereditary spastic paraparesis. J Neurol Sci 125:206–211

Brzustowicz LM, Lehner T, Castilla LH et al. (1990) Genetic mapping of chronic childhood-onset spinal muscular atrophy to chromosome 5q11.2–13.3. Nature 344:540–541

Budka H, Sluga E, Heiss WD (1976) Spastic paraplegia associated with Addison's disease: adult variant of adreno-leukodystrophy. J Neurol 213:237–250

Bundey S (1985) Genetics and neurology. Churchill Livingstone, Edinburgh, London, Melbourne, New York

Burck U, Goebel HH, Kuhlendahl HD, Meier C, Goebel KM (1981) Neuromyopathy and vitamin E deficiency in man. Neuropediatrics 12:267–278

Chamberlain S, Shaw J, Rowland A et al. (1988) Mapping of mutation causing Friedreich's ataxia to human chromosome 9. Nature 334:248–250

Cote F, Collard JF, Julien JP (1993) Progressive neuronopathy in transgenic mice expressing the human neurofilament heavy gene: a mouse model of amyotrophic lateral sclerosis. Cell 73:35–46

Durr A, Brice A, Serdaru M et al. (1994) The phenotype of "pure" autosomal dominant spastic paraplegia. Neurology 44:1274

Figlewicz DA, Krizus A, Martinoli MG et al. (1994) Variants of the heavy neurofilament subunit are associated with the development of amyotrophic lateral sclerosis. Hum Mol Genet 3:1757–1761

Fink JK, Sharp GB, Lange BM et al. (1995a) Autosomal dominant, familial spastic paraplegia, type I: clinical and genetic analysis of a large North American family. Neurology 45:325–331

Fink JK, Wu CT, Jones SM et al. (1995b) Autosomal dominant familial spastic paraplegia: tight linkage to chromosome 15q. Am J Hum Genet 56:188–192

Fournier B, Smeitink JAM, Dorland L, Berger R, Saudebray JM, Poll-The BT (1994) Peroxisomal disorders: a review. J Inherit Metab Dis 17:470–486

Geoffroy G, Barbeau A, Breton A et al. (1976) Clinical description and roentgenologic evaluation of patients with Friedreich's ataxia. Can J Neurol Sci 3:279–286

Gilliam TC, Brzustowicz LM, Castilla LH et al. (1990) Genetic homogeneity between acute and chronic forms of spinal muscular atrophy. Nature 345:823–825

Gispert S, Santos N, Damen R et al. (1995) Autosomal dominant familial spastic paraplegia: reduction of the FSP1 candidate region on chromosome 14q to 7 cM and locus heterogeneity. Am J Hum Genet 56:183–187

Harding AE (1981) Friedreich's ataxia: a clinical and genetic study of 90 families with an analysis of early diagnositc criteria and intrafamilial clustering of clinical features. Brain 104:589–620

Harding AE (1984) The hereditary ataxias and related disorders. Churchill Livingstone, Edinburgh, London.

Harding AE (1993) Hereditary spastic paraplegias. [Review]. Semin Neurol 13:333–336

Harding AE, Thomas PK (1980) Hereditary distal spinal muscular atrophy. J Neurol Sci 45:337–348

Hazan J, Lamy C, Melki J, Munnich A, de Recondo J, Weissenbach J (1993) Autosomal dominant familial spastic paraplegia is genetically heterogeneous and one locus maps to chromosome 14q. Nat Genet 5:163–167

Hentati A, Bejaoui K, Pericak-Vance MA et al. (1994a) Linkage of recessive familial amyotrophic lateral sclerosis to chromosome 2q33–q35. Nat Genet 7:425–428

Hentati A, Pericak-Vance MA, Hung WY et al. (1994b) Linkage of "pure" autosomal recessive familial spastic paraplegia to chromosome 8 markers and evidence of genetic locus heterogeneity. Hum Mol Genet 3:1263–1267

Hentati A, Pericak-Vance MA, Lennon F et al. (1994c) Linkage of a locus for autosomal dominant familial spastic paraplegia to chromosome 2p markets. Hum Mol Genet 3:1867–1871

Kane JP, Havel RP (1995) Disorders of the biogenesis and secretion of lipoproteins containing the B apolipoproteins. In: Scriver CR, Beaudet AL, Sly WS (eds) The metabolic and molecular bases of inherited disease, vol 2. McGraw-Hill, New York. pp 1853

Kennedy WR, Alter M, Sung JH (1968) Progressive proximal spinal and bulbar muscular atrophy of late onset. A sex-linked recessive trait. Neurology 18:671–680

Kobayashi T, Yamada T, Yasutake T, Shinnoh N, Goto I, Iwaki T (1994) Adrenoleukodystrophy gene encodes an 80 kDa membrane protein. Biochem Biophys Res Commun 201:1029–1034

La Spada AR, Wilson EM, Lubahn DB, Harding AE, Fischbeck KH (1991) Androgen receptor gene mutations in X-linked spinal and bulbar muscular atrophy. Nature 352:77–79

La Spada AR, Roling DB, Harding AE et al. (1992) Meiotic stability and genotype-phenotype correlation of the trinucleotide repeat in X-linked spinal and bulbar muscular atrophy. Nat Genet 2:301–304

Lefebvre S, Burglen L, Reboullet S et al. (1995) Identification and characterization of a spinal muscular atrophy-determining gene. Cell 80:155–165

Lewin B (1995) Genes for SMA: multum in parvo. Cell 80:1–5

Melki J, Abdelhak S, Sheth P et al. (1990a) Gene for chronic proximal spinal muscular atrophies maps to chromosome 5q. Nature 344:767–768

Melki J, Sheth P, Abdelhak S et al. (1990b) Mapping of acute (type I) spinal muscular atrophy to chromosome 5q12–q14. The French spinal muscular atrophy investigators. Lancet 336:271–273

Morrison KE Harding AE (1994) Disorders of the motor neurone. In: Harding AE (ed) Genetics in neurology, vol 3. Bailliere Tindall, London pp 431–445

Moser HW (1995) Adrenoleukodystrophy. Curr Opin Neurol 8:221–226

Moser HW, Smith KD, Moser AB (1995). X-linked adrenoleukodystrophy. In: Scriver CR, Beaudet AL, Sly WS (eds) The metabolic and molecular bases of inherited disease, 7th edn, vol 2. McGraw-Hill, New York, pp 2325–2350

Mosser J, Lutz Y, Stoeckel ME et al. (1994) The gene responsible for adrenoleukodystrophy encodes a peroxisomal membrane protein. Hum Mol Genet 3:265–271

Mulder DW, Kurland LT, Offord KP, Beard CM (1986) Familial adult motor neuron disease: Amyotrophic lateral sclerosis. Neurology 36:511–517

Muller DPR, Lloyd JK, Wolff OH (1983) Vitamin E and neurological function. Lancet i:225–228

Munsat TL (1991) Workshop report. International SMA collaboration. Neuromuscul Disord 1:81

Navon R, Khosravi R, Korczyn T et al. (1995) A new mutation in the HEXA gene associated with a spinal muscular atrophy phenotype. Neurology 45:539–543

Osawa M, Keiko S (1991) Werdnig-Hoffmann disease and variants. In: Vinken PJ, Bruyn GW Klawans HL Handbook of Clinical Neurology, vol 15. Elsevier, Amsterdam, pp 51–80

Ouahchi K, Arita M, Kayden H et al. (1995) Ataxia with isolated vitamin E deficiency is caused by mutations in the α-tocopherol transfer protein. Nat Genet 9:141–145

Pearn J (1978a) Autosomal dominant spinal muscular atrophy: a clinical and genetic study. J Neurol Sci 38:263–275

Pearn J (1978b) Segregation analysis of chronic childhood spinal muscular atrophy. J Med Genet 15:418–423

Pearn J, Hudgson P (1979) Distal spinal muscular atrophy. A clinical and genetic study of 8 kindreds. J Neurol Sci 43:183–191

Pearn JH (1973) The gene frequency of acute Werding–Hoffmann disease (SMA Type I) a total population survey in North East England. J Med Genet 10:260–265

Pearn JP, (1978) Incidence, prevalence and gene frequency studies of chronic childhood spinal muscular atrophy. J Med Genet 15:409–413

Polo JM, Calleja J, Combarros O, Berciano J (1991) Hereditary ataxias and paraplegias in Cantabria, Spain. An epidemiological and clinical study. Brain 114:855–866

Polo JM, Calleja J, Combarros O, Berciano J (1993) Hereditary "pure" spastic paraplegia: a study of nine families. J Neurol Neurosurg Psychiatry 56:175–181

Powers JM (1985) Adreno-leukodystrophy (adreno-testiculo-leukomyelo-neuropathic-complex). Clin Neuropathol 4:181–199

Rader DJ, Brewer H Jr (1993) Abetalipoproteinemia. New insights into lipoprotein assembly and vitamin E metabolism from a rare genetic disease. JAMA 270:865–869

Rosen DR (1993) Mutations in Cu/Zn superoxide dismutase gene are associated with familial amyotrophic lateral sclerosis. Nature 364:362

Rowland LP (1994) Amyotrophic lateral sclerosis. Curr Opin Neurol 7:310–315

Roy N, Mahadevan MS, McLean M et al. (1995) The gene for neuronal apoptosis inhibitory protein is partially deleted in individuals with spinal muscular atrophy. Cell 80:167–178

Sarde CO, Mosser J, Kioschis P et al. (1994) Genomic organization of the adrenoleukodystrophy gene. Genomics 22:13–20

Sharp D, Blinderman L, Combs KA et al. (1993) Cloning and gene defects in microsomal triglyceride transfer protein associated with abetalipoproteinaemia. Nature 365:65–69

Siddique T, Figlewicz DA, Pericak-Vance MA et al. (1991) Linkage of a gene causing familial amyotrophic lateral sclerosis to chromosome 21 and evidence of genetic-locus heterogeneity. N Engl J Med 324:1381–1384

Sobrevilla LA, Goodman ML, Kane CA (1964) Demyelinating central nervous system disease, macular atrophy and acanthocytosis (Bassen–Kornzweig syndrome) Am J Med 37:821–828

Strong MJ, Hudson AJ, Alvord WG (1991) Familial amyotrophic lateral sclerosis, 1850–1989: a statistical analysis of the world literature. Can J Neurol Sci 18:45–58

Troost J (1991) Spinal muscular atrophy of infantile and juvenile onset, due to metabolic derangement. In: PJ V, Bruyn GW Klawans HL (eds) Handbook of Clinical Neurology, vol 15. Elsevier Science Publishers, Amsterdam, pp 97–105.

Vuopala K, Ignatius J, Herva R (1995) Lethal arthrogryposis with anterior horn cell disease. Hum Pathol 26:12–9

Wallis J, Shaw J, Wilkes D et al. (1989) Prenatal diagnosis of Friedreich ataxia. Am J Med Genet 34:458–461

Wanders RJ, van Roermund CW, Lageweg W et al. (1992) X-linked adrenoleukodystrophy: biochemical diagnosis and enzyme defect. J Inherit Metab Dis 15:634–644

Willems PJ (1994) Dynamic mutations hit double figures. Nat Genet 8:213–215

Xu Z, Cork LC, Griffin JW, Cleveland DW (1993) Increased expression of neurofilament subunit NF-L produces morphological alterations that resemble the pathology of human motor neuron disease. Cell 73:23–33

Zierz S, Zerres K (1991). Wohlfart–Kugelberg–Welander disease. In: PJ V, Bruyn GW Klawans HL Handbook of Clinical Neurology vol 15. Elsevier Science Publisher, Amsterdam, pp 81–96

Chapter 27

Deficiency Diseases of the Spinal Cord

R.A. Shakir and L.A. Bindoff

The spinal cord can be affected in many nutritional deficiencies, the best recognized is subacute combined degeneration of the spinal cord due to cobalamin deficiency. Folic acid deficiency may lead to a similar neurological problem. Other vitamin deficiencies can also cause spinal cord dysfunction.

Vitamin B$_{12}$ Deficiency

Vitamin B$_{12}$ (cobalamin) is converted into coenzymes, and as methylcobalamin, is concerned with conversion of homocysteine into methionine, and, as deoxyadenosylcobalamin, with the conversion of methylmalonyl-CoA into succinyl-CoA. The active coenzymes are essential for cell growth and replication. Transmethylation is a vital step for DNA synthesis and maintenance of myelin basic protein. Cobalamin cannot be synthesized by humans, although it is produced by bacteria in the intestine the production is too distal for any absorption to occur. The daily requirement for cobalamin for an adult is 3 μg; the body stores are around 4–5 mg mostly in the liver. The brain is relatively rich in cobalamin, the maximum concentration being found in the choroid plexus (Ordonez 1977). The concentration of cobalamin in the CSF is 10–30 times less than the serum, with a concentration ranging from 2.1 to 22.9 pmol/l (5–95% confidence limits) with a mean of 8.7 pmol/l. The serum to CSF ratios are similar in both sexes and do not change with age (Nijst et al. 1990). Cobalamin is transported in the blood bound to a protein (transcobalamin II) which releases the vitamin when required. The amount of unsaturated cobalamin in the blood is 3–4 times that of the CSF. In an ambulatory geriatric population 3%–7% were reported to have low serum B$_{12}$ levels (Marcus et al. 1987). It is, therefore, imperative that, in patients with suspected neurological symptoms of cobalamin deficiency, in addition to the measurement of total serum cobalamin level, other parameters of cobalamin metabolism should be carefully sought. The presence of multilobulated polymorphonuclear neutrophils is perhaps the most universal indicator, but in addition red blood cell cobalamin, serum and urinary methylmalonic acid, total serum homocysteine and CSF S-adenosyl methionine are all indicative of cobalamin metabolism (Allen et al. 1990; Bottiglieri et al. 1990; Beck 1991).

Pathophysiology

Cobalamin deficiency results in two main systemic abnormalities. The haemopoetic one leads to a megaloblastic picture and defective proliferation of fast dividing cells with glossitis and hypospermia. The second major manifestation is neurological. Classically neurological sequelae start late, after the haematological ones. This sequence is not always seen, as many patients who present with cobalamin deficiency-induced neurological disorders, do not have anaemia or macrocytosis. A substantial number present atypically, 28% did not have anaemia or a raised MCV in one large series (Lindenbaum et al. 1988). A fifth of patients with low serum cobalamin, abnormal Schilling test or intrinsic factor (IF) antibodies did not have anaemia and 33% did not have macrocytosis; of the 14% without anaemia and macrocytosis, 60% had significant neurological symptoms (Carmel 1988a).

Aetiology

Addisonian pernicious anaemia (PA) with deficiency of a gastric IF due to an autoimmune mechanism remains the classical and commonest cause of the neurological syndrome of cobalamin deficiency. IF is a glycoprotein produced by the parietal cells of the fundus of the stomach; it binds with cobalamin to allow its absorption. The presence of parietal and IF antibodies leads to gastric mucosal atrophy, achlorhydria and IF deficiency. PA is associated with other autoimmune disorders and is usually familial.

Conditions associated with loss of gastric mucosa can also cause IF deficiency; total gastrectomy and to a lesser degree partial gastrectomy, chronic atrophic gastritis and gastric tumours can all be responsible for parietal cell destruction. Hereditary disorders including "R" binder deficiency presenting with myelopathy and defective posterior column involvement (Carmel and Herbert 1969; Carmel et al. 1987; Carmel 1988b; Sigal et al. 1988). In those with defective IF, the presentation is usually in early childhood with developmental delay including myelopathy (Yang et al. 1985). Imerslund–Grasbeck syndrome is due to defective cobalamin transport by the enterocytes with decreased serum cobalamin, normal IF, TC II and absent IF antibodies. The condition starts early with rare neurological involvement (Burman et al. 1985). Absent transcobalamin II usually presents in infancy with a severe megaloblastic picture and failure to thrive; neurological involvement may occur late (Hall 1992). A defective transcobalamin II has been reported in adults. It leads to a functional cobalamin deficiency with normal or high serum cobalamin levels but with high homocysteine and methylmalonic acid (Reynolds et al. 1993). There are several intracellular cobalamin utilization defects which generally present in infancy and childhood, including methylmalonic aciduria and homocysteinuria (Rosenblatt and Cooper 1987; Shevell and Rosenblatt 1992).

Drugs may interfere with cobalamin absorption, e.g. cholestyramine, neomycin, and to a certain degree alcohol. Ileal diseases can impair absorption, e.g. Crohn's disease and lymphoma. Increased gut consumption of cobalamin can occur by bacteria in blind loop syndromes and with fish tape worm infestation. Dietary deficiency is rare except in vegans who rarely have neurological sequelae. The administration of folic acid to cobalamin-deficient patients may precipitate or aggravate neurological complications of cobalamin deficiency (Schwartz et al. 1950; Reynolds 1979). Similarly, administration of nitrous oxide anaesthesia has been reported to induce neurological manifestations in borderline cobalamin deficient patients. Nitrous oxide neutralizes active cobalamin and can result in a myeloneuropathy (Schilling 1986; Holloway and Alberico 1990). It has, therefore, been extensively used in producing animal models of cobalamin deficiency and the study of the consequent neuropathy and spinal cord disease (Metz 1992). It should be remembered that a low serum cobalamin and a neurological syndrome do not always imply a causal relationship (Pallis and Lewis 1974).

Neuropathology

The term subacute combined degeneration of the spinal cord was introduced by Russell et al. (1900), but the association of spinal cord disease and PA was known previously and was thought to be due to tabes dorsalis (Leichtenstern 1884). Lichtheim (1887) was the first to point out that the spinal cord lesions of patients with PA were different from tabes dorsalis. This was followed by Minnich (1892) who showed some degeneration of the lateral and posterior columns of the spinal cord in patients with PA.

Although the neurological syndrome of cobalamin deficiency is termed subacute combined degeneration of the spinal cord, the commonest and earliest neurological involvement is a peripheral neuropathy. This was recognized early on (Woltman 1919; Woltman and Heck 1937; Adams and Kubik 1944) and confirmed repeatedly (Pallis and Lewis 1974; Cox-Kalzinga and Endtz 1980). The pathology of peripheral nerve involvement is not absolutely clear; demyelination and axonal loss have been reported (Pant et al. 1968; Victor 1984). In some studies no axonal loss was noted, whereas in others loss of myelinated nerve fibres with no evidence of demyelination on examining teased nerve fibres was noted (McCombe and McLeod 1984).

Spinal cord pathology is that of myelin loss with "degeneration" of the white matter. The process usually starts in the thoracic spinal cord and spreads rostrally and caudally, coalescing with other areas of degeneration. The upward ascent stops at the level of the medulla (Lampkin and Saunders 1969). Retrograde changes of the Betz cells and wallerian degeneration may occur later. Demyelination and disappearance of myelin sheaths and axis cylinders leaves vacuolated spaces separated by a thin glial framework. A honeycomb appearance due to discontinuance degeneration of myelin sheaths is said to be characteristic. The fibres adjacent to the grey horns are spared, but the whole spinal cord is involved later. The degeneration gets less towards the cervical cord where the posterior columns are more affected and also in the lumbar cord where the lateral columns are predominantly involved. The brunt of the process therefore involves the posterior and lateral columns and the spinocerebellar tracts (Mancal 1989).

Clinical Features

Cobalamin deficiency mainly affects middle-aged and elderly individuals with an average age of onset in the early 50s. The onset is insidious and symptoms vary according to the main site of pathological involvement. The earliest symptoms are peripheral sensory ones with paraesthesiae affecting the toes and later the fingers. Paraesthesiae ascend from the toes and spread to the legs and a "sock and glove" sensory loss to pain, temperature and touch are noted. Stabbing and girdle pains are also noted. The posterior column loss is more marked in the legs initially, with loss of proprioception and vibration senses. Motor weakness, hypotonia and ataxia develop usually after the sensory symptoms, but the picture can be dominated by a spastic ataxic paraparesis with a positive Romberg's sign. Deep tendon reflexes vary; ankle jerks are usually absent and knee jerks may be absent later. Plantar responses are usually extensor and even if they are flexor early they become extensor eventually. Impotence may be seen early in those with spinal cord involvement along with bladder dysfunction. Other neuropsychiatric symptoms include optic atrophy, nystagmus, cerebellar ataxia and a whole host of psychiatric symptoms, including confusion, hallucinations, mood changes, poor recent memory, personality changes and dementia (Fine and Soria 1991).

Achlorhydria, macrocytic anaemia and megaloblastic bone marrow are seen in cases associated with addisonian PA. Glossitis is usually associated with the anaemia rather than the neurological involvement.

Diagnosis

Low serum cobalamin, achlorhydria, macrocytosis, megaloblastic bone marrow, hypersegmented neutrophils, high lactate dehydrogenase (LDH) and bilirubin are fairly straightforward indicators. Unfortunately, the case is rarely as clear. Patients with neurological disorders which may be due to a cobalamin deficiency but do not have the classical features are the ones usually encountered in clinical practice. The normal serum cobalamin level is 200–2000 nmol/l. Levels below 100 nmol/l are diagnostic of neurological cobalamin deficiency. Those in between will need further evaluation to establish the significance of the cobalamin level. Looking at the metabolites which require cobalamin action as a coenzyme for their conversion is an excellent way of detecting cobalamin deficiency. Total serum homocysteine (normal range 5.4–16.2 nmol/l) and serum methylmalonic acid (normal range 73–271 nmol/l) as well as urinary excretion of the latter are raised in cobalamin deficiency (Allen et al. 1990; Fine et al 1990; Lindenbaum et al. 1990). Red cell cobalamin is more useful as it suggests the amount of unsaturated cobalamin in the system. These tests are valuable in the appropriate patient.

The value of the Schilling test is perhaps important when there is strong clinical suspicion of PA with positive parietal cell antibodies and achlorhydria. The one-stage Schilling test utilizing two different types of cobalt radioisotope can be misleading. The more cumbersome standard Schilling test or the modified Schilling test (protein-bound absorption test) are rarely required (Schilling 1982; Carethers 1988).

Parietal cell antibodies are present in the vast majority of patients with PA but are also present in those with gastric atrophy without PA. IF antibodies are specific but not sensitive as they are present in 50%–75% of PA patients. Achlorhydria is not always associated with IF deficiency and PA, and is a common finding in the elderly. Neurophysiological abnormalities including features of denervation on electromyography with slow nerve conduction and abnormal evoked potentials can be seen even in subtle cobalamin deficiency (Krumholz et al. 1980; Karnaze and Carmel 1990).

Treatment

It is important to emphasize that it is vital not to delay treatment while trying to confirm the diagnosis, as important as that may be. The aim of therapy is to quickly replenish body stores of cobalamin of 3000 μg by daily intramuscular hydroxycobalamin initially for 7–10 days, followed by three monthly injections. There are a few exceptional cases due to an abnormal transcobalmin II, where a more frequent dosage is recommended (Reynolds et al. 1993).

Prognosis

It is always possible to prevent neuropathy and other neurological manifestations in patients with PA. In those with established neurological dysfunction, disease progression can be halted with recovery of function occurring in the peripheral nervous system through peripheral nerve regeneration. In a report of 153 episodes of cobalmin deficency leading to neurological disorders, follow-up was adequate in 121 episodes to assess neurological response to cobalamin therapy. There was initial deterioration in four, but all patients responded and in 47.1% recovery was complete. The severity scores as judged by the investigators as improved by 50% or more, was reported in 91% of patients. Long-term disability was only noted in 6.3%. The authors concluded that in modern practice, neurological disorders of cobalamin deficiency respond well and early diagnosis and commencement of cobalamin therapy are most important in preventing permanent disability (Healton et al. 1991).

Folate Deficiency

The metabolism of folic acid is closely related to that of vitamin B_{12}. Methylfolate donates its methyl group to homocysteine to form methionine where cobalamin acts as a coenzyme. Methionine passes the methyl group to S-adenosylmethionine which is the only methyl donor in the brain (Reynolds et al. 1984; Carney 1986).

The clinical manifestations of folate deficiency are generally similar to cobalamin deficiency. Neurological involvement is perhaps only seen in its "pure" form in those with an inborn error of folate metabolism (Niederweiser 1979), those using antifolate drugs, e.g. methotrexate, trimethoprim and triamterene (Bleyer et al. 1973; Lambie and Johnson 1985) and also in newborns with spinal tube defects in whom folic acid was not used during gestation. Long-term anticonvulsant use has been well documented to lead to a macrocytic anaemia and peripheral neuropathy due to folate deficiency.

Inborn errors of folate metabolism cause an early and severe neurological syndrome. Marked leukoencephalopathy with perivascular demyelination and a picture of subacute combined degeneration of the spinal cord was reported in a 2 year old who died with 5,10-methylenetetrahydrofolate reductase deficiency (Clayton et al. 1986). This supports the idea that defective 5-methylenetetrahydrofolate is the link between cobalamin deficiency and subacute combined degeneration.

The commonest cause of folate deficiency is dietary or as a result of malabsoption. The initial neurological symptoms are neuropathic with paraesthesiae and spinal cord involvement may or may not occur (Crellin et al. 1993).

The diagnosis is made by measuring serum and more importantly red cell folate in suspected individuals. Folic acid treatment improves the neuropathic symptoms as well as the neurophysiological parameters as was demonstrated in epileptic patients who had a folate deficiency and a peripheral neuropathy (Martinez-Figuroa et al. 1980).

Pellagra

Niacin deficiency causes the classical triad of dermatitis, diarrhoea and dementia. The neurological manifestations are late and result from chromatolysis. They include polyneuritis, cerebellar ataxia, spasticity, retrobulbar neuritis and deafness. Mental changes predominate including manic depression states and progressive dementia.

The spinal cord histologically shows central chromatolysis of the anterior horn neurones without proliferation of neuroglia. Degeneration of the lateral and posterior columns is a feature of pellagra which is histologically different from that of cobalamin deficiency with the absence of the characteristic honeycomb appearance. The appearance in pellagra resembles that of wallerian degeneration with involvement of the posterior and anterior roots. Both central and peripheral lesions may occur together or separately but it is usually a mixture in the context of multiple vitamin and calorie deficiency.

Vitamin E

Deficiency of vitamin E is rare. Vitamin E is important in maintaining nervous system function (Muller et al. 1983; Harding 1987; Muller and Gross-Sampson 1989). Alpha tocopherol has a role as an antioxidant and is used in this context in clinical practice.

Chronic fat malabsorption due to reduced concentration of bile salts may be associated with vitamin E deficiency. Isolated vitamin E malabsorption has been reported as an inborn error of metabolism (Sokol 1989). Abetalipoproteinaemia was first described by Bassen and Kornzweig (1950). As a result of a defect of chylomicrons, low density and very low density lipoprotein synthesis, there is a failure of intestinal absorption and plasma transportation of vitamin E, leading to low plasma levels and acanthocytosis. Further detailed description of vitamin E deficiency is in Chapter 27.

In conclusion, the main deficiency disease affecting the spinal cord is due to cobalamin deficiency. Its recognition is dependent on familiarity with cobalamin metabolism and performing the correct investigations in the appropriate clinical circumstances.

References

Adams RD, Kubik CS (1944) Subacute combined degeneration of the brain in pernicious anaemia N Engl J Med 23:1–9

Allen RH, Stabler SP, Savage DG, Lindenbaum J (1990) Diagnosis of cobalamin deficiency I: Usefulness of serum methylmalonic acid and total homocysteine concentrations. Am J Hematol 34:90–98

Bassen FA, Kornzweig AL (1950) Malformation of the erythrocytes in a case of atypical retinits pigmentosa. Blood 5:381–387

Beck WS (1991) Neuropsychiatric consequences of Cobalamin deficiency. Adv Intern Med 36:33–56

Bleyer WA, Drake JC, Chambner BA (1973) Neurotoxicity and elevated cerebrospinal fluid methotrexate in meningeal leukaemia. N Engl J Med 289:770–773

Bottiglieri T, Godfrey P, Carney MWP, Toone BK, Reynolds EH (1990) CSF 5-adenosylmethionine in neurological and psychiatric patients: effects of treatment with parenteral and oral S-adenosylmethionine. In: Linnell JC, Bahtt HR (eds). Biomedicine and physiology of vitamin B₁₂. Children's Medical Charity, London, pp 167–174

Burman JF, Walker WJ, Smith JA et al. (1985) Absent ileal uptake of IF-bound-vitamin B₁₂ in the Imerslund–Grasbeck syndrome (familial vitamin B₁₂ Malabsorption with proteinuria). Gut 26:311–314

Carethers M (1988) Diagnosis of vitamin B₁₂ deficiency, A common geriatric disorder. Geriatrics 43:89–112

Carmel R (1988a) Pernicious anaemia: the expected finding of very low serum cobalamin levels, anaemia and macrocytosis are often lacking. Arch Intern Med 148:1712–1714

Carmel R (1988b) Plasma R Binder deficiency. N Engl J Med 318:1401

Carmel R, Herbert V (1969) Deficiency of vitamin B₁₂ binding alpha globulin in 2 brothers. Blood 33:1–12

Carmel R, Sinow RM, Karnaze DS (1987) A typical coblamin deficiency. Subtle biochemical evidence of deficiency is commonly demonstrable in patients without megaloblastic anaemia and is often associated with protein-bound cobalamin malabsorption. J Lab Clin Med 9:454–463

Carney MWP (1986) Neuropharmacology of S-adenosylmethionine. Clin Neuropharamcol 9:235–243

Clayton PT, Smith I, Harding B, Hyland K, Leonard JV et al. (1986) Subacute combined degeneration of the cord, Dementia and parkinsonism due to an inborn error of folate metabolism. J Neurol Neurosurg Psychiatry 49:920–927

Cox-Klazinga M, Endtz LJ (1980) Peripheral nerve involvement in pernicious anaemia. J Neurol Sci 8:611–612

Crellin R, Bottiglieri T, Reynolds EH (1993) Folate and Psychiatric disorders. Clinical potential. Drugs 45:623–636

Fine EJ, Soria ED (1991) Myths about vitamin B₁₂ deficiency. South Med J 84:1475–1481

Fine EJ, Soria ED, Paroski MW, Petryk D, Thomasula L (1990) The neurophysiological profile of vitamin B₁₂ deficiency. Muscle Nerve 13:158–164

Hall CA (1992) The neurologic aspects of transcobalamin II deficiency. Br J Haematol 80:117–120

Harding AE (1987) Vitamin E and the nervous system. CRC Clin Rev Neurobiol 3:89–103

Healton EB, Savage DG, Burst JCM, Garrett TJ, Lindenbaum J (1991) Neurologic aspects of cobalamin deficiency. Medicine 70:229–245

Holloway KL, Alberico AM (1990) Postoperative myeloneuropathy: A preventable complication in patients with B₁₂ deficiency. J Neurosurg 72:732–736

Karnaze DS, Carmel R (1990) Neurologic and evoked potential abnormalities in subtle cobalamin deficiency states, including deficiency without anaemia and with normal absorption of free cobalamin. Arch Neurol 47:1008–1012

Krumholz A, Weiss DH, Goldstein PJ, Harris KC (1980) Evoked responses in vitamin B₁₂ deficiency. Ann Neurol 9:407–409

Lambie DG, Johnson RH (1985) Drugs and folate metabolism. Drugs 30:145–155

Lampkin BC, Saunders EF (1969) Nutritional vitamin B₁₂ deficiency in an infant. J Pediatr 75:1053–1055

Leichtenstern O (1884) Progressive perniciose anamie bei tabeskranken. Disch Med Wochenschr 10:849–850

Lichtheim (1887) Zur kenntniss der perniosen anamie. VCI 6:84–99

Lindenbaum J, Healton EB, Savage DG et al. (1988) Neuropsychiatric disorders caused by cobalamin deficiency in the absence of anaemia or macrocytosis. N Engl J Med 318:1720–1728

Lindenbaum J, Savage DG, Stabler SP, Allen RH (1990) Diagnosis of cobalamin deficiency II. Relative sensitivities of serum cobalamin, methylmalonic acid and total homocysteine concentrations. Am J Hematol 34:99–107

Mancal EL (1989) Subacute combined degeneration of the spinal cord. In: Rowland L (ed) Houston Merritt's textbook of neurology. Lea and Fabiger, Philadelphia, pp 691–694

Marcus DL, Shadick N, Crantz J, Gray M, Hernandez F, Freedman ML (1987) Low serum B₁₂ levels in a haematologically normal elderly subpopulation. J Am Geriatr Soc 35:635–638

Martinez-Figueroa A, Johnson RH, Lambie DG, Shakir RA (1980) The role of folate deficiency in the development of peripheral neuropathy caused by anticonvulsants. J Neurol Sci 48:315–323

McCombe PA, McLeod JG (1984) The peripheral neuropathy of vitamin B_{12} deficiency. J Neurol Sci 106:117–126

Metz J (1992) Cobalamin deficiency and the pathogenesis of nervous system disease. Annu Rev Nutr 12:59–79

Minnich W (1892) Kenntnis der im verlaufe der perniciosen anamie beobachteten spinalerkrankungen. Z Klin Med 21:264–314

Muller DPR, Goss-Sampson MA (1989) Role of vitamin E in neural tissue. Ann N Y Acad Sci 570:146–155

Muller DPR, Lloyd JK, Wolff OH (1983) Vitamin E and neurological function. Lancet i:225–228

Niederweiser A (1979) Inborn errors of pterin metabolism. In: Boetz MI, Reynolds EH (eds) Folic acid in neurology psychiatry and internal medicine. Raven Press, New York, pp 349–384

Nijst YQ, Wever RA, Schoonderwaldt HC, Hommes OR, De Haan AFJ (1990) Vitamin B_{12} and folate concentrations in serum and cerebrospinal fluid in neurological patients with reference to multiple sclerosis and dementia. J Neurol Neurosurg Psychiatry 53:951–954

Ordonez LA (1977) Control of the availability to the brain of folic acid, vitamin B_{12} and choline. In: Wurtman RJ, Wurtman JJ (eds) Nutrition and the brain. vol 1. Raven Press, New York, pp 205–248

Pallis CA, Lewis PD (1974) The neurology of the gastrointestinal disease. In: Walton JN (ed) WB Saunders, London, pp 30–97

Pant SS, Asbury AK, Richardson EP Jr (1968) The myelopathy of pernicious anemia. Acta Neurol Scand 44(suppl 35): 1–36

Reynolds EH (1979) Folic acid, Vitamin B_{12} and the nervous system: historical aspects. In: Boetz MI, Reynolds EH (eds) Floic acid in neurology, psychiatry and internal medicine. Raven Press, New York, pp 1–5

Reynolds EH, Carney MWP, Toone BK (1984) Methylation and mood. Lancet ii:196–198

Reynolds EH, Bottiglieri T, Laundy M et al. (1993) Subacute combined degeneration with high serum vitamin B_{12} level and abnormal vitamin B_{12} binding protein. A new cause of an old syndrome. Arch Neurol 50:739–742

Rosenblatt DS, Cooper BA (1987) Inherited disorders of vitamin B_{12} metabolism. Blood Rev 1:177–182

Russell JSR, Batten FE, Collier J (1900) Subacute combined degeneration of the spinal cord. Brain 23:39–110

Schwartz SO, Kaplan SR, Armstrong BE (1950) The long-term evaluation of folic acid in the treatment of pernicious anaemia. J Lab Clin Med 35:984–988

Schilling RF (1982) Vitamin B_{12}: Assay and absorption testing. Lab MGT 31–37

Schilling RF (1986) Is nitrous oxide a dangerous anaesthetic for vitamin B_{12} deficient patients. JAMA 225:1605–1606

Shevell MI, Rosenblatt DS (1992) The neurology of cobalamin. Can J Neurol Sci 19:472–486

Sigal SH, Hall CA, Antel JP (1988) Plasma R binder deficiency and neurologic disease. N Engl J Med 318:1330–1332

Sokol RJ (1989) Vitamin E and neurologic function in man. Free Radic Biol Med 6:189–207

Victor M (1984) Polyneuropathy due to nutritional deficiency and alcoholism. Peripheral neuropathy. In: Dyck PJ, Thomas PK, Lambert EH, Bunge R, (eds) WB Saunders, Philadelphia, pp 1899–1940

Woltman HW (1919) The nervous system in pernicious anemia: an analysis of one hundred and fifty cases. Am J Med Sci 173:400–409

Woltman HW, Heck FJ (1937) Funicular degeneration of the spinal cord without pernicious anemia. Arch Intern Med 60:272–300

Yang Y-M, Ducos R, Rosenberg AJ et al. (1985) Cobalamin malabsorption in three siblings due to abnormal intrinsic factor that is markedly susceptible to acid and proteolysis. J Clin Invest 76:2057–2065

Chapter 28

Vertebral Body Collapse

J.P.R. Dick

Vertebral collapse is not an uncommon finding post mortem, present in 20%–30% of autopsies when sought (Fornasier and Czitrom 1978; Sartoris et al. 1986) and may be due to many aetiologies. In general, collapse of the anterior structures of the vertebral body is due either to infection or neoplasms, usually metastatic, or to a more generalized process causing osteopenia, e.g. metabolic or inflammatory disorders. In these conditions minor trauma may finally precipitate vertebral fracture. Involvement of the posterior vertebral structures by infection (Roberts 1988) or neoplasia is uncommon as metastatic disease usually involves the vascular tufts just deep to the end plate (Waldvogel et al. 1970).

Pathology

In a study of 659 consecutive autopsies from a general hospital and a hospital specializing in the treatment of cancer, Fornasier and Czitrom (1978) found 133 spines with vertebral collapse: an incidence of 17.3% from the general hospital and 24% from the cancer hospital. Using radiographic and histological techniques they studied from T3 downwards and found 372 collapsed vertebrae; the thoracic spine was involved twice as often as the lumbar spine and most commonly involved T12 and T6 and least frequently T3 and T4. Of the 133 involved spines, 75 cases had cancer and 58 cases did not; however, malignant disease was over-represented in this series as, in another study (Sartoris et al. 1986), 70% of cases of vertebral collapse were due to benign disease. In half of the 58 cases of non-malignant disease collapse was considered to be due primarily to osteoporosis and in two there was histological evidence of osteomalacia. In the remainder, collapse was due to serious degenerative disc disease in the lumbar spine with end plate erosion and collapse. End-plate erosion is commoner in rheumatological conditions such as rheumatoid arthritis (RA) than in purely degenerative conditions such as osteoarthritis (Heywood and Meyers 1986) but as the latter is so common it tends to account for a high proportion of cases.

Rheumatic diseases (RA, Still's disease, ankylosing spondylitis), developmental conditions (Scheuermann's disease, spondylolisthesis) and traumatic vertebral body collapse are dealt with elsewhere in this book. Here we shall deal with collapse due to osteoporosis, neoplasia and vertebral osteomyelitis.

Radiology

Typically, benign osteopenic conditions show a generalized decrease in bone density with a tendency for vertebral collapse in the low thoracic spine. Apart from erosion of a single pedicle, which has a high degree of specificity for neoplasia, the radiological features of malignant collapse are non-specific. In most cases there are multiple osseous deposits which are lytic with or without sclerotic margins. As sclerosis around end plate deformities can occur around healing fractures its presence is non-specific.

To establish criteria which might reliably differentiate benign from malignant vertebral collapse Sartoris et al. (1986) studied 300 nearly consecutive routine autopsies. They found vertebral collapse in 99 spines, 30 due to neoplastic disease and 69 due to benign metabolic bone disease (osteoporosis, osteomalacia, osteitis fibrosa cystica). They found that neither disc space narrowing nor diffuse involvement of the end plate region reliably differentiated between benign and malignant groups. However, the presence of angled end plates occurred in 64% of malignant cases but in less than 25% of benign cases ($P < 0.001$). By contrast, a benign collapse was predicted by anterior wedging of the vertebral bodies at T6/7, or by vertebral collapse with an even concavity of both superior and inferior end plates in a low thoracic vertebra (cod fish vertebra). This is seen in osteopenic spines as the major mechanical forces of body weight are transmitted through the axis of the vertebral body (apex of the concavity) where the end plate tends to be more porous due to the presence of the nucleus pulposus (Schmorl and Junghanns 1971). In some cases of benign disease more angulated end plates were explicable by recent local trauma.

Using CT, the presence of an epidural or paraspinal soft tissue mass is suggestive of malignant vertebral collapse. The presence of a vacuum phenomenon within a vertebra and a fracture line in the cancellous bone but not in the cortical bone is suggestive of benign collapse (Laredo et al. 1995).

Metabolic Bone Disease

Osteoporosis

Osteoporosis is the commonest metabolic disorder associated with vertebral collapse though its coexistence with osteomalacia or hyperparathyroidism should be considered (Fornasier and Czitrom 1978). The classical radiological features of osteitis fibrosa cystica (primary hyperparathyroidism) are seen better in the hands than in the spine but over the last 50 years the pattern of bone disease in hyperparathyroidism has changed. This is probably due to earlier treatment of primary hyperparathyroidism and the greater prevalence of secondary hyperparathyroidism due to renal failure. This gives a picture of diffuse osteopenia similar to osteoporosis though less homogeneous (Fairney 1983).

Osteoporotic vertebral collapse may be asymptomatic but usually is associated with back pain, often after trivial injury. As a consequence patients may lose height and develop back deformity which if progressive can lead to a hunched thoracic spine and protuberant abdomen. Osteoporosis is defined as a decrease in bone mineral density of 2.5 standard deviations from that of young adult bone; lesser degrees of demineralization is termed osteopaenia. Two patterns of osteoporosis are recognized. In the first cancellous bone rather than cortical bone is demineralized, this type of osteoporosis is associated with vertebral crush fractures. In the other type, cortical bone also is demineralized, possibly as a result of defective 1,25-dihydroxyvitamin D production by the kidney; in this type long bones, as well as vertebrae, tend to fracture (neck of femur, distal radius). The propensity to fracture requires trauma for its full expression and the wide variety of hormonal influences that are thought to be involved with the pathogenesis of osteoporosis may well also influence a patient's strength and stability (Raisz 1988). It is rare to develop myelopathic features consequent to osteoporotic collapse (Parfitt and Duncan 1982) though delayed neurological decline can occur if retropulsed fragments of vertebra come to compress the spinal cord (Kaneda et al. 1992).

Osteoporosis is commoner in women than men (7:1 for vertebral collapse), in white or Asian than blacks and becomes more prevalent with age in both sexes, being particularly related to the female menopause. It may be prevented by the administration of oestrogens in women and is probably related to insufficient levels of androgen and testosterone in men as it is more prevalent in hypogonadal males. It has been associated with a wide range of endocrine disorders (primary/secondary/tertiary hyperparathyroidism, hyperthyroidism, hypercortisolism, steroid therapy, acromegaly, hyperprolactinaemia) as well as with disordered homeostasis of calcium and vitamin D (dietary deficiency and renal disease). Surprisingly, osteoporosis is not directly correlated with abnormal parathormone (PTH) activity or vitamin D status (1,25-dihydroxyvitamin D). Serum concentrations of bioactive PTH increase with age but the levels are not correlated with decreased bone mass (Raisz 1988) and, although a primary excess of PTH is associated with an increase of long bone fractures, it is not associated with an increased incidence of vertebral fractures (Raisz 1988). Serum levels of 1,25-dihydroxyvitamin D decrease with age and patients with vertebral crush fractures have lower mean levels than age-matched normals; however, the values are not particularly low and remain within the normal range. In addition, although older patients have decreased intestinal absorption of calcium, and the administration of 1,25-dihydroxyvitamin D can reverse this abnormality, it does not reverse osteoporosis.

Other Metabolic Bone Diseases

Osteomalacia typically presents with bone pain, often in the back and may be associated with a cod fish spine on X-ray. The differential diagnosis from osteoporosis may be difficult, if routine testing of calcium homeostasis is not abnormal, and may require bone biopsy. A wide variety of conditions predispose to osteomalacia (e.g. dietary deficiency, malabsorption, anticonvulsant medication, chronic renal diseases and chronic liver disease especially after transplantation); often osteoporosis and osteomalacia coexist (Fairney 1983). Rarely, Paget's disease of bone (osteitis deformans) may cause compression of the spinal cord or nerve roots though involvement of the skull is more usual (Fairney 1983).

Cancer

Primary

Of the three common primary malignant tumours of bone (myeloma, osteosarcoma and Ewing's sarcoma), only myeloma typically affects the spine. Osteosarcoma and Ewing's sarcoma affect the metaphyseal areas of long bones (Schajowicz and Araujo 1983). Myeloma has a particular propensity to affect the spine where it may cause diffuse osteopenia and vertebral collapse or cause epidural compression due to florid focal activity.

Secondary

Pathology

The skeleton, and in particular the vertebral column, is the third commonest site for distant metastases after lung and liver (Boland et al. 1982). This conclusion is based on autopsy data which may underestimate the real incidence of bony metastases (BMs), as it is rare to examine all vertebrae (Fornasier and Czitrom 1978). Jaffe's (1958) study showed that, of all patients with cancer 70% had BMs though only 30% had clinically evident BMs; he found that 10% of all cancer patients had pathological vertebral fractures from BMs, half of whom had a compressive myelopathy. The commonest site for BMs was the thoracic spine and the body of each vertebra was more often affected than were the arches, pedicles or spines. Radiological assessment tends also to underestimate the true incidence of BMs as 50% of trabecular bone must be destroyed before loss is discernible by conventional radiographic techniques (Edelestyn et al. 1967).

The commonest tumour types encountered have been breast, bronchus and lymphoma (Gilbert et al. 1978; Boland et al. 1982) though other tumours have a predilection for the spine (e.g. myeloma and prostatic carcinoma). Tumours of the gastrointestinal (GI) tract are seen more frequently than expected as they are common tumours. Gilbert et al. (1978) analysed 235 patients with surgically managed spinal cord compression due to malignant disease at the Memorial Sloan Kettering Cancer Center, New York over a nine-year period. Primary intraspinal tumours (sarcomata) accounted for 9% of cases and metastatic disease for the rest (breast 20%, lung 13%, lymphoma 11%, prostate 9%, kidney 7%, myeloma 4%, melanoma 3%, GI 4%, female reproductive tumour 2%, embryonal cell carcinoma 2%, neuroblastoma 2%). About 68% of tumours were in the thoracic spine though this figure was skewed by the high incidence of breast metastases. In none of their cases did they report intramedullary deposits; these are 20 times less common than epidural deposits (Edelson et al. 1972).

Tumours of breast and bronchus metastaisize preferentially to the spine (Gilbert et al. 1978) and this may be related to the system of valveless vertebral veins which communicate with intercostal and lumbar veins (Batson 1940). This anatomical feature is well recognized in the pelvis and accounts for the high incidence of vertebral metastases from prostatic carcinoma (Fornasier and Czitrom 1978). It is suggested that marantic emboli enter the vertebral venous system, particularly during periods of raised intra-abdominal pressure, such as coughing. This has been demonstrated experimentally by the injection of rat femoral veins with malignant cells. Normally 100% of metastases are pulmonary; however, with 15–60 seconds light abdominal pressure vertebral metastases become frequent (Coman and Delong 1951).

Clinical Presentation

Although osteoporotic vertebral collapse in the thoracic spine may be asymptomatic, pathological fractures due to BMs presented with severe local pain in 216 of 235 cases in one series (Gilbert et al. 1978). It was a constant severe pain, exacerbated by coughing or sneezing and was noticed particularly when rolling over in bed at night. Metastases in the cervical (72%) or lumbar spine (90%) were more commonly associated with a radiculopathy than those in the thoracic spine (55%) and the site of the pain usually localized the tumour accurately (Gilbert et al. 1978). Radiculopathy in the thoracic spine tended to be bilateral. Occasionally, pain was more diffuse (32%) but passive neck manipulation (cervical tumours), local percussion (thoracic tumours) and straight leg raising (lumbosacral tumours) help localize the site of the lesion clinically. Myelopathy developed after the onset of pain in all but two of this series; however, only 77% complained of weakness at presentation. Sensory and autonomic features developed subsequently, being present at the initial examination in 51% and 57% respectively. Gait ataxia, an unusual clinical manifestation, was seen in 9% of cases and was the main presenting complaint, in the absence of sensory or motor features, in only two patients (Gilbert et al. 1978).

   Plain radiographs of the spine may be normal at a time when a bone scan is abnormal but usually they show an absent pedicle and a mixture of lytic and sclerotic lesions; the apperances in myeloma, lymphoma or highly anaplastic tissue are predominantly lytic whereas those in Hodgkin's disease, prostatic carcinoma and carcinoid tumour are predominantly sclerotic. A bone scan shows multiple deposits in 90% of cases. In the presence of myelopathy further investigation either by myelography and CT or by MRI is essential. The latter is non-invasive, shows the entire length of the vertebral canal, demonstrates paraspinal and epidural disease more clearly and is preferable; when compared with myelography/CT it provided additional information in 13 of 22 patients (Smoker et al. 1987).

Treatment

Management of spinal cord compression due to malignant disease poses a significant problem as a one-year survival rate of 30% is not unusual (Gilbert et al. 1978). The most important criterion defining outcome has been the extent of neurological deficit at presentation and the speed of appropriate referral (Findlay 1984). In the series of Gilbert et al. (1978), 15% of cases were paraplegic at the time of diagnosis, half of whom had had a precipitate course. In none of these was a haemorrhagic tumour found at operation, none improved after surgery and it was assumed that cord infarction had occurred. It is therefore important to initiate therapy as early as possible. Establishing that vertebral collapse is due to a malignant condition and not due to a metabolic bone disease or infective osteomyelitis may require biopsy. This can be done via a percutaneous route in the absence of cord compromise. However, if there is a myelopathy, then a more aggressive approach is indicated.

There was a vogue for decompressive laminectomy but the results of this approach proved singularly disappointing (Findlay 1984). Brice and McKissock (1965) noted that no patient with a severe neurological deficit and vertebral collapse improved after laminectomy and Findlay (1987) analysing 37 patients with a myelopathy due to malignant vertebral collapse found that laminectomy was associated with a significant neurological deterioration in 18 and improvement in one. Laminectomy has therefore fallen into disfavour and other treatment regimes have evolved.

Based on experimental work in the rodent, Posner's group in New York initiated treatment with radiotherapy alone (Ushio et al. 1977). After a phase of pulsed, high-dose dexamethasone therapy which substantially ameliorated pain, they gave an initially intense burst of local radiotherapy followed a few days later by a maintenance course. Their results were slightly better than those from surgery and radiotherapy and as a result radiotherapy alone became the standard treatment for metastatic disease of the spine (Greenberg et al. 1980).

However, surgical therapy may often be necessary for tissue diagnosis or in the face of clinical deterioration despite radiotherapy. As spinal instability had occurred following posterior surgical approaches and recalling experience from the management of chronic osteomyelitis, anterior decompression with or without stabilization was investigated (Siegal and Seigal 1985; Moore and Uttley 1989, Sundaresan et al. 1991). Although a 30% postoperative mortality from the chest complications of thoracotomy (pneumonia and pulmonary emboli) was reported, the ability to walk returned in one series for 10 of 16 patients who could not walk preoperatively. This improvement was maintained till death an average of 7 months later (Moore and Uttley 1989). With the better surgical results of the anterior approach, Sundaresan et al. (1991) in a prospective study suggest that a combined surgical and radiotherapy approach is the current management of choice.

Infection

Pyogenic Osteomyelitis

Osteomyelitis develops following septicaemia and tends to involve two adjacent vertebrae and a vertebral disc. This is due to the embryological origin of the arterial supply; a single segmental artery supplies the lower half of one vertebra and the upper half of the next vertebra. As a result, disc space narrowing is common. This radiographic finding is important in differentiating osteomyelitis from malignant collapse.

It is commoner in children than adults (Waldvogel et al. 1970); however, bacterial seeding in this group is to the actively growing ends of long bones. In one study of osteomyelitis there was involvement of the femur or humerus in 63%, the tibia in 19% and the vertebrae in 19% (Waldvogel et al. 1970). A bimodal age distribution was observed, the first peak in childhood and a second peak in the sixth decade; a high proportion of patients in the second peak had vertebral osteomyelitis. Seeding in these cases seems to be to the richly vascularized bone of the vertebral end plates (Waldvogel and Vasey 1980).

Patients complain of constant spinal pain, exacerbated by mechanical manoeuvres, that has been present for weeks or months. Although they may be afebrile with normal peripheral white blood cell count, the ESR is usually markedly elevated, particularly in pyogenic infections (Harris 1983). Plain radiographs of the spine may be unhelpful as several weeks are necessary before bone changes are seen in vertebral osteomyelitis. Radionuclide bone scanning is more effective in the early detection of bony lesions (Boland et al. 1982).

An unequivocal source of infection is found in 40% of cases with pyogenic and mycobacterial infection. This is slightly less than in acute spinal epidural abscess, and has a different topography (Ross and Fleming 1976). Thus, in order of frequency, infection may be derived from the genitourinary tract, the skin and the respiratory tract. *Staphylococcus aureus* is the commonest organism accounting for 60% of identified cases but Enterobacteriaceae are more prominent than in acute spinal epidural abscess (Sapico and Montgomerie 1979; Waldvogel and Vasey 1980) and in the veretebral osteomyelitis of drug abusers Gram-negative aerobic bacilli account for 92% of infections (Sapico and Montgomerie 1980). *Pseudomonas* infection can occur, being observed most commonly in heroin addicts (Kaufman et al. 1980; Waldvogel and Vasey 1980). Occasionally unusual organisms are encountered. For example, *Brucella abortus* is a well-recognized cause of subacute, pyogenic vertebral osteomyelitis in the Middle East and 12% of cases develop signs of cord compression (Harris 1983; Cordero and Sanchez 1991); fungal species may affect patients with diabetes, impaired immunity or those who abuse intravenous drugs. Fungal osteomyelitis occurs in less than 1% of patients with candidaemia and has a predilection for the spine (Harmon 1984).

Untreated, the osteitis leads to vertebral collapse and angulation with progressive deformity. Infection may spread to adjacent tissue, and, if partially treated, may lead to chronic osteomyelitis which may result in anaemia and secondary amyloidosis. Confirmation that vertebral collapse is due to infection requires tissue and in the absence of neurological phenomena this may be undertaken by needle biopsy of the infected vertebra. Bed rest and antibiotics while monitoring spinal pain and the ESR are the mainstays of therapy for acute vertebral osteomyelitis and, as cortical bone is thin, sequestrum formation is uncommon in pyogenic osteomyelitis (Harris 1983). As a result surgical management is rarely necessary. However, if chronic osteomyelitis develops or it becomes necessary surgically to debride necrotic tissue, an anterior approach is used though fixation by bone graft is usually unnecessary (Harris 1983).

Vertebral Osteomyelitis due to Tuberculosis

The spine is involved in about 50% of patients with bone and joint tuberculosis and is complicated by kyphoscoliosis which may lead to respiratory difficulties, and by paraplegia (Harris 1983). It is commoner in young adults and in the third world. Paraplegia occurs in about 20% of patients with spinal tuberculosis (Tuli 1975). It is associated with a greater tendency to local spread, e.g. psoas abscess, sinus formation and epidural abscess (Kaufman et al. 1980). Paraplegia may be either early when it is related to an expanding mass of infective tissue, or late when either the infection has been rekindled or chronic deformity has caused slowly progressive damage due to mechanical factors. Paraplegia due to the latter cause tends to respond poorly to surgical intervention though some improvement even after two years of paraplegia may occur. The best results are seen with anterior decompression and fixation by bone grafts or mechanical prostheses (MRC 1982).

References

Batson OV (1940) The function of the vertebral veins and their role in the spread of metastases. Ann Sug 112:138

Boland PJ, Lane JM, Sundaresan N (1982) Metastatic disease of the spine. Clin Orthop 169:95–102

Brice J, McKissock W (1965) Surgical treatment of malignant extradural spinal tumours. Br Med J i:1341–1344

Coman DR, Delong RP (1951) The role of the vertebral venous system in metastasis of cancer to the spinal column: experiments with tumour cell suspensions in rats and rabbits. Cancer 4:610–618

Cordero M, Sanchez I (1991) Brucellar and tubercular spondylitis: a comparative study of their clinical features. J Bone Joint Surg 73B:100–103

Edelestyn GA, Gillespie PJ, Grebbell FS (1967) The radiological demonstration of osseous metastases: experimental observations. Clin Radiol 18:158–162

Edelson RN, Deck MDF, Posner JB (1972) Intramedullary spinal cord metastases: clinical and radiographic findings in 9 cases. Neurology 22:1222–1231

Fairney A (1983) Metabolic bone disease. In: Harris NH (ed) Postgraduate textbook of clinical orthopaedics. Wright, Bristol, pp 307–338

Findlay GFG (1984) Adverse effects of the surgical management of malignant spinal cord compression. J Neurol Neurosurg Psychiatry 47:761–768

Findlay GFG (1987) The role of vertebral body collapse in the management of malignant spinal cord compression. J Neurol Neurosurg Psychiatry 50:151–154

Fornasier VL, Czitrom AA (1978) Collapsed vertebrae a review of 659 autopsies. Clin Orthop 131:261–265

Gilbert RN, Kim JH, Posner JB (1978) Epidural spinal cord compression from metastatic tumour: diagnosis and treatment. Ann Neurol 3:40–51

Greenberg HS, Kim JH, Posner JB (1980) Epidural spinal cord compression from metastatic tumour: results with a new treatment protocol. Ann Neurol 8:361–366

Harmon DC (1984) Case records of the Massachussets General Hospital. N Engl J Med 311:455–462

Harris NH (1983) Bone and joint infections In: Harris NH (ed) Postgraduate textbook of clinical orthopaedics. Wright, Bristol, pp 339–396

Heywood AWB, Meyers OL (1986) Rheumatoid arthritis of the thoracic and lumbar spine. J Bone Joint Surg 68B:362–368

Jaffe WL (1958) Tumors and tumorous conditions of bones and joints. Lea and Febiger, Philadelphia

Kaneda K Asano S Hashimoto T Satoh S Fujiya M (1992) The treatment of osteoporotic-posttraumatic vertebral collapse using the Kaneda device and a bioactive ceramic vertebral prosthesis. Spine 17 (8 suppl):S295–S303

Kaufman DM, Kaplan JG, Litman N (1980) Infectious agents in spinal epidural abscesses. Neurology 30:844–850

Laredo JD Lakhhdari K Bellaiche L Hamze B Janklewicz P Tubiana JM (1995) Acute vertebral collapse CT findings in benign and malignant non-traumatic cases. Radiology 194:41–48

Medical Research Council working party on tuberculosis of the spine (1982) A 10 year assessment of a controlled trial comparing debridement and anterior spinal fusion in the management of tubercolosis of the spine in patients on standard chemotherapy in Hong Kong. J Bone Joint Surg 64B:393–401

Parfitt J Duncan AM (1982) Metabolic bone disease affecting the spine In: Rothman RH Simeone FA (eds) The Spine Vol II, 2nd edn. WB Saunders, Philadelphia, pp 828–830

Moore AJ, Uttley D (1989) Anterior decompression and stabilization of the spine in malignant disease. Neurosurgery 24:713–717

Raisz LG (1988) Local and systemic factors in the pathogenesis of osteoporosis. N Engl J Med 318:818–828

Roberts WA (1988) Pyogenic vertebral osteomyelitis of a lumbar facet joint with associated epidural abscess: a case report with a review of the literature. Spine 13:948–952

Ross PM, Fleming J (1976) Vertebral body osteomyelitis: spectrum and natural history, a retrospective study of 37 cases. Clin Orthop 118:P190–198

Sapico FL, Montgomerie JZ (1979) Pyogenic vertebral osteomyelitis: report of nine cases and a review of the literature. Rev Infect Dis 1:754–776

Sapico FL, Montgomerie JZ (1980) Vertebral osteomyelitis in intravenous drug abusers: report of three cases and review of the literature. Rev Infect Dis 2:196–206

Sartoris DJ, Clopton P, Nemcek A, Dowd C, Resnick D (1986) Vertebral collapse in focal and diffuse disease: patterns of pathologic processes. Radiology 160:479–483

Schajowicz F, Araujo EH (1983) Cysts and tumours of the musculoskeletal system. In: Harris NH (ed) Postgraduate textbook of clinical orthopaedics. Wright, Bristol, pp 605–639

Schmorl G, Junghanns H (1971) The human spine in health and disease, 2nd edn. (EF Bersemann trans.) Grune and Stratton, New York

Siegal T, Seigal T (1985) Surgical decompression of anterior and posterior malignant epidural tumours compressing the spinal cord. Neurosurgery 17:424–432

Smoker WR, Godersky JC, Knutson R, Keyes WD, Norman D, Bergman W (1987) The role of MR imaging in evaluating metastatic spinal disease. AJR 149:1241

Sundaresan N, Digiacinto GV, Hughes JEO, Cafferty M, Vallejo A (1991) Treatment of neoplastic cord compression: results of a prospective study. Neurosurgery 29:645–650

Tuli SM (1975) Results of treatment of spinal tuberculosis by "middle path" regime. Br J Surg 169:29

Ushio Y, Posner R, Kim JH, Shapiro WR, Posner JB (1977) Treatment of experimental spinal cord cord compression by extradural neoplasms. J Neurosurg 47:380–390

Waldvogel FA, Vasey H (1980) Osteomyelitis: the past decade. N Engl J Med 303:360–370

Waldvogel FA, Medoff G, Swartz MN (1970) Osteomyelitis: a review of clinical features therapeutic considerations and unusual aspects. N Engl J Med 282:198–206; 316–322

Chapter 29

Spinal Epidural Abscess

J.P.R. Dick

In an editorial describing his clinical experience of spinal epidural abscess, Heusner (1948) reminds us that "… the decisive factor in the outcome of most cases is the celerity with which the first physician suspects the probable nature of the ailment and summons expert aid". On pathological grounds he recognized three presentations: (1) an acute metastatic presentation which evolves over hours to days and where the epidural abscess cavity contains frankly purulent material; (2) a subacute presentation evolving over days to weeks where the epidural abscess cavity comprises granulation tissue without significant quantities of necrotic material; (3) a chronic presentation, most often associated with osteomyelitis. The last accounted for only 10% of his series and involved a broader differential diagnosis. In more recent series (Hlavin et al. 1990; Nussbaum et al. 1992; Darouiche et al. 1992; Corboy and Price 1993) this classification has been less distinct with the acute variety predominating.

Anatomy

Infection is usually confined to the adipose tissue of the dorsal epidural space between the ligamenta flava where there is a rich venous plexus (Batson 1940). Thoracic and lumbar sites have been equally represented in most series, cervical sites being less frequent. However, with increasing abuse of intravenous drugs cervical epidural abscesses are being seen more frequently. Infection usually extends vertically over 4–5 vertebral segments and may become circumferential, reaching the anterior epidural compartment, particularly in the lumbar region. Early reports commented on the rarity of extension to the anterior epidural space but Danner and Hartman (1987) observed several patients with anterior epidural collections following low back surgery. The dura mater limits the further spread of sepsis and subdural or intraspinal abscesses are unusual (Fraser et al. 1973; D'Angelo and Whisler 1978); however, epidural infection can spread to the paravertebral muscles or subcutaneous tissues if left untreated (Dandy 1926). Paradoxically, autopsy studies often fail to show substantial compression of the cord and histological examination shows pan-necrosis with little or no inflammatory response suggesting infarction rather than infection (Hassin 1928); this mechanism probably accounts for the precipitate course of the myelopathy.

Clinical Presentation

Acute Metastatic Epidural Abscess

This is the commonest syndrome in most series (Heusner 1948; Hancock 1973; Baker et al. 1975; Danner and Hartman 1987; Hlavin et al. 1990; Nussbaum et al. 1992; Darouiche et al. 1992) and requires the greatest speed of clinical response. Several authors describe a typical clinical progression of initial backache, often with radicular radiation, followed by myelopathic symptoms; however, errors of initial diagnosis are not infrequent (Heusner 1948; Hancock 1973; Baker et al. 1975; Danner and Hartman 1987; Darouiche et al. 1992). Typically, the patient presents with exquisite localized back pain associated with tenderness to percussion; in 2 of 39 cases reported by Baker et al. (1975) its severity was great enough to be associated with a florid behavioural syndrome leading, erroneously, to a psychiatric diagnosis. Epidural abscesses in the lumbar region may be associated with severe local and radicular pain but little neurological symptomatology (Adams and Victor 1989) and can be confused with musculoskeletal pain or disc prolapse. However, the presence of headache with neck stiffness and the systemic signs of sepsis, such as an elevated temperature, ESR and peripheral white blood cell count should help differentiate these conditions. Other alternative diagnoses have been recorded, particularly intra-abdominal sepsis and transverse myelitis (Findlay 1987). The latter usually prompts urgent radiological investigation and is not often as painful as an epidural collection of pus nor is it associated with such striking local tenderness. Although severe abdominal pain and the systemic features of sepsis may simulate an intra-abdominal abscess, abdominal examination usually differentiates an epidural from an intra-abdominal abscess. By the second or third day of the illness, a recognizable clinical syndrome will have evolved with radicular pain in the absence of a vesicular rash and root signs and investigation (radiological and bacteriological) should be undertaken urgently.

Plain radiographs of the spine are usually normal and urgent MR scanning and/or myelography should be undertaken. Since infection is usually confined to the dorsal epidural space, spinal puncture may be hazardous and is best undertaken by an experienced radiologist. There is usually a complete block to the flow of dye at the upper border of the abscess and in order to delineate the upper and lower limit of the abscess, a second spinal puncture may be necessary. However, in view of the risks and the difficulty of such a puncture in a patient with rigid paraspinal muscles, MR imaging is currently the preferred method of investigation (Angutaco et al. 1987). CSF is abnormal and this will help differentiate an epidural abscess from osteomyelitis where it is normal (Darouiche et al, 1992). Typically there is an elevated protein concentration with a modest lymphocytic pleocytosis and a normal sugar. If the sugar is depressed an associated meningitis should be suspected.

Once the diagnosis has been made, urgent neurosurgical intervention should be undertaken to avoid clinical progression and for bacteriological confirmation.

Clinical deterioration may occur at any time and the patient will suddenly develop an ascending paralysis with double incontinence. The interval between presentation and the onset of myelopathy in Hancock's (1973) series of 49 patients ranged from 1 to 23 days and in Darouiche's series was as short as hours in two patients. This change may be precipitous and once spinal cord damage has occurred is irreversible. Experimental data suggest that the early symptoms (backache, radicular pain) reflect the sequelae of local mechanical compression but later complications (cord weakness, urinary incontinence) are associated with venous congestion and cord infarction leading to myelomalacia (Feldenzer et al. 1988).

Although the mainstay of therapy is an adequate course of antibiotics, cure of an epidural abscess can rarely be achieved without surgical drainage (Findlay 1987). As the main collection of infected tissue is likely to be posterior, laminectomy is usually performed with antiseptic irrigation of the adjacent segments by soft catheter. There is debate as to whether the wound should be closed with or without drainage. Recent series have focused on the possibility of managing patients whose neurology is relatively slight with antibiotics alone. Although, their outcome (65% ambulant, Corboy and Price 1993) is similar to those of surgical series, the latter start with more neurologically damaged individuals and in several patients precipitate declines are recorded while awaiting surgery despite full dose antibiotics (Hlavin et al. 1990; Nussbaum et al. 1992; Darouiche et al. 1992).

The acute presentation is most frequently associated with haematogenous spread of infection from a distant focus, such as a furuncle, wound infection or decubitis ulcer, though in 40% of cases no source can be identified (Danner and Hartman 1987). Characteristically, the causative organism is *Staphylococcus aureus* which can be grown from blood cultures. In 40% of cases blood cultures are negative and culture from the abscess cavity is required for bacteriological diagnosis.

Danner and Hartman (1987) point out that the incidence of spinal epidural abscesses in New York City has increased from 0.18/100 000 during the period 1971–1973 to 2.8/100 000 for the calendar year 1982. They suggest that this is not only due to the greater prevalence of intravenous drug abuse but also to the greater frequency of invasive medical procedures. A wide variety of organisms causing spinal epidural abscess have been recorded (*Staph. aureus* 103/166, aerobic streptococci 14/166, aerobic Gram-negative rods 30/166, anaerobic organisms 3/166, *Staph. epidermidis* 4/166). These infections are seen more often in the immunosuppressed population and often present subacutely. Since *Staph. aureus* is no longer the sole infecting organism as was the case in Heusner's (1948) series, they suggest that it would be prudent, pending further bacteriological data, to give antibiotic cover for Gram-negative organisms and *Staph. epidermidis* (Danner and Hartman 1987).

Subacute Osteomyelitic Epidural Abscess

This syndrome is similar but more variable than the acute syndrome. It is seen in the immunocompromised, in the diabetic and in the partially treated. The course may be protracted and merge with the chronic syndrome or may progress over two weeks merging with the acute syndrome. Baker et al. (1975) and Darouiche et al. (1992) make no distinction between acute and subacute presentations. Although the subacute patients usually present with spinal and radicular pain, and with signs suggestive of radicular and cord disease (Phillips and Jefferson 1979), diagnostic difficulties are more frequent than with the acute presentation (Darouiche et al. 1992). In their series Danner and Hartman (1987) note that, due to a toxic confusional state, several patients failed to give any history of back pain whereas in others spinal tenderness was minimal (see also Hancock 1973); thus 64% of patients had no neurologic deficit on admission and in 43% of cases the initial diagnosis was unrelated to the spine. In the series reported by Baker et al. (1975) 10 of 39 patients had an initial diagnosis unrelated to the back though 34 of 39 had root signs. One can anticipate difficulty in confused patients in whom there are no clinical or radiographic findings and in drug abusers, whose only symptom may be pain, whose only sign a mild pyrexia, and from whom a history may be unreliable. Koppel et al. (1988) describe their experience with this group of patients: they tend to have prolonged histories (1–2 months), prominent pain and little fever. As is seen in other series (Kaufman et al. 1980) there is a slight excess of patients with recent back trauma which may confound the issue. Whether the increase in incidence of epidural sepsis in drug abusers is due to impaired host immunity or due to the introduction of infection by frequent needling is not clear; the former is likely as there is an undue prevalence of cervical osteomyelitis in heroin abusers (Sapico and Montgomerie 1980). The bacteriology is similar to that seen in individuals with normal immunity (Heusner 1948) though different from that seen in the vertebral osteomyelitis of drug abusers (Sapico and Montgomerie 1980) where Gram-negative aerobic bacilli account for 92% of infections. Plain radiographs are more helpful in this group and may show disc space narrowing or end plate erosion though the latter is best appreciated on tomography. Although, radionuclide scanning can be helpful in locating the site of the abscess and its extra axial extent (Koppel et al. 1988), urgent myelography with CT scanning or MR imaging remain the investigations of choice (Berns et al. 1989). Once epidural infection has been demonstrated surgical decompression is necessary.

Chronic Epidural Abscess

This syndrome usually complicates pyogenic vertebral osteomyelitis (Findlay 1987) or tuberculous epidural cord compression (Kaufman et al. 1980). However, only 17% of patients with osteomyelitis develop neurological phenomena. This figure is similar for pyogenic osteomyelitis (Sapico and Montgomerie 1979), infection due to *Mycobacterium tuberculosis* (Waldvogel and Vasey 1980) and vertebral osteomyelitis in drug abusers (Sapico and Montgomerie 1980). By contrast, of patients with acute or subacute presentations, less than 35% had radiographic features suggestive of vertebral osteomyelitis (Baker et al. 1975; Danner and Hartman 1987).

The duration of history is usually more than 6 weeks (Heusner 1948; Kaufman et al. 1980) and patients may be relatively asymptomatic; however, once neurological complications have started they may proceed rapidly (Kaufman et al. 1980). Autopsy studies suggest thrombotic infarction of the cord occurs in these circumstances. If vertebral osteomyelitis is left untreated, osteitis may spread to involve the intervertebral disc, or the patient may develop vertebral collapse and kyphotic angulation. Waldvogel and Vasey (1980) suggest that neurological involvement in patients with tuberculous spondylitis is due to mechanical probems rather than epidural infection (chapter 28).

Confirmation of diagnosis requires tissue and in the absence of neurolgical phenomena this may be undertaken by needle biopsy of the infected vertebra; however, if epidural disease is evident, surgical intervention is usually necessary. Bed rest and antibiotics while monitoring spinal pain and the ESR are the mainstays of therapy for vertebral osteomyelitis. With neurological involvement, usually consequent to anterior epidural disease, anterior decompression with debridement is current practice; fixation is rarely necessary (Harris 1983) unless associated with tuberculous spondylitis (MRC 1982).

References

Adams RD, Victor M (1989) Principles of neurology, 4th edn. McGraw-Hill, New York, pp 168, 728

Angutaco EJC, McConnell JR, Chadduck WM, Flanigan S (1987) MR imaging of spinal epidural sepsis. AJR 149:1249–1253

Baker AS, Ojemann RG, Swartz MN, Richardson EP (1975) Spinal epidural abscess. N Engl J Med 293:463–468

Batson OV (1940) The function of the vertebral veins and their role in the spread of metastases. Ann Surg 112:138

Berns DH, Blaser SJ, Modic MT (1989) Magnetic resonance imaging of the spine. Clin Orthop 244:78–100

Corboy JR Price RW (1993) Myelitis and toxic, inflammatory and infectious disorders. Curr Opin Neurol Neurosurg 6:564–570

Dandy WE (1926) Abscesses and inflammatory tumours in the spinal epidural space (so-called pachymeningitis externa). Arch Surg 13:477–494

D'Angelo CM, Whisler WW (1978) Bacterial infection of the spinal cord and its coverings. In: Vinken PJ, Bruyn GW, Klawans HL (eds) Handbook of clinical neurology 33:187–194

Danner RL, Hartman BJ (1987) Update of epidural abscess: 35 cases and a review of the literature. Rev Infect Dis 9:265–274

Darouiche RO Hamill RJ Greenberg SB Weathers SW Musher DM (1992) Bacterial spinal epidural abscess. Review of 43 cases and literature survey. Medicine 71:369–385

Findlay (1987) Compression and vascular disorders of the spinal cord. In: Miller JD (ed) Northfields surgery of the central nervous system. Blackwell Scientific, Oxford, pp 745–748

Fraser RAR, Ratzan K, Wolpert SM, Weinstein L (1973) Spinal subdural empyema. Arch Neurol 28:235–238

Feldenzer JA McKeever PE Schaberg DR Cambell JA (1988) The pathogenesis of spinal epidural abscess: microangiopathic studies in an experimental model J Neurosurg 69:110–114

Hancock DO (1973) A study of 49 patients with acute spinal epidural abscess. Paraplegia 10:285–288

Harris NH (1983) Bone and joint infections. In: Harris NH (ed) Postgraduate textbook of clinical orthopaedics. Wright, Bristol, pp 339–396

Hassin GB (1928) Circumscribed suppurative (non-tuberculous) peripachymeningitis. Arch Neurol Psychiatry 20:110–127

Heusner AP (1948) Non tuberculous spinal epidural infections. N Engl J Med 239:845–854

Hlavin ML Kaminski HJ Ross JS Ganz E (1990) Spinal epidural abscess: a ten year perspective Neurosurgery 27:177–184

Kaufman DM, Kaplan JG, Litman N (1980) Infectious agents in spinal epidural abscesses. Neurology 30:844–850

Koppel BS, Tuchman AJ, Mangiardi JR, Daras M, Weitzner I (1988) Epidural spinal infection in drug abusers. Arch Neurol 45:1331–1337

Medical Research Council working party on tuberculosis of the spine (1982) A 10 year assessment of a controlled trial comparing debridement and anterior spinal fusion in the management of tuberculosis of the spine in patients on standard chemotherapy in Hong Kong. J Bone Joint Surg 64B:393–401

Nussbaum ES, Rigamonti D, Standiford H, Numaguchi Y, Wolf AC, Robinson WL (1992) Spinal epidural abscess: a report of 40 cases and review Surg Neurol 38:225–231

Phillips GE, Jefferson A (1979) Acute spinal epidural abscess. Observations from 14 cases. Postgrad Med J 55:712–715

Sapico FI, Montgomerie JZ (1979) Pyogenic vertebral osteomyelitis: report of nine cases and a review of the literature. Rev Infect Dis 1:754–776

Sapico FL, Montgomerie JZ (1980) Vertebral osteomyelitis in intravenous drug abusers: report of three cases and review of the literature. Rev Infect Dis 2:196–206

Waldvogel FA, Vasey H (1980) Osteomyelitis: the past decade. N Engl J Med 303:360–370

Chapter 30

Spinal Tumours

N.T. Gurusinghe

In 1753, Lecat made the first surgical attempt to remove an intraspinal tumour (Lecat 1765). Over a century later, in 1887, Sir Victor Horsley performed the first successful operation to remove a spinal intradural tumour which had caused cord compression (Horsley and Gowers 1888). In the following century significant advances were seen in the diagnosis and treatment of spinal tumours. Positive contrast myelography, computed axial tomography and magnetic resonance imaging techniques have enabled the radiological demonstration of spinal neoplasms. Safer, modern neuroanaesthesia combined with advanced microneurosurgical techniques and spinal stabilization methods have reduced the surgical morbidity and considerably improved the prognosis. This section will describe the basic pathology and special clinical features and treatment of individual spinal tumours excluding vascular malformations and tumours associated with spinal dysraphism. The methods of radiological diagnosis are mentioned only briefly as they are dealt with in Chapter 9. Treatment is outlined under the individual tumour types and special aspects emphasized in the section on management.

Incidence

Spinal tumours are less common than cerebral neoplams, the reported ratios varying from 1:4 (Nittner 1976) to 1:9 (Gudmundsson 1970). It is difficult to establish their true incidence in the general population. A population-based survey carried out in Norway revealed the annual incidence of primary intraspinal neoplasms as five per million for females and three per million for males (Helseth and Mork 1989).

The relative frequency of different types of spinal tumour in a reported series is not necessarily an index of the natural order in the population, the figures being biased by the local patterns of case referral as well as the criteria of patient selection of the neurosurgical department concerned. Table 30.1 compares the conclusions of a comprehensive review of 29 series by Nittner (1976) with to two large series within that analysis (Sloof et al. 1964; Nittner 1968). The inclusion or exclusion of paediatric patients and/or those with spinal metastatic tumours are factors which determine the variations in incidence figures.

Table 30.1. Incidence of adult spinal tumours. Nittner (1976) devised a composite analysis of 29 published series of primary and metastatic tumours including those of Sloof' (1964) and Nittner (1968). Helseth's series contained primary spinal tumours only but included children. The author's series analyzed intradural tumours in a predominantly adult population

	Incidence (%)				
	Sloof (1964) 1322 cases	Nittner (1968) 513 cases	Nittner (1976) 4885 cases	Helseth (1989) 467 cases	Gurusinghe and Perera (1994) 141 cases
Extradural metastasis	None	9	6	None	None
Sarcoma	12	8	8	None	None
Intradural Extramedullary					
Schwannoma	29	21	23	11	43
Meningioma	26	22	22	47	32
Intramedullary					
Astrocytoma	22	9	13	32	5
Ependymoma		6	3		5
Vascular tumours and Angiomas	6	7	7	4	3
Others	5	18	18	6	12

As cancer is a common disease and the spine is the commonest site of cancer spread, metastatic tumours are the most common neoplasms of the spine encountered in clinical practice. About 10% of cancer patients develop symptomatic spinal metastases.

The incidence of paediatric spinal tumours is discussed later in the chapter.

Classification

The traditional method is to divide spinal tumours according to their anatomical relationship to the dura and spinal cord.

1. Extradural
   (a) Primary tumours of the axial skeleton
   (b) Metastatic tumours
2. Intradural
   (a) Extramedullary, i.e. situated outside the cord
   (b) Intramedullary, i.e. situated inside the cord
3. Transdural – these tumours occupy the extradural and intradural spaces
4. Juxtamedullary – these tumours are situated within and without the cord.

Metastatic tumour, myeloma and lymphoma are very frequent causes of extradural spinal cord compression encountered in clinical practice. Meningioma and schwannoma are the most frequently encountered intradural extramedullary neoplasms. Astrocytoma and ependymoma are the commonest of the intra-

Table 30.2. Classification of spinal neural tumours (adapted from WHO system)

Type of tissue	Examples of tumour
1. Neuroepithelial	Astrocytoma, ependymoma, oligodendroglioma, ganglioglioma, neuroblastoma
2. Nerve sheath cells	Schwannoma, neurofibroma
3. Meninges and related tissue	Meningioma
4. Lymphocytes	Malignant lymphoma
5. Blood vessels	Haemangioblastoma
6. Germ cells	Teratoma
7. Malformative tumours and tumour like lesions	Epidermoid cyst, Dermoid cyst, Enterogenous cyst, Lipoma
8. Vascular malformations	Cavernous haemangioma, Arteriovenous malformation
9. Notochord	Chordoma
10. Chemodectomas	Paraganglioma
11. Metastatic tumours	Carcinoma, lymphoma
12. Unclassified tumours	

medullary tumours. The best example of a transdural tumour is the schwannoma. Haemangioblastoma and true lipomas of the cord are usually intramedullary but may encroach on to the surface. A more detailed clinical frequency classification will be given under each category later.

In 1990, The World Health Organisation (WHO) agreed a system of histological typing of central nervous system (CNS) tumours based on the tissue or origin of the tumour (Zulch 1979). Table 30.2 shows a classification adapted from the WHO system indicating the position of common neoplasms of CNS origin encountered in the spinal canal.

Radiological Diagnosis

A brief general account of the available radiological methods and possible findings will be helpful prior to the description of individual tumour types. The area to be studied must be determined by a careful clinical examination. Also, it is a very wise practice to view the examinations with the radiologist and correlate the clinical and radiological findings. It is important to remember that the site of a spinal tumour is identified according to the vertebral level ("Radiological level").

Plain radiographs of the spine are very useful when investigating a malignant spinal neoplasm because the axial skeleton is invariably affected by the disease. It may reveal wedge collapse or pathological fractures of the vertebral body and/or erosion of the pedicles caused by extradural metastatic disease. By contrast the chances of finding a diagnostic abnormality are much reduced in benign tumours which produce changes in the skeleton only in the late stages when the lesion is large. Intradural tumours including intramedullary tumours may cause enlargement of the canal diameter with scalloping of the posterior vertebral border, widening of the interpedicular distance and erosion of the pedicles. Calcification of the neoplasm is a very useful clue if seen on plain films. A dumb-bell neurofibroma will expand

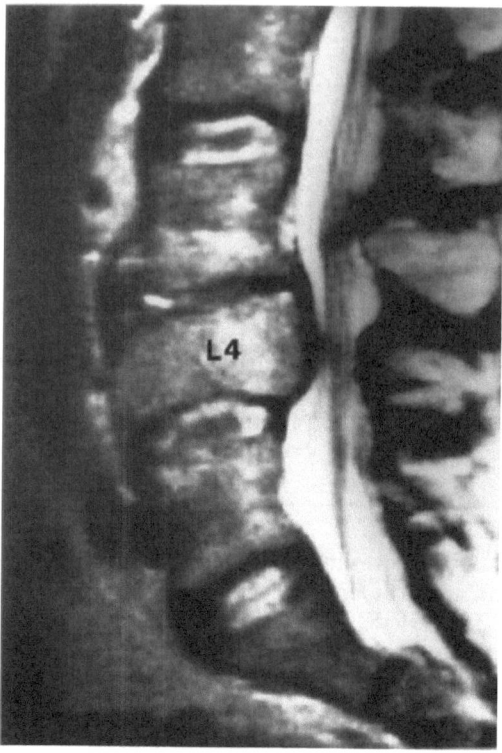

Fig. 30.1. MR scan (T2 image) of lumbar region demonstrating an extradural tumour involving the body of the L4 vertebra causing compression of the cauda equina (diagnosis: myeloma). The patient was a 65-year-old man who presented with low back pain and right anterior thigh pain (L4 root pain).

the intervertebral foramen and is best seen in oblique views. Congenital vertebral abnormalities are associated with intradural dermoid and epidermoid cysts, lipomas and enterogenous cysts. It behoves the clinician to proceed to more detailed imaging techniques when the clinical suspicion of a tumour is present.

An X-ray of the chest is essential, especially in the investigation of metastatic disease.

Magnetic resonance imaging (MRI) is the most convenient and non-invasive method of studying the entire length of the spine and spinal cord. It has superseded myelography and CT as the investigation of choice and can be performed as an out-patient with excellent results in detecting extradural or intradural tumours (Figs 30.1–30.3). The ability to view the spine in the sagittal and coronal planes enables MRI to identify the relationship of the tumour to the cord. The T2 weighted scans depict CSF as a hyperdense signal similar to the contrast-filled subarachnoid space seen in myelography. MRI is by far the best method to detect the morphological anatomy of intramedullary neoplasms. The site and extent of solid and cystic components are demonstrated extremely well by this method. Paramagnetic substances (gadolinium) injected intravenously will enhance the signal from the solid component. Some patients require sedation or general anaesthesia as they are unable to tolerate the noise and the confined space of the scanning chamber.

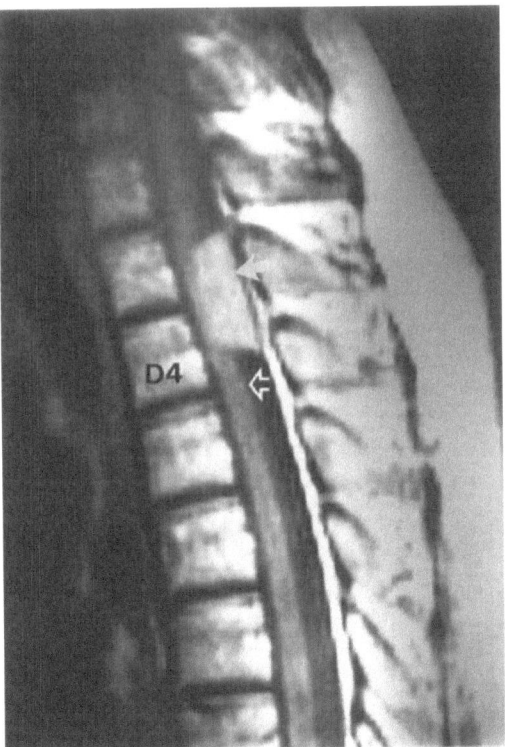

Fig. 30.2. MR scan (T1 post-gadolinium image) demonstrating a posteriorly placed intradural extramedullary meningioma (*solid arrow*) at D3/4 causing severe compression of the spinal cord (*open arrow*). The patient was a 30-year-old woman presenting with a spastic paraparesis and initially diagnosed as suffering from multiple sclerosis.

Conventional myelography is now performed only when MRI is not available or as an additional method of obtaining information regarding the anatomy of the tumour. The contrast medium may outline a tumour as a filling defect or the flow will become obstructed partially or completely by the tumour. The pattern of the defect can be used to identify whether the lesion is extradural, intradural/extramedullary or intramedullary in position. An intramedullary tumour causes expansion of the spinal cord with the contrast thinning out around the narrow subarachnoid gutters. The contrast is held up either completely or partially at the polar end of a tumour.

Computed tomography (CT) scans do not demonstrate the morphology of intradural tumours as well as MRI. On the other hand, the bone destruction and paravertebral extensions of extradural lesions, primary osseous tumours and calcified intradural tumours are well demonstrated on axial scans. Axial CT combined with conventional myelography (CT myelography) is very useful in indicating the relationship of a tumour to the dural sac and spinal cord if MRI cannot be performed.

Isotope bone scans demonstrate the presence of benign and malignant tumours involving the vertebral column even when they are not visualized on plain

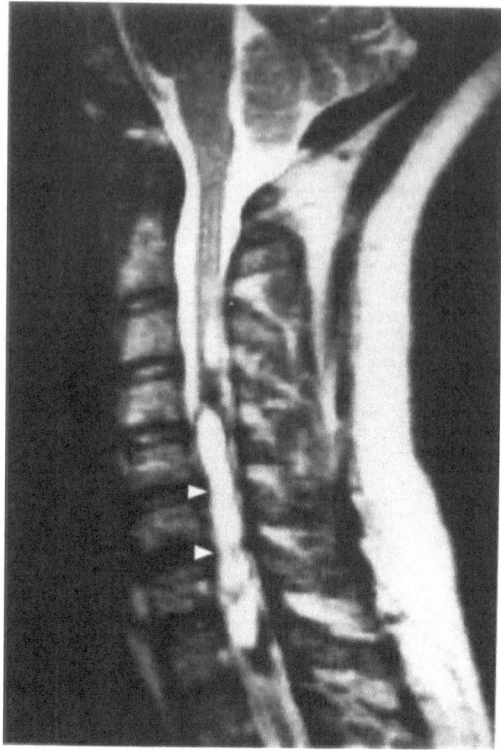

Fig. 30.3. MR scan (T2 image) of cervical intramedullary ependymoma (*arrowheads*). The patient was a 50-year-old woman presenting with walking difficulty. The tumour was completely removed at operation.

radiographs or CT scans. It is a very useful method of detecting metastatic cancer and myeloma.

Spinal angiography can be used to investigate the blood supply and venous drainage pattern of haemangioblastomas prior to undertaking surgery.

Extradural Spinal Tumours

A classification of extradural tumours according to incidence is shown in Table 30.3.

Metastatic Tumours

The spine is the commonest site for metastatic cancer. Virtually all (secondary) deposits involving the spine are situated in the extradural, vertebral/paravertebral compartments. Intradural metastatic lesions are rare except in tumours such as medulloblastoma, ependymoma and cerebral lymphoma which can produce spinal

Table 30.3. Classification of extradural tumours according to incidence

Common	Less common	Uncommon
Metastatic carcinoma	Haemangioma	Aneurysmal bone cyst
Myeloma	Chordoma	Sacrococcygeal tumours
Non-Hodgkin's lymphoma	Osteoblastoma	Primary lymphoma
	Osteochondroma	

seedlings spread by the CSF pathways. These most often lodge in the subarachnoid space of the lumbar–sacral canal due to gravitational forces.

The increased life expectancy of cancer patients has enhanced the prevalence of spinal metastatic disease. About 10% of all cancer patients develop symptomatic spinal extradural metastases but a much higher incidence is noted in those who die of cancer. Extradural malignant tumour is the commonest neoplasm encountered in the spinal epidural space. The resulting clinical syndrome of spinal cord compression is one of the commonest emergency conditions referred to a neurosurgical department.

Some tumours exhibit a selective spread into bone (osteotropism) and the common sites of primary disease are lung (17%), breast (16%), prostate (11%) and kidney (9%) but thyroid and gastrointestinal tract malignancy as well as malignant melanoma are also well-recognized sources. Lymphoma (5%) also accounts for a significant number (see below). Myeloma in the spine is grouped under metastatic lesions in most studied series and is an important cause of extradural spinal cord compression (Gilbert et al. 1978; Connolly 1982).

The commonest mode of spread into the epidural tissues is via the bloodstream, either through the arterial system or the vertebral extradural venous plexus, the latter being especially incriminated in the dissemination of prostatic cancer into the spine. Direct spread to the vertebrae can occur from mediastinal, retroperitoneal and pelvic growths. Occasionally the neoplastic cells spread from the paravertebral tissues via the intervertebral foramen into the epidural space traversing along the lymphatics and/or the perineurium.

The anatomically long thoracic region is most commonly affected (60%) followed by the lumbosacral segment (26%) and cervical region (14%). The tumour vertebral segment is involved in up to 85% but the tumour may lie entirely within the extradural space in many cases (15%). The vertebral body and pedicle are the sites commonly affected but the laminae and spinous processes can be occasionally affected. One to three contiguous vertebrae are usually diseased but multiple separate sites are common. The disc and vertebral end plates are unaffected and this is an important diagnostic feature on plain films to distinguish the bone destruction of metastatic disease from that of osteomyelitis. Wedge collapse of the vertebral body, pathological fracture, erosion of pedicles and a paraspinal soft tissue mass may be seen on plain films and scans.

In the majority of instances, the tumour mass is sited anterior, anterolateral or lateral to the spinal canal. This feature determines the direction of the compression force on the spinal cord or cauda equina. Vertebral collapse can propel a fragment of bone into the spinal canal causing further neural embarrassment. Occasionally the tumour is entirely posterior to the cord or encircles the dural sheath circumferentially. These pathological features dictate the modern surgical approaches designed to excise the tumour and decompress the neural structures.

Vertebral metastases are asymptomatic in the early stages and detected by chance or routine radiology. In 10% of patients spinal neural compression may be the initial manifestation of the malignant process the primary site being unknown at the time of first presentation with cord symptoms and may remain so even after systemic investigations (Macdonald 1990). Whilst no age is exempt, the disease is more common in the high cancer risk ages of 40–65 years. The onset of symptoms can be acute or insidious. Back pain is the commonest initial symptom and is present in virtually all patients at the time of diagnosis. Radicular pain occurs when a nerve root is compressed by tumour involving the pedicle. Spinal pain in a cancer sufferer must be considered to be due to metastatic disease until otherwise proved. Neurological symptoms commence about 6–8 weeks after onset of pain but may be earlier or later. At the time of diagnosis nearly 80% of patients have weakness, 50% have sensory symptoms and 50% sphincter dysfunction. About 50% of patients have a severe neurological disability on presentation and are unable to walk, and 15% are paraplegic. Anterior cord compression is associated with weakness and loss of spinothalamic function with preservation of posterior column sensation. The predominant loss of the latter modality signifies a posteriorly situated tumour mass. When the cord compression is in a lateral direction the neurological deficits are symmetrical and a Brown–Séquard pattern is recognized. With an acute onset of paralysis (i.e. within 24 hours) flaccidity may be a feature even though the cord itself is affected. The neurological findings depend on the spinal region affected and conform to the general description given earlier in this chapter. In 20% of patients neurological deterioration occurs during the time between diagnosis and definitive treatment.

In addition to the radiological investigations mentioned previously, the ESR, serum protein, electrophoresis, serum acid phosphatase and bone marrow biopsy will yield very useful diagnostic information. Treatment is by surgical decompression and/or biopsy combined with radiotherapy and/or chemotherapy.

Lymphoma

The lymphomas can be classified into three types:

1. Primary central nervous system lymphoma
2. Systemic non-Hodgkin's lymphoma
   (a) Nodular type
   (b) Diffuse type
3. Hodgkin's lymphoma

Primary Central Nervous System Lymphoma (PCNSL)

There is no true lymph tissue within the brain or spinal cord. Primary CNS lymphoma was an uncommon disease but is being diagnosed more frequently due to the increasing incidence of immune deficiency states. It is the second commonest tumour of the CNS in patients with AIDS. Probably the commonest effect of lymphoma on the CNS is a paraneoplastic syndrome without the presence of a true neoplasm. PCNSL arises from the microglial cells which are the equivalent of lymphoreticular cells elsewhere. The tumour occurs in multiple sites within the CNS and is much more common in the brain than in the spinal cord. Occurrence is commoner in immune deficiency states (congenital or acquired) and an association with Epstein–Barr virus infection has also been recognized. The tumours represent proliferating B cells of the immune system in the absence of T-cell suppression which is normally present. Spinal tumours can occur either as intrameduallary tumours which expand the cord or as diffuse meningeal seedlings from a cerebral lymphoma (Hochberg and Millar 1988). They cause weakness and sensory symptoms in the lower limbs. The lesions can be detected on MRI scans. It is unusual to find evidence of lymphoma elswhere in the viscera or lymph nodes. The CSF may show lymphoma cells on careful cytological examination. There is a dramatic clinical and radiological improvement with corticosteroids. The tumour is radiosensitive.

Systemic Non-Hodgkin's Lymphoma (SNHL)

This type primarily involves viscera, bone marrow and lymph nodes. It occurs mostly unrelated to PCNSL but the two can coexist. SNHL incorporates tumours previously called giant follicular lymphoma, lymphosarcoma, reticulum cell sarcoma and lymphoblastic lymphoma. Foci of intramedullary parenchymatous lymphoma occur rarely in the spinal cord. A diffuse lymphomatous leptomeningitis may cause the spinal nerve roots to become thickened. Of SNHL cases 5% are associated with extradural spinal tumours which invariably cause cord compression. (Grant et al. 1986). The tumour may be confined to the extradural space with no evidence of vertebral involvement in two thirds of patients.

The "metastatic" origin of the lymphoma in the extradural space is disputed. There is no well-recognized lymph tissue in the extradural compartment. The tumour may arrive by haemotogenous spread into the fat or from direct extension of adjacent vertebral disease. Paravertebral lymphoma may extend into the spinal canal via the foramen (Haddad et al. 1976). In a few instances (termed primary spinal epidural lymphoma) there is no evidence of visceral or nodal disease and the extradural tumour is the only manifestation of lymphoma. Systemic involvement can develop later but cord compression is the first sign of the disorder. SNHL is usually histologically different from PCNSL. The tumour does not occur in the intradural space. The clinical and radiological features are those typical of extradural cord and nerve root compression. In extradural lymphoma the vertebral involvement may be confined to the laminae and spinous process rather than to the vertebral body. MRI is an excellent method of diagnosis.

SNHL has a relatively good prognosis because the tumour is often of low grade malignancy and is radiosensitive. This emphasizes the importance of establishing a histological diagnosis by biopsy in any unknown neoplastic cause of extradural cord compression. Treatment is by surgical decompression or biopsy combined with steroids and radiotherapy.

Neural compression from an extradural metastatic tumour can occur in Hodgkin's lymphoma. It is always secondary to disease in the vertebrae, mediastinum or retroperitoneal lymph nodes.

Vertebral Myeloma and Solitary Plasmacytoma

Neoplasms of the mature immunoglobulin secreting B lymphocyte are characterized by destructive (osteolytic) bone lesions. They include a number of diseases grouped under the term "Plasma cell dyscrasias". These can be divided into two types depending on the presence or absence of bone involvement. The former constitute conditions such as benign monoclonal gammopathy and Waldenstrom's macroglobulinaemia. The second group consists of solitary plasmacytoma of bone and multiple myeloma.

Solitary Plasmacytoma of Bone (SPB) is a tumour of plasma cells in the bone marrow within the bone affected. It is commoner in men around the sixth decade. The spine is affected in up to 50% of patients. Midline spinal and radicular pain is followed by neurological symptoms due to spinal compression. The osteolytic lesions can be demonstrated on CT and MRI scans. Abnormal paraproteins may be present in the blood but considerably less than in multiple myeloma. (Wiltshaw 1976). A percutaneous or open biopsy of the bone lesion may be required to confirm the diagnosis. Light microscopy reveals well and poorly differentiated plasma cells.

Multiple myeloma is caused by malignant proliferation of plasma cells chiefly in the bone marrow. It spreads to the adjacent bone and then to other bones, blood and viscera in the later stages. It involves marrow containing parts of the skeleton such as the spine, skull, sternum and ribs. Neoplastic cells produce a variety of abnormal paraproteins (including Bence-Jones protein) which can be detected in the serum and/or urine. It occurs in adults around the sixth to seventh decade and affects men and women with equal frequency. Midline back pain and radicular pain are the common initial symptoms when the spine is affected. The affected bone undergoes osteolytic change and pathological fractures occur causing severe back pain due to wedge collapse of vertebrae. The tumour mass can extend into the spinal canal by direct extension and is a well recognized cause of malignant extradural spinal cord compression. The lower dorsal and lumbar segments are more often affected. The lesions can be detected on plain radiographs, isotope bone scans, CT and MRI (Fig. 30.1). The condition is associated with anaemia, markedly elevated ESR, uraemia, proteinaemia and hypercalcaemia. The degree of systemic involvement is expressed by a staging system (Durie and Salmon 1975). The diagnosis can be confirmed by bone marrow examination.

Treatment of SPB and myeloma consists of a combination of surgical decompression of the cord, local radiotherapy and systemic chemotherapy. Surgical decompression is indicated when progressive neurological deterioration is evident with radiological features of spinal compression. Stabilization of the spine may be neces-

Table 30.4. Tumours and "tumour-like" conditions of the spinal column

Benign	Malignant	"Tumour-like" conditions
Enchondroma	Metastases (carcinoma)	Vertebral haemangioma
Osteochondroma	Lymphoma	Aneurysmal bone cyst
Osteoid osteoma	Myeloma: solitary/multiple	Eosinophilic granuloma
Osteoblastoma	Chordoma	
Chondroblastoma	Osteosarcoma	
Giant cell tumour	Chondrosarcoma	
	Ewing's sarcoma	
	Fibrous histiocytoma	

sary following the decompression or due to vertebral instability caused by the disease. SPB is a very radiosensitive tumour and may be successfully treated entirely with radiotherapy if detected early. The treatment of multiple myeloma is determined according to the stage of the disease and consists of excision (total or partial), combined with radiotherapy and chemotherapy. The most effective are cyclophosphamide, BCNU, CCNU and melphalan. Despite treatment, the average survival after diagnosis is about two years.

Tumours of Spinal Column

Tumours arising primarily from the vertebrae can be benign or malignant (Table 30.4). Primary osseous tumours whether benign or malignant are important causes of back pain in adults, adolescents and children. Certain conditions, e.g., aneurysmal bone cyst, benign osteoblastoma, Ewing's sarcoma and eosinophilic granuloma are commoner in the younger age groups. The likelihood of a neoplasm involving the vertebrae must always be considered in patients with persistent undiagnosed back pain. Most of the tumours have characteristic plain x-ray appearances but are better demonstrated with MRI, CT or isotope bone scans the last being a particularly good screening test for both benign and malignant vertebral neoplasms. Whilst the vertebral body is the commonest part afffected, pedicles, laminae, spines and transverse processes can be involved. With continued growth these tumours can extend to the spinal canal or intervertebral foramen and cause extradural neural compression. Primary bone tumours are usually the province of the orthopaedic surgeon but when the spine is involved and neurological features are present, a combined orthopaedic and neurosurgical team effort is essential. A few common examples are described below.

Vertebral Haemangioma

This is one of the commonest primary tumours affecting the spinal column. It is usually sited in the dorsal or lumbar region. Most are asymptomatic discovered incidentally on a radiograph or at autopsy. The tumour is commoner in women over 40 years of age. Usually, only a single vertebra is involved and the disc is unaffected pathologically and radiologically. It is a cavernous haemangioma, effectively an arteriovenous shunt fed by the intercostal and lumbar arteries. All the components of the vertebra can be affected. The clinical presentation is back pain, paraparesis or radicular symptoms. The typical plain radiograph appearance consists of vertical trabeculae (honeycomb appearance) in the vertebral body which is reduced in height but has preserved end plates. The lesion is detected on CT, MRI and angiography. Asymptomatic lesions can be kept under observation. Radiotherapy has been a traditional treatment for symptomatic lesions and is effective in reducing the size of the lesion. Excision can be hazardous due to the intense vascularity of the tumour. Preoperative embolization of the tumour mass with small particles helps to reduce the blood flow facilitating surgical removal. Vertebral body replacement and other stabilization methods are necessary to maintain alignment and stability after tumour resection.

Chordoma

The notochord appears in the fourth week of embryonic life and the spinal column develops almost entirely from condensations of mesenchyme formed around the notochord. This tumour arises from remnants of primitive notochord and is a slow growing, locally invasive malignant tumour which can extend into the extradural space causing cord compression (Sundaresan et al. 1979). They account for about 20% of malignant primary tumours of bone. The majority of spinal chordomas occur in the sacrococcygeal region but other parts of the spine can be affected. It has recently been recognized to have the capacity to metastasize to distant sites.

Despite the embryonic origin, the tumour is symptomatic usually between 40 and 60 years of age. Sacral tumours present chronic sacral back pain, or urinary/bowel symptoms due to a pelvis mass. The tumour is palpable on rectal examination. Other vertebral chordomas manifest as chronic spinal pain later associated with paraparesis or radicular symptoms. Plain radiographs show an expanding, destructive lesion within the bone often with calcification and a paraspinal soft tissue mass. CT scans can demonstrate the extent of bone involvement, extradural extension or the size of a pelvic tumour component. Total surgical excision is the treatment of choice but the extent of the tumour at the time of diagnosis and the patient's general medical condition may preclude radical surgery. If so, surgery is confined to partial excision and achieving some degree of decompression of the neural structures. The tumour is known to be resistant to radiotherapy but this method can be used to obtain palliative pain relief and as an adjunct to subtotal excision. Chemotherapy has not proved to be effective in achieving tumour regression.

Aneurysmal Bone Cysts

This is a rare but interesting lesion. Its aetiology is uncertain and it is probably not a true neoplasm. There is a soft, fleshy, trabeculated highly vascular mass within the vertebra any component of which can be affected. The "cyst" contains engorged vascular spaces lined by endothelium. The sufferer is usually under 20 years old and women are more commonly affected. It can occur in any region of the spine but the lumbar area is a frequent site. The usual symptoms are back pain, paraparesis and radicular complaints. Other cystic lesions which may undergo haemorrhage include giant cell tumour, osteoclastoma and osteoblastoma. The diagnosis can be established by percutaneous biopsy under X-ray control. Plain radiographs show a rounded, rarefied area with septa within an expanded vertebra. Radical surgery is fraught with hazard due to severe bleeding but decompression with partial excision is usually possible. Radiotherapy has been described as effective.

Osteoid Osteoma

This is a benign neoplasm which occurs usually in males under 30 years. About 10% of the lesions occur in the spine. Midline spinal pain localized to the area of the tumour is the commonest symptom. Radicular pain also occurs depending on the site of the tumour. This lesion must be excluded in all young patients with unexplained back and sciatic type radicular pain because the lumbar spine is the commonest region to be affected. Cord compression and myelopathy is uncommon. The lesion may be missed on MRI and plain radiographs. An isotope bone scan is the best method of demonstrating the tumour initially. This can be followed by a detailed CT examination of the region. Surgical excision is the treatment of choice in symptomatic patients. Asymptomatic lesions can be treated conservatively because there is no risk of malignant transformation.

Benign Osteoblastoma

This is an unusual tumour (Myles and Macrae 1988). About 40% occur in the spine and the presentation is predominantly in the first and second decades. The tumour affects the posterior elements of the vertebra rather than the body. It is a cause of back pain, scoliosis and sciatica as well as limb weakness. The tumour may be missed on plain radiograph and an isotope scan is essential for diagnosis. Myelography will reveal the extent of neural compression. Complete excision will relieve symptoms and remove the risk of possible malignant change later. Partial removal and radiotherapy is an alternative but the tumour is not very radiosensitive.

Osteochondroma

This is probably the commonest benign tumour of bone. It occurs at multiple sites, has a familial tendency and is therefore called hereditary multiple exostoses. The lesions occur most commonly at the ends of long bones and are often bilateral and symmetrical. The vertebral lesions can encroach into the spinal canal causing neural compression and/or back pain (O'Connor and Roberts 1984). The disease is transmitted as an autosomal dominant and there is a strong male preponderance. If symptomatic, the only treatment is excision because the tumour is radioresistant.

Sacrococcygeal Masses

A variety of neoplastic and non-neoplastic lesions can present as a mass in this region. The capacious sacral canal and presacral space accommodates the "tumour" allowing it to reach a large size before symptoms occur. The commonest complaint is low back pain, sciatic pain, constipation, rectal symptoms or fullness in the perineum. The mass may be visible as a unilateral swelling of the buttock or palpable on rectal examination. Neural compression within the sacral canal or the sacral plexus outside the canal causes features of a low cauda equina lesion. Plain radiographs of the sacrum though usually abnormal are difficult to interpret. CT is the most useful radiological examination. In adults, the common lesions encountered are: chordoma, schwannoma, ependymoma, osseous tumours of all types and anterior sacral meningocele. In neonates and children, teratomas, meningoceles, lipomas and neuroblastoma are common causes. Meningoceles communicate with the CSF space and therefore increase in tension on straining or crying.

Table 30.5. Classification of intradural extramedullary tumours according to incidence

Common	Less common	Rare
Schwannoma	Lymphoma	Secondary carcinoma
Meningioma	Seedlings from CNS	Lipoma
Neurofibroma	malignant tumours	Dermoid cyst
Ependymoma	Paraganglioma	Epidermoid cyst
	Arachnoid cyst	

Intradural Extramedullary Tumours

Table 30.5 shows a classification of intradural extramedullary tumours according to incidence.

Schwannoma and Neurofibroma

Schwannoma is the commonest intradural extramedullary neoplasm. In the past, many authors have incorrectly grouped them together as "neurinoma", "neurilemmoma" or simply "neurofibroma". They are now recognized as "nerve sheath tumours" and comprise about 25% of all primary intradural spinal neoplasms. It has been postulated that both tumours originate from the perineural (Schwann) cell (Russell and Rubinskein 1989). However, they have distinctive microscopic features. The schwannoma has a mixture of packed (Antoni type A) or loose (Antoni type B) cellular elements but is almost devoid of nerve fibres whereas a neurofibroma has a loose myxoid stroma containing numerous nerve fibres. The tumours have a special relationship to the neurofibromatoses (NF). Together with meningioma they constitute about 90% of tumours in this spinal compartment

The neurofibromatoses are genetically determined disorders (Barker et al. 1987). Two types are recognized with distinct genetic, clinical and pathological features. Neurofibromatosis type I (NF I) is the entity classically described by von Recklinghausen (1882). It is an autosomal dominant disease occurring 1 in every 4000 live births due to a defect of the "neurofibromin" gene on chromosome 17 (Marchuk et al. 1991) and is characterized by the presence of any two or more of the features in Table 30.6. There is no family history of the disease in half the affected individuals indicating a high incidence of spontaneous mutation. The sufferers are

Table 30.6. Criteria for diagnosis of neurofibromatosis type I

TWO or more of the following features:
Multiple neurofibromas of one plexiform neurofibroma
Six or more cafe au lait spots each >15mm in postpubertal and >5mm in prepubertal patients
Axillary or inguinal freckling
Two or more Irish hamartomas (Lisch nodules)
Optic pathway glioma
Bone changes of neurofibromatosis (sphenoid dysplasia, thinning of long bone cortex)
Neurofibromatosis type I in a first degree relative

Table 30.7. Criteria for diagnosis of neurofibromatosis type II

ONE of the following features:
Bilateral 8th cranial nerve schwannomas
NF II in a first degree relative + unilateral 8th cranial nerve tumour
NF II in a first degree relative + two of the following:
    neurofibroma, meningioma, glioma, schwannoma, juvenile posterior subscapular lenticular opacity

prone to develop multiple neurofibromas. The spinal tumours have the histopathological features of a neurofibroma. Most of them occur in the cervical region and
commonly extend into the extradural compartment producing "dumb bell" or "hour
glass" tumours.

Neurofibromatosis type II (NF II) is characterized by multiple cranial or spinal
intradural tumours, the commonest being bilateral Vestibular schwannomas. It is an
autosomal dominant disease with a prevalence of 0.1 per 100 000 population and
therefore much less common than NF I. The locus for NF type II is on the long arm
of chromosome 22. The features of NF II are indicated in Table 30.7.

The majority of benign spinal nerve sheath tumours are schwannomas and occur
in individuals without the features of NF (Seppala et al. 1995). Seppala et al. (1995)
reviewed the records of 283 patients with spinal nerve sheath tumours and identified
195 schwannomas (including eight of the cellular type), 32 neurofibromas and six
malignant nerve sheath tumours. In all, only three patients had NF II and four had
features of NF I. It has been observed that tumours which occur in patients with NF I
are predominantly neurofibromas and in NF II schwannomas (Halliday et al. 1991).
However, this is not a strict rule and schwannomas can occur in patients with NF I
or II. They usually arise from dorsal (sensory) roots and less commonly from anterior (motor) roots.

In addition to nerve sheath tumours, both NF I and II show a predilection for the
development of tumours of glial and meningeal origin. This tendency is less
apparent in NF I where the classical association is optic nerve glioma. NF II is,
however, frequently associated with cranial and/or spinal meningiomas, astrocytomas and ependymomas or a diffuse gliomatosis of the pia-arachnoid of the brain
or spinal cord. Neural sheath tumours can undergo malignant change and even
metastasize into distant sites (Chandler et al. 1994).

In adults, nerve sheath tumours represent 23% of primary spinal tumours
(Nittner 1976). The incidence is virtually equal to that of spinal meningiomas. Both
sexes are equally affected although a slight female preponderance has been suggested by certain authors. The mean age of presentation is in the fifth decade
although rather earlier in men and in those with cervical region tumours. Over half
the tumours occur in the dorsal region and the others are equally distributed
between the cervical and lumbar regions. The distribution is compatible with a
uniform incidence irrespective of region when considering the relative length of
each area of the spine. Cervical and lumbar region tumours have the longest duration of symptoms prior to diagnosis. This may reflect the relatively smaller space
available for tumour expansion in the dorsal region before causing cord
compression.

Most tumours (72%) are intradural/extramedullary in site. Purely intramedullary
lesions have been described in a few rare instances (less than 1%). Transdural
tumours, i.e. intradural lesions with extradural extension (dumb-bell or hourglass

type) are as common (13%) as the purely extradural lesions (14%) and the latter may extend into the paravertebral tissues. The waist of an hourglass tumour lies within the enlarged intervertebral foramen and a surgeon who encounters an apparently extradural tumour should open the dura to exclude any intradural extension. The extradural/paravertebral component can be larger than the intradural part and may be palpable in the neck. Some dorsal neurofibromas are associated with lateral extraspinal meningoceles which can be seen as a mediastinal mass on a chest x-ray.

As nerve sheath tumours commonly arise from a dorsal root they are invariably sited posterolateral in relation to the cord and dorsal to the plane of the dentate ligament. Occasionally, a tumour can arise from a ventral root and is then sited anterior or anterolateral to the cord. The root involved is very closely adherent or attached to the tumour and has to be divided to achieve radical excision of the lesion. The sensory root involved can be sacrificed with impunity but section of a ventral root may cause a significant motor deficit in the cervical or lumbar region. In practice, the surgeon is pleasantly surprised at the absence of even a sensory deficit after dorsal root division and this is probably due to the overlap of cutaneous supply by adjacent roots. If more than one dorsal root is sacrificed, sensory loss is invariable and this can be troublesome if the hand, foot or genital area is involved.

An intradural tumour is usually a pinkish-yellow mass 2–3 cm in size, sausage-shaped and often lobulated but some, especially those in the lumbar region, can be much larger. They have a firm consistency and the cut surface has a yellow "lipomatous" appearance. Contrary to common belief, most are quite vascular making surgical excision difficult. A few contain tumour cysts but calcification is rarely found. The mass lies entirely in the subarachnoid plane and the nerve root of origin is attached to the rostral and caudal poles of the tumour. The spinal cord is displaced and moulded around the tumour and the adjacent nerve roots draped around it. Small tumours especially those in the cauda equina can be mobile but larger lesions are wedged firmly between adjacent tissues.

Radicular pain is the commonest early presenting symptom. However, severe cord compression and neurological disability can occur without pain. Weakness and pyramidal signs follow the onset of root pain and sensory symptoms occur thereafter. Sphincter disturbance is the last major symptom to appear (Levy et al. 1986). About half the patients are diagnosed within two years of the onset of symptoms. The lumbar CSF protein may exceed 5 g/litre, well in excess of that expected with a spinal block. This feature may cause impairment of CSF absorption and contribute to the occasional syndrome of raised intracranial pressure described in association with many spinal tumours (Ridsdale and Moseley 1978).

Plain radiographs may show an enlarged intervertebral foramen and/or widening of the interpedicular distance. These changes are more common in neurofibromas than in spinal meningiomas. MRI is the best means of diagnosis (See Fig. 29.4). The treatment is surgical excision of symptomatic lesions. There is no place for radiotherapy unless as an adjunct to surgical treatment especially when malignant change has occurred.

Meningioma (Fig. 30.2)

Meningiomas also form nearly 25% of all primary spinal neoplasms. They are of mesodermal descent and commonly arise from arachnoid cells situated in the dura near the root exit. The tumour is therefore usually situated lateral to the cord and firmly attached to the dura at the point of origin. Their growth is related to sex hormones, perhaps explaining the marked female preponderance (80%) of the tumour (Levy et al. 1982). Oestrogen and progesterone receptors have been identified in meningiomas (Poisson et al. 1983) which is obviously linked to the increased rate of growth observed during pregnancy. Cranial meningiomas are four to five times commoner than their spinal counterpart probably due to the greater available dural surface for tumour origin.

Although they may occur in any part of the spine, 75% are found in the dorsal region. Also over 80% of the tumours in females occur in this area (Levy et al. 1982). The tumour is much less common in the lumbosacral area (8%). The age at presentation is 40–70 years with a peak incidence in the sixth decade. A middle-aged or elderly female presenting with features of gradual cord compression related to the dorsal area must be assumed to have a meningioma until proved otherwise. The dorsal predilection is not observed in male patients. Most tumours are intradural/extramedullary in position. Intramedullary meningiomas have not been described. Intradural/extradural lesions occur (7%) and some of these can have a typical dumb-bell appearance. Meningiomas occur in the upper cervical region and at the foramen magnum. In this situation the tumour is usually situated anterior or anterolateral to the cord. Cervical tumours are commoner in men (Levy et al. 1982). A more interesting observation is that tumours sited above C7 are invariably anterior and those at or below C7 have a greater likelihood of being posterior to the dentate ligament. Purely extradural tumours are also well recognized (8%); they are more vascular, grow more rapidly and can erode the bone.

The meningeal origin can be small or broad based, the latter conferring a degree of immobility to the tumour. The main blood supply arises from enlarged extradural arteries resulting in hypervascularity of the adjacent extradural space usually near the insertion of the dentate ligament in proximity to the exit zone of the spinal root. Therefore, most meningiomas are sited lateral, posterolateral or anterolateral to the cord. Only a small proportion of tumours are truly anterior or posterior to the cord. The classical "en plaque" tumour with a very broad osseous attachment is a rare finding in the spine.

An intradural meningioma will enlarge displacing the arachnoid membrane towards the cord. This protective layer of arachnoid is very useful to the surgeon engaged in excision of the tumour. The pinkish grey or purple mass is about 2–3 cm, either rounded or oval shaped and lobulated only occasionally. The consistency is firm and numerous blood vessels are seen on the surface. The cut surface has a granular appearance and gritty areas of calcification occur. The occasional heavily calcified or even ossified tumour is an arduous challenge to the surgeon because the tissue cannot be fragmented by ordinary methods of tumour removal. Additional manipulation of the tumour and cord required to excise these lesions leads to a poor functional result after excision. Cyst formation and haemorrhage are uncommon but oedema, cystic change and myelomalacia of the adjacent cord may occur. Most meningiomas are totally benign tumours of the transitional or fibroblastic type but the occasional aggressive angioblastic variant is found in pure extradural growths.

Radicular pain occurs much less commonly than in neurofibroma (21%). Midline back pain is the commonest early complaint and may precede other symptoms by several months. Sensory symptoms (ascending numbness) follow the pain and motor and bladder symptoms appear later. The average duration of symptoms prior to diagnosis is two years and about 50% come to surgery within a year of onset. About 80% of patients have motor or sensory features at the time of diagnosis.

Table 30.8. Comparison of clinical, pathological and radiological features of schwannoma and meningioma

	Neurofibroma	Meningioma
Number	Usually single	Usually single
Age at presentation	Fifth decade	Sixth decade
Sex	Equal	Females × 4 dorsal
		Males × 7 cervical
Spinal level	Equal distribution considering length of each region	75% dorsal
Usual relationship to cord	Posterolateral	Lateral/Posterolateral
Radicular symptoms	>80%	20%
Midline pain	Late	Early
CSF protein	>500 mg%	<500 mg%

Misdiagnosis can occur in some who present with a fluctuating course when multiple sclerosis is naturally the first consideration. A rapidly growing angioblastic extradural meningioma with a short history of neurological evolution, pedicle erosion on plain radiograph and an extradural mass on the scans can be mistaken for a metastatic deposit. The rare syndrome of raised intracranial pressure which has been described with spinal tumours occurs but is less likely because the elevation of CSF protein is less than with schwannomas.

Plain radiographic changes are found in less than 20% of patients. Pedicle erosion is the commonest and calcification occurs in about 3%. Hyperostosis akin to the skull changes seen in cranial meningiomas does not occur in the spinal tumours. MRI or conventional myelography combined with CT scanning are the main methods of radiological diagnosis. A comparison of the main clinical and radiological features of schwannoma and meningioma is given in Table 30.8. The ideal treatment is surgical excision of the tumour along with the dural attachment. The recurrence rate is very low after such radical excision. Radiotherapy has a place following subtotal excision especially in the aggressive angioblastic variety. Sex hormone treatment is being used to control the growth of some inoperable cranial meningiomas and may also be useful in the spinal variety for residual tumour after surgical excision.

Intramedullary Tumours

These tumours are not uncommon and comprise about 10%–20% of adult primary neoplasms (Sloof et al. 1964). There is a much higher (50%) incidence of intramedullary tumours in children's series because neurofibroma and meningioma are less frequent in younger age groups. The commonest intramedullary tumours are astrocytomas and ependymomas both arising from cells of neuroepithelial origin. The ependymoma is commoner in adults and benign astrocytoma in children. The association with NF I and II has already been mentioned. A practical clinical classification is shown in Table 30.9.

Table 30.9. Classification of intramedullary tumours according to incidence

Common	Less common	Uncommon
Ependymoma	Malignant astrocytoma	Secondary carcinoma
Benign astrocytoma	Dermoid cyst	True lipoma
Haemangioblastoma	Epidermoid cyst	Schwannoma
	Cavernous haemangioma	Enterogenous cyst

Astrocytoma

Intraspinal astrocytomas are rarer than their cerebral counterparts. In adults, they form about 8% of all primary spinal tumours (Sloof et al. 1964) and about 30% of intramedullary tumours. In children's series, astrocytomas are commoner comprising about 60% of intramedullary tumours (Reimer and Onofrio 1985; Rotisch et al. 1990). The tumour occurs mostly in the cervical and dorsal regions of the cord. Cervical tumours may extend to or be an extension of a brainstem astrocytoma.

Astrocytomas are usually slow-growing, histologically benign neoplasms. Cyst formation is common (nearly 50%) and may be situated at either end of a solid tumour component or even extend to involve the entire length of the spinal cord (holocord tumours). Such lesions are commoner in children and young adults. The cysts contain xanthochromic proteinaceous fluid, have smooth walls and do not contain neoplastic cells. Macroscopically, the cord is enlarged but the tumour is not usually visible on the surface. The posterior nerve roots are wider apart and the cord may have a pale grey appearance. These benign astrocytomas are pale, relatively avascular tumours which usually have an identifiable plane of separation from the cord. They can be of the pilocytic or non-pilocytic (diffuse fibrillary) types on microscopic examination. More rarely, a benign astrocytoma expands the cord but the tumour cells intermingle with nerve cells without a defined plane of cleavage (infiltrating type).

Symptoms run a slow, subtle course over months or years, often with long periods of stability. The pattern may mimic the symptomatology of multiple sclerosis causing diagnostic error. There is a slight male preponderance with a peak incidence in the second and third decades. Scoliosis is a feature in children and adolescents. Midline spinal or central pain occurs in half the patients. Paraesthesiae eventually evolve into the typical dissociated sensory loss pattern. Limb paralysis is very subtle at first, perhaps affecting only one limb and progressing gradually to affect others sequentially.

As for other intramedullary lesions MRI is the best imaging technique for diagnosis. Paramagnetic contrast media will enhance the solid component. It is very important to identify the presence and extent of a tumour cyst and the exact segmental location of the solid component in order to decide the exact length of the surgical exposure. This can be achieved by MRI preoperatively or by ultrasonography peroperatively (see below). Myelography merely demonstrates an expanded spinal cord over the area of the tumour. CT scan imaging is very unhelpful in the diagnosis of intramedullary lesions.

In current surgical practice surgical excision is attempted in most patients. Surgical intervention is often accompanied by neurological deterioration with partial recovery in most patients. Excision of the tumour is very unlikely to improve an established deficit. Therefore, early surgical intervention which is associated with a reduced neurological morbidity is advised by most authors (Cristante and Herrmann 1994). Another recent series (Minehan et al. 1995) indicated a better prognosis in pilocytic astrocytoma. Aggressive tumour resection was not associated with improved survival but adjunct radiotherapy was associated with a better outcome particularly in the non-pilocytic type.

Malignant Astrocytoma

This neoplasm is seen only rarely and comprises about 7.5% of all spinal cord astrocytomas in adults and occurs even less frequently in children. The sexes are affected equally and the tumour is symptomatic within the first three decades of life. There is a rapidly progressive course of neurological deterioration with pain, paralysis and sensory impairment. The radiological evidence is similar to the benign variety. The solid tumour has a reddish colour, is more vascular and is not well demarcated from the cord. Tumour cysts containing xanthochromic fluid are present. Microscopic appearances are akin to Grade 3 or 4 cerebral astrocytomas. The tumour can spread to other areas along the CSF with leptomeningeal involvement of brain and spinal cord. Despite aggressive surgical treatment with resection, radiotherapy and chemotherapy, the prognosis is extremely poor (Cohen et al. 1989). There is little benefit in resorting to aggressive surgical excision in these patients.

Ependymoma (Fig. 30.3)

Intraspinal ependymomas are also less common than the cerebral counterparts. They form about 5% of all primary CNS tumours, only a third occurring within the spinal canal. Nearly 60% of the spinal ependymomas occur in and around the cauda equina (Sloof et al. 1964). Of the remainder the majority occur in the cervical region. (McCormick et al. 1990). In adults, ependymomas comprise the majority of intramedullary tumours accounting for nearly 85%. It is the commonest (88%) primary tumour in the region of the conus/cauda equina (Norstrom et al. 1961). Some conus intramedullary ependymomas are juxtamedullary because they have an exophytic extramedullary component extending into the lumbosacral spinal canal.

Males are more commonly afflicted. The mean age of presentation is about 35 years for both sexes but the tumour is uncommon below 20 years. It originates from the ependymal lining of the central canal or filum terminale and is histologically benign with a slow rate of growth and very little capacity to infiltrate the cord. A soft red or purple solid tumour mass expands the cord often separating the proprioceptive columns and presenting beneath the pial surface in the midline posteriorly. Rostral tumour cysts (polar cyst) with xanthochromic fluid are described. The cyst wall is non-neoplastic. The tumour, though unencapsulated, has a layer of gliotic tissue around it which facilitates tumour excision. On microscopic examination the tumours around the conus and cauda equina are invariably of the benign myxopapillary variety. Malignant cerebrospinal ependymomas may produce subarachnoid seedlings via CSF dissemination.

The symptoms are of gradual onset and progress slowly. The average duration before diagnosis is about 14 months (Epstein et al. 1993). There is good preservation of neurological function even with extensive tumours because of the protracted slow growth. Back pain, worse at night, and radicular pain, invariably of a sciatic distribution, are very common. Dysaesthesiae are a common feature. Sudden haemorrhage into the tumour may cause acute sciatic pain (Fincher's syndrome). The pattern of paralysis and sensory change will depend on the site of the tumour being either a central cord or cauda equina syndrome. Plain radiographs show an enlarged spinal canal in about one third of patients. MRI is the best method of diagnostic imaging and demonstrates a discrete mass with gadolinium enhancement of the upper and lower poles. A polar cyst is seen in about 30% of patients. Myelography demonstrates either an enlarged cord or a filling defect in the cauda equina depending on the site and extent of the lesion.

Total excision can be achieved in the majority of patients (Epstein et al. 1993). Subtotal excision is combined with radiotherapy but this is not necessary when a total removal has been performed. The prognosis is very good following total excision.

Haemangioblastoma

These tumours occur most commonly in the cerebellum either sporadically or as a manifestation of the von Hippel–Lindau syndrome (Neumann et al. 1989). They occur, although less frequently, in the spinal cord mostly as intramedullary or juxtamedullary tumours and more rarely as pure extradural tumours (Murota and Symon 1989). Any part of the cord can be affected but thoracic lesions are commoner probably due to the anatomical extent of the region. The syndrome is associated with retinal haemangioblastoma, hepatic and pancreatic cysts and renal carcinoma.

The solid part of the tumour is a reddish orange mass with tortuous arterial channels on its surface and large draining veins situated in a polar position. This arrangement is very similar to that of an arteriovenous malformation and surgical removal is tedious because of the intense vascularity. Associated tumour cysts are well described. These contain clear lemon-yellow fluid rich in erythropoietin. The solid tumour is situated on the inner wall of the cyst (mural nodule). A family history of von Hippel–Lindau disease may be elicited and the patient may have been treated previously for a cerebellar tumour of the same type.

Clinical features depend on the site of the lesion and usually consist of a progressive neurological disturbance with limb weakness and sensory deficit. Multiple tumours are common. MRI demonstrates a solid tumour or a cyst with a mural nodule. The vessels around the lesion will appear as low signal flow voids. It is imperative to scan the whole spine and the cranial cavity because multiple lesions occur. Myelography will merely reveal an expanded cord but the presence of enlarged blood vessels around it as filling defects will provide the clue to the possible diagnosis. This appearance may also occur with an arteriovenous malformation situated within the cord. Spinal angiography provides useful information before contemplating surgical attack on these extremely vascular lesions but may cause neurological deterioration. This may reveal tumour nodules in relation to a large cyst which may have been undetected with other radiology methods. Magnetic resonance angiography may be able to demonstrate the vasculature adequately. Excision is the best treatment but the vascularity of the tumour renders the operation tedious. Yet, the results following excision are extremely good with 85% symptomatic improvement (Xu et al. 1994).

Table 30.10. Classification of cystic spinal lesions

Extradural	Intradural/extramedullary	Intramedullary
Meningeal cysts types I and II	Dermoid cyst	Astrocytoma
Synovial cysts	Epidermoid cyst	Ependymoma
Ganglion cysts	Meningeal cyst type III	Haemangioblastoma
	Teratoma	Dermoid cyst
		Epidermoid cyst
		Enterogenous cyst
		Teratoma

Other Cystic Spinal Lesions

A variety of neoplastic and non-neoplastic cystic extradural or intradural lesions of differing aetiology occur in relation to the spinal cord, nerve roots and meninges (Table 30.10). These will be conveniently described here even though some are not intramedullary tumours. Many are a result of maldevelopment and are therefore present at birth. They cause symptoms in childhood or in early adult life. Although some are harmless and invariably asymptomatic most cause neurological disease due to spinal neural compromise. The term cyst implies that the contents are fluid but certain notable exceptions contain solid material. Meningoceles, parasitic cysts and syringomyelia cysts are outside the scope of this chapter. Neoplastic cysts associated with spinal astrocytoma, ependymoma and haemangioblastoma have already been mentioned.

Dermoid and Epidermoid Cysts

These are invariably developmental lesions which are well recognized but relatively uncommon. They account for about 1%–2% of primary adult spinal tumours (Sloof et al. 1964). In paediatric series incidences of 4.5% (Rand and Rand 1960) and 13% (Lunardi et al. 1989) have been reported. They arise from ectodermal tissue destined to become skin which is implanted within the neural tube during its closure. Such implantation can rarely occur following trauma or lumbar puncture. A small number of cases are therefore iatrogenic in origin and follow repeated spinal taps for the diagnosis and treatment of meningitis (Choremis et al. 1956).

Epidermoid cysts originate from epidermal elements only. The cyst has a glistening grey white external surface thus acquiring the description of pearly tumour. The wall is lined with stratified squamous epithelium and the creamy white, cheese-like material within arises from dead desquamated epidermal cells. Keratin breakdown produces an abundance of cholesterol and stearine-like compounds which produces shiny lipid droplets when the cyst contents float in water at operation. This tumour has also acquired the confusing misnomer cholesteatoma since the contents resemble the chronic inflammatory masses which occur in the middle ear.

Dermoid cysts originate from both epidermal and dermal elements. The wall has stratified squamous epithelium as well as hair follicles, sweat glands and sebaceous glands. The contents resemble an epidermoid but, in addition, hair is commonly seen and, very rarely, teeth are found. Both dermoids and epidermoids occur invariably as intradural lesions, extradural occurrence is rare. The intradural lesions are either intramedullary or juxtamedullary in situation. As a group they are more common in the region of the conus than elsewhere in the spine. Intramedullary epidermoids are more common in the thoracic region whereas intramedullary dermoids occur more often at the conus. The cervical region is relatively less affected by both tumours.

Being present at birth, initial presentation is usually in childhood but due to their slow rate of enlargement the diagnosis may be made only in adult life. A slight male preponderance is recognized for both lesions. There is an association with spina bifida occulta and the cutaneous stigmata of this condition (naevus, dimple, tuft of hair) may be present over the lumbosacral region. More importantly, dermoids can be associated with a dermal sinus which may communicate with the spinal subarachnoid space, lending a vulnerability to meningitis which may be the mode of initial presentation. The usual clinical picture is a gradually progressive neurological syndrome specific to the location of the cyst. The most common is a conus/cauda equina lesion with back pain, saddle anaesthesia, leg weakness and sphincter disturbance.

Plain radiographs may show localized enlargement of the spinal canal, congenital vertebral abnormalities and, rarely, teeth. MRI demonstrates the tumour extremely well as a high signal lesion within the cord on T2 weighted images. Myelography combined with CT reveals an intradural mass enlarging the cord. MRI is also useful to exclude associated congenital abnormalities of the spinal cord which may be present.

The best treatment is excision. However, total excision is often impossible and hazardous because the capsule is very adherent to the cord. The results of surgery are usually gratifying even with only partial excision creating sufficient tumour debulking to relieve neural compression. The edges of the cyst wall can be "marsupialized" to the dural surface so that tumour material which recurs does not cause cord compression. Recurrence only occurs after several years and with a prudent surgical approach the patient can be given years of independent mobility, continence and satisfactory sexual function. Radiotherapy is ineffective.

Teratomas

These developmental tumours of germ cell origin are less common than dermoid and epidermoid cysts. Their incidence is higher in children than in adults. The lumbar region is affected most frequently and the tumour is either intradural/extramedullary or intramedullary in position. The contents may be cystic or solid and, histologically, cartilage, bone, smooth and skeletal muscle are recognized. The lining of the wall consists of columnar or cuboidal epithelium. The bony elements cause radiographic opacities which are diagnostic. Some tumours are malignant and produce remote seedlings via the CSF. Teratomas and seminomas (germ cell tumours) of the mediastinum can cause epidural metastatic deposits due to direct or bloodstream spread. Teratomas can occur anterior to the sacrum or coccyx often associated with a dermal sinus which opens near the anal verge. These so-called sacrococcygeal tumours are much commoner in children. The treatment is total or subtotal excision.

Neurenteric (Enterogenous) Cysts

The neurenteric canal joins the primitive yolk sac to the amniotic cavity. The canal splits the developing vertebrae and spinal cord in the early stages of fetal life. Persistence of any part of this canal in the fully formed fetus is a developmental defect. In the worst type, the entire neurenteric canal is patient and the stomach and intestines herniate onto the dorsal surface of the fetus. The condition is very rare and survival is unknown. A persistent intradural (less commonly extradural) neurenteric canal can produce an expanding cystic lesion with resultant cord compression. The thoracic spine is most often affected. The cysts contain either clear colourless fluid or a viscous, mucoid material. Associated vertebral anomalies such as spina bifida occulta or anterior defects of the vertebral body occur in the region of the cyst. The tumour is commoner in young adult males and the usual presentation is back pain, root pain and a progressive neurological disturbance. The best treatment is excision but the tumour capsule is adherent to the cord and radical removal may be difficult and hazardlous. Percutaneous or operative cyst drainage provides good symptomatic benefit in recurrent tumours. Radiotherapy is not effective.

Spinal Meningeal Cysts

These are not true neoplasms and often asymptomatic incidental findings. They can sometimes become clinically significant by causing cord or nerve root compression. Most are congenital and a result of meningeal maldevelopment but a few may be traumatic in origin. A confusing array of terms has arisen in their classification but a simple method based on anatomical features was suggested by Nabors et al. (1988) (Table 30.11).

Extradural Meningeal Cyst (Type I)

The type IA cysts occur typically in the thoracic spine of adolescent males (Cloward and Bucy 1937). The cyst is situated either in the posterior midline or posterolaterally in relation to the dura covering the dorsal root. The cyst is essentially an evagination or herniation of the arachnoid layer and contains clear fluid (Gortvai 1963). The opening is usually situated near the entrance of the dorsal root. It enlarges gradually probably due to a valve-like effect at the neck or pedicle which passes through

Table 30.11. Classification of spinal meningeal cysts

Type	Description
I	Extradural meningeal cyst without nerve fibres
IA	"Extradural meningeal cyst" = "Extradural arachnoid cyst"
IB	"Sacral meningocele" = "occult sacral meningocele"
II	Extradural meningeal cyst with spinal nerve root fibres
	("Tarlov's perineural cyst" = "spinal nerve root diverticulum")
III	Spinal intradural meningeal cysts (= "intradural arachnoid cyst")

the dural hiatus. Smaller cysts are often multiple and asymptomatic. Large lesions eventually cause neural compression, the characteristic feature of which is a spastic paraparesis with a sensory level. A fluctuating course is possible because the cyst may empty intermittently. The contrast used in myelography may or may not fill the sac. CT myelography is much more likely to demonstrate the communication. MRI scans will demonstrate the cyst very well in T1 and T2 images. Treatment is by excision with ligation of the pedicle.

Type IB cysts usually occur in the sacral region. They are commoner in adults. The presentation is sacral radicular pain and sphincter dysfunction. The radiological features are similar to type IA lesions. Ligation of the ostium is sufficient to relieve symptoms.

Type II Meningeal Cysts (Syn: Tarlov's Cysts)

These are subarachnoid cysts sited in relation to a nerve root which is either within the cyst wall or lying free in the fluid. They occur in the lumbar and sacral regions in relation to the posterior roots and are usually multiple and bilateral (Tarlov 1938). The cyst contains clear fluid and fills with contrast medium during myelography appearing as dilated root sleeves. CT myelography demonstrates the lesions very well. MRI coronal sections are very useful to show multiple bilateral lesions. Most are asymptomatic and clinicians as well as radiologists have a tendency to disregard them as incidental findings. However, the associated root can become compressed by the cyst causing sciatic pain and cauda equina symptoms and the relevance to the clinical problem must be carefully evaluated. Treatment by excision is not possible due to the absence of a pedicle. Simple aspiration of the fluid leads to recurrence. Therefore, the aim of surgery is to partially excise the wall and oversew the remainder to reduce the size. The treatment of symptomatic lesions gives gratifying results.

Intradural Arachnoid Cyst (Type III)

These rare lesions occur in the posterior midline anywhere along the spine. They are often multiple and asymptomatic. The cyst contains clear fluid and causes cord compression if sufficiently large. A common symptom is back pain which increases on standing and is relieved on lying supine. Spastic paraparesis with a sensory level occurs in dorsal lesions. Myelography reveals a filling defect posterior to the cord. CT myelography will demonstrate a communication with the subarachnoid space if the cyst fills slowly. Sagittal MRI will show the extra-axial lesion of CSF signal density compressing the cord from behind. Treatment is drainage with excision of the outer arachnoid covering.

Synovial and Ganglion Cysts (Syn: Juxta-Articular Cysts)

These cysts arise from the capsule of the facet joints. They are commonly found in the lumbar region. The exact mechanism of causation is unknown but may be related to trauma to the joint resulting in a herniation of the synovium through the capsule. Synovial cysts are lined by reactive synovial cells. Ganglion cysts have a wall consisting of fibrous tissue and chronic inflammatory cells. Although uncommon they may cause symptoms and must be considered in the differential diagnosis of extradural neural compression (Friedberg et al. 1994). Myelography reveals an extradural filling defect. CT myelography and MRI will demonstrate the relationship to the facet joint. Treatment is excision of symptomatic lesions.

Spinal Lipomas

Lipomatous tissue can occur within the spinal canal in two distinct conditions. The commonest is the lipomyelomeningocele which is a lesion associated with spinal dysraphism. The intradural lipoma is within the conus of a low lying cord and continuous with an extradural and subcutaneous lipoma. This condition is described in the relevant chapter and will not be discussed here.

True intramedullary lipomas (without the association of dysraphism) are exceedingly rare (Sloof et al. 1964). The sex incidence is equal. Symptoms begin in the first three decades of life but may be present even at birth. They are found in the cervical and thoracic levels (Lee et al. 1995). The tumour capsule is very adherent to neural tissue and at operation, the intradural mass expands the thecal sac into a taut, non-pulsatile lump. The tumour itself is yellow, rubbery and lobulated. Multiple tumours may be present involving other cranial or spinal neural tissue. Associated malformations of the vertebrae are found in one third of cases. The typical clinical picture is a slow progressive spastic paraparesis and sensory ataxia followed by incontinence. Root pain is rare. Plain radiographs of the spine reveal a widened canal and congenital vertebral anomalies may be seen. MRI is an excellent technique to demonstrate the tumour because of the distinctive signal characteristics of fat. Myelography merely reveals a localized expansion of the cord. Total excision is rarely possible due to the adherence of the capsule to the spinal cord. Partial excision with tumour debulking is sufficient to obtain good symptomatic benefit. Radiotherapy is not helpful. The neurological outcome is not very optimistic (Lee et al. 1995).

Intradural extramedullary lipomas have been described. These also become symptomatic early in life. Purely extradural lipomas are very uncommon (Ehni and hove 1945). They form large extradural fatty lumps on the posterior aspect of the dura in the dorsal region. The fat is reddish-yellow or brown in colour, loosely attached to the dura and can be removed easily at operation. The clinical history of cord compression is of short duration. Plain radiographs of the spine are usually normal. MRI is diagnostic. Excision produces good symptomatic benefit.

Some Unusual Tumours

Epidural Hibernoma

The lipomas described above contain white or yellow adipose tissue. Brown fat is an important source of non-shivering heat production under cold stress in animals who hibernate. This tissue is relatively underdeveloped in man for obvious reasons. Fat-cells contain steroid receptors and dexamethasone binds to these strongly. Steroids deplete white fat by lipolysis but increase the mass of brown fat by enhancing the metabolism of glycogen and lipid. Patients on long-term steroid therapy are known to develop centripetal fat deposition. This increase may occur in the epidural space and the condition epidural lipomatosis is a recognized complication of steroid therapy (Perling et al. 1988). The excess fat can produce spinal neural compromise manifesting as a neurological syndrome of a myelopathy, radiculopathy, cauda equina syndrome or neurogenic claudication. Unless the aetiology is recognized the steroid dose may be increased when the cord syndrome occurs thus worsening the situation. Laminectomy and excision of the fatty mass may be necessary if the symptoms do not improve with tailing off the steroids.

Paraganglioma

This neoplasm arises from cells of neuroendocrine origin associated with the autonomic nervous system. The nomenclature and classification is complex but currently the term paraganglioma is applicable to all tumours arising from chromaffin tissues of adrenal or extra-adrenal sites. They are related to phaeochromocytomas and chemodectomas. The extra-adrenal paragangliomas are usually benign and non-secretory. Common examples are carotid body tumour and glomus jugulare tumour. Paraganglioma is a well-described tumour within the lumbosacral canal occurring as an intradural lesion which can produce a cauda equina syndrome (O'Sullivan et al. 1990). It probably arises from neuroblast cells which are capable of differentiating into chemoreceptor cells or ganglion cells. The sex incidence is equal and the tumour occurs in late adult life. It is attached to the filum terminale or a nerve root of the cauda equina, is well encapsulated and can be excised easily. It is not pharmacologically active but may contain dopamine, adrenaline and noradrenaine. MRI reveals an intradural/extramedullary mass. The treatment is excision and results are excellent.

Calcifying Pseudoneoplasms

Recent literature has revealed unusual granulomatous fibrochondro-calcifying masses which can occur within the spinal canal which can cause neural compression (Bertoni et al. 1990). Their aetiology is unknown and they are probably nonneoplastic lesions. There is neither a sex predilection nor an age pattern but the described cases have been in adults. The patients with spinal lesions presented with spinal pain. Similar lesions within the cranial cavity have been described in the same series. Plain radiographs reveal a calcified mass within the spinal canal. Myelography and CT confirm an intraspinal tumour which is difficult to distinguish from a prolapsed calcified disc protrusion. Treatment is by excision. Histopathology examination revealed a granulomatous tissue with foci of calcification.

Extradural Haematopoiesis

In thalassaemia and myelosclerosis compensatory haematopoiesis can occur in sites remote from the marrow, liver and spleen. Extradural masses of such haematopoietic tissue can produce spinal cord compression (Jackson et al. 1988). The diagnosis is by bone scan or MRI and treatment is excision and/or radiotherapy.

Table 30.12.   Incidence of spinal cord tumours in children

	Rand and Rand (1960) (65 cases)*	Matson (1969) (135 cases)*	Till (1975) (68 cases)*	O'Sullivan et al. (1994) (31 cases)*
Intramedullary				
Astrocytoma	14%	18%	3%	48%
Ependymoma	12%	4%	6%	35%
Other Gliomas	5%	0%	15%	17%
Extramedullary				
Meningioma	3%	2%	3%	Nil
Neurofibroma	8%	4%	9%	
Seedlings	6%	3%	4%	
Extradural				Nil
Metastases		13%		
Sarcoma	15%	1%	6%	
Neuroblastoma	8%	18%	25%	
Primary Bone Tumours	12%	2%	6%	Nil
Developmental Tumours	11%	27%	16%	Nil
Others	6%	6%	6%	Nil

Paediatric Spinal Tumours

Incidence

The annual incidence of primary tumours of the spinal cord in children is about 1 per million (O'Sullivan et al. 1994). Similar to adults, childhood spinal tumours are much less common than cerebral neoplasms. There are many benign intraspinal neoplasms seen in paediatric practice. Metastases, schwannomas and meningiomas occur much less frequently in comparison to adults. In contrast to adults, intramedullary tumours are commoner (25%) and astrocytoma is commoner than ependymoma. Malignant extradural spinal compression is relatively uncommon. Sarcoma and neuroblastoma, are the commonest extradural lesions (Klein 1991). Intradural seedlings from cranial malignant neoplasms such as medulloblastoma, ependymoma, pinealoma and choroid plexus papilloma occur. Developmental tumours are commoner in the lumbosacral and cervical regions. The relative incidence of the various tumours is shown in Table 30.12.

Clinical Features

The basic neurological disturbances caused by a spinal neoplasm are similar to those described in adults. However, diagnostic difficulties arise for a variety of reasons. Many tumours being benign and slow growing produce a subtle and gradual neurological evolution. Very young children are unable to complain and even the older child is not usually prone to do so unless pain is a feature. Pain is not an early symptom of intramedullary tumours which are the commonest neoplasms seen in children. The low incidence of spinal tumours in children renders an element of impaired vigilance in the inexperienced clinician. Therefore, diagnostic errors are made, confusing the clinical picture with other neurological or orthopaedic disorders. In an infant, the only manifestation of pain may be irritability, being off feeds or incessant crying. In older children, root pain may be mistaken for joint disease or visceral pain.

A rigid spine with paraspinal spasm is always sinister. Weakness of a limb may only be noted by a parent as a limp, reluctance to run or play, or a sudden change of dexterity when an upper limb becomes weak. Sensory examination is difficult and requires tact and patience. Examination with a pin should be kept to the last in the routine. Incontinence in a child who had previously acquired sphincter training is significantly abnormal. Scoliosis, kyphosis, torticollis and foot deformities such as talipes should alert the clinician to the possibility of neurological dysfunction. Recurrent meningitis may be caused by infection of a dermal sinus communicating with the subarachnoid space. Symptoms of raised intracranial pressure or hydrocephalus may be the first sign of a spinal neoplasm (Ridsdale and Moseley 1978). When a family history of neurofibromatosis or von Hipper–Lindau disease is present there is a greater vulnerability to develop spinal tumours. The presence of cutaneous stigmata of spina bifida should alert the clinician to the potential possibility of an intraspinal tumour.

Diagnosis

The fundamental concepts are similar to those noted in adults. Plain radiographs will show canal widening, congenital anomalies or scoliosis. MRI is the most useful examination especially because the majority of tumours are intramedullary in situation. It can be used to screen the entire central nervous system in a search for multiple lesions. Axial CT is an excellent method for investigation of extradural lesions. Myelography is not tolerated well by children because a needle puncture is necessary. With MRI becoming universally available myelography is performed only infrequently. CT myelography is useful in extradural and extramedullary lesions. Young children will require sedation or general anaesthesia to achieve a technically satisfactory examination.

Intramedullary Astrocytoma

These comprise about 4% of CNS tumours in childhood. They are histologically benign with low or moderate cellularity belonging to the fibrillary of pilocytic varieties of astrocytoma. The common presenting symptoms are weakness, scoliosis and gait disturbance. The treatment is outlined below.

Malignant Epidural Tumours

A number of solid malignant neoplasms which are rare in adults can produce spinal metastatic disease in children. The commonest are Ewing's sarcoma, rhabdomyosarcoma and soft tissue sarcomas. Neuroblastoma is a malignant tumour of the adrenal medulla or sympathetic ganglia in the retroperitoneal tissues (Wilson and Draper

1974). It spreads by direct extension via the intervertebral foramen into the spinal canal to produce an extradural mass. Severe and rapidly progressive spinal neural compromise occurs. The majority of neuroblastomas arise in children less than four years old. It is probably the commonest malignant tumour in childhood. Treatment is by partial excision, radiotherapy and chemotherapy.

Ewing's Sarcoma

This is a malignant tumour of bone seen in the first two decades of life. The primary tumour is usually extraspinal. Metastatic lesions in the spine are common. Apart from the neurological features due to cord compression the patients present with low grade fever, anaemia, raised sedimentation rate and leucocytosis. The mainstay of treatment is radiotherapy and chemotherapy. Surgical decompression and vertebral stabilization have been described (Friedlaender 1982).

Eosinophilic Granuloma

This is a benign lesion resembling a tumour with a peak incidence in the first decade of life. The tissue is characterized by the presence of histiocytes and eosinophils. The spinal lesion may be part of Letterer–Siwe and Hand–Schuller–Christian disease which are the systemic forms of the condition. Thoracic back pain is the common presentation. Spinal neural compression is uncommon. The systemic form is treated with chemotherapy but the disease is self-limited. The spinal lesion can be managed conservatively with a supportive brace to reduce pain.

Medulloblastoma

This is a malignant neoplasm which occurs in and around the fourth ventricle. Tumour cells can spread via CSF pathways into the spinal subarachnoid space. These seedlings are initially asymptomatic and often multiple. Back pain, root pain, weakness and sensory loss are common symptoms. It is customary to perform a spinal MRI in all patients with a posterior fossa medulloblastoma. Most radiotherapists administer full craniospinal radiotherapy even if there is no clinical or scan evidence of metastatic disease in the spinal subarachnoid space. The spinal lesions can be treated with radiotherapy and chemotherapy. Surgery has a place for discrete lesions which are causing severe cord compression.

Management of Spinal Tumours

Delay in Diagnosis

Spinal compression due to a neoplasm is one of the commonest conditions requiring urgent treatment in a neurosurgical department. Compression can evolve slowly or rapidly. When the time course is gradual there is greater opportunity for diagnostic assessment and the institution of definitive treatment to avoid the catastrophe of permanent neurological disability. Rapidly progressive compression is a surgical emergency and delay in treatment will alter the prognosis significantly. The latter clinical scenario may expose inherent drawbacks of even the most comprehensive health care system.

Despite the availability of modern sophisticated techniques of radiological diagnosis a number of tumours are detected long after the onset of symptoms. Early diagnosis of a spinal neoplasm is essential to achieve a good outcome following appropriate treatment. Diagnostic error is the main cause of delay at the family doctor level. Failure of the patient to seek early medical help is not a significant factor. The main avoidable delays at the referring hospital consist of failure of diagnosis as a result of poor neurological assessment and misinterpretation of the clinical picture, the failure to realize the urgency of the condition or a delay in obtaining the appropriate medical opinion. Neurological deterioration, including worsening paralysis and loss of sphincter control, occurs during the process of diagnostic delay and lethargy of referral (Maurice-Williams and Richardson 1988). This was further highlighted by a retrospective analysis of spinal intradural tumours treated in the Department of Neurosurgery at Preston over a period of 35 years. (Fig. 30.4). There was a marked deterioration of neurological condition between onset of symptoms and surgical treatment (Gurusinghe and Perera 1994). Sensory symptoms increased from 13% to 43% (trebled), motor symptoms from 12% to 50% (quadrupled) and sphincter dysfunction from 3% to 24% (eightfold increase).

The avoidance of diagnostic pitfalls is primarily achieved by the capability of family practitioners and hospital doctors to recognize or at least suspect the condition and then refer the patient to an appropriate department for further evaluation. In most instances this will be the local neurosurgical unit and all cases of spinal compression should at least be initially referred for an opinion to a neurosurgeon.

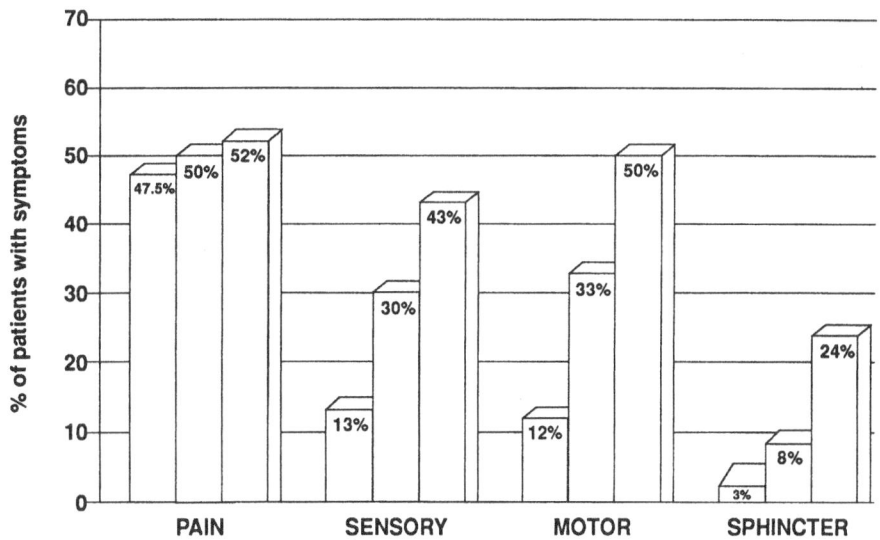

Fig. 30.4. Symptoms of intradural spinal tumours (141 patients) depicting neurological deterioration from onset to surgical treatment. The four major symptoms are represented. The three columns in each group indicate symptoms noted on first presentation to the family doctor (left), specialist (middle) and neurosurgeon (right). The numbers are percentages of the total (Gurusinghe and Perera 1994).

Constant clinical vigilance is essential. Back pain in a patient known to have a history of carcinoma must be investigated. Similarly, chronic back pain associated with lumbar paraspinal muscle spasm is always of sinister significance in a child. Vascular accidents of the cord are uncommon and demyelinating disease rarely produces a steady progressive cord disturbance in the initial stages. Neither condition is commonly associated with back pain or radicular pain at the onset. If symptoms and signs cannot be explained on a rational clinical basis further investigation and opinion should be sought expediently. Careful documentation of neurological findings is important so that the attending neurosurgeon can determine the rate of evolution of the neurological deterioration.

General Treatment

The control of pain is an important aspect of treatment. Pain can be severe especially in extradural tumours and regular opiate analgesia may be required. Analgesics must be prescribed in adequate dosage but modified according to the needs of the individual patient. Patient controlled opiate analgesic pumps are extremely useful particularly in the postoperative period. Bed rest is an effective method of pain control and mobilization must be commenced only when the patient is able to cope with the discomfort involved. Electrically operated beds minimize discomfort when nursing procedures are carried out. Patients with acute retention or dribbling incontinence require an in dwelling urinary catheter. Active and passive physiotherapy to paralysed limbs will help maintain joint mobility and muscle tone. The general care of anaesthetic skin areas is essential to prevent pressure sores. A bed cradle will facilitate free lower limb movement which should be encouraged in the pre- and postoperative periods.

Dexamethasone is commonly used to gain neurological stability until definitive treatment is carried out and for a short while thereafter. Often a dramatic improvement to neurological function is seen within a few hours of commencing the medication. Dexamethasone reduces cerebral oedema (Yamade et al. 1979) and the mechanism of action on the compromised spinal cord may be similar. Very high doses of steroids have been shown to enhance spinal cord blood flow after injury (Braughler and Hall 1983). A specific antimitotic effect of steroids has also been postulated and the dramatic effect of dexamethasone in reducing the size of a lymphoma is well recognized. The standard dose used in routine practice is 16 mg per day given in divided doses but high bolus dose administration over a short period is feasible in severe cases of cord compression.

All non-ambulant patients should wear anti-embolism stockings and receive subcutaneous heparin as prophylaxis against deep venous thrombosis. Ambulant patients should commence this regime 24 hours prior to surgery and continue after the operation until a normal ambulatory pattern is achieved.

Surgical Treatment

Aims

The patient with a symptomatic spinal tumour usually has three main aspects of concern and disability. They are (1) pain, (2) difficulty in walking and (3) lack of sphincter control. The aims of treatment are therefore to relieve pain, restore mobility and normal sphincter function. Fortunately, many patients are ambulant and continent when the diagnosis is made and remain so after tumour excision.

The best and most effective treatment of a spinal tumour is total excision. This ideal cannot always be attained and the extent of possible excision is mainly determined by the relationship of the tumour to the neural structures and/or to the extent of involvement of the spinal column and paraspinal structures. It is relatively easy to excise an intradural/extramedullary schwannoma or meningioma or even to remove a well-encapsulated intramedullary astrocytoma but not so to achieve radical excision of an extensive extradural metastasis involving the vertebral column. The ambition to achieve a total excision must always be tempered by an awareness of the hazards of surgery with inevitable worsening of existing neurological function. The age and general medical condition of the patient is an essential consideration in the decision regarding surgical treatment.

Methods of Access

Surgical access to a spinal tumour is determined by the location of the lesion in relation to the spinal cord, meninges and vertebral column (Fig. 30.5). Whichever

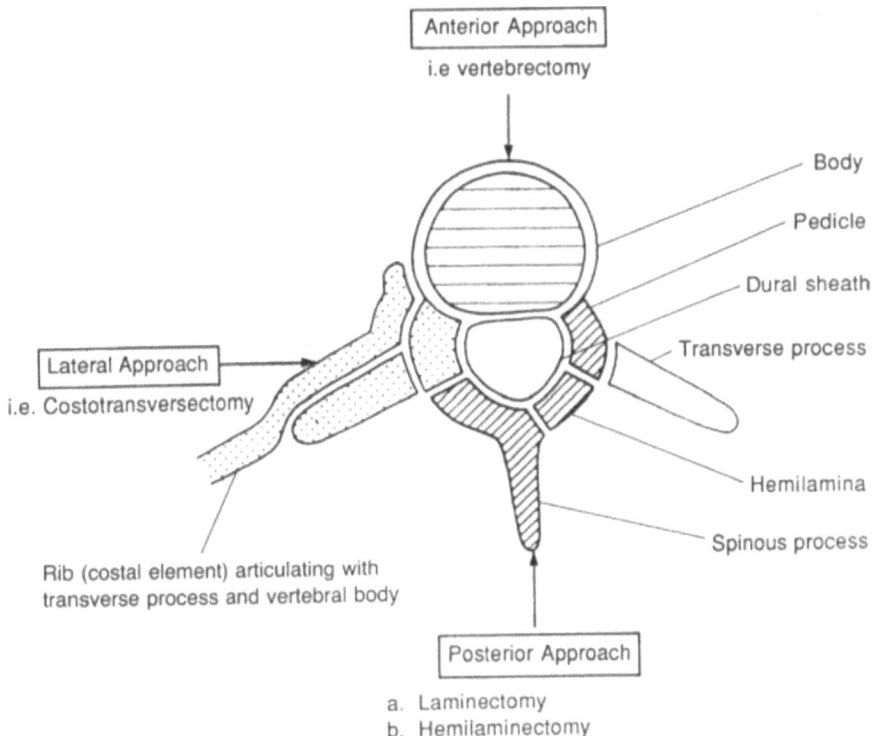

Fig. 30.5. Surgical approaches to spinal tumours. Shaded areas represent bone removal necessary for access depending on the approach used. ▤ anterior approach; ▨ lateral approach; ▨ posterior approach.

approach is used it is important to identify the level of the tumour in relation to the vertebrae so that the surgical incision is placed accurately. Posterior, posterolateral and a few anterolateral tumours are approached by removal of the overlying spinous processes and laminae (laminectomy or hemilaminectomy). This is by far the commonest route of surgical access to a spinal tumour. A laminostomy is a preferred method in children and young adults especially if several vertebral levels need to be exposed. In this method the the spinous processes and laminae are removed in continuity and replaced and wired into place after tumour removal. This procedure increases the duration of the operation but probably reduces the likelihood of postoperative spinal deformities.

Anterior and most anterolateral tumours are difficult to approach in this manner because the spinal cord intervenes between the surgeon and the tumour and tumour visualization involves excessive cord manipulation. Such tumours situated in the thoracic region can be reached by the anterolateral exposure called a costotransversectomy. This operation involves excision of the relevant rib, transverse process and pedicle to gain access into the spinal canal. There are two specific hazards of this surgical approach. The exposed pleura may be injured during the operation resulting in a pneumothorax. In the thoracolumbar region, especially on the left side, the artery of Adamkiewicz is endangered. The resultant ischaemic disturbance to the cord can be catastrophic. Nevertheless this route is very useful especially to deal with extradural benign and malignant tumours. An anterolateral approach can be used in tumours situated in the upper cervical and foramen magnum region.

Anterior approaches to the spine have become increasingly popular and safer. Tumours involving the vertebral body are best visualized and dealt with from this approach. The commonly used routes are transoral (C1, C2 levels), transcervical (C3 – C7 levels), transthoracic (T3 – T10 levels) and extraperitoneal/transabdominal methods to reach the anterior aspect of the lumbar vertebrae or sacrum. All these methods are most suitable for extradural tumours. A vertebral body involved with tumour can be excised (vertebrectomy). If the dura is breached or deliberately opened, suture repair of the defect is very difficult and closure is best achieved by a patch graft using artificial dura or fascia and sealed with tissue glue. If a water-tight closure is not obtained, CSF can leak into the wound with the potential risk of meningitis or extradural abscess.

The midline incision for laminectomy (or hemilaminectomy) is centred just above the tip of the spinous process corresponding to the vertebral level of the tumour, recognizing the slope of the spinous element to the laminae especially in the thoracic region. The laminectomy is extended to expose the cranial and caudal poles of the tumour and widened up to the vertebral facet joints. Usually, about three laminae are removed but more may be necessary depending on the size of the tumour. A posterior or posterolateral extradural tumour will be immediately visible. Absence of extradural fat in the region of any tumour is useful in recognizing the site and extent of an intradural lesion. The tumour will be seen as a tense, non-pulsatile localized expansion of the dura which is firm to gentle palpation. The dura is opened in the midline usually beginning below the lower pole of the tumour. The operating microscope must be used at this stage to obtain good illumination and magnification. When the arachnoid is opened a gush of CSF will occur from the subarachnoid space.

Removal of the tumour is best achieved by piece-meal excision. The central part of the lesion is removed first so that the peripheral part and capsule can be systematically peeled away from the neural structures. It is important to avoid or minimize manipulation of the cord and nerve roots. The Ultrasonic aspirator will disintegrate and remove the tumour without causing significant disturbance to adjacent neural structures. Constant irrigation of the operation field is important to prevent heat generated from the ultrasonic tip causing damage to the adjacent neural tissue. Laser excision is also useful in dealing with spinal intramedullary tumours (Epstein and Epstein 1982).

Somatosensory evoked potentials can be used to monitor cord function during the operation to alert the surgeon of cord manipulation, However, the system may prove too sensitive and therefore impractical. Electrophysiological monitoring of the cauda equina can be used to detect manipulation of the roots during tumour excision and also to differentiate between motor and sensory nerves (Kothbauer et al. 1994). The cord which is distorted and displaced by a tumour will begin to pulsate gently after tumour debulking. The dural edges are sutured following tumour removal after ensuring haemostasis. The laminae and spinous processes are replaced if a laminostomy exposure has been used. Infiltration of the paraspinal muscles with dilute local anaesthetic (marcaine) reduces postoperative pain. The muscles must be resutured in two or three layers to achieve good haemostasis and to prevent a CSF leak from the wound.

Intradural Extramedullary Tumours

The primary aim is total excision of the tumour with the tissue of origin and attachment.

Nerve Sheath Tumours The excision of an intradural schwannoma or neurofibroma inevitably involves sacrifice of the nerve root which is attached to the tumour. This will result in a neurological deficit determined by the function of the root involved. When dealing with a dumb-bell tumour the dural sleeve is opened in the direction of the intervertebral foramen to expose the extradural portion. In addition, the pedicle and articular facets may need to be removed. A large extradural/extraspinal extension may be best dealt with at a separate second stage procedure via a more lateral approach. When multiple tumours are present the aim should be to remove the tumour identified as being responsible for the current symptoms on the basis of careful clinical assessment. If precise identification is impossible the largest tumour which is the most likely culprit should be removed. Prophylactic excision of other lumps in the vicinity at the same operation is sensible but the choice must be limited by the nature of the associated obligatory neurological deficit.

Meningioma The aim is to remove the tumour as well as the portion of dura which lends attachment and origin to the lesion. The latter achieves a true radical excision and minimizes the possibility of tumour recurrence. If the dural origin is in the posterior or posterolateral circumference of the dura, excision is not technically difficult. Anterior attachments are awkward to excise and can instead be dealt with by heavy bipolar coagulation instead. The excised dura can be replaced by a patch of cadaver dural graft which can be sutured or glued into place. Watertight repair will prevent the recurrence of a CSF leak from the wound or the formation of a pseudomeningocele. A calcified tumour can prove to be a tedious technical challenge especially when placed in the anterior quadrants of the canal. Often even the ultrasonic aspirator will fail to disintegrate a hard tumour. In these circumstances, cord manipulation is unavoidable and increases the hazard to existing neurological function.

Intramedullary Tumours

The primary aim is surgical excision of the tumour.

Astrocytoma and Ependymoma For many years, intramedullary astrocytomas and ependymomas were treated with a wide decompressive laminectomy, tumour biopsy, cyst aspiration followed by radiotherapy. In current neurosurgical practice, the primary treatment for these tumours is surgical excision of the solid tumour along with drainage of the cyst followed by radiotherapy in appropriate cases. This trend has evolved in the realization that excision is technically feasible, that radio-therapy has only little benefit to offer the majority of patients and that radical surgery improves neurological function and increases survival time (Epstein and Epstein 1982). A more optimistic efficacy of radiotherapy treatment has been reported with 20-plus year survival in 67% of children receiving irradiation for primary spinal cord tumours (O'Sullivan et al. 1994).

The cord is exposed by a laminectomy which is limited to the extent of the solid tumour only. Polar cystic components can be drained whilst dealing with the solid part without extending the laminectomy. The tumour is reached by an incision on the dorsal midline of the cord (myelotomy) which can be extended over the entire length of the tumour. The lesion is excised by debulking the central core and then gradually separating it from the surrounding expanded cord leaving a shallow trench-like tumour bed. The capsule of a dermoid, epidermoid cyst, enterogenous cyst or lipoma can be very adherent to the spinal cord making radical excision difficult and dangerous.

Extradural Malignant Tumours

The main options of aggressive treatment are surgery, radiotherapy and chemother-apy used singly or in combination. Rapidly progressive neurological deterioration due to extradural metastatic compression has a poor prognosis whatever method of treatment is adopted. The management of these patients presents a multitude of controversies including the role of surgery in the treatment. The clinician is invari-ably confronted with a patient who has developed pain, paralysis and incontinence or retention. The expected survival time is short, being determined by the nature, extent and response to treatment of the primary tumour rather than the secondary deposit in the spine. Therefore, the treatment of the spinal lesion is usually palliative rather than curative. The goals of treatment are to return the patient to a reasonably pain free, ambulant and continent status. The attainment of these ideals is especially relevant to a patient with malignant disease because quality of life is paramount when longevity is reduced. The method of treatment used must be judged primarily in terms of possible benefit in improving symptoms but modulated by the risk of producing neurological deterioration as well as the discomfort and the distress caused to the patient.

Many patients with malignant cord compression are elderly with either cardiores-piratory compromise, other systemic diseases or malignant cachexia. Primary lung carcinoma has a notoriously bad prognosis whereas lymphoma, prostate and breast cancer patients have better outcomes and longer survival. Many are poor surgical risks, prone to postoperative infections as well as impaired wound healing. Therefore the physical age (rather than the actual age), and general medical condition of the adult patient may dictate the choice of treatment method. In children, an aggressive policy of treatment is more readily accepted. After an overall assessment of the patient and the primary disease, a certain group will be much better served with conservative treatment. These are usually patients with complete cord transection, multiple levels of spinal metastatic disease and those with advanced and widespread disseminated tumour. Pain control is the mainstay of treatment combined with good basic nursing care usually in a hospice or home environment.

It is good clinical practice to establish the diagnosis of metastatic cancer by tissue examination especially when the site of the primary cancer is unknown. A percutaneous needle biopsy will provide excellent diagnostic material. Alternatively, a hemilaminectomy will achieve the dual purpose of tumour decompression and diagnostic biopsy without jeopardizing spinal stability significantly. These simple procedures can be performed safely and quickly even in poor risk patients. It seems reasonable to accept the concept that neural structures which are being mechanically compressed will benefit from surgical decompression. This is best achieved by excision of the tumour, as in the case of benign intradural tumours. However, most malignant extradural lesions are extensive at clinical presentation and total excision is not possible. Traditionally, decompression was achieved by a laminectomy at the tumour site. This procedure is relatively simple technically and therefore quickly performed, thus conferring an advantage when dealing with poor risk, elderly patients. However, in most instances the tumour is sited anteriorly or anterolaterally and only a limited excision or diagnostic biopsy is possible via a laminectomy. Being considered a neurosurgical emergency, decompressive laminectomy (DL) was often carried out late at night by junior surgeons operating on poor risk patients. Not surprisingly, the operation gradually became unpopular due to an unsatisfactory outcome and associated complications. Although neurological improvement occurred in some, less than 5% of those who were unable to walk before surgery became ambulant. More importantly, only 50% of those who were able to walk before operation retained this ability after surgery (Findlay 1984). The predominant cause of neurological deterioration following DL was anterior vertebral collapse due to removal of posterior supporting elements when the anterior spinal column was already diseased by tumour (Bryce and McKissock 1965). The results were better when DL was combined with radiotherapy although about 30% of patients deteriorated despite the treatment (Findlay 1984). Several studies have shown that radiotherapy combined with steroids has a similar beneficial response as DL plus radiotherapy, with ambulation rates of 46% and 40%, respectively (Black 1979; Barcena et al. 1984; Findlay 1984). These studies gradually led to the concept that surgical decompression was not the ideal initial treatment for malignant spinal compression and established radiotherapy as the primary therapy.

Surgical excision was reconsidered in the treatment of recurrent tumours or those which did not respond to radiotherapy. During the same period, the methods of spinal stabilization also became more advanced. An aggressive approach in the surgical treatment of spinal metastatic disease is beginning to emerge on the basis that more patients can be made ambulatory and the quality of life improved during the period of survival (Sundaresan et al. 1991). Since most extradural metastases are sited anterior or anterolateral to the cord the most logical method of tumour debulking is via a costotransversectomy or anterior approach. The tumour can be removed under direct vision and a greater extent of debulking can be achieved. In solitary vertebral body disease almost a total excision is possible. Ambulation rates of 70%–80% have been reported (Siegal et al. 1985) by this method and the recovery to ambulatory status of paraplegic patients is far higher than with DL (Findlay 1984). Anterior decompression produces a potentially unstable spinal column and most patients require a spinal stabilization procedure (see below). The operation is thus a major surgical exercise and not easily tolerated by elderly and poor risk patients.

The unpopularity of DL was predominantly related to the indiscriminate use of the procedure for all patients with spinal metastases irrespective of the site of the tumour. DL is still the ideal surgical approach when the tumour is situated in the posterior or even posterolateral quadrants of the canal but it should be combined with a stabilization procedure whenever the stability of the spine is in question.

The correct choice of patient is therefore all important in achieving therapeutic goals whichever method is used. The indications for surgery can be summarized as follows:

1. Diagnosis – when primary tumour is unknown (options hemilaminectomy or needle biopsy)
2. Decompression of cord when:
   a) Tumour is radioresistant
   b) When deterioration occurs during radiotherapy
   c) When vertebral collapse has caused bone fragments to collapse into spinal canal causing cord compression.
   d) Recurrent cord compression by tumour after maximal radiotherapy doses
   e) Single body disease with significant anterior cord compression.
   Anterior decompression is the ideal method.
3. Spinal stabilization

The definite indications for radiotherapy are:

1. Radiosensitive tumours (especially without significant anterior collapse or cord compression), e.g. lymphoma, neuroblastoma, Ewing's sarcoma, myeloma
2. Stable, ambulant patients with known primary tumour who present with pain and/or minor neurological deficit
3. Postoperatively in de novo cases
4. Advanced, generalized disease
5. Refusal of, or medically unfit for major surgery

Primary Spinal Tumours

These lesions may be benign or malignant. The common presentation is midline spinal pain. Tumour excision is difficult because of the adjacent neural structures. The best approach is anterior or anterolateral. The spine will be rendered unstable following extensive resection. Therefore, a stabilization procedure will be necessary in the majority of patients.

Spinal Stabilization

Whatever method of cord decompression and tumour removal is used, it is sound surgical practice to aim for stability of the spinal column. If anterior disease is absent and posterior bone removal did not involve bilateral facet joint excision, the stability will be acceptable without added instrumentation. In most other instances, an internal stabilization procedure must complement the decompression whether the latter is performed from an anterior or posterior approach. Instability of the spine will result in deformity, pain and neurological disability due to neural compression and distortion.

A variety of complex spinal instrumentation methods are available. Posterior stabilization is achieved by using metal rods or rectangular metal prostheses which are fixed across the weakened area of the spinal column with wires or screws at a minimum of two levels above and below the level of the decompression. Anterior stabilization is achieved by using vertebral prostheses. Acrylic vertebral body prostheses are available to replace a single vertebral body involved with tumour (Moore and Uttley 1989). Alternatively, the space can be filled with methyl methacrylate supported by metal pins inserted into the adjacent bones (Sundaresan et al. 1991).

In children, severe spinal deformities (kyphosis/scoliosis) can occur as a result of laminectomy for spinal tumours. This is common in children under two years of age or when the laminectomy involves more than three consecutive vertebral levels. The cervical spine is especially vulnerable. The cause is muscle weakness due to neurological deficit, loss of posterior support to the vertebral column and radiation growth arrest of the vertebral body. External supports do not usually help and eventually anterior or posterior internal fixation becomes necessary (Holmes and Hall 1978). Gross deformities of the neck may require anterior corpectomy and plate fixation (Herman and Sauntag 1994). The deformities can be prevented by limiting the laminectomy to the level essential for tumour excision, preservation of facet joints at surgery or performing en bloc excision (laminostomy) and replacement of the laminae. It is better to perform the stabilization procedure as part of the initial surgical exercise when it is anticipated that spinal deformity may occur as a result of the bone and tumour excision.

Radiotherapy

The vast majority of benign intradural/extramedullary tumours can be excised totally and do not require additional treatment.

The role of radiotherapy (RT) has already been mentioned under the individual tumours. It may be used as the primary treatment or as an adjunct to surgery. If total tumour excision can be achieved RT is rarely necessary. Reduction of tumour bulk facilitates the efficacy of RT. When radical resection is not feasible the residual tumour should be treated with RT to reduce tumour growth. In essence, the indications for RT are:

1. Malignancy
2. Incomplete resection
3. Poor surgical risk
4. Refusal of surgery
5. Recurrence

Therefore, RT plays an important role in the treatment of primary and metastatic malignant tumours of the spinal column. RT is the treatment of choice in radiosensitive tumours such as Ewing's sarcoma, primary lymphoma and solitary plasmacytoma (Suit and Austin-Seymour 1990). The role of radiotherapy in extradural malignant and metastatic lesions has already been described. Meningiomas of the aggressive type or those treated with partial excision or when the dural origin is not removed, can be administered local irradiation treatment in order to reduce the likelihood of recurrence. In medulloblastomas, spinal irradiation is used as a prophylactic measure or when seedlings are known to be present. A number of spinal tumours are relatively radioresistant. Radionecrosis of the cord is an uncommon but recognized complication. This causes a delayed relentless neurological deterioration. In intramedullary tumours radiotherapy is used when tumour excision is incomplete and/or when the neoplasm is malignant.

Chemotherapy

Chemotherapy is usually an adjunct to surgery and RT. It is particularly useful in diseases such as myeloma associated with systemic spread. However, it is becoming increasingly relevant in the control of certain malignant spinal tumours. For instance, it is the ideal treatment for leukaemia involving the spine. Chemotherapy alone is not effective in the treatment of solid tumour masses because of limited penetration into the tumour and the occurrence of drug-resistant tumour cells. The intravenous route will achieve a more effective blood level of the drugs than oral therapy. It is common practice to use combinations of drugs for greater efficacy.

Certain spinal tumours, e.g. osteosarcoma and Ewing's sarcoma, are sensitive to chemotherapy (Harmon 1990). Antimitotic chemotherapy is used as standard treatment in the management of myeloma and lymphoma. The best drug for the treatment of myeloma is melphalan which reduces the systemic spread and complications of the disease especially when combined with prednisolone. The role of steroid therapy in the treatment of spinal compression has already been discussed.

There is no evidence of a superior survival when chemotherapy is used in malignant astrocytomas of the cord. Optimistic results are being reported especially in intramedullary malignant ependymomas. Immunotherapy with intrathecal monoclonal antibodies may become useful in the treatment of subarachnoid seedlings of medulloblastoma and other primitive ectodermal tumours.

The demonstration of oestrogen and progesterone receptors in cerebral meningioma cells has led to the belief that synthetic steroids may be beneficial in the treatment of these tumours especially those at relatively inaccessible sites. Mifepristone and gestrinone have been considered to be the most suitable (Davis 1995). Such receptors have also been demonstrated in primary spinal tumours particularly neurinomas and ependymomas (Concolino et al. 1984). Therefore, hormonal treatment may be a suitable adjuvant treatment option to be considered for residual or recurrent spinal meningiomas. The same may apply in the future to other receptor positive spinal tumours. Dopamine D1 receptors have also been found in cerebral meningiomas (Schrell et al. 1992). Therefore drugs such as bromocriptine may become useful in the treatment of cerebral and spinal meningiomas.

Recovery and Rehabilitation

Following successful tumour excision neurological recovery is dependent on several factors, the most important of which is the degree of initial disability. Patients with mild deficits recover better and complete reversal of paraplegia is uncommon but not unknown. Children and young adults show a greater potential for regaining normal function. The general health of the patient is important and poor nutrition and intercurrent infections impair recovery. Those who show signs of regaining function in the early stages are more likely to continue to do so. It is reasonable to allow about 18–24 months for the recovery process to continue before accepting that the residual neurological disability is unlikely to improve further.

During this period there is immense benefit in intensive, supervised physiotherapy. Formal programmes of rehabilitation are ideal and should include bladder retraining and teaching of self-catheterization if necessary. Control of pain, spasticity and dysaesthesiae may require regular medication and provide a significant improvement in the quality of life.

The vast majority of patients who undergo excision of a benign intradural tumour return to a normal independent life. The unfortunate few who retain a severe residual deficit need to be cared for in special institutions. Some with moderate disability will be able to manage at home with the provision of special domestic adaptations and the support of social services, friends and relatives.

References

Barcena A, Lobato RD, Ruivas JJ et al. (1984) Spinal metastatic disease: analysis of factors determining functional prognosis and the choice of treatment. Neurosurgery 15:820–827

Barker D, Wright K, Nguyen L (1987) Gene for von Recklinghausen's neurofibromatosis is in the pericentric region of chromosome 17. Science 236:1100–1102

Bertoni F, Unni MK, Dahlin D (1990) Calcifying pseudoneoplasms of the neural axis. J Neurosurg 72:42–48.

Black P (1979) Spinal metastases: current status and recommended guidelines for management. Neurosurgery 5:726–746

Braughler JM, Hall ED (1983) Lactate and pyruvate metabolism in injured cat's spinal cord before and after a single large intravenous dose of methylprednisolone. J Neurosurg 59:256–261

Bryce J, McKissock W (1965) Surgical treatment of malignant extradural spinal tumours. Br Med J i:1341–1344

Chandler CL, Uttley D, Wilkins PR et al. (1994) Primary spinal malignant schwannoma Br J Neurosurg 8:341–345

Choremis C, Oelonomos D, Papadatos P, Gargoulas A (1956) Intraspinal epidermoid tumours (cholesteatomas) in patients treated for tuberculous meningitis. Lancet ii:437–439

Cloward RB, Bucy PC (1937) Spinal cyst and kyphosis dorsalis juvenalis. AJR 28:681–706

Cohen ARM, Wisoff JH, Allen JC, Epstein F (1989) Malignant astrocytoma of the spinal cord. J Neurosurg 70:50–54

Concolino G, Liccardo G, Conti C et al. (1984) Hormones and tumours in central nervous system. (CNS) Steroid Receptors in primary spinal cord tumours. Neurol-Res 6/3:121–126

Connolly ES (1982) Spinal cord tumours in adults. In: Youman JR (ed) Neurological surgery vol 5. WB Saunders, Philadephia, pp 3196–3214

Cristante L, Herrmann HD (1994) Surgical management of intramedullary spinal cord tumours: functional outcome and sources of morbidity. Neurosurgery 35:69–76.

Davis C (1990) Meningiomas and sex hormones. Eur J Cancer 26:859–860

Davis C (1995) Symptomatic meningiomas. Br J Neurosurg 9:295–302

Durie BJM, Salmon SE (1975) A clinical staging system for multiple myeloma. Correlation of measured cell mass with presenting clinical features, response to treatment and survival. Cancer 36:842–854.

Ehni G, Love JG (1945) Intraspinal lipomas. Report of cases: review of the literature and clinical and pathologic study. Arch Neurol Psychiatry 53:1–28

Epstein F, Epstein N (1982) Surgical treatment of spinal cord astrocytomas of childhood. A series of 19 patients. J. Neurosurg 75:685–689

Epstein FJ, Farmer J, Freed D (1993) Adult intramedullary spinal cord ependymomas: the result of surgery in 38 patients. J Neurosurg 79:204–209

Findlay G (1984) Adverse effects of the management of malignant spinal cord compression. J Neurol Neurosurg Psychiatry 47:767–788

Friedberg SR, Fellows T, Thomas CB et al. (1994) Experience with symptomatic spinal epidural cysts. Neurosurgery 34:989–993

Friedlaender GE, Southwick WO (1982) Tumours of the spine. In: Rothman RH, Simeone FA (eds) The spine. Saunders, Philadelphia, pp 1022–1040

Gilbert RW, Kim JH, Posner JB (1978) Epidural spinal cord compression from metastatic tumours. Diagnosis and treatment. Ann Neurol 3:40–51

Gortvai P (1963) Extradural cysts of the spinal cord. J Neurol Neurosurg Psychiatry 26:223–230

Grant JW, Kaech D, Jones DG (1986) Spinal cord as the first presentation of lymphoma: a review of 15 cases. Histopathology 11:1191–1202

Gudmundsson KR (1970) A survey of tumours of the central nervous system in Iceland during the 10 year period 1954–1963. Acta Neurol Scand 46:538–552.

Gurusinghe NT, Perera S (1994) Spinal intradural tumours: Preston experience. JN Neurol Neurosurg, Psychiatry (abstract) Vol 57, No 9, p 1156

Haddad P Thaell JF, Kelly JM et al. (1976) Lymphoma of the spinal extradural space. Cancer 38:1862–1864

Halliday AL, Sobel RA, Martuza RL (1991) Benign spinal nerve sheath tumours: their occurrence sporadically and in neurofibromatosis types 1 and 2. J Neurosurg 74:248–253

Harmon DC (1990) Chemotherapy. In: Sundaresan N, Schmidek HH, Schiller AL, Rosenthal DI (eds) Tumours of the spine. Diagnosis and clinical management. WB Saunders Philadephia, pp 92–98

Helseth A, Mork SJ (1989) Primary intraspinal neoplasms in Norway 1955 to 1986 – a population based survey of 467 patients. J Neurosurg 71:842–845

Herman JM, Sonntag VKH (1994) Cervical corpectomy and plate fixation for post-laminectomy kyphosis. J Neurosurg 80:963–970

Hochberg FH, Millar DC (1988) Primary CNS lymphoma. J Neurosurg 68:835–853

Holmes JC, Hall JE (1978) Fusion for instability and potential instability of the cervical spine in children and adolescents. Orthop Clin North Am 9:923

Horsley V, Gowers WR (1888) A case of tumour of the spinal cord. Trans R Med Chirug Soc Glasgow 79:377

Jackson DV, Randall ME, Richards F (1988) Spinal cord compression due to extramedullary haematopoiesis in thalassaemia: long term follow up after radiotherapy. Surg Neurol 29:389–392

Klein SL (1991) Paediatric spinal epidural metastases. J Neurosurg 74:70–75

Kothbauer K, Schmid UD, Seiler RW et al. (1994) Intraoperative motor and sensory monitoring of the cauda equina. Neurosurgery 34:702–707.

Lecat CNL (1765) Traite de l'existence, de la nature et des proprietes du fluide des nerfs et principalement de son action dans le mouvement musculaire. Ouvrage coutonne en 1753, par l'Academic de Berlin: suivi des dissertations sur la sensibilite des meninges, des tendons, etc., l'insensibilite du cervaux, la structure des nerfs, l'irritabilite hallerienne. Berlin

Lee M, Rezai AR, Abbott R et al. (1995) Intramedullary spinal cord Lipomas. J Neurosurg 82:394–400

Levy WJ, Bay J, Dolm D (1982) Spinal cord meningiomas. J Neurosurg 57:804–812

Levy WJ, Latchew J, Halm JF et al. (1986) Spinal neurofibromas. A report of 66 cases and a comparison with meningiomas. Neurosurgery 18:331–334

Lunardi P, Missori P, Gagliardi FM, Fortuna A (1989) Long term results of the surgical treatment of spinal dermoids and epidermoid tymours. Neurosurgery 25:860–864

Macdonald DR (1990) Clinical manifestations. In: Sunderesan N, Schmidek H, Schiller A, Rosenthal A (eds) Tumours of the spine. Diagnosis and clinical management. WB Saunders, Philadelphia, pp 6–21

Marchuk DA, Saulino AM, Tavakkol R et al. (1991) cDNA cloning of the type I neurofibramatosis gene: complete sequence of the NFI gene product. Genomics 11:931–940

Matson D (1969) Neurosurgery of infancy and childhood, 2nd edn. Thomas. Springfield, II

Maurice-Williams RS, Richardson PW (1988) Spinal cord compression: delay in the diagnosis and referral of a common neurosurgical emergency, Br J Neurosurg 2:55–60

McCormick PC, Torres R, Post KD, Stein B (1990) Intramedullary ependymomas of the spinal cord. J Neurosurg 72:523–532

Minehan KJ, Shaw EG, Scheithauer BW et al. (1995) Spinal cord astrocytoma: pathological and treatment considerations. J Neurosurg 83:590–595

Moore A, Uttley D (1989) Anterior decompression and stabilisation of the spine in malignant disease. Neurosurgery 24:713–717

Murota K, Symon L (1989) Surgical management of haemangioblastoma of the spinal cord. A report of 18 cases. Neurosurgery 25:699–708

Myles ST, Macrae ME (1988) Benign osteoblastoma of spine in childhood. J Neurosurg 68:884–888

Nabors MW, Pait TG, Byrd EB et al. (1988) Updated assessment and current classification of spinal meningeal cysts. J Neurosurg 68:366–377

Neumann HPH, Eggert HR, Weigel K et al. (1989) Haemangioblastomas of the central nervous system. J Neurosurg 70:24–30

Nittner K (1968) Discussion zy den Vortragen von Jellinger U.von Piscol. Bericht uber die Jahresfagung der Dtcsch. Ges fur Neurochirugie (13–16 Sept 1967 Bad Harzburg). Loew F (ed). Acta Neurochir (Wien) 19–91

Nittner K (1976) Spinal meningiomas, neurinomas and neurofibromas and hour-glass tumours. In: Vinken PJ, Bruyen BW (eds) Handbook of clinical neurology, vol 20. Elsevier, Amsterdam, pp 177–322

Norstrom CW, Kernohan JW, Love JG (1961) One hundred primary caudal tumours. JAMA 178:1071–1077

O'Connor GA, Roberts TS (1984) Spinal cord compression by osteochondroma. J Neurosurg 60:420–423

O'Sullivan MG, Keohane C, Buckley TF (1990) Paraganglioma of the cauda equina: a case report and review of the literature, Br J Neurosurg 4:63–68

O'Sullivan C, Jenkin RD, Doherty MA et al. (1994) Spinal cord tumours in children: long term results of combined surgical and radiation treatment. J Neurosurg 81:507–512

Perling LH, Laurent JP, Cheek WR (1988) Epidural hibernoma as a complication of corticosteroid treatment. J Neurosurg 69:613–616

Poisson M, Pcrtuiset BF, Hauw JJ et al. (1983) Steroid hormone receptors in human meningiomas, gliomas and brain metastases. J Neurooncol 1:179–189

Rand RW, Rand CW (1960) Intraspinal tumours of childhood. Thomas, Springfield, II

Reimer R, Onofrio M (1985) Astrocytomas of the spinal cord in children and adolescenets. J Neurosurg 63:669–675

Ridsdale L, Moseley I (1978) Thoracolumbar intraspinal tumours presenting features of raised intracranial pressure. J Neurol Neurosurgery Psychiatry 41:737–745

Rotish E, Zeidman SM, Burger PC et al. (1990) Clinical and pathological analysis of spinal cord astrocytomas. Neurosurgery 27:193–196

Russell DS, Rubinstein LJ (1989) Pathology of tumours of the nervous system, 5th edn Williams and Wilkins Baltimore

Seppala MT, Haltia MJJ, Sankila RJ et al. (1995) Long term outcome after removal of spinal neurofibroma. J Neurosurg 82:572–577

Siegal T, Topya P, Siegal T (1985) Vertebral body resection for epidural compression by malignant tumours. Results of 47 consecutive operative procedures. J Bone Joint Surg 67A:375–382 .

Schrell UMH, Nomikos P, Fahlbusch R (1992) Presence of dopamine D1 receptors and absence of dopamine D2 receptors in human cerebral meningioma tissue. J Neurosurg 77:288–294

Sloof JL, Kernohan JW, McCarty CS (1964) Primary intramedullary tumours of the spinal cord and filum terminale. Saunders, Philadephia, pp 124–129

Suit HD, Austin-Seymour M. (1990) The role of radiation therapy. In: Sundaresan N, Schmidek HH, Schiller AL, Rosenthal DI (eds) Tumours of the spine. Diagnosis and clinical management. Publisher WB Saunders Philadelphia, p 86–91

Sundaresan N, Galicich JH, Chu FCH, Huvos AG (1979) Spinal chordomas. J Neurosurg 50:312–319

Sundaresan N, Digiacinto GV, Hughes JEO et al. (1991) Treatment of neoplastic spinal cord compression: results of a prospective study. Neurosurgery 29:645–650

Tarlov IM (1938) Perineural cysts of the spinal nerve roots. Arch Neurol Psychiatry (Chicago) 40:1067–1074

Till K (1975) Paediatric neurosurgery for paediatricians and neurosurgeons. Blackwell Scientific, Oxford, pp 193–204

Von Recklinghausen F (1882) Uber die multiplen Fibrome der Hant und ihre Bezichung zu den multiplen Neuromen. Fetschrift zur Feier des funfundzwanzigjahrigen Bestehens des pathologischen Instituts ze Berlin, (Herrn Rudolf Virchow dargebracht). Hirschwald, Berlin

Wilson LMK, Draper GJ (1974) Neuroblastoma – its natural history and prognosis: a study of 487 cases. Br Med J 3:301–307

Wiltshaw E (1976) The natural history of extramedullary plasmacytoma and its relation to solitary myeloma of bone and myelomatosis. Medicine 55:217–238

Xu Qi-Wu, Bao Wei-Min, Mao Ren-Ling et al. (1994) Magnetic resonance imaging and microsurgical treatment of intramedullary haemangioblastoma of the spinal cord. Neurosurgery 35:671–676

Yamada K, Bremer AM, West CR (1979) Effects of dexamethasone on tumour induced brain oedema and its distribution in the brain of monkeys. J Neurosurg 50:361–367

Zulch KJ (1979) Histological Typing of Tumours of the Central Nervous System. International Histological Classification of Tumours No. 21, p 19. World Health Organisation, Geneva

Chapter 31

Trauma and Paraplegia

T.T. Lee and B.A. Green

Introduction

This chapter deals with traumatic injury to the thoracic and upper lumbar regions, which results in paraplegia when the neural elements are involved. The anatomy and biomechanics of the upper/mid thoracic (T2–T10) and thoracolumbar junction (T11–L3) are different, and will be discussed below in the Anatomy section.

The goal of treatment of thoracolumbar spinal injury is to maintain neurological function, stabilize haemodynamic and pulmonary function, restore spinal alignment and stability, and preserve life. There is not a single best approach to the management of these patients, however, the general philosophy and treatment methods do show great similarities. In this chapter, the authors present their approach to the injuries of the thoracolumbar spines.

Epidemiology

Vertebral column fracture and spinal cord injury carry substantial morbidity, mortality, and economic impact in the United States and the world. Vertebral column fractures result in physician visits and cause physical activity restrictions for 162 000 Americans every year (Grazier et al. 1984) Thoracolumbar spine region is the predominant site of such injuries. Of these patients, approximately 2.9% become paraplegic.

There are multiple aetiologies for the thoracolumbar spine fracture, of which trauma is the single most frequent cause. The mechanism can be blunt (motor vehicle accident, fall, assault, etc.) or penetrating (gunshot wound, knife or other sharp object). Osteoporosis, especially in elderly females, causes a significant number of fracture. Tumours, both primary and metastatic may cause pathological fracture of the vertebral column. This chapter will focus on blunt trauma to the thoracolumbar region, and briefly discuss penetrating trauma at the end.

History

The earliest written record of spinal injury dates back to 3000 BC in the Edward Smith Papyrus (Breasted 1930). Celsus described the difference between cervical and thoracolumbar trauma (Bick 1937). He noted that cervical spine fracture led to respiratory problems and vomiting, whereas thoracolumbar trauma caused paraplegia and urinary incontinence. Manual extension for spinal deformity reduction was described.

Extended bedrest had long been prescribed as the treatment for vertebral fractures, and numerous foreseeable complications arose as a result, including pneumonia, sepsis, deep vein thrombosis and ischaemic ulcers. Guttman (1973) emphasized the role of closed reduction of fractures in spinal trauma. Davis (1929) used a pulley system to raise lower extremities to produce hyperextension and aid reduction for an anaesthetized patient in a prone position. More theories on reduction and stabilization were proposed by Boehler (1932). He advocated spine reduction by hyperextension, then placement of the patient in a body cast postreduction. Muscle training and ambulation were also stressed in the recovery process. Watson-Jones (1943) continued to emphasize extension cast treatment and early mobilization.

After World War II, Holdsworth and Harvey (1953) devised a surgical stabilization system with spinous process plating for unstable fractures; however, inadequate stability was provided by this system alone. The era of antibiotics preceded the popularization of these surgical procedures. Harrington (1962) initially devised the distraction rod and laminar hook system for treatment of scoliosis, but later used this posterior instrumentation system for post-traumatic spinal stabilization. A double-rod distraction system was used. His system has been modified many times, and multiple other posterior instrumentation devices have since been invented, but the Harrington system still serves as the original standard of treatment for thoracolumbar fractures against which all other devices are measured.

The benefits of internal fixation of spinal fractures are early mobilization, shorter hospital stay, stabilization and prevention of spinal deformity and complications from immobilization (Convery et al. 1978). Rehabilitation time has been reduced by surgical intervention (Rimoldi et al. 1992). Neurological recovery from such surgical procedures is minimal when compared to prolonged immobilization (Bedbrook 1980; Jacobs et al. 1980; McAfee et al. 1985). However, in certain cases, spinal cord and nerve root decompression could lead to some neurological improvement.

Anatomy

The human spine consists of seven cervical, twelve thoracic, five lumbar, and one fused sacrococcygeal vertebrae. The line of gravity in the thoracic and lumbar regions runs anterior to the vertebral column. Therefore anterior compression and posterior ligament tension/distraction are the predominant components of stress. The anatomy and biomechanical support for the typical thoracic vertebrae (T1–T10) are different from that of the thoracolumbar vertebral (T11–L2), and they are discussed separately below.

The thoracic spine contains a natural kyphotic angle, with 91% of the healthy population having an angle between 18 and 51 degrees (Stagnara et al. 1982). The thoracic vertebral bodies are generally wedge-shaped with longer posterior height, and larger in terms of posterior width, which contribute to the natural kyphosis. The diameter of the thoracic spinal canal is also narrower than the lumbar region. At midthoracic levels, the canal shape is almost circular, with a diameter of 16 mm, which is narrower than the average cervical and lumbar-sacral canal by 7–10 mm (Louis 1983). Therefore, any mal-alignment or protrusion of disc or bony fragment is more likely to cause neurological symptoms of cord compression. However, the general stability of the thoracic vertebrae is greater than that of the cervical or lumbar area. The facet joint plane is more sagittal than the cervical spines, but more coronal than the typical lumbar spines. These factors protect against rotational injury, and allow somewhat more axial rotation. The rib cage and costovertebral ligament afford an additional element of stability, when compared to either the cervical or the thoracolumbar junction. As a result, more force is required to produce a fracture in the thoracic spine region. Instability is not as great a concern for fracture in the upper and midthoracic vertebrae than elsewhere in the human spine (White and Panjabi 1990). The vascular supply of the spinal cord comprises the single anterior spinal artery, paired posterior spinal arteries and the segmental radicular arteries. The anterior spinal artery supplies the anterior two-thirds of the cord and posterior spinal arteries supply the posterior third of the cord. In the cervical cord, the main vascular supplies come from the spinal arteries, but in the thoracic and lumbar regions, the segmental radicular arteries are the major contributors of blood supply. In the upper thoracic cord, the vascular supply may be sparse, especially between the fourth and eighth vertebrae, creating the "critical zone" (Louis 1983).

At the thoracolumbar junction and distally, the vertebral bodies allow a greater degree of motion than elsewhere in the spine. The facet joints in the lumbar region are almost entirely sagittal, as compared to the more coronal orientation of the thoracic spine. This transition occurs from T10 to T12. Because of the alteration of the facet plane, the lowest thoracic vertebrae have a range of mobility similar to that of the lumbar vertebrae (White and Panjabi 1990). The lack of rib cage support, the more room for flexion/extension, and the change in disc size and shape may all contribute to the relatively greater mobility. However, the additional degree of mobility at the thoracolumbar junction, especially T11 to L2, makes it more susceptible to injury than other adjacent portions of the spine. In fact, almost half of all vertebral body fractures occur from T11 to L2. The normal conus medullaris usually begins at T11 and ends at L1–2 disc space, and could be compromised by an injury at this level. The vascularity in the thoracolumbar junction is more consistent than the upper thoracic region (Parke 1982; Louis 1983).

A vertebral column fracture always raises the issue of spine stability. Clinical instability is defined by the loss of the ability of the spine under physiological loads to maintain its pattern of movement so that there is no initial or additional neurological deficit, no major deformity and no incapacitating pain (White and Panjabi 1990). This may be, but is not necessarily, related to the degree of retained neurological function. For instance, a transverse process fracture associated with nerve root injury can produce a deficit, whereas an unstable fracture can occur in patients with an intact neurological examination.

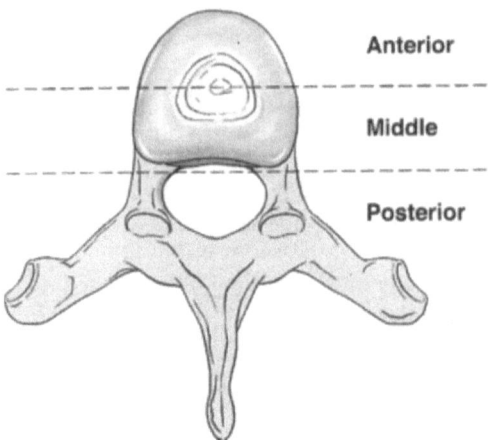

Fig. 31.1. The original Denis classification of the three columns of the vertebral body. The anterior column consists of the anterior half of the annulus fibrosis, nucleus propulsus, and vertebral body, plus the anterior longitudinal ligament. The middle column includes the posterior half of the annulus fibrosis, nucleus propulsus and vertebral body, as well as the posterior longitudinal ligament. The posterior column includes the posterior osseous arch and the multiple ligamentous structures.

Nicoll (1949) considered the most important factor of stability to be the integrity of the interspinous ligament. He proposed anterior and lateral wedge fractures to be stable, and fracture subluxation and fracture dislocation to be unstable. Holdsworth (1963) classified stability based on the two-column model. The anterior weight-bearing column was defined as the vertebral body and the intervertebral disc, and the posterior column as the bony arches with ligaments. The integrity of the posterior osseous components and posterior ligamentous structures (interspinous, supraspinous, ligamentum flavum) was proposed to be the major determinant of stability. Flexion–rotational injury was considered the most unstable, as it disrupts the posterior column. Experimental data, however, did not support the primary importance of the posterior column in determining stability (Nicoll 1949; Holdsworth 1963). Bedbrook (1975, 1979) believed that anterior disc and vertebral body were the primary determinants of stability.

The current concept of stability is based largely on the "three-column" theory proposed first by Denis (1983). This is further defined by the advent of computerized tomography, which visualizes the vertebral body in axial views, and is also capable of reconstructing images in sagittal and coronal orientations. The three columns are: anterior, middle, and posterior (Fig. 31.1). The anterior column consists of the anterior half of the vertebral body, anterior half of the annulus fibrosis, and the anterior longitudinal ligament. The middle column consists of the posterior half of the vertebral body, the posterior half of the annulus fibrosus and the posterior longitudinal ligament. The posterior column consists of the posterior arch, interspinous ligament, supraspinous ligament and ligamentum flavum. A fracture which causes the disruption of the middle column is termed a burst fracture. A combination of anterior and middle, or middle and posterior columns results in an unstable injury. Stable injuries include minimal and moderate compression features with an intact posterior and middle column, which prevents abnormal forward flexion.

White and Panjabi (1990) recommended a systematic approach to stability, and devised a checklist to determine it (Table 31.1). Because more variables are taken

Table 31.1. Checklist for determination of stability of thoracic and thoracolumbar spine. (Adapted from *White and Panjabi* (1990))

Element	Point value
Anterior element destroyed/unable to function	2
Posterior element destroyed/unable to function	2
Disruption of costovertebral articulation	1
Plain film radiographic criteria	4
1. Sagittal plane displacement > 2.5 mm (2 point)	
2. Relative sagittal plain angulation (2 point)	
Spinal cord/cauda equina damage	2
Anticipated dangerous loading	1
Total of > 5 points = unstable	

into consideration, they believe it to be a more accurate system. The system aims to prevent the unnecessary treatment of stable injuries and to protect against neurological complications. A patient having a total score of 5 or higher is considered to have a clinically unstable spine.

There are also other radiographic signs that should alert the physician to the presence of instability. These include: (a) widened interlaminar or interspinous distance observed in facet joint and posterior ligament injury; (b) vertebral displacement which implicates a three-column injury; (c) increased interpediculate distance suggesting three-column injury and in burst fracture; (d) mis-aligned posterior vertebral body line suggesting injury to the anterior and middle column (Roberts and Curtis 1970 Daffner et al. 1990; El-Khoury et al. 1992). In addition to the CT scan, the authors presently utilize magnetic resonance imaging (MRI) to assess cord intraparenchymal and paraspinous soft tissue/ligamentous injuries.

Mechanisms of Injury

The forces responsible for a spinal column injury are: axial compression, flexion, extension, rotation, shear, distraction or a combination of these forces (Eismont et al. 1993; Lebwohl and Starr 1993). The forces of vectors are depicted in Figs. 31.2 and 31.3. The combined use of plain radiographs, CT scans, and MRIs delineates the osseous as well as ligamentous injuries, and consequently allows for a more precise definition of the forces causing the injury. Unstable injury can be identified this way and proper surgical intervention can be taken.

Axial Compression

The anatomical kyphosis of the mid and upper thoracic spine, axial compressive forces are usually converted into an anterior flexion load on the anterior vertebral body (Fig. 31.2). The result is a wedge compression fracture of vertebral body, the same injury caused by a pure flexion force. Axial load in the thoracolumbar junction results in pure axial compressive force on the vertebral body. End-plate fracture

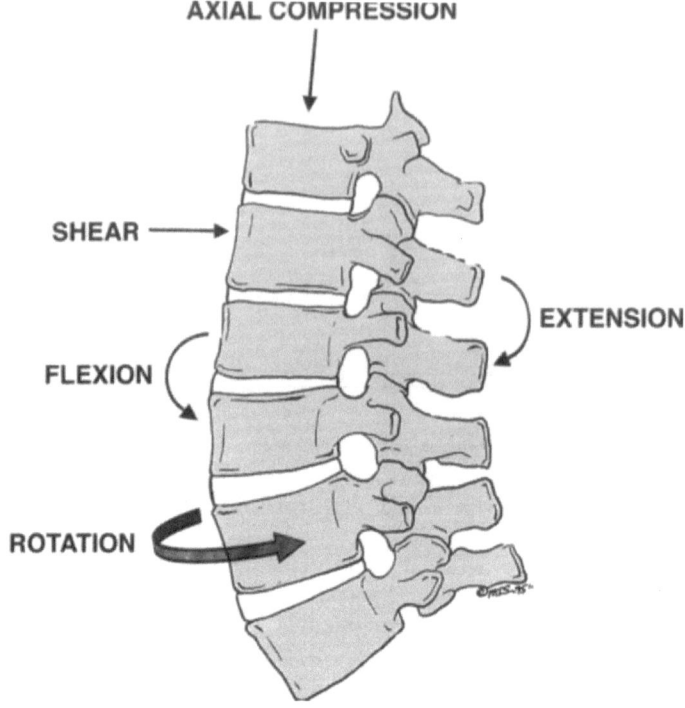

Fig. 31.2. The forces of spinal injury. Depicted here are axial compression, flexion, extension, rotation, and shear.

followed by vertebral body compression may occur. When sufficient force is present, vertical fracture through the vertebral body will produce a breakdown of the middle column, creating a "burst fracture" (Eismont et al. 1993). Pedicles and eventually posterior elements may be involved with progressively greater forces.

Extension

Forced posterior movement of the head or upper trunk is the predominant force in this injury (Fig. 31.2). The majority of problems stem from the fractures of the posterior osseous elements (facet, lamina, spinous process). A pure extension injury is generally stable. But if associated anterior injury occurs, the retrolisthesis of superior vertebral body is possible. This would then become an unstable injury.

Flexion

Flexion and associated anterior compression produce a compressive vector on the anterior vertebral body and a tensile force on the posterior column. An anterior wedge compression fracture with an intact posterior vertebral body (intact middle column) generally results in a stable fracture. This is not associated with spinal cord injury. When the anterior wedge exceeds 50%, posterior ligamentous or facet joint disruption may be assumed, causing an unstable injury. A facet joint fracture or capsule injury can cause the superior vertebral body to sublux on the inferior body, leading to a fracture-dislocation.

Flexion–Rotation

This injury pattern is caused by a combination of flexion and rotation forces (Fig. 31.2). The injury caused by flexion, as described above, results in anterior vertebral body compression fracture. The rotational force, on the other hand, causes ligament and facet capsule rupture. Retropulsion of bony element into the canal is possible (Lebwohl and Starr 1993). An unstable fracture pattern develops, with ruptured joint capsules and posterior ligaments and a disrupted anterior column. This is frequently associated with neurological deficits.

Shear

The forces can be directed in any direction along the longitudinal axis of the spine (Fig. 31.2). Severe ligamentous tears similar to those observed in flexion–rotation are found. These forces cause the superior vertebral body to sublux on the inferior vertebral body, most commonly anteriorly. When the anterolisthesis of the superior vertebral body disrupts the pars interarticularis or the pedicles, the neural elements may be "decompressed" and spared from severe neurological deficit (White and Panjabi 1990).

Flexion–Distraction

This type of lesion, also known as "seat-belt" injury, was first described by Chance (1948). The mechanism was not fully understood until later. Denis (1983) reclassified this type of injury as a category of fracture–dislocation. The axis of rotation is shifted anteriorly to the vertebral column by having the seat belt restrain the trunk anteriorly (Fig. 31.3). A flexion movement causes tensile forces on the middle and posterior column, as well as compressive force on the anterior column. Both ligamentous or osseous disruption could arise from such an injury. The annulus is

FLEXION DISTRACTION

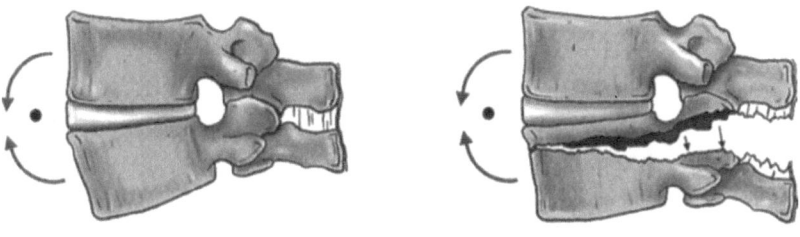

● = center of rotation

Fig. 31.3. Flexion–distraction injury. Left, the centre of the axis of rotation of a flexion–distraction injury lies anterior to the spinal column. Right, a chance fracture could result from such an injury.

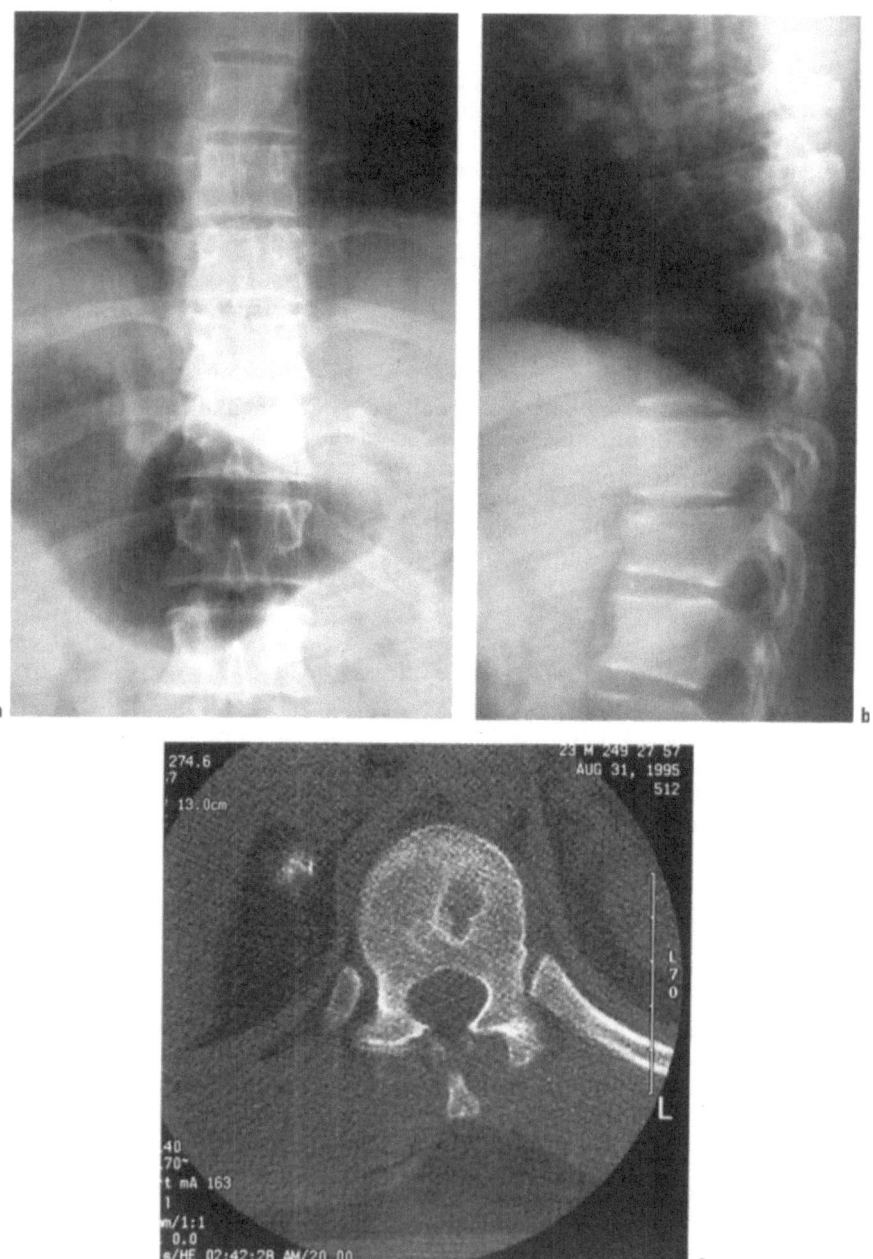

Fig. 31.4. This was a 18-year-old male who was involved in a motor vehicle accident. Plain films (**a,b**) show a T11 anterior wedge compression fracture, with slight reduction of column height. **c** CT scan demonstrated preservation of the middle column and the canal.

disrupted and the anterior longitudinal ligament is torn away from the inferior vertebral body, causing anterior column failure. A horizontal fracture beginning in the spinous process, and extending through the lamina, transverse process, pedicle and eventually vertebral body, could occur. Bilateral facet dislocation in the thoracic and thoracolumbar spine has been described by Eismont et al. (1993).

Classification of Thoracolumbar Injury

Many classifications have been proposed to define the types of spinal injury. Although more comprehensive systems have been described (Magerl et al. 1989), the most widely utilized system presently is that described by Denis (1983). Denis developed his system based on the review of 412 patients with major thoracic and lumbar injuries. The four major types of injuries are compression, burst, seat-belt type injury and fracture–dislocation.

Compression Fracture

This is a fracture of the anterior column with middle column intact (Fig. 31.4). This is the most frequently seen lesion, as 47.8% of Denis' patients belong to this group. The fracture is generally stable, as the middle column is intact. Neurological deficit is rare. Fractures may involve both end-plates (type A), superior end-plate only (type B), the inferior end-plate only (type C), or disruption of anterior column with intact end-plates (type D). When the anterior body collapses, the intact middle column acts as a hinge, imposing tensile force on the posterior ligamentous structures. However, if the anterior vertebral column height reduction is 50% or greater, the likelihood of posterior column failure is significant (Maiman and Pintar 1990). If the kyphotic angle is greater than 30°, the vertebral body height decrease is greater than 50%, or if the patient undergoes subsequent laminectomies, there has been a report of increased long-term deformity (Bohlman 1985). A stabilization is recommended for the above circumstances. A posterior stabilization system such as the Harrington distraction rod system, or one of the newer universal segmental fixation systems will suffice for the stabilization and resist further compression and kyphosis.

Burst Fracture

In such a fracture, the predominant mechanism is axial loading. Combination with flexion or rotation causes the characteristic patterns seen with burst fractures. A characteristic feature of this type of injury is the failure of the middle column, which is not present in a compression fracture (Fig. 31.5). Posterior column fractures may also be associated, which make this type of fracture even more unstable. The subtypes (A–E) of burst fractures are classified similarly to compression fractures in subtypes A to C. Type D is a middle column burst fracture combined with rotation, resulting in lateral displacement or tilt. This is best seen on anteroposterior plain radiographs. Type E burst fracture is seen with an asymmetric anterior column compression.

Denis (1983) proposed several key features to burst fractures: (a) comminution of the vertebral body; (b) loss of posterior vertebral body height; (c) retropulsion of bony and ligamentous/disc material into the spinal canal; (d) fracture of the lamina; (e) increase in interpediculate space. The initial degree of canal compromise was reported (Lemons et al. 1992) to correlate directly with the degree of neurological deficit, though other reports disputed this claim. About 47% of the patients with a burst fracture sustained neurological deficits. These injuries are generally unstable and should be stabilized, especially if there is an associated injury to the facets, pars interarticularis, ligaments, or if there is associated neurological deficit.

Seat Belt Type Injury

The use of seat belts (most commonly with a lap belt without associated shoulder belt) fixes the lower spine against the seat, and the upper spine flexes anteriorly

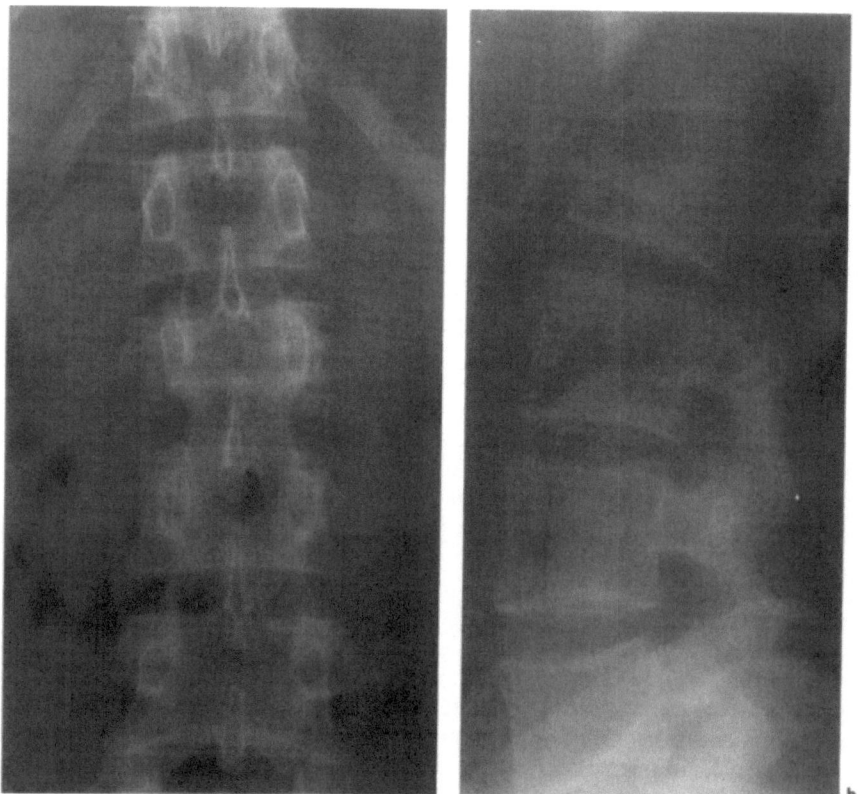

Fig. 31.5. This was a 34-year-old female involved in a motor vehicle accident. She was neurologically intact. **a,b** Plain radiographs demonstrated compression of vertebral body height at L2. Lateral radiograph (**b**) showing buckling of the posterior vertebral cortex into the canal. **c** CT scan showing the burst fracture, with moderate bony retropulsion into the canal. **d** Sagittal T2-weighted MRI image showing the bone fragment impinging on the dural sac and the subarachnoid CSF space.

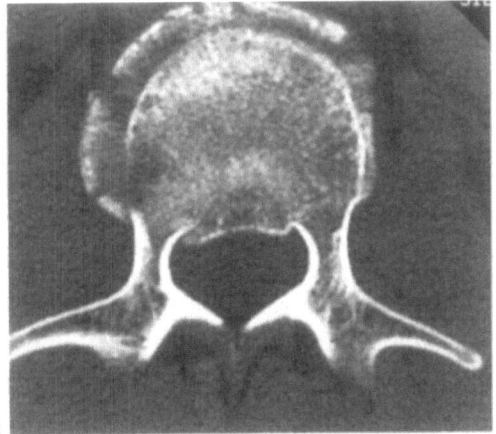 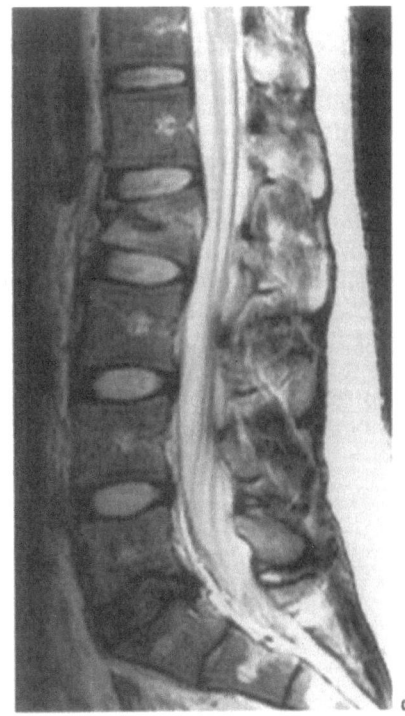

Fig. 31.5. *(Continued)*

around a pivot point near the anterior abdominal wall. Such a change in the axis of rotation with the flexion force results in spinal distraction. The posterior and middle columns are distracted with anterior column usually intact.

The subtypes of seat belt type injuries are defined according to osseous vs. ligamentous involvement, and single vs. two level vertebral involvement. The posterior element failure through the osseous structures at a single vertebral body level is seen in type A, as type B injury involves single-level ligamentous injuries. Two-level injuries involving the osseous and ligamentous structures are type C and D, respectively.

Of note is that none of the 19 patients in Denis' series with seat belt type injury developed any neurological deficit related to the fracture. Incidences are generally low, in the vicinity of 5%–10% for neurological sequelae from the injury. By the virtue of the involvement of both the middle and posterior columns, such injuries are unstable and stabilization is recommended.

Fracture–Dislocation

Such fractures are characterized by the failure of all three columns (Fig. 31.6). The forces involved may be compression, rotation, tension, extension or shear. Such an injury is most frequently associated with a spinal cord pathology and neurological deficit (Denis 1983). Three subtypes of fracture–dislocations have been described.

Type A injury is the result of combined flexion/rotational forces. Though initially described in mining accident victims (Holdsworth 1963), this may also occur as a result of a fall or an ejection from a motor vehicle accident. The characteristic CT scan picture shows the superior and inferior vertebral bodies to be rotated on axial images. Facet disruption, canal compromise, as well as articular surface fracture are frequently observed.

Type B fracture–dislocation is caused by the force of shear across the horizontal plane. Both anterolisthesis and retrolisthesis of the superior vertebral body are possible, depending on the direction of the impact. When the posterior osseous arch is fractured, the neural elements may be "decompressed" from such "laminectomy", resulting in less severe neurological injury. Of the twelve patients from Denis' series, all suffered spinal cord injuries, and most had complete injuries. The anterior longitudinal ligament was disrupted in each of these patients, rendering the failure of the Harrington distraction system. A simultaneous compression rod with the two distraction rods to provide segmental fixation, or a segmental fixation system (Cotrel–Doubousset or TSRH) may be used to provide adequate stabilization without over-distraction (Denis and Burkus 1992).

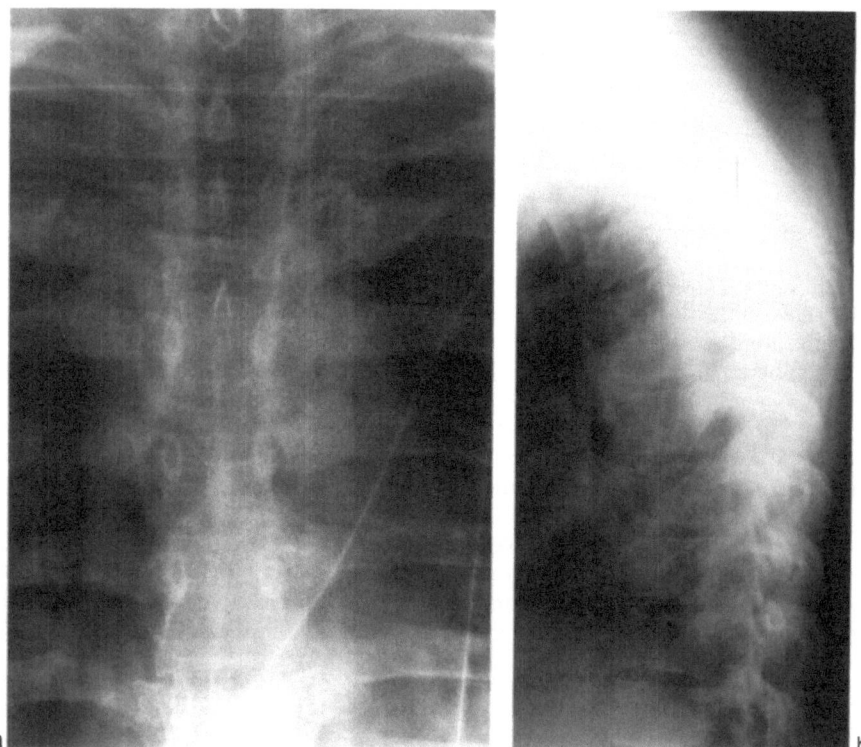

Fig. 31.6. A fracture–dislocation injury in a 24-year-old male involved in a motorcycle accident. He sustained immediate paraplegia. **a,b** Radiographs showing anterior subluxation of T4 vertebra on T5, as well as compression of column height at these levels. **c** CT scan showing the anterior overlap of vertebral body images on this axial CT. Associated posterior element fractures were also revealed. **d** A T2-weighted MRI image showing severe indentation of the dural sac and transection of the spinal cord. The patient underwent posterior decompression and reduction of the fracture. He remained paraplegic postoperatively.

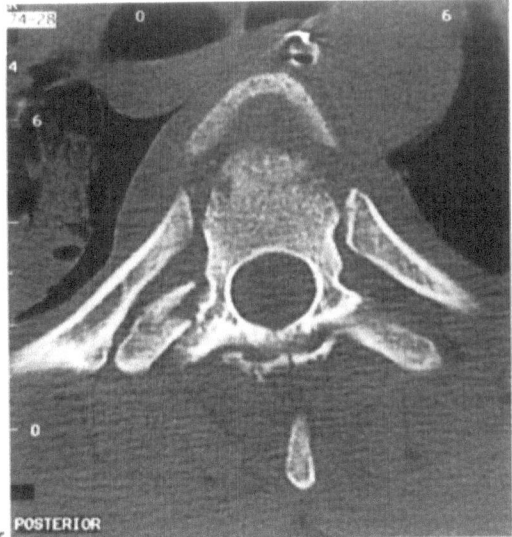

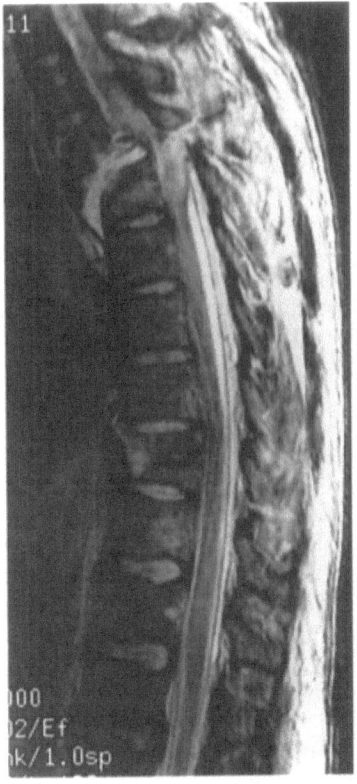

Fig. 31.6. *(Continued)*

Type C injury is a bilateral facet dislocation caused by the flexion–distraction mechanism. It resembles the seat belt type injury, but associated anterior column failure is also present. The anterior column failure most frequently involves the intervertebral disc or the anterior vertebral body. The anterior longitudinal ligament is stripped but not torn (Denis 1983), as significant superior vertebral subluxation can occur. Levine et al. (1988) advocated a discectomy prior to the placement or a stabilization system, citing the incompetency of the posterior annulus and the possibility of a compression construct forcing disrupted disc herniation into the canal. Further neurological deficit may result from such further intervertebral disc herniation.

Initial Management of a Thoracolumbar Spine Fracture

High index of suspicion for a spinal cord injury must be undertaken by medical personnel who come into initial contact with a traumatized patient (which, in most cases, would be paramedics). Any motor or sensory signs, pain, incontinence or external sign of trauma should be documented. A rigid cervical collar in combination with backboard should be used to immobilize the spine and to expedite transport to the emergency room. Continuous movement of an injured spinal cord could inflict further damage, causing neurological deterioration (Green and Eismont 1984; Green et al. 1987). This guideline should also be followed in patients with altered mental status, as a spinal neurological deficit may not be immediately apparent. Spinal shock and respiratory muscle (diaphragm, intercostal muscles) failure should be considered in patients with cervical or high thoracic injuries. The "sympathectomy" syndrome from a cervical or thoracic lesion generally causes hypotension and bradycardia because of unopposed vagal tone. Fluid support, appropriate haemodynamic monitoring, which includes a pulmonary artery catheter and arterial line, and pressors may be necessary for optimal management. In the emergency department, a spinal cord injury (cervical, thoracic, lumbosacral) must be ruled out. Once the patient is haemodynamically and respiratorily stabilized and the neurological status assessed, plain radiographs of cervical, thoracic and lumbosacral spine should be obtained. Computerized tomography (CT) can be utilized to image areas poorly visualized by the plain films and areas of suspected injury on the plain film. Magnetic resonance imaging (MRI) or computerized tomography (CT) with myelography may be needed to assess soft tissue/cord injury.

If the patient shows any sign of a spinal cord injury, the high-dose methylprednisolone protocol outlined by the National Spinal Cord Injury Study II is recommended (Bracken et al. 1990). It should only be administered if the loading dose can be given within 8 hours of the onset of injury. In the first hour, 30 mg/kg of methylprednisolone is given as slow bolus followed by 5.4 mg/kg/h infusion for 23 h. In the study conducted by Bracken et al. (1990), the benefit of high-dose steroid was observed in incomplete spinal cord injury, as complete motor injury with or without sensory sparing did not show major improvement. This study, however, excluded patients who subsequently underwent decompression and stabilization. The benefit of the steroid should also be weighed against the possible complication of infection and gastrointestinal haemorrhage.

Grading Scales

Various systems for grading spinal cord injuries have been developed, including the Frankel classification (Frankel et al. 1969), motor index score (Lucas and Ducker 1979), Sunnybrook cord injury scale (Tator et al. 1982), and the spinal cord injury severity scale (Bracken et al. 1990). All these systems aim to assess the initial neurological status and to follow the neurological status after the treatment is initiated.

The Frankel classification is shown in Table 31.2. It is simple, widely utilized, and well known. The grading system assesses the extent of motor and sensory injuries,

Table 31.2.   The Frankel grading system for spinal injury

A:	Complete neurological injury
B:	Incomplete: preserved sensation only
C:	Incomplete: non-functional motor
D:	Incomplete: functional motor
E.	Complete recovery (abnormal reflexes allowed)

but does not take into account the significance of bowel or bladder function. A patient with paraplegia is classified into the same category as a patient with quadriplegia. Furthermore, neither grade C nor D is sensitive to the degree of improvement within the defined category.

The Sunnybrook system is an extrapolation of the Frankel system, and aims to address some of the problems mentioned above. A total of ten grades are described, mostly from subdividing the grades C and D of the Frankel system. Sensory loss is subdivided into incomplete and complete. Bowel and bladder functions are not assessed. The system is obviously not as simplified as the Frankel grading system.

The motor index score which was originally defined by Lucas and Ducker (1979), was subsequently modified by the American Spinal Injury Association (ASIA) into a 100-point system. Muscle strength of the brachial and lumbosacral plexi are assessed with the traditional 0–5 motor strength scale. Nerve root motor function of C5 – T1, and L2 – S1 is assessed bilaterally (10 total nerve roots on each side) The deficiency still lies in the exclusion of sphincter function assessment.

Newer grading systems, such as the one proposed by Esses and Botsford (1990), attempt to incorporate sphincter functions into the traditional motor and sensory examinations. When applied routinely, such systems may more accurately document patients' clinical progression. They are, however, not as simplified as the Frankel classification.

Surgical Management in Thoracolumbar Spine Injury

The treatment of thoracolumbar fractures has been at the centre of controversy. In the earlier description of treatment, prolonged bedrest played a prominent role in the management of such patients. The evolution of decompression and stabilization surgeries relied heavily on the development of anaesthesia, aseptic/sterile technique and condition, antibiotic and successful management of spinal shock syndrome.

Decompressive laminectomy has increased the level of instability of spinal fractures on certain lesions, as it destabilizes the posterior column by reducing both the ligamentous and osseous elements (Braakman et al. 1991). With the introduction of the Harrington distraction system and other newer instrumentations, surgical intervention plays a more important role in the management plan of these patients. Neurological improvement has been documented in patients presenting with incomplete spinal injury, through anterior or posterior decompression. The timing and approach of spinal decompression remains controversial. Bohlman et al. (1984) and Krengel et al. (1993) advocated late anterior and early (< 24 h) posterior stabilization, respectively. With delayed anterior decompression, Bohlman et al. reported an improvement of 2.0 Frankel grades in each patient, whereas Krengel et al. reported a 2.2 Frankel grade improvement in their series.

With non-surgical management in thoracolumbar spinal injury, neurological deterioration can occur. Denis et al. (1984) advocated surgical treatment for patients with burst fractures, as 18% showed deterioration in his series. Frankel et al. (1969), on the other hand, reported only a 0.5% incidence of deterioration with postural reduction and strict bedrest alone. Due to conflicting past reports, it is unclear whether the correction of bony anatomy improves the neurological symptoms

(Nicoll 1949; Soreff et al. 1982). Most authors, however, agree that surgical stabilization shortens the hospitalization time of paralysed patients (Dickson et al. 1978; Jacobs et al. 1980). Early mobilization and a rehabilitation programme can follow stabilization of an unstable spinal fracture (Rimoldi et al. 1992; Place et al. 1994). The complication rate of prolonged immobilization, including infectious, pulmonary and thromboembolic phenomenon can be reduced by early surgical intervention.

There is no "standard" surgical therapy for the thoracolumbar spine injury, as any specific treatment regimen should be tailored for each individual patient's injury. Different treatment plans may be available and equally effective. The eventual outcome depends also on the surgeons' techniques, perioperative management and rehabilitation. It is the authors' opinion that a patient with spinal cord injury be transferred to a regional spinal cord injury centre because of the complexity of the problem and the available resources. Such an approach may facilitate the planning and progress of the spinal cord injury patient rehabilitation. (Heinemann et al. 1989). Most surgeons would decompress and stabilize a patient with neurologically incomplete injury. There has been no consensus regarding stabilizing a patient with complete neurological injury. The authors advocate aggressive posterior stabilization of such injuries to facilitate the rehabilitation process and to avoid prolonged immobilization.

Multiple measures are taken preoperatively and prior to incision to ensure the optimal intraoperative condition. Baseline preoperative somatosensory evoked potential (SSEP), motor evoked potential (MEP), and spontaneous electromyography should be obtained as appropriate. Intraoperative SSEP and MEP monitoring, as well as portable ultrasonography, should be available. If the patient's injury is neurologically complete, monitoring is not necessary. The high-dose methylprednisolone protocol should be continued within the first 24 hours of injury, or restarted on a prophylactic basis. Perioperative intravenous antibiotic is given. After intubation, the patient is log rolled into a lateral decubitus position for transthoracic or retroperitoneal procedure, or a prone position on the Relton–Hall scoliosis operating frame (Imperial Medical Ltd, Markham, Ontario, Canada) for posterior or posterolateral decompression/stabilization. Careful positioning is essential in avoiding brachial plexus or meralgia paresthetica. Awake intubation is utilized for patients with incomplete injury and an unstable spine. Anaesthesia is composed of a balanced nitric oxide–narcotic combination, where spinal cord monitoring is implemented. Even a low concentration of inhalational anaesthetics may alter or diminish the evoked potential waveforms (Calancie et al. 1991). The employment of the Mayfield three-point skull clamp (Ohio Medical Instrument Co, Cincinnati, OH) allows optimal positioning, prevention of globe (eye) injury, and decubitus ischaemic ulcer. The sequential Compression Device (Kendall Healthcare Products, Mansfield, MA) is used to reduce lower extremity venous pooling and stasis. The Cell Saver system (Haemonetics, Raintree, MA) is routinely utilized at our institution to minimize the total amount of blood loss, and to allow for autotransfusion, as needed.

Intraoperative ultrasonography is routinely performed through a laminectomy or vertebrectomy near the site of fracture to assess the degree of neural compression by bone, disc, or ligament. A scanner with 7.5 MHz or greater should be utilized to optimize resolution. Air bubbles, blood, antibiotic solution, or debris should be minimized, as they distort the images. Both axial and sagittal images should be obtained.

The aim of the instrumentation is eventual bony fusion. Therefore, a generous amount of autologous bone graft is harvested from the iliac crest if possible. In posterior fusion, facet arthrodesis and decortication of the transverse process, pars interarticularis and lamina are performed prior to laying the bone graft. Cadaveric allograft is utilized at our institution only for anterior vertebral body decompression, and is supplemented with autograft whenever possible. It must be stressed that a bony fusion must be performed with the instrumentation.

Posterior Instrumentation Systems

The following section discusses specific instrumentation systems, and operative techniques for thoracolumbar spine fractures. The description is not intend to be all-inclusive, but merely offers a representative overview of the various instrumentation devices. The following instrumentation systems are discussed: Harrington distraction system, universal segmental fixation system and the pedicle screw system.

Harrington Distraction System

The Harrington distraction rod fixation system (Zimmer Johns and Assoc., Warsaw, IN) was initially used to treat postpoliomyelitis scoliosis in 1949, but it was soon used to reduce and internally stabilize the fractured thoracic and lumbar spine (Riebel et al. 1993; Harrington 1967). This system provided reduction of the spinal deformity, which is balanced against 15.5% overall instrumentation-related complications (Riebel et al. 1993; Dickson et al. 1978; McEvoy and Bradford 1983), to be discussed later.

Reduction of the vertebral body fracture relies partially on the distraction forces created by the Harrington rods and hooks. Three- or four-point fixation is needed by the rods to pull the hooks posteriorly at levels cephalad and caudal to the fracture site. Constant anterior force at the level of fracture is also provided this way. The end result is the reduction of anterior vertebral deformity and closure of posterior disruption. The Harrington distraction rod may be used to reduce and stabilize burst fracture, and compression fracture associated with posterior column injury. The Harrington construct tends to increase extension and lateral bending stability, but resistance to flexion and torsion is not as significant (McAfee 1985) Sublaminar wires may increase the rotatory stability of the system. (Asher et al. 1988). Experimental models utilizing crosslinking of the rods augment the stability of the simple rod/hook construct three-to fourfold. The combined technique of segmental wiring and crosslinking provides tremendously increased resistance to torsion.

Several complications are possible with this instrumentation. Dislodgement at the rod–hook junction, fracture of the rachet–rod junction, and separation at the hook–laminar junction are the most common. Sublaminar wiring decreases the incidence of these complications by increasing the resistance to torsion and flexion.

Different opinions exist regarding the number of spinal levels to instrument. Earlier recommendations suggested instrumenting two segments above and below the injured site. All levels between the cephalad and caudal instrumentations were fused, and the device left in place unless a problem necessitated its removal. By placing the superior hooks three levels above and the inferior hooks two levels below the fracture, better resistance to flexion could be achieved (Purcell et al. 1981). Others have instrumented three levels above and below the fracture, fused only the fractured site, and removed the instrumentation after one year (Jacobs et al. 1980). They reported 1.9 levels of fusion with a 9% loss of the correction of kyphosis. Benzel (1993) described a short-rod/two-claw technique for treating thoracic and lumbar fractures. The compression mode maintained the kyphotic angle much better than the distraction mode. (1.6 vs. 18.3 degrees loss). Increased incidence of degenerative changes has been observed in instrumented but unfused levels (Jacobs et al. 1980; Kahanovitz et al. 1984) More recent reports using long Harrington's rods and short arthrodesis and fusion found no degeneration or fusion at the levels that were instrumented but not fused (Dekutoski et al. 1993). The authors recommend

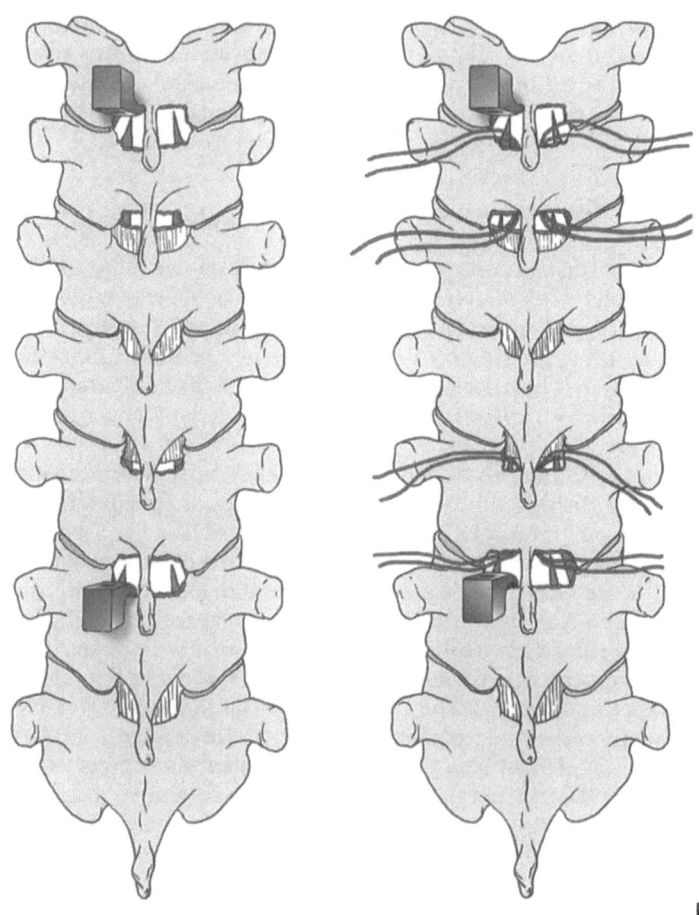

a   b

Fig. 31.7. The placement of the Harrington distraction instrumentation system. The standard posterior midline incision and subperiosteal dissection had been completed to expose the lamina. **a** 5 mm-wide square laminotomies were made to accommodate the insertion of Edwards hooks. **b** Sublaminar wires were passed bilaterally at the levels immediately inferior to the cranial hooks, and immediately superior to the caudal hooks. **c** The rod was secured with a rod holder and threaded through the hooks as demonstrated. **d** After a Gaines distractor was used to distract the fracture, the sublaminar wires were tightened and cut.

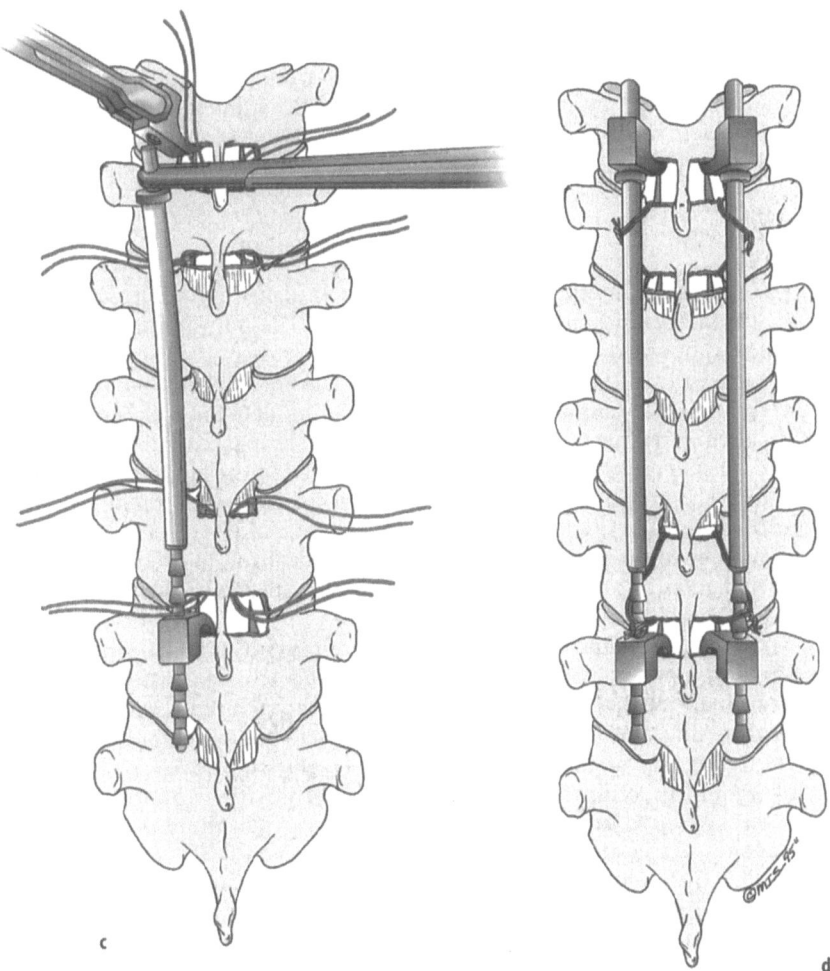

c

d

Fig. 31.7. *(Continued)*

instrumentation from three levels above to two levels below the fracture segment. Autologous bone graft fusion is routinely performed over the entire length of the construct. The instrumentation is removed only if a problem arises requiring its removal. A review of the literature revealed that contoured rods have an average final follow-up kyphosis of 16.4° (Eismont et al. 1993). The authors recommend that the Harrington rods are not contoured if possible, and that sublaminar cables be placed immediately below the superior hooks and immediately above the inferior hooks for further rod stabilization. Edwards' Anatomic Hooks (Zimmer-Johns and Assoc. Warsaw, IN) are used by the authors because they have a wider contact surface to engage the posterior laminar surface. This is supported by the report by Levine et al. (1988), who noted that the above modification decreased hook dislodgement by 1.3%. The authors also utilize the Edwards Sleeves (Zimmer-Johns and Assoc. Warsaw, IN) to provide the pivot point for the correction of kyphosis.

Because the Harrington construct is essentially a distraction system, the authors now utilize the universal system more frequently for the stabilization of thoracic and lumbar spine fractures in general. Denis and Burkus (1992) have noted that the Harrington distraction system alone does not help the spine that had a fracture dislocation to heal in anatomic position.

Surgical Procedure

After the anaesthesia is induced and the patient is placed in the prone position on the Relton frame, a midline skin incision is made. The paraspinous muscle is dissected away subperiosteally to expose the lamina and transverse processes three levels above and two levels below the fracture. The square laminotomies and ligamentum flavum resections are carried out to accommodate the appropriate Edwards hooks (Fig. 31.7a). The titanium cables can then be passed sublaminarly to be secured to the rods (Fig. 31.7b). The hooks are placed in the laminotomy site with a hook holder. The rachet end of the rod is threaded through the inferior hook and a hook holder is used to insert the rod into the rostral end (Fig. 31.7c). A Gaines distractor (Zimmer Johns and Assoc., Warsaw, IN) is utilized to gradually extend the rachet mechanism in order to distract the injured site. The sublaminar wires are then tightened and cut (Fig. 31.7d).

The end of both the superior and inferior tips of the rod should extend about 1 cm beyond the last hook to avoid hook dislodgement and skin penetration/erosion. The authors routinely perform a small laminotomy at the fractured segment to allow for intraoperative ultrasonography. Intraoperative plain radiographs are obtained to verify the reduction of the fracture and detect any sign of over-distraction. A crosslink should be utilized for an unstable fracture with a rotatory component. Edwards sleeves could act as a pivot against kyphotic deformity. Autologous bone grafts are laid to facilitate osseous fusion. Postoperatively, a thoraco-lumbar-sacral orthosis (TLSO) should be worn whenever the patient is out of bed for three to six months, depending on the success of the osseous fusion.

This instrumentation system includes a compression rod that can be used for an acute flexion–distraction injury, as long as the anterior column is intact. In general, only one level above and below the fracture is needed for an acute injury, and two levels above and below the fracture is instrumented in a chronic injury (Eismont et al. 1993). The Harrington compression rod is threaded, and multiple hooks can be placed over the lamina or transverse process. Laminotomy is performed for direct visualization of the hook insertion. Sublaminar wires are not recommended for the compression system, as the hooks may be driven into the canal.

Universal Segmental Fixation System

The Cotrel–Dubousset instrumentation (Sofamor Danek USA, Memphis TN) was designed to improve on the shortcomings of the Harrington distraction system and the Luque rod/rectangle system. The problem of rotational instability is specifically addressed. When multiple vectors of forces are involved in an injury, such an instrumentation system can help with the reduction of the fracture, stability and correction of scoliosis. Cotrel et al. (1988) use hooks at the end of the rod in a particular fashion to fix the rod to the spinal column. This consists of placing one hook each superior and inferior to the vertebral lamina at each level to be instrumented. Additional hooks are placed at the intervening levels to correct any local deformity, and provide additional stability and support. Reduction of an abnormal curvature can also be achieved, as two rods parallel to each other are fixed to each side of the lamina. Pedicle hooks placed into the facet joint can lock onto the inferior surface of the pedicle, and replace the need to place the infralaminar hooks. Similarly, transverse process hooks can be used to replace the supralaminar hooks. Crosslinks can be used to lock the two rods together, which in turn increase the resistance to rotation (Cotrel et al. 1988; Ashman 1993) This system has been shown to effectively restore physiological thoracic and lumbar postural contours (Benli et al. 1994), and stabilize thoracolumbar fracture (McBride 1993).

The TSRH (Texas Scottish Rite Hospital) spinal instrumentation system (Sofamor Danek USA, Memphis, TN) incorporated the ideas of crosslinking the two parallel rods and improvement of the Harrington distraction system in terms of more flexibility for the directions of corrective forces (Ashman 1993). Benzel et al. (1991) has reported good results with the TSRH instrumentation system, with no dislodgement, pseudoarthrosis, or instability in a series of 28 patients. Both the Luque and the TSRH systems have a wide selection of hooks. The hooks can be placed under the pedicle or over the transverse process. Segmental wiring is not used with these two systems. The Isola (Acromed Corp., Cleveland OH) system (Asher et al. 1992) has a more limited selection of hooks than the C-D or TSRH systems. It incorporates the concept of segmental wiring (transforaminal or sublaminar).

These universal segmental fixation systems have mostly replaced the use of the Luque or the Harrington systems for the treatment of spinal injuries. They provide segmental stabilization, better alignment of the spine, increased resistance to rotation, and the ability to use pedicle screws in the lumbar region. These benefits come at the cost of increased operating time and more spine manipulation.

Different patterns of hooks can be placed. Many possible permutations of sublaminar, pedicle, and transverse process hooks exist, but the final pattern should be individualized for the specific injury. In general localized compression and contralateral distraction are used for the correction of scoliosis. Near the ends of the construct, short segments of "clawing" are utilized. At the thoracolumbar junction at or below T11, pedicle screw system could be incorporated into the construct. Such arrangements would allow for distraction of superior and inferior ends of the rod, and compression of the fracture site. The authors generally avoid placing two sublaminar hooks at the same laminotomy level to avoid narrowing the canal excessively and injuring the the neural elements.

Surgical Procedure

The standard exposure for posterior instrumentation has been described in the previous sections. Additional hook sites for sublaminar, transverse process, or pedicle hooks need to be prepared. For the inferior laminar edge, the authors clean off the ligamentum flavum and perform a small laminotomy for better hook fitting. When utilizing a pedicle hook in place of a upward-facing sublaminar hook, the superior facet needs to be trimmed with an osteotome to facilitate hook insertion. The authors recommend the osteotomy site should be 5 mm from the centre of the facet, and 4 mm inferior to the transverse process and facet junction (Roach et al. 1990).

The transverse process hook may replace a downward-facing sublaminar hook, after the transverse process has been properly cleaned. Pedicle screws are inserted as indicated.

After the appropriate hooks are placed, the rods are inserted and fixed to the rods with appropriate connectors. After they are tightened, two crosslinks are installed between the two rods to create a closed-circuit construct. The appropriate-size crosslinks should avoid lateral or medial pull on the crosslinks, so the rods will not be dislodged. The rods could be bent to fit the appropriate contour. Anteroposterior and lateral radiographs are taken to ascertain the final position of the instrumentation system. After the entire construct is in place and tightened, autologous iliac crest bone grafts are harvested and placed on the transverse process, facet and lamina.

Postoperatively, the patient is placed in a thoracolumbar orthosis whenever out of bed. The progress of fusion and alignment are followed clinically and by plain radiographs. Approximately three months of stabilization in the brace is recommended.

Pedicle Screw Fixation System

The most recent development in spinal instrumentation is the utilization of pedicle screws. It is the first device for posterior instrumentation that can fixate onto the vertebral body. The first reported case of pedicle screw use dated back to 1969, when Harrington and Tullos (1969) attempted to utilize it to reduce L5 spondylolisthesis. Pedicles screws have been utilized with the plate or rod systems. The screws were effective in achieving positional control, as long as no bone resorption or compression occurred under the plate (Blauth et al. 1987). Newer instrumentation systems, including the Cotrel–Dubousset system (Graziano 1993) and TSRH system (Dickman et al. 1992; Zdeblick 1993), have been used in conjunction with the pedicle screw fixation system for lumbosacral stabilization.

The advantage of the system is that shorter segment fixation is often made possible. The pedicle screw construct for one level below to one level above the fracture may be feasible, especially if the anterior fragmentation is minimal. A single sublaminar hook immediately below the pedicle screw can be utilized to create a "claw". The shorter construct becomes more important in the lumbar region, as shorter segment instrumentation causes less functional disability (Benzel 1993). The thoracic spines have smaller pedicles, which makes the margin of error for screw insertion smaller. Neural injury from pedicle screw insertion is more likely in the thoracic and thoracolumbar junction because of the presence of the cord or conus. The authors believe that the most appropriate levels for pedicle screw fixation to be the lumbar region, and we utilize the TSRH titanium system.

It should be noted that the only application for pedicle screw presently approved by the Food and Drug Administration (FDA) is the Danek instrumentation for grade III L5–S1 spondylolisthesis. Several studies (Dickman et al. 1992; Zdeblick 1993) have demonstrated that the pedicle screws, when combined with a universal instrumentation system, could provide good surgical results in terms of spine stabilization, alignment, and pain relief.

Surgical Procedure

The standard incision and exposure have been described previously for posterior instrumentation. Posterolateral decompression, as described later in this chapter,

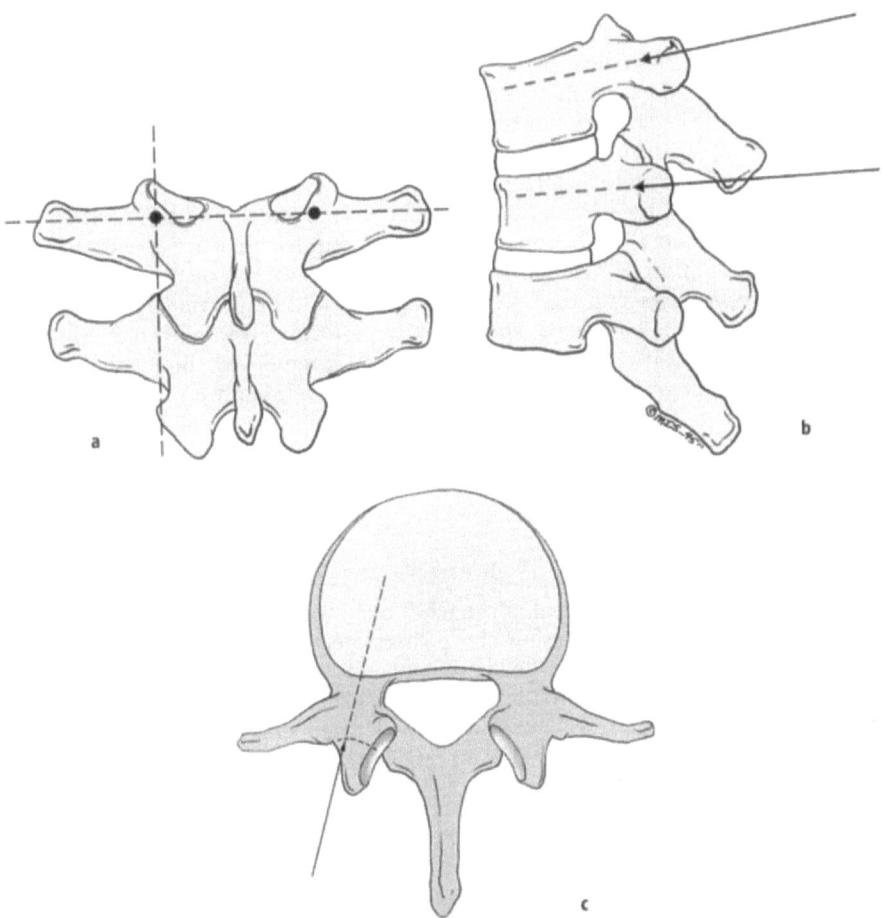

Fig. 31.8. The entry point for the pedicle screw. **a** The intersection of two lines approximate the location of the pedicle from the posterior perspective. The first line connects the two transverse processes horizontally, and the second line connects the middle of facet joints vertically. **b–c** The pedicle screw should aim 10–15° medially, and follow the pedicle anteriorly to just below to the anterior vertebral cortex. Final position could be ascertained with intraoperative fluoroscopy or plain radiograph.

should be performed as indicated. If distraction is desired, the instrumentation system should be applied as previously described. The intersection of two lines defines the point of entry for the pedicle screw (Roy-Camille et al. 1986). The first line runs horizontally through the transverse processes of the same vertebral body. The second line runs vertically and connects the facet joints (Fig. 31.8a). If a laminectomy is performed at the level of instrumentation, the pedicle could be directly identified through the laminectomy.

Once the point of entry is determined, the inferior facet is smoothened with a drill down to medullary bone. A drill is used to penetrate the pedicle and vertebral body, maintaining an approximately 10–15° medial angle and an appropriate angle in the sagittal plane (Fig. 31.8b, c) with electromyography stimulation electrode attached to the drill. The depth of penetration is determined by the measurement from the pre-operative CT scan. This process could be aided with a lateral plain radiograph, or intraoperative fluoroscopy. Each hole should be fully explored with a probe to ensure that none of the pedicle cortical surfaces has been violated. Only two or three fingers should be applied on the wrench or screw driver to avoid stripping the screw threads within the pedicle. The anterior lumbar vertebral body cortex should be preserved to avoid vascular or visceral injury. After the desired depth of insertion is achieved, the stimulation electrode should be attached on each screw to test the threshold for EMG activity. The threshold for stimulation on the pedicle screw should be recorded and should be greater than 15 mA. Sacral screws may require bicortical penetration to ensure maximal fixation (Krag et al. 1988). After the screws and instrumentation are inserted, anteroposterior and lateral radiographs should be obtained to determine the final position of the hardware. The fusion is performed over the facet joint and transverse processes, after adequate decortication is achieved. Bony fusion with autologous iliac crest graft is essential for eventual clinical stability.

Surgical Decompressions

This section describes two surgical approaches commonly used for decompression: anterior transthoracic decompression and posterolateral decompression. The posterior instrumentation systems described in the previous section provide distraction and stabilization of the spine, but do not deal with intracanalicular bony fragments, discs or foreign bodies. Neural compression can be assessed intraoperatively with ultrasonography. The following techniques allow decompression when utilized appropriately.

Anterior Transthoracic Decompression and Reconstruction

This approach is used for decompression of thoracic spine fractures which impinge on the anterior spinal canal and spinal cord from T4 to T10. Higher thoracic fractures require a midline sternotomy extending to the second intercostal space which is not described in this chapter. Slightly different approaches for the thoracolumbar (T11–L2) and mid/lower lumbar (L3–5) regions are also described. The authors' institution utilizes this procedure for neurologically intact patients, patients with incomplete spinal injury, or an old injury with fixed kyphotic deformity. Such a decompression and subsequent anterior grafting alone may be the only treatment necessary. When the reconstructed anterior column decreases in length or if there is a concurrent posterior column injury, this procedure can be combined with a posterior instrumentation procedure to allow both decompression and stabilization.

Transthoracic decompression was first described for the treatment of spine tuberculosis (Hodgson and Stock 1956). A rib resection allows for the necessary exposure. A series of eight patients with upper thoracic spine fracture (Bohlman et al. 1984), after reaching a plateau in neurological recovery, underwent transthoracic decompression and fusion for residual neural compression. All patients had anterior bone strut grafting without instrumentation. All eight improved their function postoperatively: five patients eventually ambulated independently, two ambulated with devices, and one showed increased motor function even though he was not ambulatory. Delayed anterior decompression has also been reported to reduce pain and improve neurological function (Bohlman et al. 1994).

Even with anterior bone grafting, both resistance to torsion and axial loading are markedly decreased (Gurr et al. 1988). The authors limit the graft-only procedure to patients with only anterior canal compromise and minimal associated instability. The chance of developing worsening postoperative instability warrants a posterior stabilization in most cases.

Surgical Procedure

The authors generally use a double-lumen endotracheal tube intubation for decompression of T4 to T10 level fracture. This allows for intraoperative lung collapse to facilitate exposure and minimize injury to the pulmonary and vascular structures. The left lateral decubitus position is generally chosen for the upper thoracic spine

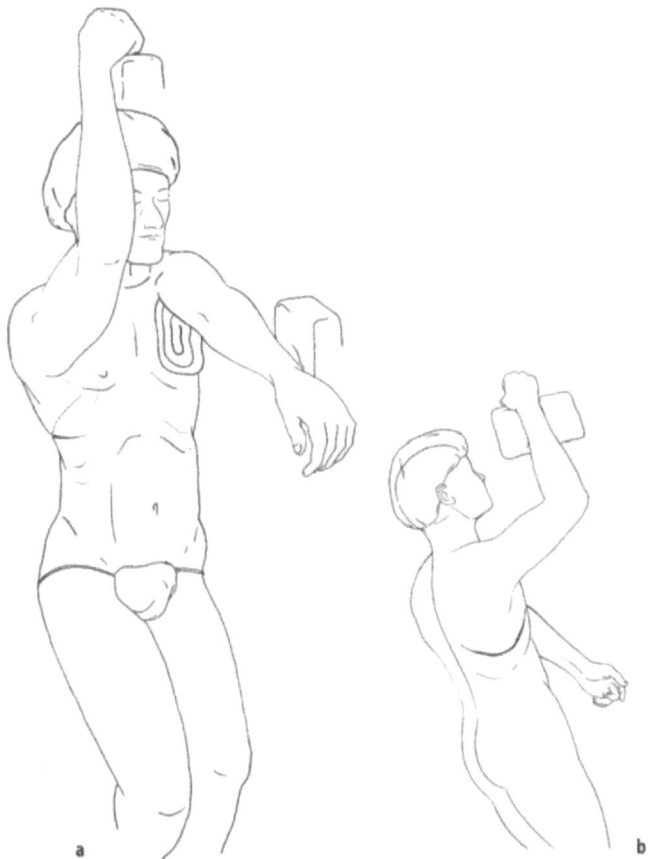

a   b

Fig. 31.9. Sequence of anterior thoracic decompression. **a** The patient is positioned approximately 45–60° up from horizontal position, with the operated side up. **b** The skin incision is as marked. **c** The skin, subcutaneous tissue and muscle are divided in layers to the level of the rib. A periosteal elevator is used to dissect the parietal pleura from the overlying rib. **d** A retractor system is inserted, and the lung is retacted medially after being deflated with the double-lumen endotracheal tube. After the level is localized with an X-ray, discectomies above and below the fracture are carried out. An osteotome is used here for the vertebrectomy. **e** Further decompression with a Kerrison rongeur is demonstrated. **f** A tibial allograft is inserted and tapped into place as a strut.

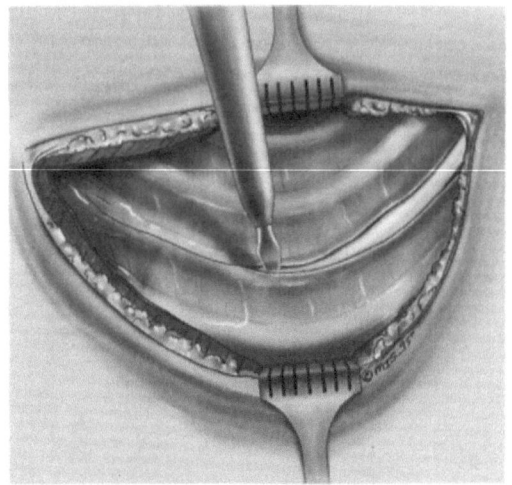

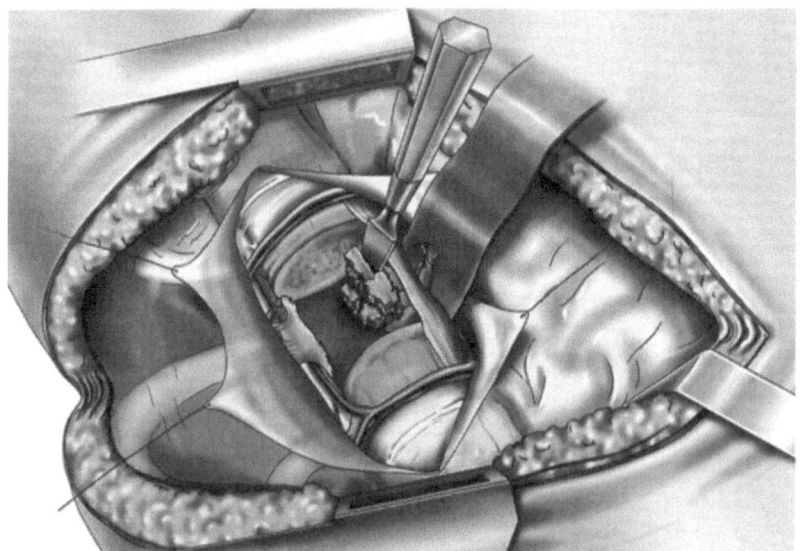

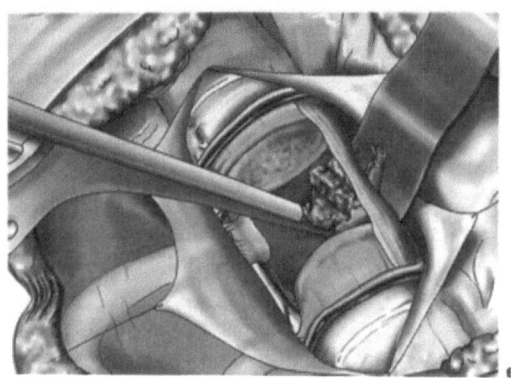

Fig. 31.9. *(Continued)*

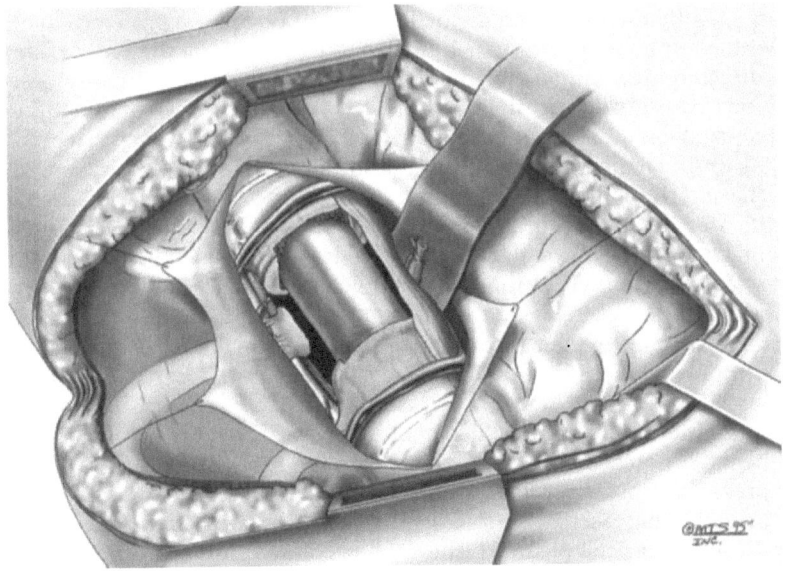

Fig. 31.9.   *(Continued)*

and the right lateral decubitus position is used for mid and lower thoracic spine lesions. A rib series radiograph, or a radiograph allowing vertebral body counting from the lumbosacral junction should be available to localize the incision.

The patient is then log rolled into position with an axillary roll, and the superior arm is held with an armrest, with the forward flexion angle of less than 90° (Fig. 31.9a). Wide adhesive tapes are used to secure the patient to the operating table. A bean bag may be helpful in maintaining position, but could cause ischaemic cutaneous lesions. The operative field should also include the possible autologous bone graft site.

For lesions from T6 to T10, the skin incision is made over the rib one to two levels cephalad to the lesion. (Fig. 31.9a,b). For higher thoracic lesions, the skin incision should incorporate from the tip of the scapula to the midpoint between the medial border of the scapula and the midline spinous processes. The incision is then deepened down through the subcutaneous tissue, fascia, and muscle serially to expose the rib (Fig. 31.9c). The rib is dissected free subperiosteally and divided. The serratus anterior muscle should be mobilized to isolate the long thoracic nerve to avoid injury to the nerve.

The ribs are next counted from inside the pleural cavity, and a self-retaining retractor system is installed. As the ipsilateral lung is deflated, full anterior view of the vertebral column covered by parietal pleura is afforded. The injured vertebral body may be identified directly, counted serially, or followed by the connection to the previously identified and resected rib. A spinal needle is inserted into the disc space, and a localizing radiograph is taken to verify the level of exposure. The parietal pleura is separated at the costovertebral junction to fully expose one level above and below the fractured site (Fig. 31.9d). Care should be taken not to penetrate the parietal pleura if possible. The intercostal vessels coursing over these three vertebral bodies are identified, ligated, and divided. The great vessels are protected by the use of a malleable retractor, as soft tissues are dissected away from the vertebral body.

Next, discectomies immediately above and below the proposed vertebrectomy level are carried out with a scalpel, curettes and rongeurs. The combination of an osteotome, rongeurs, drill and curettes should safely achieve the vertebrectomy. (Fig. 31.9d, e) Any bone fragments are saved for the subsequent reconstruction procedure. The anterior longitudinal ligament should be preserved. The dura mater can be identified at the neural foramina by a partial pedicle resection. The posterior longitudinal ligament is generally left intact, unless a residual bony fragment in the canal is strongly suspected. If this is the case, the ligament should be cut, and the epidural space explored.

The spinal column is then reconstructed using a tibial allograft packed in the centre with previously saved vertebral body fragments (Fig. 31.9f). Alternatively, autologous iliac crest may be harvested and strutted. The space between the bone graft and the anterior longitudinal ligament is packed with more autologous bone or rib fragments. A notch should be made on both the superior and inferior vertebral body to prevent the posterior displacement of the strut graft (Fig. 31.9f).

After adequate haemostasis and irrigation are completed, an attempt should be made to close the parietal pleura. A chest tube is placed. An intrapleural catheter is inserted through the chest tube or through a separate small incision to deliver local anaesthetic agents for the control of postoperative pain. Pericostal sutures are placed to aid approximating the rib. The muscles, soft tissues and skin are closed in layers.

For the thoracolumbar junction (T11–L2), the skin incision is made along the tenth rib, crossing the costochondral junction, and proceeds inferiorly along the lateral edge of the rectus abdominis sheath. The latissimus dorsi is divided to facilitate exposure of the tenth rib. The margins of the tenth rib resection are the cartilaginous attachment anteriorly, and the angle of the rib posteriorly. After the tenth rib resection, the parietal pleura, and then the diaphragm are identified. The diaphragm is freed from the peritoneum and divided from its peripheral attachment. Anteromedial retraction of the diaphragm and lateral retraction of the psoas muscle afford exposure of the desired vertebrae. The discectomy and vertebrectomy are performed as described earlier.

For lesions in the mid/lower lumbar region (L3–5), an oblique anterior incision is made from the midpoint between the anterior iliac crest and the twelfth rib to just above the pubic ramus. External oblique, internal oblique and transverse abdominis muscles are serially divided. By separating the peritoneum from the transverse abdominis muscle, accidental entry into the peritoneal cavity is avoided. The peritoneum and ureter are retracted medially and anteriorly away from the ilium and psoas muscle to expose the retroperitoneal space. The exact level can be identified by direct visualization or an intraoperative radiograph.

Posterolateral (Transpedicular) Decompression

It has been shown that the greater the delay between the time of injury and the time of posterior instrumentation, the less likely the spinal canal will be fully restored (Edwards and Levine 1986). Posterior instrumentation performed from day 3 to day 14 after the initial injury yielded improvement of canal diameter by only 23%, but early (within 2 days) instrumentation afforded an additional 32% of canal diameter restoration. Posterior instrumentation beyond two weeks did not yield any improvement of canal diameter. Therefore, if delayed instrumentation is contemplated, a posterolateral decompression is indicated if residual neural compression is present after posterior instrumentation. The posterolateral approach combined with instrumentation has been shown to effectively reduce and stabilize burst fractures (Silvestro et al. 1992). Lemons et al. (1992), however, have reported that posterolateral decompression does not affect postoperative canal dimension or neurological recovery. The advantage is obviously that anterior decompression can be achieved during the posterior instrumentation without a separate incision and procedure (Erikson et al. 1977; Edwards and Levine 1986). The disadvantage is the possibility of compromising long-term stability by removing more posterior elements. Ultrasonography can improve and assess the success of decompression. In general, good results are obtained with this particular technique.

Surgical Procedure

As stated previously, this procedure is performed prior to the posterior instrumentation. The side which is shown by computerized tomography images to have more neural compression is chosen to be the side of the posterolateral decompression. Instrumentations are placed on the opposite side of the spine. A laminectomy is performed at the level of compression to allow for ultrasonographic evaluation of the compression.

The laminotomy is extended to the pedicle, and should be cored with a high-speed power drill such as the Midas Rex system (Fort Worth, TX), but the cortical margins should be preserved (Fig. 31.10a, b). This is performed under EMG monitoring. The medial pedicle is removed, taking care not to injure the exiting nerve root. A 1 cm trough is made on the vertebral body anterior to the medial pedicle and the compressing bony fragments. Reverse angle curettes and pituitary rongeurs are used to remove the compressing fragments. Alternatively, the bone fragments may be pushed into the trough created in the vertebral body (Fig. 31.10c, d). Ultrasonography may be used to facilitate and assess the decompression. This technique can decompress up to the midline from one side. If additional decompression is needed on the contralateral pedicle, the ipsilateral side should first be instrumented. The superior disc can be removed, and bone grafts can be used to pack the vertebral body defect and the disc space.

Treatments for Specific Injuries

This section provides the outline for the treatment of a particular type of injury. The correct radiographic diagnosis is essential prior to initiating a certain course of treatment. This would also be aided by the history and neurological examination.

Spinous or Transverse Process Fracture

Direct trauma to the posterior spine can result in a spinous, transverse, or articular process fracture. In addition, extensive muscular contraction can result in a trans-

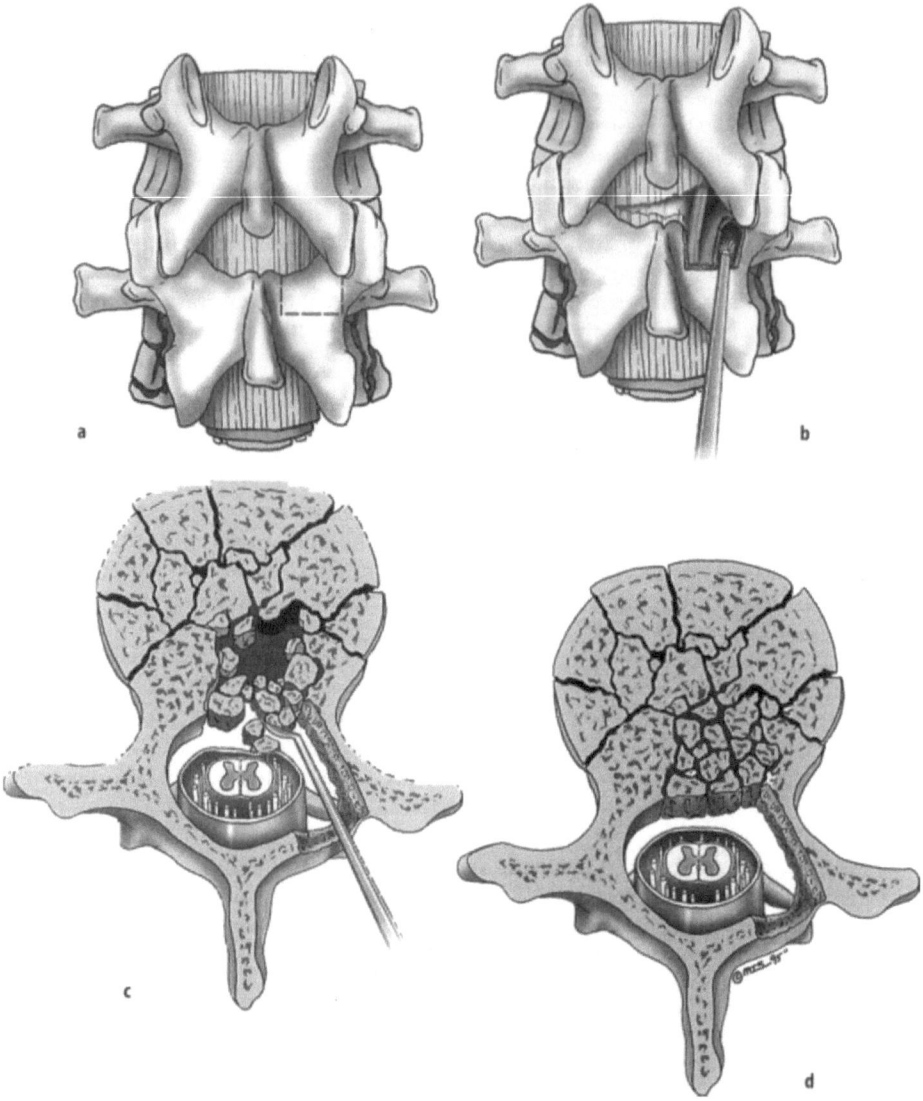

Fig. 31.10. Posterolateral decompression of a burst fracture. **a** The portion of the lamina to be drilled is marked. **b** The pedicle is drilled down centrally. **c** The medial pedicle wall is removed, and a reverse angle curette is utilized to push the bony fragments into the trough in the vertebral body. **d** Satisfactory restoration of the spinal canal is demonstrated after decompression.

verse process fracture. The use of plain radiographs and thin-cut (3 mm or thinner) computerized tomography scan through one level above and below the fracture can be used to screen any bony injury. A magnetic resonance imaging study will detect a spinal cord, soft tissue or ligamentous injury if needed. Lateral flexion-extension views of the involved segments should determine the dynamic stability of the spine. If no other abnormality other than the simple fracture is found, the patient may resume full activity as tolerated.

Traumatic Disc Herniation

The occurrence of traumatic disc herniation is rarer in the thoracic than the lumbar region, but more significant neurological deficits are noted with thoracic disc herniation, owing to the narrower diameter of the thoracic spinal canal. The patients present with pain, paraesthesias and neurological deficit. The pain may be local or radicular. An anterior cord or Brown–Séquard syndrome may be encountered. Urinary incontinence and positive Babinski's sign are not uncommon. A CT scan alone is not an adequate diagnostic modality for detection of herniated discs. A magnetic resonance imaging scan or CT-myelogram is the test of choice for such an abnormality.

The treatment of a traumatic herniated disc in a symptomatic patient is primarily surgical. For thoracic lesions, transthoracic, transpedicular or costotransversectomy should be planned for the discectomy. These approaches yielded improvements in the absolute majority of the patients (Perot and Munro 1969; Patterson and Arbit 1978; Maiman et al. 1984). Standard laminectomies are not advised, as neurological deterioration rate of 45% is reported in patients undergoing thoracic laminectomy for discectomy (Logue 1952), most likely because of the degree of spinal cord retraction and manipulation. For lumbar discs below the conus, standard laminectomies may be contemplated.

Compression Fracture

This is the wedge fracture of the anterior column, with or without posterior column involvement. The middle column is intact. The integrity of the posterior column determines the stability of the fracture. Anterior column compression of greater than 50% and anterior kyphotic angle of greater than 25° is generally associated with posterior ligamentous injury, and surgical distraction and stabilization are indicated. Otherwise, the injury can be treated conservatively with a thoracolumbar orthosis. The brace should be worn, as long as the patient is out of the supine position. In three to six months of wearing the orthosis, lateral flexion and extension radiographs should be obtained with the patient out of the brace. If there is no movement on the flexion–extension radiographs, and no progression of the degree of wedge compression or kyphosis, the use of the orthosis can be discontinued. Physical therapy to strengthen the truncal musculature should be initiated. If there is progression of the deformity or movement on the radiographs, surgical stabilization may be contemplated.

For surgical candidates, the authors generally recommend a universal system for posterior segmental stabilization. Even though a compression system may be utilized in the presence of an intact middle column, there is no advantage compared to the universal system. Furthermore, the universal system avoids inadvertent protrusion of the disc fragment into the canal. A neutralizing system such as Luque system should not be used because it does not protect adequately against axial loading, and the sublaminar wires pose a potential threat of neural element compression. Even though this type of injury does not usually require anterior decompression and grafting, compounding factors such as severe osteoporosis may necessitate a vertebrectomy and the placement of a vertebral strut graft through a retroperitoneal or thoracotomy incision.

Burst Fracture

This type of fracture is defined by the disruption of the anterior and middle columns, but the posterior elements may or may not be injured. Other factors to consider include the neurological status of the patient, degree of angulation, and canal compromise (James et al. 1994).

Burst fractures may be managed surgically, or non-surgically depending on the above factors. There has been no consensus regarding the surgical treatment of such patients. The authors advocate conservative therapy for neurologically intact patients with less than 50% canal stenosis, and kyphotic angle of less than 25°. Such patients may be treated with a thoracolumbar orthotic device alone for three to six months. Positions and postures that exacerbate the flexion deformity, such as excessive forward-bending or sleeping with too many pillows, should be avoided. The spine alignment and kyphotic angle are followed clinically and by plain radiographs. After the healing appears complete, lateral flexion–extension radiographs are obtained to ascertain stability. The brace may then be discontinued accordingly. Any clinical or radiographical deterioration should prompt an urgent re-assessment of treatment plan and planning of surgical intervention. Neurological deficits are defined as any bowel/bladder dysfunction, any motor or sensory change (including perineal sensation change), or persistent lower extremity dermatomal pain. Options for delayed stabilization include an anterior decompression with anterior or posterior fusion, or a posterior instrumentation combined with posterolateral decompression. Conversely, patients initially presenting with neurological deficits, greater than 50% canal compromise, and/or kyphotic angle of greater than 25° should be actively decompressed and instrumented.

These fractures may be stabilized posteriorly with any distraction system. Harrington rods and hooks and universal segmental fixation system can both be used. Hardaker et al. (1992) utilized bilateral transpedicular decompression and the Harrington distraction system for thoracolumbar burst fracture, and had good results with fusion and neurological improvement. After distraction, ultrasonography should be utilized to detect any residual neural compression, which should prompt a posterolateral decompression of the residual compressing elements. Silvestro et al. (1992) has demonstrated good results both with anatomical reduction, and neurological recovery with a posterolateral approach. The Luque system should be avoided, as it does not adequately protect against axial loading, which tends to exacerbate retropulsion of bony/disc material into the spinal canal. Laminectomy alone is never indicated for the treatment of such an injury (Paul et al. 1975; Bohlman et al. 1985). No anterior decompression is achieved by a laminectomy, and its destabilizing effect on a spine with disrupted anterior and middle columns could be devastating. Neurological deterioration is the common sequelae. When a laminectomy is performed to decompress a laminar fracture or facilitate a dural tear repair, a standard posterior instrumentation with posterolateral fusion should be performed.

Fracture–Dislocation

By definition, this is a highly unstable three-column injury. Neurological deficits are common. Surgical interventions are needed for the majority of these patients. Neurologically intact patients should be instrumented to provide spinal stability, and to prevent neurological deterioration. Patients with incomplete injury should undergo canal decompression and fusion to stabilize the spine and neurological functions. Patients with complete neurological injury can benefit from early mobilization if a stabilization procedure is performed.

Since the anterior longitudinal ligament is usually intact in fracture–dislocation injuries, the spine can be distracted and fixed with a posterior distraction construct. The Harrington distraction system can be used in combination with the Harrington compression system or segmental wiring to facilitate optimal distraction (avoid over-distraction) (Denis et al. 1984). The Harrington distraction system should not be used alone to treat fracture dislocations, as the paucity of residual ligamentous support renders this construct incapable of keeping the spine aligned anatomically (Denis and Burkus, 1992). The universal segmental fixation system allows for overall distraction and local compression, and is therefore the instrumentation system of choice at the authors' institution. The Luque system provides adequate rotational stability but does not restore axial stability, and should consequently not be used for reduction of flexion–dislocation injuries. A compression construct should not be used prior to distraction in a flexion–rotation or flexion–distraction injury, as the facets may have jumped and locked.

The shear type injury disrupts all three columns, including all associated ligamentous structures. The authors generally utilize the universal segmental fixation system for reduction and internal fixation, as well as posterolateral fusion with autograft to provide optimal stabilization. This type of construct is advantageous, as it does not require ligamentous support.

Even though anterior decompression is generally not needed, patients with severe anterior column injury and incomplete neurological injury may require an anterior decompression with grafting, in addition to posterior distraction and fusion. The anterior procedure decompresses the spinal canal, and the posterior procedure corrects the deformity and stabilizes the fracture.

Penetrating Injury

Gunshot wounds and other sharp object penetration of the spinal canal and vertebral column may also cause neurological deficit. Indications for decompressive procedures are based on the presence of compression. If a missile traverses the canal with no intracanalicular bony or bullet fragment, surgical intervention is generally not needed. Conversely, if a bullet or bone fragment is compressing the neural elements, decompression is warranted after the fragment is localized with a CT scan. Laminectomy of gunshot injury patients did not improve function, and may increase the incidence of spinal instability, cerebrospinal fluid leak and infection (Yashon et al. 1970; Stauffer et al. 1979). The authors utilize intravenous antibiotics (penicillin and chloramphenicol) for patients with suspected dural/thecal sac penetration.

Laminectomy is not always the appropriate procedure. If the compression is anterior, it may be best to relieve the compression anteriorly or posterolaterally with a costotransversectomy or lateral thoracotomy. Flexion–extension spine radiographs should be obtained to determine the radiographic stability of the injured segment, if

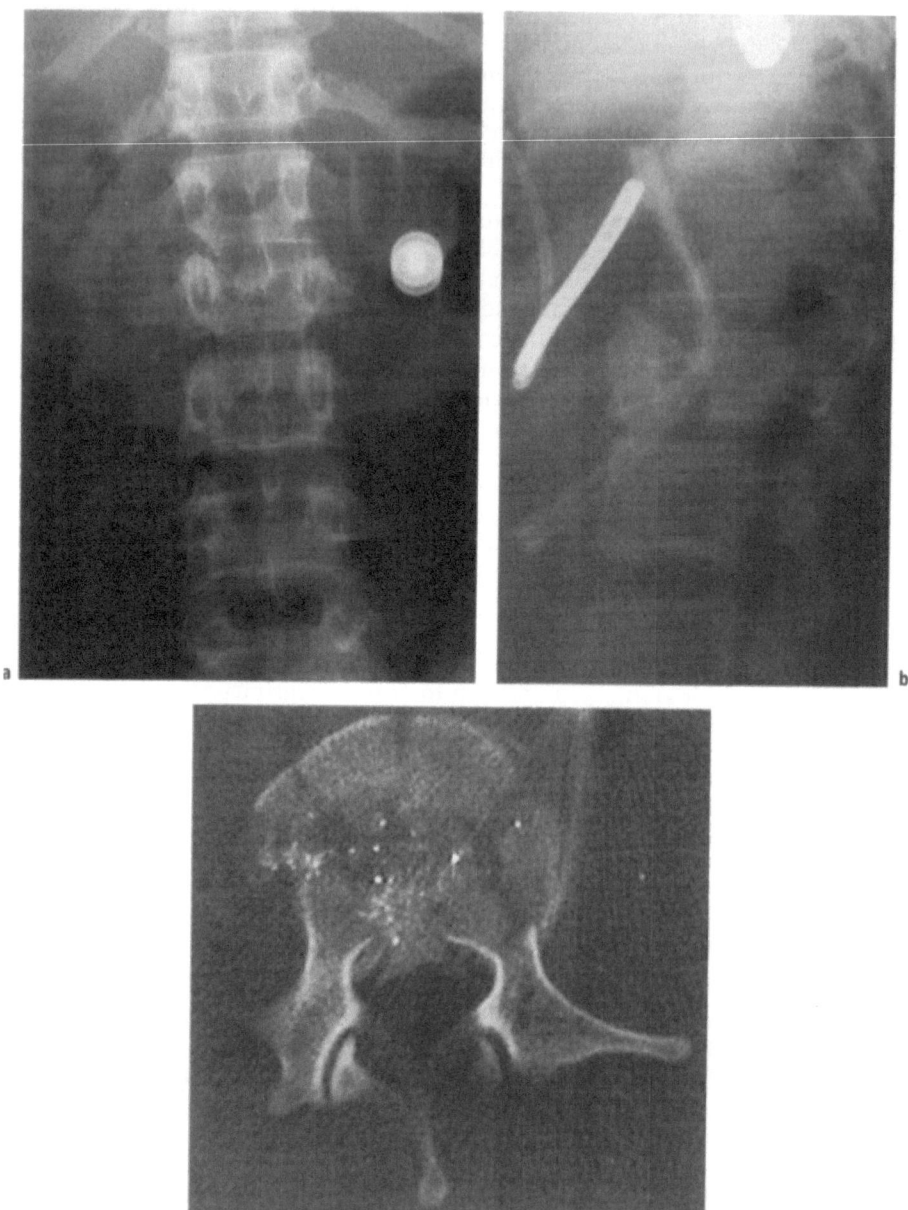

Fig. 31.11. An unstable fracture after a gunshot wound to the abdomen. The patient sustained intra-abdominal injuries and suffered from bilateral lower extremity weakness. **a,b** Plain radiographs showing a comminuted fracture of the L2 vertebral body. **c** CT scan demonstrated the "burst" fracture and the comminuted vertebral body. The patient underwent lumbar laminectomies, a transpedicular reduction of the burst fracture, and posterior stabilization procedure with the titanium TSRH system. **d,e** Postoperative plain radiographs demonstrating the instrumentation system (TSRH system with sublaminar hooks, pedicle screws at L2 and L3, and crosslinks).

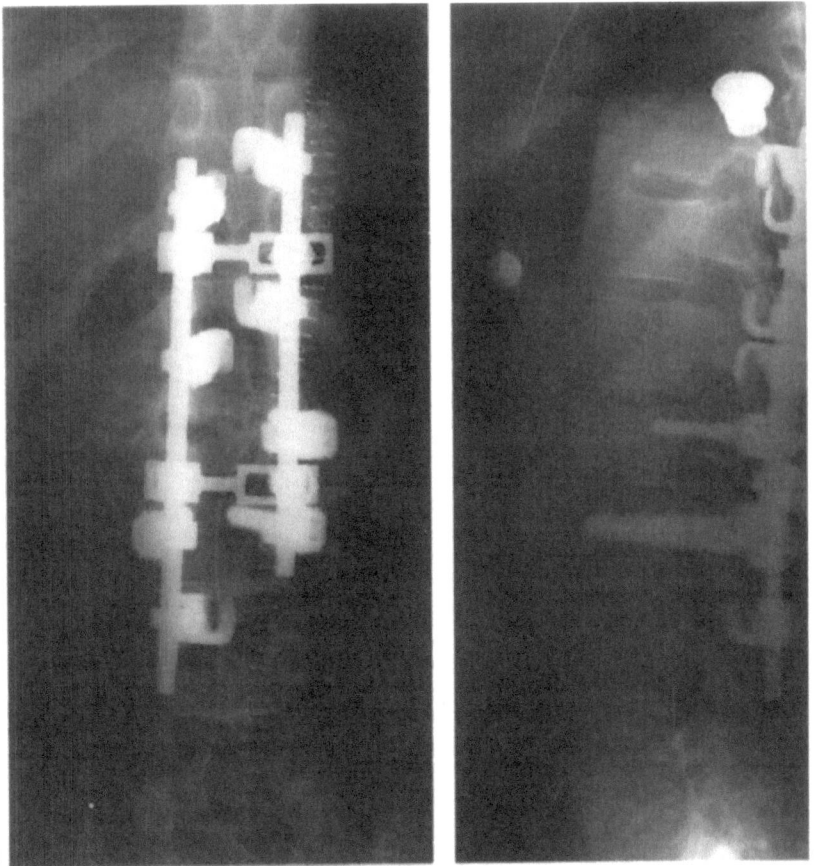

d   e

Fig. 31.11. (Continued)

the plain anteroposterior radiograph and CT scan do not suggest an unstable injury. Even though the majority of these injuries do not cause an unstable injury, posterior stabilization should be contemplated when instability is encountered. For an injury with obvious three-column injury and gross instability, instrumentation with or without decompression should be contemplated (Fig. 31.11a–c)

Complications

As with any other surgical procedure, spinal decompression and stabilization carries a certain amount of risk. Ordinary postoperative complications, such as haemorrhage, infection, pulmonary embolism and myocardial ischaemia are possible with these procedures, as well as death. Neurological deterioration associated with instrumentation is reported to be approximately 1% (Wenger and Mubarak 1989; Mueller and Larson 1991). This is usually associated with over-distraction, over-compression and direct injury to the neural element by the instrumentation, loss of reduction, or instrument dislodgement. These complications may be minimized by careful surgical techniques, ultrasonographic imaging and evoked potential monitoring. Segmental sublaminar wires (King 1984; Luque 1986) and Luque, sublaminar hooks, and pedicle screws may impinge on and injure neural elements, and should be used with great care.

Dural tear may also result from either the initial trauma, or inadvertently during the procedure. Any bony spikes should be removed, and the dura should be carefully inspected. Primary repair with muscle/fascia grafting as needed, should be performed.

References

Asher M, Carson W, Heining C et al. (1988) A modular spinal linkage system to provide rotational stability. Spine 13:272–277

Asher MA, Strippgen WE, Heinig CF et al. (1992) Isola spinal implant system: principles, design and applications. In: An HS, Cotler JM (eds) Spinal instrumentation. Wiliams and Wilkins, Baltimore, pp 325–351

Ashman RB (1993) History and development of the TSRH system. In: Ashman RB, Herring JA, Johnston CE et al. (eds) TSRH Universal Spinal Instrumentation. Hundley and Associates, Inc., pp 1–7

Bedbrook GM (1975) Treatment of thoracolumbar dislocation and fractures with paraplegia. Clin Orthop 112:27–43

Bedbrook GM (1979) Spinal injuries with tetraplegia and paraplegia. J Bone Joint Surg 61B:267–284

Bedbrook GM (1980) Recovery of spinal cord function. Paraplegia 18:315–323

Benli IT, Tandogan NR, Kis M et al. (1994) Cotrel–Dubousset instrumentation in the treatment of unstable thoracic and lumbar spine fractures. Arch Orthop Trauma Surg 113:86–92

Benzel EC (1993) Short-segment compression instrumentation for selected thoracic and lumbar spine fractures: the short-rod/two-claw technique. J Neurosurg 79:335–340

Benzel EC, Kesterson L, Marchand EP (1991) Texas Scottish Rite Hospital rod instrumentation for thoracic and lumbar spine trauma. J Neurosurg 75:382–387

Bick EM (1937) Source book of orthopaedics. Williams and Wilkins, Baltimore

Blauth M, Tscherne H, Haas N (1987) Therapeutic concept and results of operative treatment in acute trauma of the thoracic and lumbar spine: the Hannover experience. J Orthop Trauma 1:240–252

Boehler L (1932) Behandlung der wirbelbruche. Laugenbecks Arch Klin Clin 173:843–847

Bohlman HH (1985) Treatment of fractures and dislocations of the thoracic and lumbar spine. J Bone Joint Surg 76A:165–169

Bohlman HH, Freehafer A, Dejak J (1984) The results of treatment of acute injuries of the upper thoracic spine with paralysis. J Bone Joint Surg 67A:360–369

Bohlman HH, Kirkpatrick JS, Delamarter RB, Leventhal M (1994) Anterior decompression for late pain and paralysis after fractures of the thoracolumbar spine. Clin Orthop Rel Res 300:24–29

Braakman R, Fontijne WPJ, Zeegers R et al. (1991) Neurological deficit in injuries of the thoracic and lumbar spine: a consecutive series of 70 patients. Acta Neurochir 111:11–17

Bracken MB, Shepard MJ, Collins WF et al. (1990) A randomized, controlled trial of methylprednisolone or naloxone in the treatment of acute spinal-cord injury. Result of the second National Acute Spinal Cord Injury Study. N Engl J Med 322:1405–1411

Breasted JH (1930) The Edwin Smith papyrus. University of Chicago Press, Chicago

Calancie B, Klose KJ, Biaer S, Green BA (1991) Isoflurane-induced attenuation of motor evoked potentials caused by electrical motor cortex stimulation during surgery. J Neurosurg 74:897–904

Chance CQ (1948) Note on a type of flexion fracture of the spine. Br J Radiol 21:452–453

Convery FR, Minteer MA, Smith RN (1978) Fracture dislocation of the dorsal lumbar spine; acute operative stabilization by Harrington Instrumentation. Spine 8:576–582

Cotrel Y, Dubousset J, Guillaumat M (1988) New universal instrumentation in spinal surgery. Clin Orthop 227:10–23

Daffner RH, Beeb ZL, Goldberg AL et al. (1990) The radiologic assessment of post-traumatic vertebral stability. Skeletal Radiol 19:103–108

Davis AG (1929) Fractures of the spine. J Bone Joint Surg 11:133

Dekutoski MB, Conlan ES, Salciccioli GG (1993) Spinal mobility and deformity after Harrington rod stabilization and limited arthrodesis of thoracolumbar fractures. J Bone Joint Surg 75A:168–176

Denis F (1983) The three column spine and its significance in the classification of acute thoracolumbar spinal injuries. Spine 8:817–831

Denis F, Burkus J (1992) Shear fracture-dislocations of the thoracic and lumbar spine associated with forceful hyperextension (lumberjack paraplegia). Spine 17:156–161

Denis F, Armstrong GWD, Searls K, Matta L (1984) Acute thoracolumbar burst fractures in the absence of neurological deficit. Clin Orthop 189:142–149

Dickman CA, Fessler RG, McMillan M, Haid RW (1992) Transpedicular screw-rod fixation of the lumbar spine: operative technique and outcome in 104 cases. J Neurosurg 77:860–870

Dickson JH, Harrington PR, Erwin WD (1978) Results of reduction and stablization of the severely fractured thoracic and lumbar spine. J Bone Joint Surg 60A:799–805

Edwards CC, Levine AM (1989) Complications associated with posterior instrumentation in the treatment of thoracic and lumbar injuries. In: Garfin S (ed) Complications of spine surgery. Williams and Wilkins, Baltimore, pp 164–199

Edwards CC, Levine AM (1986) Early rod-sleeve stabilization of the injured thoracic and lumbar spine. Orthop Clin North Amer 17:121–145.

Eismont FJ, Garfin SR, Abitol J (1993) Thoracic and upper lumbar spine injuries. In: Browner BD, Jupiter JB, Levine AM et al. (eds) Skeletal trauma. WB Saunders, Philadelphia, pp 729–803

El-Khoury GY, Moore TE, Kathol MH (1992) Radiology of the thoracic spine. Clin Neurosurg 38:261–295

Erikson DL, Leider LL, Browno WE (1977) One-stage decompression–stabilization for thoracolumbar fractures. Spine 2:53–56

Esses SI, Botsford D (1990) Development of a new neural grading scale. Presented at the Annual Meeting of the American Spinal Injury Association. Orlando, Florida

Frankel HL, Hancock DO, Hysolop G et al. (1969) The value of postural reduction in the initial treatment of closed injuries of the spine with paraplegia and tetraplegia. Paraplegia 31:179–192

Graziano GP (1993) Cotrel-Dubousset hooks and screw combination for spine fractures. J Spine Disord 6:380–385

Grazier KL, Holbrook TL, Kelsey JL et al. (1984) The frequency of occurrence, impact, and the cost of musculoskeletal conditions in the United States. American Academy of Orthopaedic Surgeons, Chicago

Green BA, Eismont FJ (1984) Acute spinal cord injury: a systems approach. Central Nerv Sys Trauma 1:173–195

Green BA, Eismont FJ, O'Heir JT (1987) Pre-hospital management of spinal cord injuries. Paraplegia 25:229–238

Gurr KP, McAfee P, Shih CM (1988) Biomechanical analysis of anterior and posterior instrumentation systems after corpectomy: a calf spine model. J Bone Joint Surg 70A:1182–1191

Guttman L (1973) Spinal cord injuries: Comprehensive management and research. Blackwell Scientific Publications, Oxford

Hardaker Jr WT, Cook Jr WA, Friedman AH, Fitch RD (1992) Bilateral transpedicular decompression and Harriington rod stabilization in the management of severe thoracolumbar burst fractures. Spine 17:162–171

Harrington PR (1962) Treatment of scoliosis. Correction and internal fixation by spine instrumentation. J Bone Joint Surg (Am) 44:591–610

Harrington PR (1967) Instrumentation of spinal instability other than spine scoliosis. S Afr J Surg 5:7–12

Harrington PR, Tullos HS (1969) Reduction of severe spondylolisthesis in children. South Med J 62:1–7

Heinemann AW, Warkony GM, Tothe EJ et al. (1989) Functional outcome following spinal cord injury: a comparison of specialized spinal cord injury center vs. general hospital short-term care. Arch Neurol 46:1098–1102

Hodgson AR, Stock FE (1956) Anterior spinal fusion: a preliminary communication on radical treatment of Pott's disease and Pott's paraplegia. Br J Surg 44:266

Holdsworth FW (1963) Fractures, dislocations and fracture-dislocation of the spine. J Bone Joint Surg 45B:6

Holdsworth FW, Harvey AG (1953) Early treatment of paraplegia from fractures of the thoraco-lumbar spine. J Bone Joint Surg 33B:540

Jacobs RR, Asher MA, Snider RK (1980) Thoracolumbar spinal injuries: a comparative study of recumbent and operative treatment in 100 patients. Spine 5:463–477

James KS, Wenger KH, Schiegel JD et al. (1994) Biomechanical evaluation of the stability of thoracolumbar burst fractures. Spine 19:1731–1740

Kahanovitz N, Bullogh P, Jacob RR (1984) The effects of internal fixation without arthrodesis on human facet joint cartilage. Clin Orthop 189:204–208

King AB (1984) Complication in segmental spinal instrumentation. In: Luque ER (ed) Segmental spinal instrumentation. Slack, Thorofare, NJ, pp 303–330

Krag MH, Beynnon BD, Pope MH (1988) Depth of insertion of transpedicular vertebral screws into human vertebrae: effect upon screw-vertebra interface strength. J Spinal Dis 1:287–294

Krengel WF, Anderson PA, Henley MB (1993) Early stabilization and decompression for incomplete paraplegia due to a thoracic-level spinal cord injury. Spine 18:2080–2087

Lebwohl NH, Starr JK (1993) Surgical management of thoracolumbar fractures. In: Greenberg J (ed) Handbook of head and spine trauma. Marcel Dekker, New York. pp 593–646

Lemons VR, Wagner Jr FC, Montesano PX (1992) Management of thoracolumbar fractures with accompanying neurological injury. Neurosurgery 30:667–671

Levine AM, Bosse M, Edwards CC (1988) Bilateral facet dislocations in the thoracolumbar spine. Spine 13:630–640

Logue V (1952) Transthoracic intervertebral disc prolapse with spinal cord compression. J Neurol Neurosurg Psychiatry 15:227–241

Louis R (1983) Surgery of the spine. Springer-Verlag, New York

Lucas JT, Ducker TB (1979) Motor classification of spinal cord injuries with mobility, morbidity, and recovery indices. Am Surg 45:151–158

Luque ER. (1986) Segmental spinal instrumentation of the lumbar spine. Clin Orthop 203:126–134

Magerl F, Harms H, Gertzbein S, Aebi M (1989) A new classification of spinal fractures. Orthop Trans 15:728

Maiman DJ, Pintar FA (1992) Anatomy and clinical biomechanics of the thoracic spine. Clin Neurosurg 38:296–324

Maiman DJ, Larson SJ, Luck E, El-Ghatit A (1984) Lateral extracavitary approach to the spine for thoracic disc herniations: report of 23 cases. Neurosurgery 14:178–182

McAfee PC, Werner FW, Glisson RR (1985) A biomechanical analysis of spinal instrumentation systems in thoracolumbar fractures: comparison of traditional Harrington distraction instrumentation with segmental spinal instrumentation. Spine 10:204–217

McAfee PC, Bohlman HH, Wuan HA (1985) Anterior decompression of traumatic thoracolumbar fractures with incomplete neurological deficit using a retroperitoneal approach. J Bone Joint Surg 67A:89–104

McBride GG (1993) Cotrel–Douboussset rods in surgical stabilization of spinal fractures. Spine 18:466–473

McEvoy RD, Bradford DS (1983) The management of burst fractures of the thoracic and lumbar spine: experience in 53 patients. Spine 20:631–637

Mueller WM, Larson SJ (1991) Complications of spinal instrumentation. In: Tarlov EC (ed) Complications of spinal surgery, American Association of Neurological Surgeons, Park Ridge, IL, pp 15–22

Nicoll EA (1949) Fractures of the dorso-lumbar spine. J Bone Joint Surg 31B:376–388

Parke W (1982) Applied anatomy of the spine. In: Rothman R, Simeone F (eds) Spine WB Saunders, Philadelphia, pp 18–51

Patterson RH, Arbit E (1978) A surgical approach through the pedicle for protruded thoracic discs. J Neurosurg 48:768

Paul RL, Michael RH, Dunn JE, Williams JP (1975) Anterior transthoracic surgical decompression of acute spinal cord injuries. J Neurosurg 43:299

Perot PH, Munro DD (1969) Transthoracic removal of midline thoracic disc protrusions causing spinal cord compression. J Neurosurg 31:452–458.

Place HM, Donaldson DH, Brown CW, Stringer EA (1994) Stabilization of thoracic spine fractures resulting in complete paraplegia. A long-term retrospective analysis. Spine 19:1726–1730

Purcell GA, Markolf KL, Dawson EG (1981) Twelfth thoracic-first lumbar vertebral mechanical stability of fractures after Harrington-rod instrumentation. J Bone Joint Surg 63A:71–78

Riebel GD, Yoo JU, Fredrickson BE et al. (1993) Review of Harrington rod treatment of spinal trauma. Spine 18:479

Rimoldi RL, Zigler JE, Capen DA, Hu SS (1992) The effect of surgical intervention on rehabilitation time in patients with thoracolumbar and lumbar spinal cord injuries. Spine 17:1443–1449

Roach JW, Ashman RB, Allard RN (1990) The strength of a posterior element claw at one versus to spinal levels. J Spinal Disord 3:259–261

Roberts JB, Curtis PH (1970) Stability of the thoracic and lumbar spine in traumatic paraplegia following fracture or fracture–dislocation. J Bone Joint Surg 52A:1115–1130

Roy-Camille RR, Saillant G, Mazel C (1986) Internal fixation of the lumbar spine with pedicle screw plating. Clin Orthop 203:7–98

Silvestro C, Fraccaviglia N, Bragazzi R, Viale GL (1992) Near-anatomical reduction and stabilization of burst fractures of lower thoracic and lumbar spine. Acta Neurochir 116:53–59

Soreff J, Axordorph G, Bylund P et al. (1982) Treatment of patients with unstable fractures of the thoracic and lumbar spine. Acta Orthop Scand 53:369–381

Stagnara P, Demauroy JV, Drang et al. (1982) Reciprocal angulation of vertebral bodies in a sagittal plane: approach to references for the evaluation of kyphosis and lordosis. Spine 7:335–342

Stauffer ES, Wood W, Kelly EG (1979) Gunshot wounds of the spine: the effect of laminectomy. J Bone Joint Surg 61A:389–392

Tator CH, Rowed DW, Schwartz ML (1982) Sunnybrook cord injury scales for assessing neurological injuries and neurological recovery. In: Tator CH (ed) Early management of acute spinal cord injury. Raven Press, New York, pp 7–24

Watson-Jones R (1943) Fracture and joint injuries. Williams & Wilkins Baltimore

Wenger DR, Mubarak SJ (1989) Managing complications of posterior spinal instrumentation and fusion. In: Garfin SR (ed) Complications of spine surgery. Williams and Wilkins, Baltimore, pp 127–143

White AA, Panjabi M (1990) Clinical biomechanics of the spine. JB Lippincott, Philadelphia

Yashon D, Jane JA, White RJ (1970) Prognosis and management of spinal cord and cauda equina bullet injuries in sixty-five civilians. J Neurosurg 32:163–170

Zdeblick TA (1993) A prospective randomized study of lumbar fusion. Preliminary results. Spine 18:983–991

SCI Rehabilitation: Concepts, Mobility, Functional Electrical Stimulation, Spasticity

R.J. Weber and R.C. Davis

Concepts

Injuries to the vertebral column resulting in damage to the spinal cord are uncommon with an annual incidence at about 20–40 per million population and a prevalence somewhere between 183 000 and 230 000 in the United States (Go et al. 1995). Although small in number, the cost in personal terms to the individual, his family and to society in health, social and other resources is immense. Through the pioneering work of many including Riddoch and Guttman in Britain and Munro and Bors in the United States (Collins and Chehrazi 1982), management of spinal cord injury (SCI) is becoming an acknowledged medical subspecialty in its own right and preliminary efforts are underway by the American Board of Physical Medicine and Rehabilitation to create special certification in SCI management.

The purpose of medical rehabilitation is the restoration and maintenance of optimal physical, psychological and social function following injury or disease. Many rehabilitation principles were developed through experience with individuals with SCI since it presents a broad spectrum of acute and chronic medical management issues, physiological changes, and psychological and social challenges. Perhaps the two foremost of these principles are the need for early and consistent structuring of patient management away from methods which foster dependency and the attention to the broad issues which affect the individual's functioning within society. Although both acute medical/surgical and rehabilitation medicine can provide similar health care services, they differ in the principal perspective from which they are organized. Acute care is "disease" focused and medical issues predominate. It seeks to cure, and through curing, prevent residual problems and return the patient to their normal routine. Medical rehabilitation is a process in which medical principles operate within a structured milieu to support an individual whose capabilities are changed by injury or disease and to help him or her reestablish and maintain an optimal societal role. The principal concept of rehabilitation is the impact of an individual's functional status on his broadly defined societal role. Put differently, global rehabilitation outcome depends both on the disease and on the individual. This interrelationship is implicit in the international classification of impairments, disabilities and handicaps of the World Health Organization (1980):

Impairment – loss or abnormality of psychological, physiological or anatomical structure or function;

Disability – restriction or lack of the ability to perform an activity in the manner or within the range considered normal for a human being;

Handicap – disadvantage for a given individual that limits or prevents the fulfilment of a role that is normal for that individual.

In this construct, injury or disease issues operate at the impairment level while broader factors influence outcome at the disability and handicap level. Outcome varies not only between individuals with identical impairments but for a single individual at different life stages. This time-dependent outcome factor is prominent in SCI since it most commonly affects young people prior to their establishment of mature vocational and social roles.

Service Units designed to address issues across the spectrum of injury and handicap are referred to as comprehensive medical rehabilitation programmes. They are characterized by the use of a transdisciplinary team of professional staff and the reliance on a structured rehabilitation milieu. A transdisciplinary team has two strengths. First, by enabling team members to provide specific services which may be provided traditionally by another discipline, i.e. staff function outside their usual roles, the team is better able to intensively address important management issues. This is particularly true for psychosocial adjustment where continual reinforcement of behavior or attitude is most effective and in physical training where frequent repetition is required. A transdisciplinary approach ensures that there is continual attention to these issues. Secondly, the team approach to goal development tends to redirect service delivery toward practical objectives which reflect longer term needs rather than toward discipline specific, technically "hot" items. The core members of this team are rehabilitation nursing, physiatrist, psychologist, physical and occupational therapists and the social worker. Recreation therapy, dietary, respiratory therapy, orthotic/prosthetic, vocational and others often add important contributions. An important responsibility of medical leadership in comprehensive programmes is to help focus the programme on outcome-directed intervention. The growing array of surgical and technological interventions for SCI impairments must be considered in the context of their impact on more global, handicap level effects. The physiatrist role, therefore, must encompass some gatekeeper function if we are to avoid the "technically possible" overwhelming the "practical" in patients with SCI.

It is impossible to overstate the acute psychological impact of SCI. The rehabilitation milieu provides a supportive environment in which individuals with SCI can experience initial success and interact with peers. It enables the team to identify and address more readily the psychosocial factors affecting patients and their supporters. The complete integration of activities within the milieu permits the team to adjust the level of challenge encountered by the patient appropriate to his progress. Its structure permits consistent reinforcement of effective strategies and behaviour. While its environment should always be supportive, it must also promote independence and empower self-direction. However imperfect, it offers a reasonable setting in which to resolve conflict and promote effective adjustment strategies.

Rehabilitation goals and outcomes are often influenced as much by patient-related factors such as gender, psychosocial and financial resources as by the neurological level and completeness of injury. Problem categories which form the rehabilitation process include paralysis, physiological dysfunction and psychosocial disruption. Paralysis results in prominent mobility and self-care deficits and these are the factors which are most visibly addressed during comprehensive rehabilitation. They include basic skills such as positioning in bed, transferring (to chair, toilet, bath or car) and standing, the development of strength and balance, and advanced special techniques for dressing, bathing and grooming which build on the preceding elements.

The most encompassing physiological disruption in SCI is autonomic nervous system dysfunction which ultimately affects most organ systems. Loss of sympathetic drive increases the more cephalad the SCI lesion. It causes the loss of splanchnic and peripheral vasoconstriction producing general and orthostatic hypotension, the loss of cardiovascular response to exercise, and interference with temperature regulation, sweating and sexual function. In lesions above T6 the sympathetic system may be triggered through spinal reflexes, usually caused by noxious stimuli below the lesion level, to over respond. This hyperactivity results in profuse sweating, hypertension and reactive bradycardia. This is termed autonomic dysreflexia and patients must be trained to recognize and effectively manage its difficulties. Both somatic and autonomic nervous system loss contribute to the difficulties seen in neurogenic bowel and bladder. The patient must become adept at regulating stool bulk and hardness and controlling evacuation through, for example, stimulation of the rectal ampulla and the appropriate use of bowel medications. Bladder management through, for example intermittent self-catheterization is often preferred in males but requires adequate hand function or regular assistance of another individual trained to perform this procedure. Reflex voiding, indwelling catheters and urinary diversions all have roles. Spasticity from altered spinal cord reflex activity can impair function and disrupt rehabilitation progress.

More than most difficulties, sexual dysfunction presents both physiological and psychological challenges. The young male, trauma related SCI patient is most vulnerable to the psychological aspects of self-image, worth and role loss and the threat to newly emerging interpersonal relationships inherent in sexual issues. These stresses are compounded by the technical aspect of erectile and ejaculatory problems, more obvious in the male than analogous difficulties of the female, and positioning, physical performance and psychogenic arousal challenges. The rehabilitation adjustment process must address core psychological issues related to self-concept, family role change, vocational challenge and the impact of alteration in dependency. The rehabilitation process must enable the patient and supporters to gain a new, effective accommodation with their lives.

Mobility

Walking and driving come as close as any to an abbreviated description of daily life in our hypermobile society. It is not surprising that regaining these skills is of primary interest to those entering rehabilitation regardless of their impairments. The interest seems particularly acute in SCI where, for the frequently young patients, acceptance and independence were often acute concerns prior to injury.

When SCI results in an immediate, complete lesion, it is easier to predict which method of mobility is likely to be effective since significant neurological recovery of more than one neurological level is unlikely. Here, however, acceptance by the patient may be difficult. Although significantly incomplete lesion implies increased potential for neurological improvement, presence of co-morbidities may make selecting the preferred mobility method more challenging and decisions may need to be revisited. The situation is made more complicated by the fact that if practicality of function is set aside, virtually every individual with SCI can be enabled to ambulate through some technological means. Thus, mobility discussions present inherent conflict between addressing issues at an impairment and at handicap level. Wheelchair decisions also present an opportunity for conflicts of values. Mobilization of a manually powered chair is possible in all but the highest SCI levels, and use of a standard wheelchair can be made to "work" for most individuals with SCI. Yet clearly, power chairs and more technologically advanced, lighter weight manually powered chairs offer many individuals greater independence and more effective mobility.

The rehabilitation team must often broker these issues of cost, efficiency, practicality and desire through both the inexact process of adjustment and of funding. Here sensitivity and principled position are both essential in order to secure the goal of minimalizing the level of outcome handicap.

All things being equal, there are transition levels of SCI around which practical orthotic decisions pivot. Preservation of C7 provides elbow extension as well as wrist and sensory functions such that manual chair use becomes more practical. Lower lesions progressively allow improved grip, transfers and trunk balance which in turn increase the efficiency of manual chair activation and increase the benefit of innovative designs. In this era of improved alloys, only lightweight designs should be considered for prescription in SCI. The preservation of effective quadriceps function which usually accompanies L3 or lower lesions offers the potential for more practical, orthotic-assisted ambulation. Energy costs remain high but practical applications are frequent, particularly within defined settings. Lesions below L3 further improve efficiency and practicality whereas higher lesions produce the reverse. Orthotic-assisted ambulation both stresses the upper extremities and by requiring use of the hands, limits their concurrent function for useful tasks, an important consideration when planning mobility strategies.

Wheelchairs

Individuals with SCI often utilize a manual or power wheelchair for independent mobility. Recent advances in their design and construction have produced significantly lighter, stronger and more efficient models which extend user performance. "Standard" wheelchair design consists of steel frame construction, full height back with handles for attendant use, rear set main wheels with solid or pneumatic tyres, a separate hand rim attached to the main wheels for propulsion (perhaps coated or with knobs or bars projecting to assist grip; leg/foot rests which may swing away and be removed for access; removable arms of various designs permitting side entry; front caster wheels set beneath the frame. These models in theory permit a single frame design to be customized to user need. In practice, there is little advantage taken of this feature. The design is useful in situations where staff often assist and floor surfaces are ideal. The weight and geometry of the design interfere with efficient use by active individuals with SCI. Loading these chairs into an auto-mobile can tax not only the user, but individuals free from impairments. There is little, if any, justification for prescription of these chairs in SCI other than for insti-tutional purposes.

Although stronger, lighter weight alloys are essential components in new wheel-chair designs, the more significant aspect is the evolving change in concept and geometry. First, modularity has been replaced by integration of parts further reduc-ing weight and improving rigidity. Leg supports are usually integrated to the frame and hand rims integrated into the wheel structure.

Building on racing experience, the centre of gravity is lowered. This improves sta-bility which has, in turn, permitted the more forward placement of the main pro-pelling wheels. Wheel placement and changes in wheel camber improve the efficiency of manual propulsion, speed and manoeuvrability. Seat positioning incorp-orating some flexion improves trunk stability. Variations such as models with a more rigid, box frame and easy wheel removal for transport provide options for special user requirements. These chairs are now available in mass-produced ver-sions. Their typical weight of 28 pounds (12.7 kg), about half that of a standardized chair, improves mobility and transportability significantly. All users benefit from these lighter models. They should be the chair of choice for all independent users. The more active user should consider more aggressive design features permitting easier curb jumping and manoeuvrability, trading off stability.

The use of power wheelchairs is effective for injury above C7 and appropriate for many at C7 or lower. The SCI level for respirator dependence varies due to the mul-tiple root supply to the diaphragm. Most C4 (C4 root functioning) injuries can even-tually be weaned from respirators whereas most C2 injuries cannot. Needle electromyography of the diaphragm and phrenic nerve conduction studies can help predict the potential for diaphragmatic pacing. Although respirator-dependent indi-viduals do require an assistant to be available full time who could, in theory, push a manual chair, such dependency is severely limiting to both the assistant and the SCI individual. Power chairs with appropriate modifications for a portable respirator including increased battery capacity, power recline and computer-based communi-cation and environmental control devices permit an important degree of self-direction. They open some vocational and avocational options and permit much more flexibility for the care giver. This is of critical importance in permitting home care by family members.

Power chair design has also advanced. Electronic controllers now permit smooth operation, even if the user has difficulty modulating the control device. Although full-time power chairs remain heavy, requiring a van and lift for transport, convert-ible systems with easily removed power units provide use options and easier trans-port for individuals who have assistants. All-terrain models utilizing four uniform sized, directly driven wheels increase both manoeuvrability and accessibility in varied settings. Newer approaches which add powered standing features are now available. Unfortunately, battery technology remains the limiting factor in power chair development.

In very high SCI, head control is diminished. Although the intact spinal accessory and facial nerves provide for some cervical motor activity, it may be insufficient to permit wheelchair or other device activation in very high cervical SCI. The presence of a tracheostomy and respirator tubes further complicates the situation. These indi-viduals require special head supports, power recline features and special control switches.

Wheelchairs come in an assortment of sizes. Important selection elements include width, seat depth and back height. Proper width is determined not only by patient buttock size but also, on occasion, by absolute architectural constraints at home. Seat depth correlates with leg size and positioning needs whereas back height is related to trunk stability and arm mobility. Seat features and cushioning are critical to pressure ulcer avoidance. Solid seats tend to improve balance but decrease transportability. Cushions help evenly distribute weight to avoid pressure sores. Weight, durability and balance features vary among types of cushions.

Walking Aids

Assistive devices can be grouped into canes, crutches or walkers. Canes may be made of wood or metal alloy and may be three-legged (tripod) or four-legged (quad-cane) to provide greater stability. The height of a cane is of paramount importance: the handle should be level with the greater trochanter when the patient is standing erect in shoes. As most patients with spinal lesions have bilateral lower limb weakness it is often necessary for them to use two canes.

Crutches also come in various types suitable for different purposes. Axillary crutches are only suitable for short-term use. They put considerable strain on upper limb joints and muscles, particularly the shoulder joints, which can lead to osteoarthrosis or brachial neuropathy. Forearm (Lofstrand) crutches put less strain on the joints than axillary crutches but are less stable and usually need stronger arms. They are essentially walking sticks with a vertical extension to the vertical component with an arm clip. This needs to be correctly aligned and well padded to prevent pressure over the ulna. A third form of crutch is the gutter crutch, also known as platform crutch. The length of the crutch is adjusted so that the forearm rests in the gutter. This demands less of the upper arm joints. It is particularly suitable for those with weakness of the hands and wrists. They tend, however, to be heavier and less stable and manoeuvrable.

Walkers provide more support and stability than canes. The types available in addition to the standard model include gutter frames which, like gutter crutches, take weight through both forearms, which can be useful in early mobilization states, and models with wheels or rollators. Rollators may have brakes and folding models are available.

Orthoses

Support with orthoses can enable healthy young individuals with complete paraplegia to stand and ambulate. That is not to say that this is an effective answer to their mobility needs. Two orthotic approaches are available for individuals with complete, high level lesions. Long leg braces, now known as hip-knee-ankle foot orthoses (HKAFO), sometimes attached to a pelvic band to control abduction/adduction and rotation of the limb, provide knee and ankle locking necessary for weight bearing. Once standing with the brace joints locked, the individual must elevate the body using the arms and a walker or crutches and advance by swinging or dragging the legs forward to a new weight-bearing location. This is known as a two point gait.

The other approach exemplified by the Louisiana State University gait orthosis (RGO) (Beckman 1987) is to place the individual into a device similar in appearance to a HKAFO with all joints locked and with pelvic bands but with its hip joints also controlled and connected to each other by a cable. The standing user can tilt weight from one leg and, by shifting body weight, cause it to advance due to the action of the cross-leg control cable. Although similar to the HKAFO it permits easier pacing of ambulation and better freedom of the hands during standing. Individuals with cervical or midthoracic lesions usually require a spinal orthotic extension for back stabilization since adequate trunk control requires abdominal muscle function which is only fully present at T12. This and similar systems such as the ParaWalker (Butler and Major 1987) require exceptionally active users and considerable training to use.

Ambulation with no or minimal lower extremity voluntary control requires reasonable trunk control and strong shoulder depressors to lift the body forward over the orthoses. This is very difficult to accomplish with upper cervical level lesions. HKAFOs require good balance despite absent lower body proprioception, upper extremity strength and a very high work capacity. High level paraplegics have impaired respiration and cardiovascular responses which contribute to fatigue in high work situations. Doffing and donning the orthoses are difficult and time-consuming; repair and adjustment are frequent. Spasticity can make donning and use more difficult. These orthoses can be a source of skin breakdown. Mobility in them is very much slower than in a chair, it requires a significantly greater amount of energy, and prevents hand use for functional tasks. Nevertheless, they provide a means of standing, weight bearing and ambulation which have perceived benefits for a selected group of individuals and, for some, can provide the capability necessary to resume life tasks.

Although adding functional spinal levels through the thoracic and upper lumbar levels improves performance, basic orthotic factors are unchanged (other than elimination of spinal extensions). The presence of L2/3 improves hip stabilization and leg swing with ambulation utilizing HKAFOs and provides a motor (rectus femoris, iliopsoas) to directly activate leg swing in a RGO, improving energy efficiency.

The addition of L4 function adds new capability: strong knee extension sufficient to support the body (plus active hip flexion) permits more energy-efficient walking. Ambulation with ankle-foot orthoses (AFO) entails shifting the weight of the body behind the hip axis (passive hip locking support by anterior ligaments) and actively locking the knee with quadriceps on one side while on the opposite side the hip is actively and the knee is passively flexed to generate a forward step (swing phase). Energy requirements are reduced since it is no longer necessary to elevate the whole body to advance the flexed limb. Ankles are stabilized by plastic AFOs. Setting the ankle in slight dorsiflexion permits the body to roll forward over the foot during late stance phase (weight bearing) of gait. The gait is waddling due to poor hip stabilization and forearm crutches are used to compensate by providing medial-lateral stability. The addition of L5 greatly improves gait through additional hip, knee and partial ankle control and may permit elimination of all bracing. The S1 root level is necessary, however, to gain full hip and knee stability along with good push-off for a fully efficient gait.

The situation is very different in incomplete SCI. Here some neurological improvement usually occurs but its ultimate extent is unpredictable. The course of recovery is sometimes delayed and often extends more than a year beyond injury. With the pressure to shorten hospital stays, patients may still be showing neurological improvement at discharge. In such circumstances, although the neuro-logical level of the SCI remains important in determining ambulation capability and appropriate orthotic needs, the extent of sensation, proprioception, motor control and spasticity below the lesion is also critically important. These individuals are often managed best by a strategy of cardiovascular reconditioning and strengthen-ing of functional muscles linked to an initial goal of wheelchair independence – if possible, using a stand pivot transfer technique. From this point, hospital discharge can occur when adjustment and home support status permit, and efforts toward ambulation or other advanced mobility goals pursued at the appropriate pace in the outpatient centre.

Features which influence whether individuals with incomplete SCI will become community ambulatory include: trunk control, lower extremity proprioception, sen-sation, motor control of one knee, spasticity, upper extremity strength. When a number of these factors are favourable early post-injury, an initial goal of independ-ent ambulation at discharge may be elected rather than that of phased management.

An individual with incomplete SCI can require considerable orthotic aid and still be an effective community ambulator. Balance assistance from walker, forearm crutches or canes is frequently required. Bracing with single or bilateral ankle foot orthoses (to provide ankle dorsiflexion and/or to control plantar spasms) often permits effective walking. A single knee-ankle-foot orthosis (KAFO) can also prove effective. Orthotic needs beyond this level such as bilateral KAFOs or HKAFOs with pelvic bands to control the hips and spinal extensions may permit ambulation but they impose marked energy consumption and speed penalties.

Energy expenditure studies reveal that normal ambulation at a comfortable walking speed is approximately 70–80 m/min, and requires 0.83 kcal $\times$ 10^{-3}/m/kg for men and 0.76 kcal $\times$ 10^{-3}/m/kg for women (Gonzalez and Corcoran 1994). Any type of gait pathology or the use of an orthotic device markedly increases energy consumption with ambulation.

In paraplegia, deciding whether or not to make ambulation a goal is often not so clear cut, and it is mixed with emotional overtones. It has been shown by various authors that patients with lesions at T12 or below have a better chance of success, but they usually give it up by the end of the first year after training. Paraplegic ambulation was found to be 66% slower than ambulation in normal subjects with an energy cost per unit distance from 230% to 380% higher than that required for normal subject walking at their comfortable walking speeds.

Wheelchair propulsion was found to require no additional energy per unit time with only a 9% increase in energy consumption per unit distance than comfortable walking speed in normal subjects. Additionally, if light weight "sport" wheelchairs are used, energy consumption costs are decreased by 17% when compared with energy costs of propelling a conventionally designed wheelchair. Again, functional needs must be considered in selecting the method of routine mobility. Aging may require revision of a previously successful strategy if developing osteoarthritis or cardiovascular problems interfere with performance.

Driving

Next to walking, the ability to drive may be the most valuable tool for resuming independent living after SCI. Happily, all new public transportation in the United

States must be wheelchair accessible; however, most of the US is not served by public transport. Even in cities where it is available, the layout and density of the city limit its benefit. Driving is usually necessary for vocational access, health care, shopping and normal social contact.

Power-equipped vans including power wheelchair lifts and automatic wheelchair tie downs are now readily available for about $35 000. They permit driving from the individual's own wheelchair and can benefit some individuals with C5 and most with lower level injuries. There is considerable variation in the SCI level which will permit personal automobiles equipped with hand controls to be utilized. Manipulating the automobile controls is the easiest of the tasks. Trunk control behind the wheel can be aided by seating but remains challenging even in thoracic level lesions. Independent transfer into the car and, as importantly, the ability to load the wheelchair are also necessary for independent automobile use. Modern, lightweight chairs greatly assist chair loading.

Functional Electrical Stimulation

Electrical shocks have been used to cause muscle contraction since antiquity, and many newly discovered electrical sources found a momentary application as a medical treatment for paralysis (Licht 1971). Modern clinical research has focused on electrical stimulation as a means of preserving muscle "viability" pending reinnervation and on developing orthotics such as an electrical "drop foot brace" for hemiplegics (Liberson 1961). Their efforts have had minimal success in producing clinically applicable devices. Research into electrical simulation as a means of restoring motion in paralysis has been resurgent for two decades. Public interest has centred on the possibility of restoration of ambulation. Interest among knowledgeable physicians is perhaps keenest concerning its effect on the physiology of spinal cord-injured individuals. How its use alters cardiovascular deconditioning, osteoporosis, muscular atrophy, spasticity, pressure sore frequency and other sequelae of paralysis may ultimately define its usefulness as importantly as its effectiveness as a mobility aid.

Clinicians have long appreciated the principles of muscle response to electrical stimulation in paralysis. When the lower motor neurone (LMN) is intact, i.e. upper motor neurone (UMN) paralysis, a short or long duration electrical stimulation applied over the muscle triggers a muscle twitch through depolarization of the associated intramuscular nerves or end plate, i.e. a nerve mediated response. When the LMN is lost, i.e. LMN injury as in a cauda equina injury, a long duration stimulus will produce a twitch by direct muscle cell depolarization but there is no response to a short duration pulse.

Although a muscle twitch can be produced by applying an appropriate duration and intensity of shock in either upper and lower motor neurone paralysis, a single twitch does not result in a functional muscle contraction. Effective contraction occurs only during a continuous train of twitches which can adequately sustain tension in the muscle between stimulations in order to produce muscle shortening. This is easily accomplished in UMN paralysis since intact motor nerves respond with distinct depolarizations to the high frequency (20–100 Hz) stimuli. Stimulation at a single point results in spread of the depolarization signal through the branching nerve network to the whole muscle. By contrast, the isolated muscle fibres of LMN paralysis must be individually stimulated, requiring a much larger stimulating field.

Denervated muscles may respond to an electrical stimulation pulse with a tetanic contraction (low twitch to tetany ratio) rather than a single twitch. Denervated muscle has been considered unsuitable for use as a motor for electrobracing because of the difficulties in effectively stimulating it and in controlling and sustaining its response.

Conversely, steady interest in functional electrical stimulation (FES) in UMN paralysis has resulted in numerous electrical orthotic applications utilizing brief, rapid stimulation of the peripheral nerve (Glaser 1994). The earliest efforts involved peroneal nerve stimulation to control foot drop in hemiplegia. Previous research on electrical stimulation in SCI as a means of causing muscle conditioning and on its effect on the physiology of patients with spinal injuries showed limited changes. The high frequency stimulation used in many of these studies to produce a strong, tetanic contraction rapidly exhausted the muscle, blocking the contraction. The high frequency electrical stimulations applied did not emulate the normal neuromuscular functional pattern in which each motor unit fires at its own sustainable rate and in which force of contraction is increased by both the recruitment of additional units and firing rate increases for individual units. Instead it cycled all motor units at the same high, unsustainable frequency similar to normal maximal contraction conditions. Exhaustion was usually reached before significant muscle work, i.e. exercise, was accomplished. Since muscle must be metabolically stressed, i.e. worked, in order to increase its strength or endurance, the studies often showed little physiological effect from the stimulation programme.

The crudeness of stimulation control also limited progress in orthotic application: the strength that the stimulated muscle could produce was limited; the force of tetanic contraction could not be graduated; it was difficult to coordinate stimulated contractions of several muscles to produce functional limb motions. These difficulties were significantly reduced with the introduction of the microprocessor (Petrofsky 1979; Petrofsky et al. 1983a) to control stimulation and the rotary stimulation approach (Petrofsky 1978; Petrofsky and Phillips 1979). In rotary stimulation each muscle is stimulated at multiple sites asynchronously. By stimulating each muscle at, for instance, three sites each site can be stimulated at a sustainable rate of 15–20 Hz; by stimulating each site out of phase from the others the effect on the muscle as a whole is that of a fused contraction equivalent to that of a 45–60 Hz stimulation but now it is sustainable. The microcomputer permits complex manipulation of the stimulation parameters. Stimulation rates can be easily ramped up or down as can stimulation intensity, more closely mimicking natural recruitment. Similarly, stimulation parameters can be based on real-time environmental factors such as limb position and movement, and the stimulation of many muscles can be coordinated.

While developing applications for the rotary stimulation technique, the Wright State University group followed two important FES concepts. One was to re-emphasize the critical role that work, i.e. resistance, plays in reconditioning paralytic as well as normal muscle. By utilizing progressive resistive exercise techniques coupled with sustained FES, they produced significant muscle bulk and strength improvement (Petrofsky and Phillips 1984). This "improved" muscle in turn increases the functional capabilities of FES orthotic systems.

The second concept was that of real-time, feedback control of stimulation in FES (Petrofsky et al. 1984b; Phillips et al. 1984). The closed loop approach immediately improves the efficiency and safety of FES powered exercise equipment (Petrofsky et al. 1984c). Motion and position sensors can be built into the equipment. The microcomputer utilizes sensor output to monitor performance (work) and then adjusts stimulation intensity to compensate for muscle fatigue by increasing stimulation rate and intensity. This ensures completion of a maximal muscle work programme prior to halting the exercise programme at a predetermined fatigue (stimulation intensity) level. The monitoring system can also detect a sudden change in performance indicative of system trouble such as electrode failure or limb disconnection from the system and prevent injury by instituting an emergency shutdown. The same approach can be applied to FES gait systems, although the placement and maintenance of sensors along with the control logic needed to safely and effectively operate such a system is far more complicated (Petrofsky and Phillips 1983; Petrofsky et al. 1984b).

Once strong and effectively controlled muscle was available through electrical stimulation, its application to power functional tasks was an obvious goal. Paralytic muscle-powered weight-lifting machines (Petrofsky et al. 1984c), exercise bicycles (Petrofsky et al. 1983b, 1984a) muscle-powered wheelchairs (Glaser 1983), standing, ambulation (Dralj and Grobelnik 1973; Marsolais and Kobetic 1983; Petrofsky and Phillips 1983) and ambulation via muscle-powered orthoses have followed.

Dralj and Grobelnik (1973) described a simple system which combined tetanic muscle stimulation of the quadriceps to power standing and stance with the triggering of a mass flexor response through peroneal nerve stimulation to initiate the gait swing phase. The system was manually cycled by the subjects using buttons on the walker. A similar system is now commercially available. Implantable electrodes offer the promise of better control and better tolerance when sensation is present. Their invasive nature and replacement difficulties are limiting. A recently reported modification uses surface electrodes positioned in an elasticized garment which simplifies the set up process (Patterson et al. 1990). Similar systems offer promise as an alternative to braces for supervised, therapeutic standing or ambulation.

Complex FES systems utilize multiple muscle groups with stimulation coordinated by a microprocessor. These systems control all or virtually all aspects of gait via FES including joint motion and stabilization. Closed loop systems, i.e. self-monitoring with feedback supplied by joint position and movement sensors, can adjust the stimulation intensity to smooth gait and to compensate for muscle fatigue or obstacles (Petrofsky and Phillips 1983; Petrofsky et al. 1984b; Phillips et al. 1984). The feedback-driven, closed-loop FES system has considerable theoretical advantage over the open-loop system's fixed stimulation pattern in generating an efficient and safe gait. However, its requirement for a reliable, complex sensor system and control logic has hindered its development. On the other hand, Marsolais and Kobetic (1983, 1987) have made steady progress using an open-loop approach and have developed implantable electrodes which are fairly reliable (Marsolais and Koettic 1986). They have been able to demonstrate stair climbing as well as level surface ambulation. Either of these "full" FES approaches requires improved reliability and user friendliness before moving from research to clinical use. Issues of energy cost also persist, particularly in the presence of limited sympathetic drive.

The coupling of the reciprocating gait orthosis (RGO) and FES is clinically promising. The orthosis provides a reliable, safe platform to support standing and ambulation. RGO ambulation can usually be sustained for sufficient distance to be functional in certain situations and the hands can be free while standing to perform desired tasks. FES can be utilized to power standing up, i.e. quadriceps stimulation, as well as hip flexion for forward stepping. Energy consumption using FES to power ambulation in the RGO is favourable compared to the RGO alone at most speeds and energy consumption with the RGO-FES combination is much less than that of HKAFO or pure FES at all gait speeds (Hirokawa et al. 1990; Nene and Patrick 1990). Speed and practicality issues still remain.

The clinical use of FES is not yet established. It can unequivocally reverse muscle atrophy and maintain cosmetically acceptable muscle bulk in UMN paralysis. This muscle-strengthening application of FES is the greatest beneficiary of the rotary stimulation technique since that stimulation technique permits extended, heavy resistance exercise without exhaustion from excessive stimulation rates.

Improved muscle bulk may protect against pressure sores through better weight distribution but this can only be demonstrated through extensive trials. FES of the gluteal muscles during sitting appears to improve blood flow in the muscle and adjusts the gluteal contour to a more normal one (Levine et al. 1990a, b). The combination of maintaining muscle bulk with a long-term FES resistance exercise progremme and phasic gluteal FES during sitting is promising as a means of pressure sore prevention.

Although FES can slow the demineralization process in SCI (Flores 1985) it does not reverse established osteoporosis of SCI when administered at levels used for routine muscle conditioning by a commercially available FES bicycle ergonometry system (Leeds et al. 1990).

Spasticity may be briefly reduced following an FES exercise session but use of FES appears to intensify the overall difficulty of spasticity management in some SCI patients rather than reduce it as initially hoped (Petrofsky et al. 1984c). Unfortunately, strong spasms remain a contraindication to FES since the spontaneous spasm during the use of FES could cause injury by suddenly resisting the FES contraction. This study suggests that using FES may cause some individuals, who were initially appropriate, to become inappropriate for use of FES exercise because of strengthening of their spasms.

FES-powered exercise including bicycle ergonometry provides a modest cardiac conditioning challenge (Glaser 1986; Hooker et al. 1990). It is effective in direct proportion to the degree of sympathetic innervation preserved, i.e. paraplegics show a greater cardiac response than quadriplegics. FES coupled with voluntary upper extremity exercise is more effective than FES exercise along for cardiovascular conditioning. A FES-based exercise system is commercially available for bicycle ergonometry. It will be of considerable benefit to individuals with SCI if the introduction of future commercial application is preceded by a clear exposition of their benefits, limits and long-term costs.

Spasticity Management

Spasticity is a motor disorder characterized by a velocity-dependent increase in tonic stretch reflexes with exaggerated tendon jerks, resulting from hyperexcitability of the stretch reflex (Kalz and Rymer 1989). Spasticity requires that the spinal reflex area of the cord below the level of the spinal lesion be intact. In acute spinal cord injuries, flexor spasticity gradually emerges over the first few weeks to six months as the initial spinal shock with its characteristic flaccidity ends. Subsequently, extensor spasticity emerges to become predominate in most cases (Marsden 1988).

Spasticity is perhaps the most difficult of the positive signs of SCI since it influences, if not directly produces, many of the common complications of SCI. Soft tissue and joint contractures are direct results of spasticity and pressure ulcers are frequently related to positioning problems resulting from spasticity and contracture. It can inhibit bowel and bladder elimination due to pelvic floor contraction. On a functional level active spasms can interfere with virtually all aspects of daily life – positioning, transfers, mobility, self-care work and driving. Severe spasticity can render wheelchair use (or staying seated in the chair) problematic. At modest levels, it can result in preserving some muscle bulk and tone which may help prevent pressure ulcers. Its elimination through treatment has been noted to interfere with weight bearing in some cases of incomplete SCI (Marsden 1988).

The first measures to be considered in managing spasticity are those directed at factors which provoke spasms. Strategies include provision of good skin, bladder and bowel care and prevention of pressure sores, urinary tract infections, bladder or renal stones, constipation and perianal conditions such as fissures. Other intercurrent problems such as infections, deep venous thrombosis and localized lesions such as ingrowing toenails may exacerbate spasms and require prompt and thorough treatment.

A programme of frequent passive stretching of the affected muscles not only prevents joint and muscle contractures (which themselves provoke spasms) but also directly, if temporarily, reduce spasticity. Evidence is also accumulating that proprioceptive facilitation in the early stages of spinal shock may reduce the eventual degree of spasticity (Marsden 1988).

Pharmacological management with baclofen, dantrolene sodium and diazepam is moderately effective. Each has a tendency to cause drowsiness although patients may develop tolerance to this side effect. Each has occasionally produced excessive hypotonia and loss of useful extensor tone but more often excessive spasms continue despite optimization of dosages.

Baclofen is a gamma-aminobutyric acid (GABA) analogue which selectively acts on the GABA-B receptor. It primarily restricts calcium influx into the presynaptic terminal thus reducing presynaptic transmitter release, but also is thought to have a postsynaptic action which depresses neuronal activity (Ochs et al. 1989). In general it is well tolerated although in addition to drowsiness, it can cause nausea. It occasionally results in a toxic, confusional state with hallucinations and seizures, but this is usually associated with large doses and abrupt withdrawal of the drug. Baclofen is usually given two to six times a day with a total daily dose range of 10–160 mg. Users sometimes find frequent dosing at significantly higher levels helpful. Baclofen is usually the more effective of these medications and can be used in combination with diazepam. Dantrolene sodium acts on muscle, depressing calcium ion release from the sarcoplasmic reticulum. As it acts on muscle rather than centrally, it can be used in conjunction with baclofen or benzodiazepines. It can cause minor gastrointestinal symptoms such as anorexia, nausea or alteration of bowel habit as well as drowsiness. Of more significance is the risk of hepatic damage, rarely resulting in liver failure. For this reason careful monitoring of liver function is essential. It too is given in divided doses with a range of about 25–400 mg daily, starting with 25 mg/day and building up the dose over several weeks.

Benzodiazepines, most commonly diazepam, appear to increase presynaptic inhibition of the stretch reflex mechanism. The sedative action and habit-forming tendency of these agents suggest to some a limitation of their usefulness (Grundy and Russell 1986). Tolerance frequently reduces the sedative effect and a tendency to habituation should not discourage its continued use if it is effective and necessary to improve function. The hypotensive effect of benzodiazepines may also cause difficulty in individuals who have significant autonomic dysfunction in association with their spinal lesion.

The alpha-2 adrenergic agonist, clonidine, has been shown to have an antispasticity effect in SCI patients that is recognized subjectively and demonstrable neurophysiologically by restoration of vibratory inhibition of the H reflex (Nance et al. 1989). Because of its tendency to cause postural hypotension it has been used with desipramine. Its other side effects, including dry mouth and constipation, have limited its use; however, the adverse effects seem to be minimized by using the transdermal patch as a mode of delivery. In fact, Weingarden and Belen (1992) found that none of the patients in their study group experienced persistent hypotension with this route of drug administration. Further work is needed before clonidine is recognized as an agent for routine use.

When oral drug therapy is not tolerated or found to be ineffective, there may be a place for the use of intrathecal baclofen. Recent reports have described sustained beneficial effect on spinal spasticity with few adverse effects when baclofen is given by infusion via a permanent intrathecal catheter (Ochs et al. 1989; Parke et al. 1989). The advantages of intrathecal baclofen include providing a continuous steady state to the patient with virtually no central nervous system effects such as sedation. Follow-up is essential and the risk of infection and pump failure must considered.

When spasticity significantly interferes with daily life and is unresponsive to medication, interruption of the nerve supply to the offending muscles through chemical means or neurological surgery may be necessary. The motor point of a muscle can be identified neurophysiologically and then injected with the local anaesthetic bupivacaine to give a short-lived paresis. If this block improves function, a more lasting paresis can be achieved with the motor point injection of 6% aqueous phenol or 45% ethyl alcohol (Grundy and Russell 1986). This paresis should be considered permanent although some reinnervation usually occurs. The dosage that can be administered is limited because phenol is caustic. A series of injections over an extended period may best obtain the optimal level of muscle weakening. Botulinum toxin type A is a potent neuromuscular blocker that is used in selective motor point blocks in which individual muscles can be weakened. It inhibits release of acetylcholine presynaptically at the neuromuscular junction and reduces spasticity locally by causing flaccid paralysis of the muscle into which it is injected. Adverse effects of intramuscular injection are over-weakening of the muscle, and minimal systemic symptoms such as headache, nausea, and fatigue. The average duration of effective muscle weakening is three months. It provides a significant advantage in cases with sensory preservation since unlike neurolysis, it is neither directly painful nor can it inadvertently cause sensory nerve injury and dysaesthesia. Alternatively, the nerve supply to the muscle may be interrupted by a neurectomy, the commonest example of which is obturator neurectomy for severe hip adductor spasms. These limited procedures are seldom effective in controlling generalized spasticity.

Dorsal rootlet rhizotomy can significantly reduce intractable, disabling spasms. It consists of section of selected dorsal rootlets in the lumbosacral area which interrupts the reflex arc. After laminectomy, rootlets are stimulated and those noted to produce extensive spread of reflex muscle response (monitored via multichannel electromyography) are sectioned. Other strategies for rootlet selection exist, but prediction of postoperative, long-term outcome remains imprecise. The technique has been most utilized in cerebral palsy where it has been well tolerated and is thought to be effective (Brown 1990). Other neurosurgical procedures such as anterior rhizotomy, cordectomy and myelotomy have largely been abandoned for, although they had variable efficacy, they led to problems with subsequent skin care (Marsden 1988).

Rarely, in the presence of severe spasticity, intrathecal phenol or alcohol has been used to destroy nerve roots of the cauda equina. This technique is, however, unselective, converting an upper motor neurone lesion to a lower motor neurone disturbance with resulting interference with bladder and bowel function together with sensory loss which increases the risk of pressure sores. When spasticity results in contractures, procedures such as tenotomy, tendon lengthening or muscle division may prove necessary.

Acknowledgements I wish to thank B. Pentland co-author for the first edition whose contribution remains important to this revision and is gratefully acknowledged.

References

Beckman J (1987) The Louisiana State University reciprocating gait orthosis. Physiotherapy 73:386–392

Brown E (1990) Dorsal rhizotomy for spastic cerebral palsy: report of diagnostic therapeutic technology assessment panel of the American Medical Association. JAMA 264:2569–2574

Butler PB, Major RE (1987) The Para Walker: a rational approach to the provision of reciprocal ambulation of paraplegic patients. Physiotherapy 73:393–397

Collins WP, Chehrazi B (1982) Concepts of the acute management of spinal cord injury. In: Matthews WB, Glasor CH (eds) Recent advances in clinical neurology. Churchill Livingstone, Edinburgh, pp 67–82

Dralj A, Grobelnik S (1973) Functional electrical stimulation – a new hope for paraplegic patients? Bull Prosthet Res 10–20:75–102

Flores JH Jr (1985) Electrically induced isometric exercise as a means of preventing muscle atrophy and bone demineralization. MSc thesis, Wright State University, Dayton, OH

Glaser RM (1983) Locomotion via paralyzed leg muscles: feasibility study for leg propelled vehicle. J Rehabil R D 20:87–92

Glaser RM (1986) Physiologic aspects of spinal cord injury and functional neuromuscular stimulation. Cent Nerve Syst Trauma 3:49–62

Glaser RM (1994) Functional neuromuscular stimulation: exercise conditioning of spinal cord injured patients. Int J Sports Med 15:142–148

Go BK, DeVivo MJ, Richards, JS (1995) The epidemiology of spinal cord injury. In: Stover SL, DeLisa JA, Whiteneck GG (eds) Spinal cord injury: clinical outcomes from the model systems. Aspen, Maryland, pp 21–55.

Gonzalez EEG, Corcoran PJ (1994) Energy expenditure during ambulation. In Downey JA, Myers SJ, Gonzalez EG, Lieberman JS (eds) The physiologic basis of rehabilitation medicine. Butterworth-Heinemann, Massachusetts, pp 413–446

Grundy D, Russell J (1986) ABC of spinal cord injury: medical management in the spinal injuries unit. Br Med J 292:183–187

Hirokawa S, Grimm M, Le T et al. (1990) Energy consumption in paraplegic ambulation using reciprocating gait orthosis and electric stimulation of the thigh muscles. Arch Phys Med Rehabil 71:687–694

Hooker SP, Figoni SF, Glaser RM, Rodgers MM, Ezenwa BN, Faghri PD (1990) Physiologic responses to prolonged electrically stimulated leg-cycle exercise in the spinal cord injured. Arch Phys Med Rehabil 71:863–869

Kalz RT, Rymer WZ (1989) Spastic hypertonia, mechanisms and measurement. Arch Phys Med Rehabil 70:144–155

Leeds EM, Klose KJ, Ganz W, Serafini A, Green BA (1990) Bone mineral density after bicycle ergometry training. Arch Phys Med Rehabil 71:207–209

Levine SP, Kett RL, Cederna PS, Brooks SV (1990a) Electrical muscle stimulation for pressure sore prevention: tissue shape variation. Arch Phys Med Rehabil 71:210–215

Levine SP, Kett RL, Gross MD, Wilson BA, Cederna PS, Juni JE (1990b) Blood flow in the gluteus maximus of seated individuals during electrical muscle stimulation. Arch Phys Med Rehabil 71:682–686

Liberson WT, et al. (1961) Funtional electrotherapy: stimulation of the peroneal nerve synchronized with the swing phase of the gait of hemilegic patients. Arch Phys Med Rehabil 101–105

Licht S (1971) Electrodiagnosis and electromyography, 3rd edn. Elizabeth Licht, New Haven, CT

Marsden CD (1988) Spasticity. In: Goodwill CJ, Chamberlain MA (eds) Rehabilitation of the physically disabled adult. Croom Helm, London, pp 455–464

Marsolais EB, Kobetic R (1983) Functional walking in paralyzed patients by means of electrical stimulation. Clin Orthop 175:30–36

Marsolais EB, Kobetic R (1986) Implantation techniques and experience with percutaneous intramuscular electrodes in the lower extremities. J Rehabil R D 23:1–8

Marsolais EB, Kobetic R (1987) Functional electrical stimulation for walking in paraplegia. J Bone Joint Surg 69A:728–733

Nance PW, Shears A, Nance DM (1989) Reflex changes induced by clonidine in spinal cord injured patients. Paraplegia 27:296–301

Nene AV, Patrick JK (1990) Energy cost of paraplegia locomotion using the Para Walker-electrical stimulation "hybrid" orthosis. Arch Phys Med Rehabil 71:116–120

Ochs G, Stuppler A, Myerson BA et al. (1989) Intrathecal baclofen for long-term treatment of spasticity: a multicentre study. J Neurol Neurosurg Psychiatry 52:933–939

Parke B, Penn RD, Savoy SM, Coreas D (1989) Functional outcome after delivery of intrathecal baclofen. Arch Phys Med Rehabil 70:30–32

Patterson RP, Lockwood JS, Dykstra DD (1990) Functional electric stimulation system using electrode garment. Arch Phys Med Rehabil 71:340–342

Petrofsky JS (1978) Control of the recruitment and firing frequencies of motor units in electrically stimulated muscles in the cat. Med Biol Eng Comput 16:302–308

Petrofsky JS (1979) Digital analogue hybrid 3-channel sequential stimulator. Med Biol Eng Comput 17:421–424

Petrofsky JS, Phillips CA (1979) Constant-velocity contractions in skeletal muscle by sequential stimulation of muscles in the cat. Med Biol Eng Comput 16:302–308

Petrofsky JS, Phillips CA (1983) Computer controlled walking in the paralyzed individual. J Neurol Orthop Surg 4:153–164

Petrofsky JS, Phillips CA (1984) The use of functional electrical stimulation for rehabilitation of spinal cord injured patients. Cent Nerve Syst Trauma 1:57–73

Petrofsky JS, Heaton HH, Glaser RM, Phillips CA (1983a) Applications of the Apple as a microprocessor controlled stimulator. Collegiate Microcomputer 1:97–104

Petrofsky JS, Heaton HH, Phillips CA (1983b) Outdoor bicycle for exercise in paraplegics and quadriplegics. J Biomed Eng 5:292–296

Petrofsky JS, Phillips CA, Heaton HH, Glaser RM (1984a) Bicycle ergometer for paralyzed muscle. J Clin Eng 9:13–19

Petrofsky JS, Phillips CA, Heaton HH (1984b) Feedback control system for walking in man. Comp Biol Med 14:135–149

Petrofsky JS, Heaton HH, Phillips CA, Glaser RM (1984c) Leg exerciser for training of paralyzed muscle by closed lop control. Med Biol Eng Comput 22:298–303

Phillips CA, Petrofsky JS, Hendeshot DM, Stafford D (1984) Closed loop control for restoration of movement in paralyzed muscle. Orthopedics 7:1289–1302

Weingarden SI, Belen JG (1992) Clonidine transdermal system for treatment of spasticity in spinal cord injury, Arch Phys Med Rehabil 73:876–77

WHO (1980) International classification of impairments, disabilities, and handicap. World Health Organization, Geneva

Subject Index